Emergency Care FOURTH EDITION

MANUAL OF

Susan Budassi Sheehy, RN, MSN, CEN

Director
Air Medical Transport and Trauma
Dartmouth-Hitchcock Medical Center
Lebanon, New Hampshire
and
Instructor in Surgery
Dartmouth Medical School, Hanover, N.H.

Judith E. Lombardi, RN, MSN, CEN

Director of Nursing
Emergency Department
Dartmouth-Hitchcock Medical Center
Lebanon, New Hampshire

*with **347** illustrations*

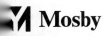
Mosby

Louis Baltimore Boston Carlsbad Chicago Naples New York Philadelphia Portland
don Madrid Mexico City Singapore Sydney Tokyo Toronto Wiesbaden

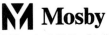
Mosby

Dedicated to Publishing Excellence

Editor: Robin Carter
Developmental Editor: Jeanne Allison
Project Manager: Gayle May Morris
Production Editor: Donna L. Walls
Manufacturing Supervisor: Karen Lewis
Book and Cover Designer: Susan Lane
Cover Photograph: © Larry Mulvehill, Science Source/Photo Researchers

FOURTH EDITION

Copyright © 1995 by Mosby–Year Book, Inc.

Previous editions copyrighted 1979, 1984, 1990

Printed in the United States of America
Composition by University Graphics, Inc.
Printing/binding by R. R. Donnelley and Sons, Inc.

Mosby–Year Book, Inc.
11830 Westline Industrial Drive
St. Louis, Missouri 63146

Library of Congress Cataloging in Publication Data

Sheehy, Susan Budassi
  Manual of emergency care / Susan Budassi Sheehy, Judith E. Lombardi. — 4th ed.
   p. cm.
  Includes bibliographical references and index.
  ISBN 0-8151-7501-9
  1. Medical emergencies—Handbooks, manuals, etc. 2. Emergency nursing—Handbooks. manuals, etc. 3. Emergency medical personnel—Handbooks, manuals, etc. I. Lombardi, Judith E. II. Title.
  [DNLM: 1. Emergency Medical Services—handbooks. WX 39 S541m 1995]
  RC86.8.S54 1995
  616.02′5—dc20
  DNLM/DLC
  for Library of Congress   94-29:
                       C

95 96 97 98 99 / 9 8 7 6 5 4 3 2 1

Contributors

The following individuals from Dartmouth-Hitchcock Medical Center contributed chapters to this edition:

Judith Boehm, RN, MSN
CHAPTER 4   Advanced Life Support

Christine DiGeronimo, RN, BSN, CURN
CHAPTER 15   Genitourinary Emergencies

Lisa Schneck Hegel, RN, BS, CEN
CHAPTER 34   Special Considerations for Geriatric Patients

Linda J. Kobokovich, RNC, MSCN
CHAPTER 29   Obstetric and Gynecologic Emergencies

Lisa McCabe, MS, RN, CCRN
CHAPTER 6   Shock and Hemodynamic Monitoring

Ingrid B. Mroz, MS, RN, CCRN
CHAPTER 6   Shock and Hemodynamic Monitoring

Delberta Murphy, RN, BS, CEN
CHAPTER 28   Domestic Violence

Carla Obar, RN, CSPI
CHAPTER 13   Toxicologic Emergencies

Sandra Thomas Ouellette, RN, CPTC
CHAPTER 35   Organ and Tissue Donation

Maureen Quigley, RN, BSN, CEN
CHAPTER 30   Pediatric Medical Emergencies
CHAPTER 31   Pediatric Trauma and Surgical Emergencies

Susan Budassi Sheehy, RN, MSN, CEN
CHAPTER 22   Chest Trauma
CHAPTER 25   Multiple Trauma
CHAPTER 32   Child Maltreatment

Lori Tucker, RN, CEN
CHAPTER 27   Sexual Assault

Kathleen Waine, RN, CEN
CHAPTER 5   Intravenous Therapy and Laboratory Specimens

Mary E. Wood, RN, MS, CDE
CHAPTER 12   Metabolic Emergencies

The following individuals from Dartmouth-Hitchcock Medical Center revised chapters for this edition:

Jorda Chapin, RN, CEN
CHAPTER 11   Blood Disorders

Jane deMoll, RN, CEN
CHAPTER 19   Spinal Cord and Neck Trauma

Deborah C. Harcke, RN, BSN, CEN
CHAPTER 33   Psychiatric Emergencies

Judith E. Lombardi, RN, MSN, ENP, CEN
CHAPTER 2   Patient Assessment, Reporting, and Documentation
CHAPTER 14   Environmental Emergencies
CHAPTER 20   Facial Trauma

Kelly F. Malmquist, RN, BSN
CHAPTER 24   Extremity Trauma

Brenda M. Moore, RN, CEN
CHAPTER 3   Basic Life Support

Tracy Pike-Amato, RN, CEN
CHAPTER 9   Neurologic Emergencies
CHAPTER 18   Head Trauma

Carol Rittenhouse, RN, CCRN
CHAPTER 8   Pulmonary Emergencies

Peggy Shedd, MSN, RN, CS
CHAPTER 1   Communicating in Crisis

Daun Smith, RN, MS
CHAPTER 21   Eye, Ear, Nose, Throat, and Dental Emergencies
CHAPTER 26   Burn Trauma

Janet L. Sudekum, RN, BSN, CCRN
CHAPTER 16   Infectious Diseases

Geoffrey Tarbox, RN
CHAPTER 7   Cardiac Emergencies

Deborah Upton, RN, CEN
CHAPTER 10   Abdominal Pain

Andrea B. Wyle, RN, ONC
CHAPTER 24   Extremity Trauma

Mary Young, RN, MSN
CHAPTER 23   Abdominal Trauma

To
John
*who gives meaning
to everything*

SBS

To
Jonah
*who taught me more
about courage
than any person*

JEL

Foreword

Every so often one comes across a resource that is useable, practical, and written in an understandable yet highly professional manner. *Manual of Emergency Care,* fourth edition is such a resource. This handbook provides state-of-the-art information that emergency care providers can use in their treatment of patients and families along the age continuum, whether they deliver care in rural or urban settings, in primary or tertiary settings, or in the field.

I have had the privilege of working directly with the manual's editors. Susan Budassi Sheehy and Judith E. Lombardi are consummate professionals who have dedicated their careers to patients and families who require emergency and trauma care. These two nurses are dedicated to creating a health care system in which the needs of patients and families are the top priority. They work diligently to foster an environment in which all providers can contribute and can feel good about their work.

The editors have brought together a group of expert authors who share cutting-edge information on clinical assessment and therapeutic approaches. Each author brings a unique perspective on emergency care and writes in a way that is readable and applicable to hands-on providers. These authors "walk the walk" of the care they write about and make a significant difference for patients and families every day. I am fortunate to work with them on a daily basis. These authors have helped to create an environment that expects excellence in the caring practices and supports individuals in their goal achievement and professional development. These nurses are well qualified to share their wealth of knowledge and experience with other emergency professionals. I am pleased that, through this handbook, you will share their expertise.

Melissa A. Fitzpatrick, MSN, RN

Vice President, Adult Critical Care Services
Dartmouth-Hitchcock Medical Center
Lebanon, New Hampshire

Preface

As we celebrate the publication of the fourth edition of *Manual of Emergency Care,* it is time to reflect on the evolution of the specialty of emergency nursing. During the 16 years since the first edition of this book, emergency nursing has attained some ambitious milestones. Perhaps the most significant has been the certification examination, where emergency nurses are able to demonstrate their attainment of a body of knowledge that allows them to bear the credential of certified emergency nurse (CEN). We have seen emergency nursing become an identified and respected nursing specialty.

Parallel to this professional recognition has come the growth of the depth and breadth of knowledge of emergency nurses. Acknowledging this trend in practice, we have restructured the fourth edition to demonstrate the expertise of a number of practicing clinical nurses. In most departments, there are individuals who have attained a level of expertise in areas of special interest above and beyond their peers. We have taken advantage of this to invite staff nurses, managers, and clinical nurse specialists to share their expertise in the many chapters of this book.

In keeping with the original intent of this manual, this edition has been written keeping the concept of collaborative practice as a main focus. It has been written using a patient-focused model of care. Also in keeping with previous editions, we have planned the manual as a "clinically usable" manual, where practicing clinicians have an easily accessible resource for use in the clinical area.

Acknowledgments

Many people have participated in the fourth edition of this book. Much credit must be given to all of the chapter authors and revisers, who did an outstanding job. Behind the scene, major credit must be given to Fred Pond, the Nursing Librarian at Dartmouth-Hitchcock Medical Center's Matthews-Fuller Health Sciences Library, who not only provided library/reference support, but also encouragement and spirit to the entire project and many of its individual participants. Also, thanks to the many DHMC Nursing Administrators who understood the need for chapter authors/revisers to have time to work on this project.

An overwhelmingly grateful thank you goes to Leta Stoddard, DHMC Trauma Registrar, who did yeoman's work on this project, ensuring that every word, every illustration, and every table was correct and that every deadline and every detail was met. This edition would never have been completed without her.

Susan Budassi Sheehy

Judith E. Lombardi

Contents

PART THREE
Trauma Emergencies

PART FOUR
Other Emergencies

PART ONE

Basic Principles of Emergency Care

CHAPTER 1

Communicating in Crisis

An unexpected and unplanned entry into the prehospital care system and/or a visit to an emergency department are experiences that produce increased anxiety in most people. The environment and faces may be unfamiliar; the patient may experience pain or other signs and symptoms that are frightening; the equipment is foreign; the surroundings are noisy; and the terminology that is heard may sound like a foreign language. The patient may also have fear of the unknown and fear of the outcome. There may be others present who are also ill or injured, or who have just died. The patient usually believes that his or her privacy is invaded when very personal questions are asked by strangers who take charge of the patient's care. The patient's family or friends may not be present or may be restricted to the waiting area, and the patient may feel very alone and helpless—a foreigner in this strange world of emergency care. So a visit to the emergency care setting is stress-producing, to say the least.

Every person involved in the delivery of emergency care should be aware of the psychological factors that surround a patient's entry into the emergency care system. The relationship between the emergency care provider and patient, family, and friends can make a difference in the patient's level of anxiety and in the overall outcome of the emergency care given. When the emergency care provider understands these factors, quality care can usually be delivered. The key word in all of patient care is *communication,* the process of sending and receiving a message, which can be verbal or nonverbal. Communication is the process through which the patient/emergency care provider relationship develops. The competence of health care delivery is based on the level of interpersonal skills possessed and demonstrated by the emergency care provider. The better the interpersonal relationship, the better the therapeutic relationship.

Here are some basic assumptions about therapeutic communications:
• All communication is learned.
• Communication of some sort is inevitable in any relationship.
• There are formal and informal channels of communication in every relationship.
• All behavior is a form of communication about the relationship.
• It is impossible *not* to communicate.
• The message sent is not necessarily the message received.

Each individual has a unique perception of the world. This uniqueness is reflected in one's behavior, language, and actions. Language is a personal attribute that reflects a person's values, beliefs, and life-style. Being aware of this fact may offer a reference point for establishing meaningful contact with the patient and may provide beneficial interventions. In emergency care it is important to talk at the patient's level, so that the patient can understand what is being said. Effective communication means that the patient must believe that he or she is being heard. Take the time to listen. Although most people talk and listen a great deal, good communication skills are not easy to acquire. Good therapeutic communication takes training, practice, and skill.

SPECIAL ASPECTS OF THERAPEUTIC COMMUNICATION

Empathy vs Sympathy

Empathy is an objective skill that allows the emergency care provider to experience an individual in such a way as to comprehend that person's feelings, but without experiencing those feelings. The emergency care provider can show respect and concern for what the patient is experiencing, while maintaining a separateness that allows the relationship to be therapeutic. *Sympathy* is subjective—it is an actual sharing of emotion with the other person. It is important to remain empathic rather than sympathetic in the emergency care setting so that a level of energy can be maintained. Sympathy can sap the caregiver's energy, and energy is necessary to be effective when helping the patient cope with the problem or crisis at hand.

Recognizing Feelings

Patients need to know that their feelings are noted and recognized as legitimate by emergency care personnel. Caregivers should never belittle or criticize feelings expressed by a patient or the patient's family and friends, because this would inhibit effective therapeutic communication. Caregivers can use verbal techniques to convey the attitude that they are willing to help the patient recognize and understand those feelings. Recognizing emotions can sometimes decrease the patient's fear of the experience to a point at which the level of anxiety becomes manageable. A statement as simple as, "It's okay to be nervous about what's happening," can do much to relieve the patient's anxiety. If the caregiver can accept the patient's feelings as legitimate, the caregiver will communicate an attitude of acceptance that encourages problem solving and promotes health.

Be careful not to try to read the patient's feelings—feelings usually cannot be read. The patient's behavior can be observed, and inferences made about why the behavior is occurring. For example, seeing a patient crying can lead to the inference that the patient is upset about something. But the patient may be crying out of relief at finding out that examination and tests rule out a myocardial infarction. Feelings are sometimes expressed as behaviors. Attempt to have the patient focus on communicating feelings verbally. This is preferable to trying to interpret behavior.

It is important for those working in emergency care to focus on their own feelings and how they affect therapeutic communication with the patient. Strive toward a climate of mutual trust and respect. This requires patience, knowledge, skill, and caring. Acceptance of a patient is recognition without value judgment; it is the commitment to treat the person as a unique human being with very individual needs.

The Need for Therapeutic Communication

Therapeutic communication is established before the initial contact with the patient. The first encounter a person has with emergency care personnel will set the tone for the entire emergency care experience. If invasive procedures must be performed immediately because of the urgency of the patient's condition, verbal contact should be used briefly to explain the procedures, gain the patient's confidence, and establish rapport. No therapeutic intervention should ever be performed without at least a brief explanation to the patient, who should know the reason for the intervention and should be made aware of any pain or discomfort the intervention will cause. Even if the patient is unresponsive, a brief explanation of the therapeutic intervention is necessary.

TECHNIQUES IN COMMUNICATION

Supportive

The supportive technique will help the patient maintain or regain self-control in the presence of anxiety. Some ways of being supportive include:
- Recognizing that the patient is an individual with special needs.
- Verbalizing support.
- Being available to listen when the patient needs to talk.
- Listening carefully (taking the time to listen).
- Accepting the patient's feelings as legitimate.
- Remaining at hand when the patient is afraid of loneliness or isolation.
- Commenting about efforts to understand what it must be like for the patient, even though the caregiver cannot really know.
- Observing and carefully commenting on behaviors or mannerisms that are clues to the patient's feelings.
- Touching the patient—hand, arm, shoulder—if it is comfortable for both the patient and caregiver.
- Initiating actions that visibly reflect a humanistic attitude; showing compassion and respect.
- Keeping close watch on personal attitudes.

Silence

Silence may be used as a therapeutic intervention. Silence is an expressive, non-verbal response.
- It is *not* the absence of activity.
- It is a natural conclusion of verbally transmitted thoughts.
- It allows time to think.
- It can help find solutions to problems and answers to questions.
- It is a way of conveying feelings.
- It promotes acceptance.
- It may indicate anxiety in both the speaker and the listener.
- It can be used for pacing, timing, closeness, alienation, resistance, or relaxation.

Listening

Listening is a way of hearing the concerns of the patient. It may relieve some of the patient's anxieties and facilitate the collection of information. The patient should be allowed to take the conversational lead whenever possible. Listening is an active, physically visible process, even when there is limited verbal activity on the part of the listener.
- A listening attitude is a learned skill.
- The patient's verbalizations should be acknowledged with active listening.
- Some comments that would encourage the patient to verbalize thoughts and feelings are, "Go on," "I see," "Uh huh," "Tell me more," "Tell me how that happened," "What made you come to the hospital today?" or "This seems really important to you."

Questions

Questions are necessary to gather specific information, but may limit therapeutic communication if the interviewer is too focused.

Types of questions

■ **LEADING QUESTION**
"Don't you know better than to skip your medications?"
- This type of question contains a suggested answer.
- It restricts the respondent.
- It implies the asker's judgment.
- It elicits nonverbal clues.

■ **NO-CHOICE QUESTION**
"You're ready for your medication, aren't you?"
- This implies a command. It shows authority and may be interpreted as "one-upmanship."

■ **CLOSED QUESTION**
"Where is your pain?"
- This type of question elicits a specific response. It asks for agreement or disagreement. One can respond to it nonverbally, which requires very little self-disclosure.
- It can narrow the focus. This may or may not be useful.

■ **LIMITED CHOICE QUESTION**
"Do you want this injection in your hip or in your arm?"
- This type of question gives the responder two choices. It implies the patient's compliance in the situation.

■ **DOUBLE QUESTION**
"Do you want something for pain? Are you allergic to morphine?"
- This type of question actually consists of two questions asked in sequence, without pausing.
- It confuses both the caregiver and the patient.
- It requires the patient to choose which question to answer.
- It allows the patient to avoid the subject.

■ **OPEN-ENDED QUESTION**
"How were you feeling just before the crash?"
- It usually begins with "what," "how," or "tell me more."
- The answer to this type of question conveys feelings and perceptions as well as thoughts.
- It encourages the patient to elaborate, describe, and compare.
- It allows freedom of response. It provides information for the assessment of reliability of the patient.

■ **INDIRECT QUESTION**
"Tell me about your medical history."
- This type of question does not seem like a question.
- It shows interest.
- It has no question mark at the end.
- It allows the patient to carry the conversational lead.

Don'ts in questioning

- Don't ask too many questions. Let the patient speak as much as possible.
- Don't ask "why" questions—they cast feelings of blame.
- Don't use "you" or "who" to begin questions.
- Don't ask double questions.
- Don't ask long, elaborate questions.
- Don't ask closed or direct questions unless you are seeking very specific information.

SPECIAL COMMUNICATION SITUATIONS

Communicating with Children

When communicating with a child, especially one who is ill or injured, a consistent, organized approach is best. Do not treat the child like a small adult. Be familiar with growth and development patterns, and deal with the child accordingly. Remember that children are individuals with special needs. How an ill or injured child is treated may have an effect on the child's development.

When communicating with a child, it is also important to communicate with the child's family or friends. It is common for parents or friends to become extremely anxious or to experience feelings of guilt when a child becomes ill or is injured. Communicate with parents and friends in a therapeutic manner.

Children react to illness or injury with anxiety, fear of separation, aversion to pain, or fear of the unknown. Encourage the child to speak openly and to express feelings appropriately. When talking with a child, speak in open, direct language. Use the child's first name frequently and don't ask too many questions. When the child asks a question, answer honestly. Speak directly and give instructions in simple comments. Whenever it can be avoided, do not ask a child to choose, because doing this may offer an unacceptable alternative. Making choices also increases the child's anxiety. Use touch to aid in communication and convey the idea of friendliness and caring.

Whenever possible, allow at least one of the parents to stay with the child. Remember that a child's way of coping with illness or injury may be to cry, sob, or scream. Always remain calm and slightly authoritative, in a way that demonstrates control.

Communicating with Victims of Trauma

When an unexpected trauma occurs, whether minor or major, the patient often appears to be in a state of crisis (Table 1-1, Guidelines for assessing patients in crisis). It should be recognized and appropriate crisis intervention should be used as early as possible. These patients may be in pain or may be afraid of disfigurement, death, or a threat to body image. They may become angry and blame themselves or someone else for the accident. They may be angry that they were hurt when others were not, or feel guilty that they were not as badly hurt as others in the accident. A type of depression in which the patient feels totally helpless and at the mercy of rescuers may develop rapidly. The language of emergency care is foreign to most people—the sound of the monitor, the banging of trays, and the feel of the equipment are new. The feeling of helplessness may be overwhelming.

People are affected in different ways by the anxiety related to trauma. Some people may narrow their focus to such a limited area that they are unaware of the serious nature of their problems. These people will require much gentle, calm repetition and explanation in order to appreciate what is happening. Then there are people who will have widened their focus of attention so much that they are overwhelmed and unable to focus on what you are saying. You will need to communicate in short, simple, direct, and repetitive phrases with these patients. Limiting extra stimulation by speaking to them in a private, relatively uncluttered area would also be helpful, as they may be distracted by extraneous sights and sounds. Your own demeanor will be very important. Keeping a calm approach will be helpful, whereas projecting a hurried, tense approach could increase the patient's anxiety.

Keep the patient informed of what is being done and why. Talk with the

TABLE 1-1 Guidelines for Assessing Patients in Crisis*

IMPACT	BEHAVIORS	EMOTIONS	COGNITION	EXAMPLES
No emotional impact				
No observable effect of the situation on the person's behavior	Questions, responses, activities are appropriate for the situation May ask questions, request information, obtain knowledge correctly Not withdrawn or anxious	Expresses that he is "all right" Feels in control of emotions Expresses concerns and reactions clearly	Evidences clear thinking Able to make decisions Plans well Is reality-oriented	Reports that "I will be OK" Reports that he can "handle it"
Mild impact				
Behavior, emotions, and cognition are only slightly affected by the situation	Questions, responses, and activities are mostly appropriate May evidence some anxiety, fear, stress May be cooperative and responsive, displays few visible signs of upset	Seems in control of emotions and is basically calm May report a little embarrassment Is able to talk about the situation	Clear, good to very good future plans	Reports some confidence that he "will be OK" Feels sure that with help "I'll handle it"

*Developed by Dr. Susan Meyers Chandler, School of Social Work and Dr. Libby O. Ruch, Sociology Department and Women's Studies Program, University of Hawaii, Honolulu, Hawaii. (From Sheehy SA: *Emergency nursing—principles and practice*, ed 3. St Louis, 1992, Mosby.)

Continued

TABLE 1-1 Guidelines for Assessing Patients in Crisis*—cont'd

IMPACT	BEHAVIORS	EMOTIONS	COGNITION	EXAMPLES
Moderate impact				
Is noticeably affected by the situation but response is not continuous or highly intense Responds to help and reassurance Can conceptualize strategies for dealing	May tear or cry a little during the examination, but visible affect or distress is minimal May display some silly or inappropriate behavior May be anxious, unable to absorb information easily, somewhat confused	May seem somewhat affected by the situation but responds to reassurance from others Expresses worry, fear, some inability to concentrate Somewhat dependent	Asks for help and has good plans and strategies for coping with the problem.	Asks for help and support Reports concern about the future impact: "Will I be OK?"
Severe impact				
Is clearly affected by the situation in one or more life areas Behavioral response occurs more than once and is somewhat intense Needs reassurance, and experiences difficulty conceptualizing strategies for future planning	Is visibly upset during part of the evaluation, yet responds to reassurance; the signs of distress can be pinpointed to certain factors (the questions about incident, the examination, the outcome and future problems)	Expresses feelings of guilt, self-blame, helplessness, either by demonstrating strong emotion or verbally expressing guilt, self-blame, or helplessness	Appears confused or disoriented Is visibly upset, yet has some plans for handling problems arising from the situation	Says he is very frightened, "doesn't want to go out anymore," or states other unrealistic plans

Very severe impact				
Has a strong reaction in one or more areas	Is visibly upset during most of the examination	Verbalizes strong reactions; may repeat responses with intensity	Very confused, disoriented, unable to comprehend situation	Reports that he will "never drive again," "never look the same," or "can't go home"
Is not incapacitated but highly affected by the situation	Crying, trembling, withdrawal evident throughout the examination	Generalized fear and/or anger	May deny responses	
Behaviors are continuous and intense	Responses occurring almost continuously–not focused only on the situation–generalized distress		No plans for the future; evidences little ability to consider alternatives or develop strategies for the future	
Seems only somewhat responsive to reassurance and is only somewhat able to conceptualize strategies for dealing with the future				
Extremely severe impact				
Is incapacitated by the situation; may be hospitalized for psychiatric observation or treatment	May be suicidal, catatonic, hysterical, or crying	Shows extreme nervous disorders, psychotic reactions	Is unable to deal with the situation or the future	Has no awareness of what happened or where he is; out of touch with reality
Behaviors are multiple, continuous, and extremely intense	May have phobias or other psychological symptoms that indicate he is incapacitated in some way		Is unable to make decisions for self	
Unaware of efforts to reassure				

*Developed by Dr. Susan Meyers Chandler, School of Social Work and Dr. Libby O. Ruch, Sociology Department and Women's Studies Program, University of Hawaii, Honolulu, Hawaii. (From Sheehy SA: *Emergency nursing—principles and practice*, ed 3. St Louis, 1992, Mosby.)

patient frequently. Allow the patient to make choices whenever possible. Even such small choices as in which arm to start the IV will help the patient feel somewhat in control. Let the patient know that it is alright to feel frightened, anxious, angry, or guilty. Help the patient verbalize feelings so that they become acceptable. Help the patient cope with feelings of guilt or frustration. Do not try to second-guess the patient. If anything the patient says is not clear, say so.

Never give a patient false assurance or false hope. Be as open and honest as possible. Sometimes it is wise to present this candor in small doses. Help the patient realize that help will be needed after the time of emergency department intervention. Help the patient plan for the future, even if it is only for short periods of time.

Patients may develop a post-trauma response[1] following a major traumatic event. This response may include flashbacks or nightmares about the event, excessive retelling of the story of the event, or survival guilt. These characteristics represent a reexperience of the event and may be a way for the person to appreciate the significance of the event. Other, more serious reactions may be emotional numbness and even life-style alterations that may become self destructive (substance abuse, suicide attempt, interpersonal difficulties, avoidance of the trauma location, general isolation, poor impulse control of behavior). Predicting the possibility of this response may reassure patients and their families if these responses occur. Patients experiencing the more serious reactions should be encouraged to seek counseling to assist in controlling these reactions. Some responses are self-limiting, but reactions that last longer than 1 month and persist in severity may develop into a psychiatric condition, post-traumatic stress disorder.[2]

This is why it is important to ensure that both patient and family receive long-term follow-up after the time of the emergency department and hospital stay.

Communicating with People Who Are Deaf or Speak a Foreign Language

An important assessment to make is the patient's or family's comprehension of your information. Be certain that they can hear and understand you. If you suspect they can't, they may be deaf or speak a foreign language.

People who are deaf may have partial or complete hearing loss. You may have to communicate by speaking in a lower tone, speaking more loudly, or allowing them to read your lips. You may even need to write your questions. Finding a quiet room may allow a partially deaf person to hear you more clearly. Some deaf people communicate through sign language; so having a list of community volunteers skilled in sign language is helpful.

Many people speak little or no English, or forget how to communicate well in English during a crisis. Different parts of our country have high populations of non-English speaking people. It would be important to have lists of volunteers available and capable of translating those languages. Sometimes family members can translate, but they may be too upset to assist reliably during the crisis of the emergency. Development of a written list of typical questions and potential answers in the common second languages in your area would be a good back-up method until translators can be obtained.

Communicating with Survivors When a Sudden Death Occurs

When a patient dies in the emergency care setting, staff involvement should go beyond the patient and reach out to the patient's family and friends. Staff personnel must become resource persons for the survivors, who will need empathy, support, and direction. The most common reaction to a sudden death is shock and disbelief. The next reactions are usually feelings of guilt, anger, and sorrow as the reality of the death of their loved one begins to set in. Finally, the survivors begin to work through their feelings of loss and return to their normal activities in life. Unfortunately for emergency care personnel, the third stage is rarely seen. Emergency care personnel are the people directly involved in the shock and disbelief and guilt, anger, and sorrow stages of the grief process. Factors that can help a family cope with sudden death include being honest with them and helping them to perceive the event realistically. It is also important to be sure that there are adequate emotional supports available, such as hospital support personnel (e.g., chaplain or social service worker), other family members, or friends. The family should be allowed to grieve in a quiet, private place whenever possible. Be able to assess the situation and intervene, using the ideas just discussed and anticipating what sort of referral or follow-up the family will need.

Bereavement assessment and intervention

As soon as it becomes evident that a patient's death is imminent or that the condition is critical, a member of the emergency care team should make contact with the family and remain with them throughout the resuscitation period, if possible. This person can either stay with the family or keep family members informed of the patient's condition frequently. If the patient is not doing well, be honest with the family. One should also consider the possibility of family presence during resuscitation. Listen to what the family is saying—they may need to talk. Be aware of the family's body language and nonverbal communication, which may also tell something about their needs. It may even be necessary to ask open-ended questions so that the family can begin to express their fears. Gently question family members about religious beliefs, because this may be important. Ask the family what happened if they were present at the traumatic event. You may also be the person who will ask the family about organ/tissue donation. (See Chapter 35.)

After the death, help the family realize that the event has actually happened, but give them a little time to react to the news. If death occurs before the family arrives, a brief description of the events leading up to the death may be appropriate. If possible, limit the number of personnel interacting with the family.

Encourage the family to talk and to support each other. Assist a family member who is alone to call someone else to come in and provide support. That other person may be family, a friend, or a pastor.

Once the patient has died and the family has been made aware of the occurrence, allow them time to perceive what has happened. Ask them if they would like to see the person who has died. A few minutes with the family member who has died will help in the grieving process. Ask them if they would like to be alone with the person, or if they would like you to accompany them, especially if other family supports have not yet arrived. If the patient was badly disfigured in an accident, the body should be covered, but the family should be allowed to see at least a part of the body that they can recognize—perhaps a hand or the face. The family may be given some item that was removed from the patient, such as a ring or necklace, so that the death becomes a reality for them.

Reactions to the death of a loved one may vary from crying and screaming to being quiet, to talking incessantly, or to any of a number of ways of showing emotion. Encourage healthy bereavement. Tell the grieving family, "It's okay to cry." Avoid giving any medication unless a person's history indicates that it would be beneficial. A person who is crying hysterically will soon be fatigued. Giving medication to a hysterical family member may only delay the grief process.

If an autopsy is necessary, help the family understand why it must be done. Tell them what is going to happen next, what kinds of papers they will have to sign, and what will happen to the body. Encourage family members to make funeral arrangements together. They may need help in calling a funeral home. Discuss some of the feelings they may experience in days to come. Encourage them to help each other. Call them in a couple of days to see how they are doing. Most important, express some of your own feelings about the death with other professionals. This will help you sustain your own emotional health.

Therapeutic, sensitive communication is essential to providing high-quality emergency care. Basic skills must be sharpened so that the emergency care providers can understand and appreciate the needs of the patient or family in crisis. Reviewing and practicing the ideas and suggestions contained within this chapter will assist the providers in developing those skills.

REFERENCES

1. North American Nursing Diagnosis Association: *Classification of nursing diagnosis: proceedings of the ninth conference,* Carroll-Johnson RM, ed. Philadelphia, 1991, Lippincott.
2. American Psychiatric Association: *Diagnostic and statistical manual of psychiatric disorders,* ed 3, rev. Washington, DC, 1987, the Association.

SUGGESTED READINGS

Aguilera DC: *Crisis intervention: theory and methodology,* ed 6. St Louis, 1990, Mosby.
Barry PD: *Psychosocial nursing assessment and intervention: care of the physically ill person,* ed 2. Philadelphia, 1989, Lippincott.

Boyle JS, Andrews MM: *Transcultural concepts in nursing care.* Boston, 1989, Scott, Foresman.

Gorman LM, Sultan D, Luna-Raines M: *Psychosocial nursing handbook for the nonpsychiatric nurse.* Baltimore, 1989, Williams and Wilkins.

Sheehy SB: Communicating with patients. In Sheehy SB: *Emergency nursing,* ed 3. St Louis, 1992, Mosby.

Smith S: *Communications in nursing: communicating assertively and responsibly in nursing: a guidebook,* ed 2. St Louis, 1992, Mosby.

Steele TW, Grover NH: Psychosocial and mental health assessment. In Sheehy SB: *Emergency nursing,* ed 3. St Louis, 1992, Mosby.

Stuart GW, Sundeen SJ, eds: *Principles and practice of psychiatric nursing,* ed 4. St Louis, 1991, Mosby.

Worden JW: *Grief counseling and grief therapy: a handbook for the mental health practitioner,* ed 2. New York, 1991, Springer.

2

Patient Assessment, Reporting, and Documentation

Rapid, accurate initial patient assessment and precise reporting and documentation, whether in the prehospital or hospital setting, are keys to effective patient care. Situations that could make assessment and/or reporting difficult are: an unconscious patient with an unknown history, poor weather or terrain conditions, loud street sounds in the prehospital setting, or an understaffed emergency department on a very busy shift.

Following patient assessment, it is crucial that the information gathered is communicated to others on the care team to ensure that care is consistent. In the scenario of prehospital care, patient information is usually reported verbally and recorded. The information given is usually interpreted by prehospital personnel and verified by hospital personnel. In many situations, prehospital personnel function under preapproved protocols or standing orders. When the information gathered is interpreted, therapeutic intervention should be instituted. This may be necessary even when information is incomplete, to correct or prevent life-threatening events.

To assess a patient accurately, one must be an astute observer and know what to look for, using eyes, ears, nose, fingers, and hands to gather data. Before assessing the patient, the caregiver must verify that the scene is secure for caregivers and safe for the patient. Occasionally it is necessary to delay patient assessment; for example, in an unsecure shooting scene, or when a patient must be removed from a burning building or other hazardous environment. After securing rescuer and patient safety, begin the initial assessment.

STEPS IN ASSESSMENT

1. The Primary Survey (*Always* begin with the primary survey.)

A = Airway

Is the airway open?
> If not, open it and clear it.

B = Breathing

Is the patient breathing? Adequately?
> Consider supplemental oxygen.
> Consider ventilatory assistance.
What is the respiratory rate, rhythm, and depth?

C^1 = Circulation

Does the patient have a pulse? Where?
> Initiate chest compressions if pulses are absent.
> Consider placing the patient on a cardiac monitor.
What is the quality, rate, and rhythm of the pulse?
What can you note regarding skin color, temperature, moisture?
Is there any obvious bleeding?
> Control bleeding by direct pressure, pressure points, or tourniquet (*last resort*).
> Consider using the pneumatic anti-shock garment (PASG) to temporarily control intraabdominal or pelvic hemorrhage.

C^2 = C-spine

Does the patient have any C-spine tenderness? (All multiple trauma patients are considered to have C-spine injury until proven otherwise.)
> *PROTECT THE C-SPINE!*

2. The Secondary Survey

General observations

What is the patient's general appearance? Note body positioning, posture, guarding or self-protection activity.
Are there any obvious problems? Any odors?
What is the patient's level of consciousness?
How is the patient's behavior?
Can the patient walk?
Can he speak? Clearly?
What is the patient's temperature?
Examine the patient from head to toe.
Check for obvious injuries.

Head and face

Check pupils for size and reactivity to light.
Consider assessing gross visual acuity.
Palpate for scalp wounds, tenderness, deformity.
Palpate facial bones for deformity, tenderness.
Inspect orifices of the head.
Check nose for bleeding or clear discharge.
Check ears for bleeding or clear discharge.
Check mouth for bleeding, obstruction, color, hydration, absent or fractured
    teeth, injured or swollen tongue.
Check for asymmetrical facial expression.

Neck

Inspect the neck:
    For wounds
    For midline trachea and presence of subcutaneous emphysema
    For jugular vein size
    For tenderness
    Auscultate carotid arteries for bruits.

Chest

Inspect for deformities, flailing, and obvious injuries.
Note rate, depth, and ease of respiratory effort.
Palpate bony areas for pain, deformities, crepitus.
Auscultate for breath sounds.
Auscultate for heart sounds.

Abdomen

Inspect for obvious injuries, discoloration, distension, masses, scars, impaled
    objects, exposed internal organs.
Auscultate for bowel sounds.
    (One minute in each quadrant)
Auscultate for abdominal aorta bruit.
Palpate for tenderness, pain, guarding, rebound, masses.
Palpate femoral pulses and aorta.
Palpate the liver.
Compress symphysis pubis and ischial wings to check for presence of pain and
    instability.

Limbs

Inspect extremities for wounds, deformities, edema or ecchymosis, and for nee-
    dle ''track'' marks.
Note distal extremity color, temperature, capillary refill, sensation.
Palpate for pain and crepitus.

Back (Log roll patient while protecting C-spine)

Check for wounds and deformities.

Palpate for tenderness or pain.

Occasionally, in the prehospital setting, it may be necessary to perform therapeutic interventions en route to the hospital because of the patient's critical nature and the need to get to the hospital as quickly as possible. In field terminology, this type of situation is usually known as a "scoop and run" or a "load and go." Patients who fall into this category are those who are rapidly losing consciousness and are in severe respiratory failure or shock from trauma. In all such cases, the patient should be stabilized en route to the hospital.

Pain assessment

If immediate transport is not necessary, perform a secondary survey at the scene. The secondary survey might include a more in-depth assessment of pain. A preferred mnemonic when assessing a patient whose chief complaint is pain is "PQRST."

P = Provokes

What provokes the pain? What makes it feel worse? Better?

Q = Quality

What does the pain feel like? Have the patient describe it. Words commonly used are dull, sharp, pressure, tearing.

R = Radiates

In what direction does the pain radiate? Is it located in one area? Does it move? Is it located in any other area?

S = Severity

How severe is the pain? On a scale of 1 to 10, with 1 being the least and 10 being the worst, ask the patient to give the pain a number.

T = Time

When did it start? How long did it last? Has the patient ever had it before? When? How long did it last?

If the patient is a trauma patient, a head-to-toe secondary survey (see Chapter 24) is appropriate. If the patient has other chief complaints, perform assessments specific to that chief complaint (see specific topic chapters for further information).

DOCUMENTATION

Be sure to obtain and record other information about the patient, such as name, age, sex, address and phone number, any medical history or allergies, the patient's approximate build and weight, and any pertinent signs (what can be observed) or symptoms (what the patient tells you he or she feels). Remember to document all findings, both positive and negative. If you are unable to assess a certain parameter (such as blood pressure), be sure to state the reason why (such as, "both arms pinned under car"). This ensures that there is an explanation for omissions. Remember that if something is not documented, it will be assumed that it did not occur.

For prehospital personnel, an organized method of presentation for your report is important. One example of a report format follows:

Prehospital Unit Name

Receiving or Base Hospital Name

Request Physician/Nurse

Type of Patient (urgent, critical, nonurgent)

Location (home, doctor's office, supermarket, street)

Age (approximate)

Weight (approximate)

Sex

Problem/Chief Complaint/Injury

Mechanism of injury/Loss of consciousness

Pertinent History/Medications

Primary Survey Results/Secondary Survey findings, including current vital signs

In the event of a multiple patient call, tell the receiver you have X number of patients. Then proceed by giving the first report on the most seriously ill or injured patient, referring to "patient number one."

In the emergency department, be sure to record detailed nurse's notes. Include a triage note that contains the time of the patient's arrival, mode of transportation (e.g., ambulance, private car), condition on arrival, initial vital signs, and the patient's statement about the chief complaint. Also include information offered by prehospital caregivers.

Record findings of the Emergency Department primary and secondary survey. Include descriptions of any therapeutic interventions that were performed and any response from these interventions. Accuracy is crucial when recording the time each event occurred. Save cardiac rhythm strips (labeled with patient's name, date, and time) to include in the patient's record. Record any lab values or x-ray results that are reported before written reports are available. Also record times phone calls/pages were made to consultants and the time consultants actually arrived in the emergency department.

Flow charts are often useful, especially if the patient being treated is in critical condition and has had multiple therapeutic interventions with documentable data points.

BIOMEDICAL COMMUNICATIONS

Biomedical communications is the term used to send medical information about a patient from one point (usually the location of the patient) to another (usually the base or receiving hospital) by radio, telephone, or television. All personnel involved in the process of biomedical communications must thoroughly understand the local EMS system policies, procedures, and protocols/patient care guidelines. There should be knowledge of the limits and liabilities of all caregivers. In addition, hospital personnel should have an understanding of and appreciation for the unique circumstances found in the prehospital care setting.

Be sure to keep accurate records on all communications, including any communication problems, mechanical or otherwise; have an alternative plan for communication should difficulties arise. When talking on the radio or telephone from field to hospital, speak clearly and use simple terms. Refer to the boxes below for information to aid you in radio transmissions (Aural Brevity Code, Frequently Used Radio Terms, and The International Phonetic Alphabet). If the Aural Brevity Code is used in your system, be familiar with it. Be as brief as possible without sacrificing information about the patient. Make sure that the message is received, and use the phonetic alphabet if it is necessary to spell a word. If using a radio, always identify yourself and the unit you are addressing with each transmission in the event that multiple runs are ongoing or multiple agencies are sending and/or receiving messages. Also, be sure to sign off at the end of the complete transmission.

If cardiac rhythm strips are sent via telemetry, transmissions should be short and intermittent. On receipt, each ECG transmission should be interpreted by concurrence by both the sender and the receiver. The diagnosis of myocardial infarction cannot be made on the basis of a single lead rhythm strip in the field.

In multiple-call situations in which more than one unit is making contact with the receiving unit at the same time, it is imperative to use proper radio communication techniques. The receiving unit will usually control the situation.

Federal Communications Commission Aural Brevity Code (the "10" codes)

10-1	Signal weak	**10-21**	Call _____ by phone
10-2	Signal good	**10-22**	Disregard
10-3	Stop transmitting	**10-23**	Arrived at scene
10-4	Affirmative (OK)	**10-24**	Assignment completed
10-5	Relay to	**10-25**	Report to _____
10-6	Busy	**10-26**	Estimated time of arrival
10-7	Out of service	**10-27**	License/permit information
10-8	In service	**10-28**	Ownership information
10-9	Repeat	**10-29**	Records check
10-10	Negative	**10-30**	Danger/caution
10-11	_____ on duty	**10-31**	Pick up _____
10-12	Stand by (stop)	**10-32**	_____ units of blood needed (specify type)
10-13	Existing conditions	**10-33**	Need help quick
10-14	Message/information	**10-34**	Time
10-15	Message delivered	**10-35**	Reserved
10-16	Reply to message	**10-36**	Reserved
10-17	En route	**10-37**	Reserved
10-18	Urgent	**10-38**	Reserved
10-19	In contact	**10-39**	Reserved
10-20	Location		

Frequently Used Radio Terms

come in   Used in asking for acknowledgment of transmission.
go ahead   Proceed with your message.
repeat/say again   The message was not understood.
OK   Used in acknowledging that the message is received and understood.
ETA   Estimated time of arrival.
spell out   Used in asking sender to spell out phonetically words that are unclear.
stand by   Please wait.
landline   Telephone communication.
over   End of message.
clear   End of transmission.

The International Phonetic Alphabet

A	Alpha	J	Juliet	S	Sierra
B	Bravo	K	Kilo	T	Tango
C	Charley	L	Lima	U	Uniform
D	Delta	M	Mike	V	Victor
E	Echo	N	November	W	Whiskey
F	Foxtrot	O	Oscar	X	X-ray
G	Golf	P	Papa	Y	Yankee
H	Hotel	Q	Quebec	Z	Zebra
I	India	R	Romeo		

The field units may not be able to hear each other. If a phone line is available, the receiving unit may request that one of the squads use the ''Land Line,'' after first ensuring that the patient's condition is not critical and there is time to do so. In such a situation, it is essential that strict attention be paid to detail. The instant a multiple-call situation occurs, all calling units should be advised of the situation. Remind each calling unit that they must be especially careful to identify themselves with each transmission. They should verify orders carefully by repeating them to the receiving unit. When sending the transmission, person- nel should state to which unit the transmission is going. Remaining calm and organized should result in the optimal handling of this potentially difficult situation.

CHAPTER 3

Basic Life Support

More than 650,000 people die from myocardial infarction each year in the United States. Almost half of these people die within the first 2 hours of the infarction. The national trend has been to educate the public regarding the warning signs of impending myocardial infarction, to train lay personnel in the skills and knowledge of basic life support, and to train paramedical and medical personnel in the skills of both basic and advanced life support. These training programs have improved the survival rate from out-of-hospital myocardial infarction that results in cardiopulmonary arrest.

THE COMPONENTS OF BASIC LIFE SUPPORT

Basic life support is the first component of advanced life support. It is the area that may be taught to all levels of personnel, from lay persons to highly skilled medical practitioners. It consists of recognizing unconsciousness, opening the airway, and maintaining the airway. The rescuer then checks for the presence or absence of breathing. If breathing is present, the rescuer must assist in maintaining an open airway. If breathing is not present, the rescuer must begin artificial respiration by giving two *slow* breaths. The rescuer must then check for the presence or absence of circulation by checking for the presence of a carotid pulse. If a pulse is present, the rescuer must continue to maintain an open airway and breathing. If a pulse is not present, the rescuer must also provide chest compressions.

Airway Management

The currently accepted method for early airway management in the patient *not* suspected of having concurrent cervical spine trauma is the **head tilt/chin lift** method (Figure 3-1). The head is tilted back with one hand, and the chin is lifted with the fingers of the other hand. In the case of a suspected cervical spine injury, the **jaw thrust** maneuver is applied, in which the head remains in a neutral position and the jaw is thrust forward using the fingers of both hands at the angle of the jaw (Figure 3-2).

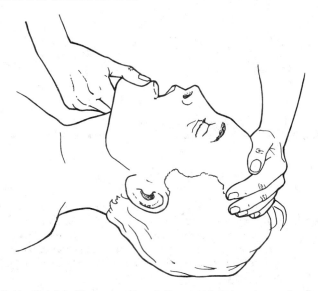

FIGURE 3-1. Head tilt/jaw thrust maneuver. Pull mandible forward using thumb and fore-fingers.

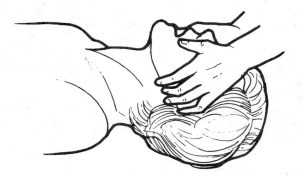

FIGURE 3-2. Jaw thrust maneuver.

Breathing

Once the airway is established, you must ensure that breathing is present. If the patient is not breathing spontaneously (one cannot see or feel the chest rising and cannot hear or feel air movement), you must assist the patient's breathing. The most rapid method of doing this is by **mouth-to-mouth** breathing, where you use your own mouth to deliver air to the patient's lungs. Instructions for

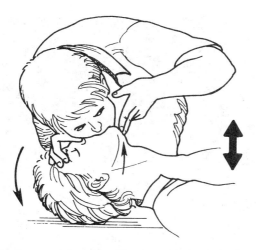

FIGURE 3-3. Mouth-to-mouth breathing. Blow into victim's mouth, observing chest rise.

this procedure follow. In an adult, place your mouth over the mouth of the patient, and pinch off the patient's nose. Forming a tight seal, force air into victim's mouth and lungs using two *slow* breaths initially of 1½ to 2 seconds each with a brief pause in between to allow for exhalation (Figure 3-3). This provides a volume of oxygen before proceeding to the next step of basic life support. When breathing into the victim's mouth, you should meet no resistance and should see the victim's chest rise.

If you cannot perform mouth-to-mouth breathing, you may elect to perform mouth-to-nose breathing; hold the patient's mouth closed and breathe into the patient's nose. In either mouth-to-mouth or mouth-to-nose breathing, you must remove your mouth from the patient's mouth or nose to allow for passive exhalation. Breathe for the patient once every 5 seconds, or in accordance with ratios determined when doing one-person or two-person CPR.

Rescuers in the field may choose or be required to use a barrier device during mouth-to-mouth ventilation. Whatever device is used, it is critical to ensure an adequate seal without air leak.

If a lone rescuer is reluctant to initiate mouth-to-mouth ventilation, due to fear of the risk of disease transmission, the rescuer should activate the EMS system, open the airway, and perform chest compressions until another rescuer arrives who is willing to ventilate.

Obstructed airway

When the rescuer attempts to breathe for a patient and finds that the patient's airway is obstructed, an attempt must be made to remove the obstruction. The rescuer should first reposition the patient's head and attempt to ventilate the patient once again. If this is unsuccessful, the rescuer must perform five abdom-

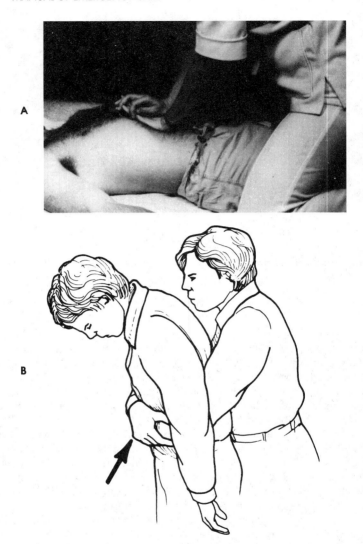

FIGURE 3-4. **A**, Abdominal thrust, lying. **B**, Heimlich (subdiaphragmatic abdominal thrust) maneuver. Place both arms around victim's waist; place fleshy part of fist below xiphoid and above umbilicus. Place other hand on top. Apply quick firm upward and inward motion.

inal thrusts (also known as the subdiaphragmatic abdominal thrust maneuver). (Chest thrust is recommended for victims in advanced pregnancy or if the patient is markedly obese.) To accomplish this maneuver when the patient is prone, straddle the patient and apply the fleshy part of the palm two finger breadths below the tip of the xiphoid process, or one finger breadth above the umbilicus, at the midline. Place the other hand on top of the first, and administer a rapid inward and upward motion (Figure 3-4, *A*). Repeat 6 to 10 times. To see if the maneuver was successful, reposition the head and attempt to ventilate the patient once again. If unsuccessful, repeat the five abdominal thrusts and follow the sequence as many times as necessary to establish an open and unobstructed airway. The Heimlich maneuver may also be accomplished if the patient is not yet unconscious or is unconscious and slumped over in a chair. Proceed as follows: Place both arms around the victim's waist, and apply the fleshy part of the fist below the xiphoid process and above the umbilicus. Place the other hand on top of the first, and administer a quick inward and upward motion (Figure 3-4, *B*). The Heimlich maneuver causes a sudden increase in intrathoracic pressure and may dislodge the foreign body if there is a total airway obstruction.

Circulation

Once airway and breathing are ensured, you must check for the presence of a pulse. Check for a pulse in the carotid area. Do *not* attempt to initiate circulation before ensuring the presence of an airway and breathing and determining the absence of a pulse. When you cannot detect a pulse, provide circulation by performing chest compressions. Ensure proper body position and hand placement before beginning chest compression. Follow this procedure: Slightly separate your knees and keep them close to the patient; keep your shoulders parallel with the axis of the patient's body. Locate the xiphoid process and place the heel of one hand two finger breadths above the xiphoid. Position the heel of the other hand on top of the first hand, locking the fingers of both hands together and ensuring that your fingers do not touch the chest. Keep your arms straight and elbows locked. Begin compressions with a smooth downward motion, compressing the sternum (Figure 3-5). The ratio of downward to upward motion should be 1:1. Avoid sharp, jabbing motions, and compress at a depth of 1½ to 2 inches or to a depth sufficient to produce a palpable carotid or femoral pulse. The ratio of compressions to breaths is 15:2 when doing one-person CPR and 5:1 when doing two-person CPR. The compression rate should be approximately 80 to 100 per minute in both one-person and two-person CPR. In two-person CPR **pause between compressions when giving the breath.** (See Tables 3-1 and 3-2.)

■ **THERAPEUTIC INTERVENTION IN INFANT CPR**

Rescuer procedure

Establish unresponsiveness.

Position the infant on its back, supporting the head and neck (Figure 3-6).

Open the airway, using the head tilt/chin lift method.

Do not hyperextend the neck because it will cause airway obstruction posteriorly.

Check for breathing by looking for chest rise, listening for air movement, and feeling the chest rise and air movement against your face.

If breathing is absent, make a seal over the infant's nose and mouth with your mouth and give two *slow* breaths 1 to 1½ seconds per breath, observing for chest rise. Allow for passive exhalation between breaths.

Check for a brachial pulse.

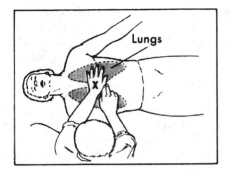

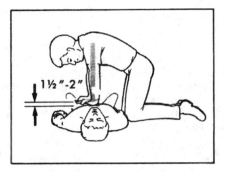

FIGURE 3-5. Body position for CPR. Rescuer should be kneeling, with knees slightly separated and elbows in straight, locked position.

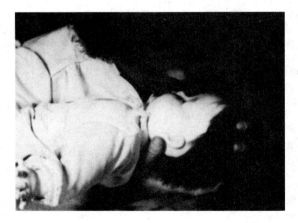

FIGURE 3-6. Infant mouth-to-mouth breathing. Place infant's head and neck in a sniffing position. Do not hyperextend infant's neck.

Feel for a pulse in the upper arm (in the brachial area) for 5 to 10 seconds. If pulses are *present*, continue to maintain the airway and breathing at 20 breaths per minute. If pulses are *absent*, prepare for chest compressions. Imagine a line between the nipples, and place two fingers one finger width below this imaginary line. Compress the chest ½ to 1 inch in an equal compression:relaxation ratio at a rate of 100 per minute (Figure 3-7, *A*, *B*). Compression to ventilation ratio should be 5:1, ensuring a pause for ventilations. Check for the return of a pulse after 1 minute. If apnea and pulselessness continue, continue CPR.

If the airway is obstructed: Reposition the head and attempt to breathe once again. If unsuccessful, place the infant head dependent and face down, and administer five blows to the back. Turn the infant supine, and administer five chest thrusts in the midsternal region. Do a jaw lift, and observe for (and remove, if present) a foreign body. Reposition the head, and attempt to ventilate. Repeat the entire procedure until the airway is unobstructed.

Notes on resuscitation of newborns. Remember that newborns are obligate nose breathers.

It is important to suction the nose first, then the mouth. If the mouth were suctioned first, the newborn would take a breath through the nose and could aspirate material in the nose.

If a newborn is breathing spontaneously, and the heart rate is over 110 beats per minute:

Suction the airway and stimulate the infant. Most infants will then begin to breathe spontaneously.

If there is still no breathing:

Begin ventilation by giving two *slow* breaths, pausing between each to allow for exhalation.

The newborn will probably begin to breathe.

If not, continue breathing for the child and check for a pulse.

Use supplemental oxygen when breathing for the child, and insert an endotracheal tube when possible.

Breaths should continue to be given at a rate of 20 to 30 per minute.

If breathing is absent or labored and the pulse rate is less than 110 beats per minute:

Open the airway.

Suction the airway.

Ventilate.

TABLE 3-1   Comparison of One-Person and Two-Person CPR

	ONE-PERSON CPR	TWO-PERSON CPR
Initial Breaths	2	2
Compression Rate	80 to 100/min	80 to 100/min
Compression: Breath Ratio	15:2	5:1
Other		Pause for breath

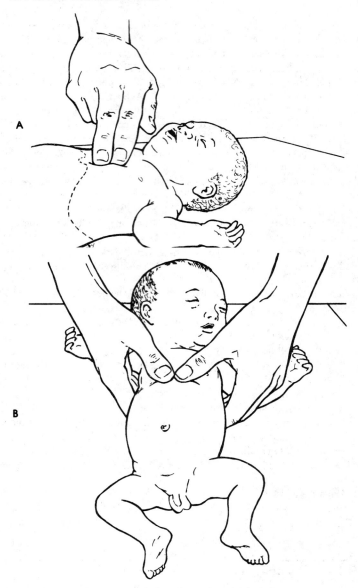

FIGURE 3-7. Infant chest compression. **A**, Two-finger technique. **B**, Thumb technique.

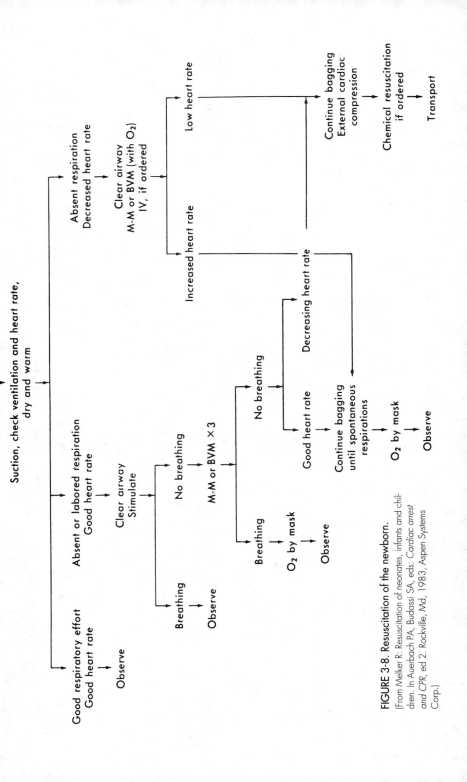

FIGURE 3-8. Resuscitation of the newborn. (From Melker R: Resuscitation of neonates, infants and children. In Auerbach PA, Budassi SA, eds: *Cardiac arrest and CPR*, ed 2. Rockville, Md, 1983, Aspen Systems Corp.)

TABLE 3-2 Differential Diagnosis in Cardiopulmonary Arrest

There are many causes of cardiopulmonary arrest in addition to primary cardiac abnormalities. It is important for the rescuer to be alert to their signs and symptoms, as identification of these may modify the type of therapeutic intervention given. Listed below are some of the conditions that may lead to cardiopulmonary arrest that are not primary cardiac abnormalities. *All therapeutic interventions listed are in addition to basic and advanced cardiac life support measures.*

CAUSES	SPECIFIC	SIGNS AND SYMPTOMS	THERAPEUTIC INTERVENTION	NOTES
Metabolic	Hypoglycemia	Physical signs of insulin or oral hypoglycemic agent usage; tachydysrhythmias; seizures; aspiration	Dextrose, 50%	Consider this a strong possibility in patients who have a history of diabetes
	Hyperkalemia	ECG: prolonged Q-T interval; peaked T waves; loss of P waves; wide QRS complexes	Calcium chloride; sodium bicarbonate	Often seen in hemodialysis and renal failure patients; also seen in patients on Aldactone
Drug-induced	Tricyclic antidepressants (e.g., Elavil, Triavil, Tofranil, Etrafon, Sinequan, Vivactil)	Tachydysrhythmias	Sodium bicarbonate (to keep pH at 7.5)	Causes direct cardiac toxicity; often delayed toxicity in adults
	Narcotics	Bradydysrhythmias; heart blocks	Naloxone (Narcan)	There is a question of direct cardiac toxicity
	Propranolol	Cardiac: Heart blocks Bradydysrhythmias, PVCs	Isuprel Atropine	PVCs may be rate-related
		Respiratory: Bronchospasm	Aminophylline	
		Metabolic: Hypoglycemia	Dextrose, 50%	
Pulmonary (any disease causing severe hypoxia)	Asthma	Severe bronchospasm causing hypoxia and respiratory acidosis; ECG: tachydysrhythmias (especially ventricular fibrillation)	Endotracheal intubation and ventilatory support	Abuse of sympathomimetic inhalants

Pulmonary embolus		Pleuritic chest pain; shortness of breath in high-risk patients (e.g., postoperative, birth control pills); syncope (recent study shows 60% have syncope as part of initial complaint); tachydysrhythmias	Good ventilatory support	Pathophysiology; acute hypoxia and cor pulmonale leading to tachydysrhythmias
Tension pneumothorax		Distended neck veins; tracheal deviation; asymmetric chest expansion; ECG: often electrical mechanical dissociation	Needle thoracotomy; chest tube	Often seen in patients with blunt chest trauma; often occurs during CPR because of chest compressions (especially in patients with COPD)
Neurogenic	Increased intracranial pressure from any cause (e.g., subarachnoid hemorrhage; subdural hematoma)	Central neurogenic breathing; decerebrate pupil(s); decorticate posturing; ECG: wide range of dysrhythmias, especially heart blocks	Central neurogenic hyperventilation (causes respiratory alkalosis which causes cerebral vasoconstriction); steroids; diuretic agents; surgery	Pathophysiology: damage to brainstem and autonomic centers
Hypovolemic	Anything that causes volume loss such as GI bleeding, severe trauma with organ damage, ruptured ectopic pregnancy, dissecting/leaking aneurysm	Tachycardia; decreasing blood pressure; skin cool, clammy, pale; obvious signs of external blood loss	IV fluids; pneumatic antishock garment (PASG); shock position; surgery	A major cause of cardiopulmonary arrest that may be unrecognized
Other cardiac causes	Pericardial tamponade	Distended neck veins; decreasing blood pressure; distant heart sounds; ECG: electrical mechanical dissociation or bradydysrhythmias; widening pulse pressure	IV fluids; PASG; atropine; Isuprel; pericardiocentesis; thoracotomy	Look for it, especially in patients with blunt chest trauma or prolonged CPR efforts

*SPECIAL NOTE FOR PREHOSPITAL CARE: Consider early transport for young patients in cardiac arrest because definitive therapeutic intervention will most likely include procedures not performed in the field situation.

From Budassi SA: JEN 7(2):79, 1981.

If respirations and heart rate continue to decrease:
Continue to ventilate the child.
If a pulse cannot be palpated:
Begin chest compressions at a rate of 100 per minute.
Institute advanced life support measures.
The initial steps in the resuscitation of a newborn (Figure 3-8) are:
1. Airway management
2. Breathing with supplemental oxygen
3. Circulation
4. Establishment of an IV line (usually via the umbilical vein)
5. Administration of sodium bicarbonate (2 mEq/kg diluted 1:1) by push
6. Administration of epinephrine (0.1 ml/kg of a 1:10,000 solution)
Remember that hypothermia can be detrimental to the resuscitation of newborns, infants, and children of all ages. *Keep the patient warm.*

■ **CHILD CPR**

Rescuer procedure. These guidelines are for children under 8 years of age. If the child is 8 years old or older, use the adult procedure for CPR.
Establish unresponsiveness.
Position the child on its back.
Open the airway using the head tilt/chin lift or jaw thrust method.
Assess for breathing by looking for chest rise, listening for air movement, and feeling for chest rise and air movement against your face. If breathing is *present*, maintain an open airway. If breathing is *absent*, make a seal over the child's mouth with your mouth and pinch off the nose. Then administer two slow breaths, 1 to 1½ seconds per breath.
Check for a pulse in the carotid area.
If a pulse is *present*, maintain an airway and breathing. If a pulse is *absent*, kneel by the child's shoulders and prepare to administer chest compressions. Place the heel of one hand two finger widths above the end of the sternum. Place the second hand on top of the first, and interlock fingers. Compress the chest at a rate of 80 to 100 per minute; compress 1 to 1½ inches. Ensure that the compression and relaxation phases are equal.
The compression:ventilation ratio should be 15:2 in one-person CPR, and 5:1 in two-person CPR. In two-person CPR, be sure to allow for a pause in chest compressions while giving the breath.
Reassess the pulse after 1 minute of compressions and ventilations.
If the airway is obstructed: Reposition the child's head and attempt to ventilate again. If unsuccessful, kneel at the child's feet and place the heel of one hand against the child's abdomen just above the umbilicus and well below the xiphoid. Place the second hand on top of the first hand. Press inward and upward quickly five times. Check for a foreign body by performing a jaw lift and attempting to visualize the foreign body. If unable to visualize, reposition the head and attempt to ventilate. Continue to repeat the procedure until the airway is unobstructed. If airway obstruction is not relieved after 1 minute, activate the EMS system.

Circulation

When initiating chest compression during cardiopulmonary resuscitation, be sure that the patient is on a firm surface. You may have to remove the victim from a bed and place him or her on the floor or another firm surface, or you may place a cardiac board under the victim in the bed. If this is not done, pressure exerted to compress the chest will be transmitted into the soft surface, and very little chest compression will occur.

SUGGESTED READINGS

American Heart Association: Adult basic life support, *JAMA* 268(16):2184, 1992.

American Heart Association: Pediatric basic life support, *JAMA* 268(16): 2251, 1992.

Cayten CG et al: Basic life support vs. advanced life support for injured patients with an injury severity score of 10 or more, *J Trauma* S 35(3):460, 1993.

Lauder GR et al: Basic life support training, *Anaesthesia* 47(11):1000, 1992.

Seidel JS et al: Education in pediatric basic and advanced life support, *Ann Emerg Med,* 22(2): 489, 1993.

CHAPTER 4

Advanced Life Support

Sudden cardiac death, or unexpected death that occurs within 1 hour of the onset of signs and symptoms of the event, accounts for approximately 400,000 deaths per year in the United States. Most sudden deaths reflect underlying coronary artery disease. The majority of persons who die suddenly initially experience ventricular tachycardia, which subsequently degenerates into ventricular fibrillation over a variable period of time.

The key to improving survival from sudden cardiac arrest is activation of a particular series of response events as rapidly as possible. Specialized knowledge and skills must be developed in all four links of this ''chain of survival.''[1] (See Figure 4-1.)

Weakness in any link lessens the chance of survival and condemns the efforts of emergency medical services to poor results. This chapter describes the care associated with the links of early defibrillation and early advanced care. The victim can survive neurologically intact if CPR is delivered within 4 minutes and defibrillation within 10 minutes of collapse. For every minute that passes without resuscitation, there is a 7% to 10% decrease in probability of patient survival even if defibrillation is achieved. *Time is of the essence.*

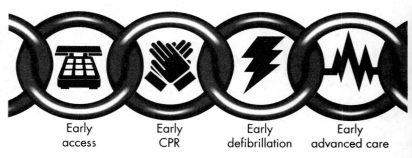

| Early | Early | Early | Early |
| access | CPR | defibrillation | advanced care |

FIGURE 4-1. Chain of survival.
(From The American Heart Association: *Guidelines for cardiopulmonary resuscitation and emergency cardiac care.* Dallas, 1992, American Heart Association.)

AIRWAY MANAGEMENT

Of supreme importance in an emergency situation are the ABCs—airway, breathing, and circulation. Because the basic positions of head tilt and chin lift for airway management have been discussed earlier, this section deals with adjuncts for airway management.

Usual Airway Adjuncts

Oropharyngeal airway (Figure 4-2)

The oropharyngeal airway is a curved piece of equipment constructed of plastic, rubber, or metal. It is inserted over the tongue and into the posterior pharyngeal area. Its primary use is to prevent the tongue from slipping back into the posterior pharyngeal area, thereby occluding the airway. It should be positioned either by inserting it upside down with the curved portion lying on the tongue, and then rotating it 180 degrees as it is advanced into the posterior pharyngeal area, or by using a tongue blade or similar piece of equipment to depress and displace the tongue while the airway is inserted right side up.

Remember that if the oropharyngeal airway is not positioned properly, it may actually cause airway obstruction. This airway is recommended for use in the unconscious patient who has an adequate respiratory effort. It should not be

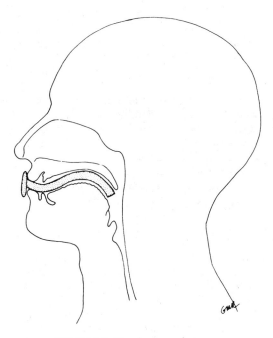

FIGURE 4-2. Oropharyngeal airway.

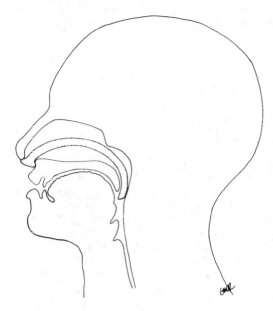

FIGURE 4-3. Nasopharyngeal airway.

used in the conscious patient with an intact gag reflex. Once the airway is in place, strict attention must be paid to maintenance of proper head tilt, chin lift, or jaw thrust maneuver.

Nasopharyngeal airway (Figure 4-3)

The nasopharyngeal airway (trumpet tube) is a soft rubber tube about 6 inches long. It is inserted through a nostril, using a topical anesthetic lubricant. Then it is gently slid backward (behind the tongue) in line with the base of the ears, with the bevel against the septum, to the posterior pharyngeal area. If inserted too deep, the tip may stimulate laryngospasm or enter the esophagus. This airway is tolerated by the alert, oriented patient and is particularly useful when there has been considerable facial trauma. Potential complications include epistaxis, laryngospasm, and vomiting.

Endotracheal intubation (Figure 4-4)

An endotracheal tube is passed directly into the trachea. Endotracheal intubation requires a great deal of technical skill and may be accomplished in the prehospital situation (in accordance with state laws) or in the hospital by trained, skilled individuals. The endotracheal tube is open at both ends.

■ **EQUIPMENT**
Cuffed tube with a standard 15-mm adapter for use with a bag-valve or other type of resuscitation device

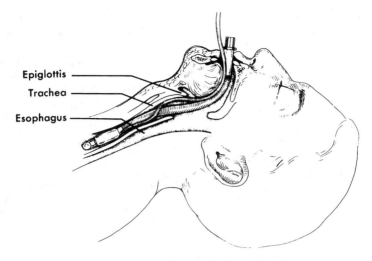

Epiglottis

Trachea

Esophagus

FIGURE 4-4. Endotracheal tube in place.

Malleable stylet
Laryngoscope handle with curved or straight blade
Suction equipment
■ **INSERTION**
  1. Prepare the equipment.
     a. Inflate the cuff of the tube to make sure it is intact, then deflate the cuff.
     b. Insert the malleable stylet into the tube and shape it to the configuration desired, ensuring that the stylet does not slip beyond the end of the tube.
     c. Prepare the laryngoscope by connecting the blade to the handle, ensuring that the batteries are charged and the light is working.
     d. Ready the suction equipment.
     e. Ready the bag-valve device or respirator.
  2. Remove the patient's dentures.
  3. Hyperventilate the patient with 100% oxygen.
  4. Align the three axes of the mouth, pharynx, and trachea to allow for visualization of the vocal cords by placing the patient's head in a "sniffing position." Put a small pillow under the occiput of the patient. (Do *not* hang the head over the end of the bed or table.)
  5. Using the left hand, insert the laryngoscope blade just to the right of the midline into the mouth, following the natural curves of the upper airway.
  6. Lift up on the laryngoscope to elevate the tongue and shift it to the left side of the mouth. The blade should be in the midline position.
  7. Advance the laryngoscope until the glottic opening can be seen by placing the curved laryngoscope blade into the space between the base of the

tongue and the epiglottis (the vallecula) or by placing the straight laryngo-scope blade under the epiglottis. Do *not* pull up on the laryngoscope against the upper teeth.

8. Advance the endotracheal tube with the right hand from the right side of the mouth into the trachea until the cuff rests just below the vocal cords.
9. Remove the laryngoscope carefully.
10. Inflate the balloon and blow into the airway to check proper positioning; watch to see that the chest rises symmetrically and auscultate bilateral breath sounds.
11. Attach an end-tidal CO_2 detector and confirm proper positioning of the tube. Confirm tube placement using a lighted stylet.
12. Attach the tube to the bag-valve device or the respirator.
13. Secure the tube to the patient's face, using adhesive tape, umbilical tape, or a device designed for this purpose.
14. Insert an oropharyngeal airway or bite block.
15. Obtain a portable anterior/posterior chest x-ray film to ensure proper positioning of the tube. If the tube is found in the right mainstem bronchus, pull back on the tube slightly.

If the patient has had spontaneous respirations for 8 hours, and the arterial blood gases are at an acceptable level, the patient may be weaned from the ventilator, and the endotracheal tube removed.

■ **REMOVAL**
1. Suction the tube and the patient's mouth and posterior pharyngeal area.
2. Deflate the cuff.
3. Withdraw the tube. (*Never* withdraw the tube without deflating the cuff.)
4. Always have a suction apparatus ready.
5. Monitor the patient for cardiac dysrhythmias.

■ **ADVANTAGES**
The tube provides control of the airway.
The patient is protected from aspiration.
Intermittent positive pressure breathing with 100% oxygen can be given.
The trachea is easy to suction.
It causes less gastric distension.
Chest compressions can be continued after insertion.
It provides access for drug administration.

■ **DISADVANTAGES**
The tube can easily pass into the esophagus.
A skilled technician is required to place it.
It may cause hypoxia during prolonged insertion. (Patient should be unventilated for no longer than 15 to 20 seconds.)
Chest compressions must be interrupted during insertion.

Tactile Endotracheal Intubation

Tactile or digital endotracheal intubation is an alternative method of intubation that may be used when the vocal cords are visually obstructed or there is a strict need to maintain the head and neck in alignment. Do not use this method unless the patient is deeply comatose.

1. Prepare the endotracheal tube by inserting a stylet and making an open-ended "J" at the end of the tube.
2. Face the patient. Insert the index and middle finger of the gloved, nondominant hand along the side of the patient's tongue, moving the tongue out of the way as the fingers are advanced to the anterior pharyngeal region.
3. Advance the fingers until the epiglottis or opening of the trachea can be palpated.
4. Grasp the endotracheal tube in the dominant hand and insert it into the patient's mouth.
5. Advance the tube to the posterior pharyngeal area until the tip of the tube can be felt by the fingers of the nondominant hand.
6. Slip the tube into the larynx.
7. Remove the stylet and advance the tube simultaneously.
8. Force air into the tube, observing for chest rise and listening for breath sounds bilaterally.
9. Proceed with the remaining steps to secure the tube, as in any other type of intubation procedure.

Alternate invasive airways

Endotracheal intubation is the preferred method of managing the airway invasively during cardiopulmonary arrest. But in some settings endotracheal intubation is not permitted, or practitioners have little experience with it. Alternative airways in use that involve blind passage are (1) the esophageal obturator airway (EOA), (2) the esophageal gastric tube airway (EGTA), and (3) the pharyngotracheal lumen (PTL) airway. With all of these there is increased risk of complications compared to endotracheal intubation. Problems seen with esophageal airways include:

Esophageal laceration and rupture

Inadvertent placement into the trachea

Inadequate seal at the face

If the patient arrives with one of these alternative invasive airways in place, it should be removed as soon as possible. Because emesis often occurs on removal of the alternate airway, an endotracheal tube should first be inserted.

■ **REMOVAL OF THE ESOPHAGEAL AIRWAY**
1. Have suction apparatus available and functioning.
2. If the patient is unable to maintain his or her own respirations, insert an endotracheal tube around the esophageal airway. If the patient has effective spontaneous respirations and a gag reflex, turn the patient on his or her side. (This is not necessary if an endotracheal tube is in place.)
3. Deflate the cuff.
4. Withdraw the airway. (*Never* withdraw it without first deflating the cuff.)

Techniques for Managing the Difficult Airway

Difficulty in obtaining an airway can lead to direct airway trauma and morbidity from hypoxia and hypercarbia. The American Society of Anesthesiologists recommends use of a specific algorithm for management of the difficult airway[2] (Figure 4-5). Three of these techniques are described.

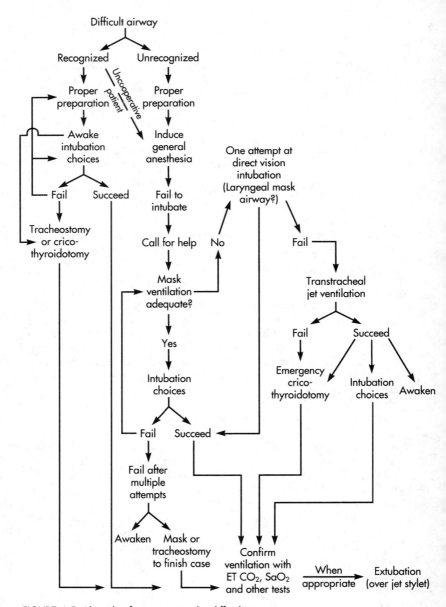

FIGURE 4-5. Algorithm for managing the difficult airway.

(From Benumof JL: Management of the difficult adult airway, *Anesthesiology* 75:1090, 1991.)

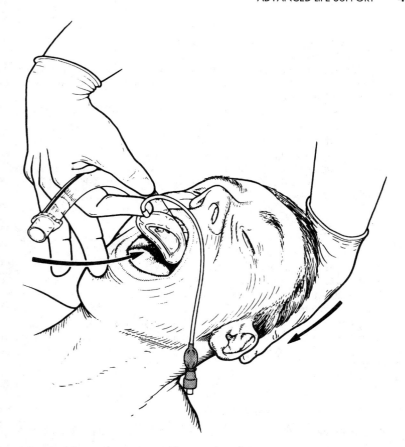

FIGURE 4-6. Technique for insertion of laryngeal mask airway.
(From Brain AIJ: The Intavent laryngeal mask instruction manual. Berkshire, UK, 1992, Brain Medical Ltd.)

Laryngeal Mask Airway (Figure 4-6)

The laryngeal mask is a new device that is intermediate in design and function between a mask/oropharyngeal airway and an endotracheal tube. It provides a safe and swift airway by sealing the outside of the laryngeal inlet with an inflatable cuff. The larynx does not need to be visualized for insertion, and little training is necessary to learn the technique. It can only be inserted when reflexes are sufficiently depressed and stomach contents are not present.

■ **EQUIPMENT**
Laryngeal mask
Lubricant
Syringe
Gauze sponges

■ **PROCEDURE**

1. Make sure that the mask is fully deflated
2. Lubricate the mask well.
3. Place the nondominant hand underneath the patient's head; using this hand extend the head and flex the neck forward. Keep the hand in place under the head during insertion.
4. Have an assistant place several fingers on the patient's lower jaw to open the mouth.
5. Insert the mask tip into the patient's mouth with the dominant hand, pressing the mask against the hard palate to flatten it.
6. Advance the mask into the pharynx using the index finger while pressing upward until resistance (upper esophageal sphincter) is felt.
7. Grasp the tube with the other hand and withdraw the index finger.
8. Inflate the mask with the recommended volume of air.
9. Ventilate the patient.
10. Use rolled gauze sponges as bite blocks and place on either side of the tube in the patient's mouth.
11. Tape the tube and gauze in place.

■ **ADVANTAGES**

The laryngeal mask provides rapid access when the trachea cannot be intubated with an endotracheal tube.

It is inserted blindly without direct visualization of the airway.

The patient can breathe spontaneously through the tube or be ventilated continuously.

■ **COMPLICATIONS**

Laryngeal spasm

Aspiration of stomach contents

Incorrect placement causing obstruction

Percutaneous transtracheal ventilation (needle cricothyrotomy) (Figure 4-7)

If the airway is obstructed, a rapid means of access to the airway is via needle cricothyrotomy. Ventilation by this method should not continue longer than 1 to 2 hours.

■ **EQUIPMENT**

14-gauge (or larger) over-the-needle catheter

3 ml syringe

Alcohol swabs

3.0 or 3.5 endotracheal tube tapered adapter

High pressure oxygen source

■ **PROCEDURE**

1. Locate the cricothyroid membrane.
   a. It extends from the thyroid cartilage to the cricoid cartilage.
   b. Palpate by placing a finger on the cricoid cartilage and moving the finger upward 2 cm.
2. Prepare the area with alcohol or other antiseptic solution.
3. Stabilize the larynx with the nondominant hand.

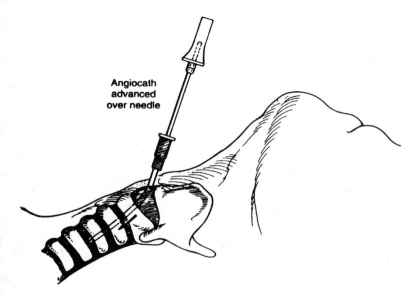

Angiocath
advanced
over needle

FIGURE 4-7. Technique for insertion of catheter-over-needle for percutaneous transtracheal ventilation.
(From Wilkins E: *Emergency medicine scientific foundations and current practice.* Baltimore, 1989, Williams and Wilkins, p. 1000.)

4. Perforate both skin and membrane with the over-the-needle catheter attached to the syringe, directing the catheter down and toward the feet at a 45 degree angle.
5. To verify entrance into the trachea, aspirate air with the syringe.
6. Remove the syringe and needle while manually stabilizing the catheter. Advance the catheter as needed.
7. Attach the catheter to the narrow tip of the endotracheal tube adapter.
8. Connect the wider end of the adapter to a bag-valve device or a high-pressure oxygen delivery device (preferred) and oxygenate the patient.
9. Secure the catheter in place.
   NOTE: Secretions in the patient's upper airway are blown out of the mouth and nose during insufflation, so stand back and wear protective garb.

■ **ADVANTAGES**
Percutaneous transtracheal ventilation is simple and relatively safe to perform. It provides rapid access to the airway when the patient cannot be intubated or ventilated by mask.

■ **COMPLICATIONS**
Subcutaneous and/or mediastinal emphysema
Hemorrhage
Posterior tracheal wall puncture
Kinking or blockage of catheter
Aspiration

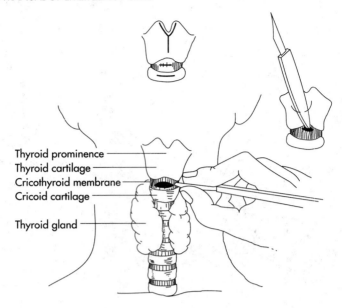

Thyroid prominence
Thyroid cartilage
Cricothyroid membrane
Cricoid cartilage

Thyroid gland

FIGURE 4-8. Cricothyrotomy incision, frontal view.
(From Miller RH, Cantrey JR: *Textbook of emergency medicine.* St Louis, 1975, Mosby.)

Surgical cricothyrotomy

Surgical cricothyrotomy is an alternate method of quick access to a blocked airway in which a scalpel or other such instrument is used to perforate the cricothyroid membrane to create an opening into the airway.

■ **EQUIPMENT**
Antiseptic solution
Scalpel and blade
Tracheal dilator or hemostat
Suction device
Small airway tube (or other such instrument)

■ **PROCEDURE**
1. Identify the cricothyroid membrane.
2. Prepare the skin with antiseptic solution.
3. Spread the overlying skin to make it taut.
4. Using the scalpel, make a small incision over the membrane through the skin.
5. Once the skin is invaded, make a horizontal puncture hole through the cricothyroid membrane into the trachea. (A little bleeding may occur, but usually it is not excessive.) (See Figure 4-8.)
6. Enlarge the space with the scalpel handle, a tracheal dilator, or hemostat.
7. Insert a small tube, such as a No. 6 tracheostomy tube, into the opening. (If a tube is not available, use whatever means are available to maintain an opening.)

8. Supply oxygen via the opening. (If the patient is apneic, there is need for a cuffed tracheostomy tube and positive pressure breathing.)

■ **ADVANTAGES**

Surgical cricothyrotomy provides rapid entrance into an obstructed airway.

A cuffed tracheostomy tube can be placed quickly for the apneic patient.

An endotracheal tube can be placed while the patient is being ventilated continuously.

■ **COMPLICATIONS**

Hemorrhage

Laceration of the esophagus

Incorrect tube placement

Subcutaneous and/or mediastinal emphysema

Vocal cord injury

Aspiration

Infection

Tracheal stenosis (later)

Tracheostomy

Tracheostomy is performed when other attempts at ventilation have failed and when one has been unable to obtain control of the airway, usually because of laryngeal edema, foreign body, or tumors.

Tracheostomy is rarely performed in the emergency department; it is usually done in surgery, in a controlled environment.

■ **EQUIPMENT**

Tracheostomy tube of appropriate size (available in French sizes 13 to 38 and Jackson sizes 00 to 9)

Tracheostomy tape

20-ml syringe

Scalpel handle and blade

Kelly clamp with rubber-coated tips

Scissors

Hemostats

Vein retractor

Suture materials

Tissue forceps

Sterile 4 × 4 inch gauze

Sterile drapes

Suction

Gloves, mask, gown, goggles, and cap

Antiseptic solution

Crash cart (including monitor and defibrillator)

■ **PROCEDURE**

1. Position the patient with a pillow under his or her shoulders and the neck in extension.
2. Ventilate the patient via an endotracheal tube, cricothyrotomy, or other method.
3. Prepare the skin (chin to nipples).

4. Drape the patient.
5. Locate the area for the incision, usually the third or fourth tracheal ring in an adult.
6. Make an incision into the skin. It may be a flap, or a horizontal or vertical incision; usually a vertical incision is used to avoid arteries, veins, and nerves on the lateral borders of the trachea.
7. Control the bleeding.
8. Dissect down through the subcutaneous fat and platysma muscle.
9. Retract the midline muscle.
10. Expose the tracheal rings. Retract the thyroid isthmus cephalad.
11. Inject local anesthesia into the tracheal lumen to decrease the cough reflex.
12. Create a stoma by removing 1 square centimeter of cartilage.
13. Continuously suction to remove blood and secretions.
14. Insert the tracheostomy tube.
15. Ensure correct tube position by checking for air movement.
16. Attach the tube to a ventilation device.
17. Auscultate the lungs.
18. Inflate the cuff.
19. Suture the corners of the incision loosely.
20. Secure the tube with tracheostomy tape.
21. Dress the wound.
22. Obtain a follow-up chest x-ray film.

■ **ADVANTAGES**

Tracheostomy reduces physiologic dead space.

It allows for prolonged positive pressure breathing.

There is direct access to the respiratory tract for secretion removal.

■ **COMPLICATIONS**

Inaccurate tube placement

Laceration of arteries, veins, and nerves

Hemorrhage

Pressure necrosis from cuff

Perforation of the esophagus

Subcutaneous emphysema

Mediastinal emphysema

Oxygen Therapy Devices

Several different devices are available for the delivery of oxygen to a patient. One should be familiar with the various types and be able to select the proper device for an individual patient's needs (Table 4-1).

Nasal cannula

The nasal cannula is the most commonly used oxygen delivery device. It can be used on the patient who is breathing spontaneously. If the oxygen flow rate is adjusted to 2 to 6 L/min, one can achieve an oxygen concentration of 24% to 44%. Its value is reduced if the person is a mouth breather.

TABLE 4-1 Summary of Oxygen Therapy Devices

TYPE OF BREATHING DEVICE	OXYGEN FLOW RATE	OXYGEN CONCENTRATIONS	ADVANTAGES	DISADVANTAGES
Nasal cannula	2-6 L/min	24%-44%	No rebreathing of expired air	Can only be used on patients breathing spontaneously; actual amount of inspired oxygen varies greatly.
Face mask	5-10 L/min	40%-60%	Higher oxygen concentration than nasal cannula	Not tolerated well by severely dyspneic patients; can only be used on patients who are breathing spontaneously
Partial rebreather mask	8-12 L/min	50%-80%	Higher oxygen concentration than nasal cannula or face mask	Must have tight seal on mask; can only be used on patients breathing spontaneously; actual amount of inspired oxygen varies greatly
Nonrebreather mask	12-15 L/min	85%-100%	Highest oxygen concentration available by mask	Must have tight seal on mask; do not allow bag to collapse; can only be used on patients breathing spontaneously
Venturi mask	2-12 L/min	24%-50%	Fixed oxygen concentration	Can only be used on patients breathing spontaneously
Resuscitation mask	10 L/min	50%	Avoids direct contact with patient's mouth; may add oxygen source; may be used on apneic patient; may be used on children; can obtain excellent tidal volume	Rescuer fatigue
Bag-valve-mask	Room air 12 L/min	21% 40%-90%	Quick; oxygen concentration may be increased; rescuer can sense lung compliance; may be used on both apneic and spontaneously breathing patients	Air in stomach; low tidal volume
Oxygen-powered breathing device	100 L/min	100%	High oxygen flow, positive pressure	Gastric distention; overinflation; standard device cannot be used in children without special adapter

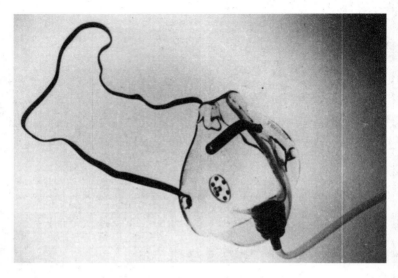

FIGURE 4-9. Oxygen face mask.

Face mask (Figure 4-9)

Face masks are tolerated fairly well in most individuals, except those who are experiencing severe dyspnea, when the face mask may make them feel like they are suffocating. This device must also be used on the spontaneously breathing patient. At a flow rate of 5 to 10 L/min, an oxygen concentration of 40% to 60% can be achieved.

Partial rebreather mask (Figure 4-10)

The face mask is attached to a reservoir bag that allows the patient to inhale the oxygen-rich air from the bag. It can provide 50% to 80% oxygen concentration with the flow at 8 to 12 L/min to patients who have adequate spontaneous respirations.

Nonrebreather mask (Figure 4-11)

The nonrebreather mask is similar to the partial rebreather mask except that (1) a one-way valve lies between the mask and reservoir bag, preventing exhaled air from entering the bag, and (2) one-way valves on the side exhalation ports allow gas to leave the mask during exhalation and prevent room air from entering during inspiration. Increase the oxygen flow rate between 12 and 15 L/min to keep the reservoir bag inflated during maximal inspiration and expiration. With this mask, it is possible to deliver a high oxygen concentration of 85% to 100%. Make sure that the reservoir bag is not pinched off or the inhalation valve obstructed, for then carbon dioxide can accumulate.

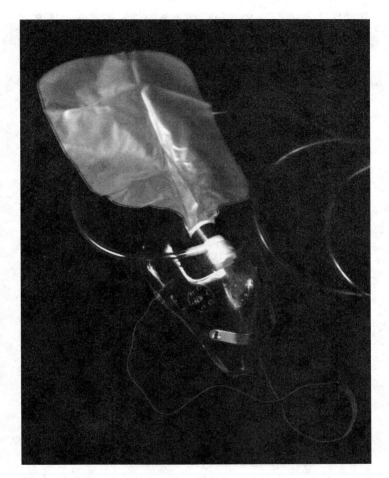

FIGURE 4-10. Partial rebreather mask.

Venturi mask (Figure 4-12)

If a victim has a history of chronic obstructive lung disease and is currently experiencing respiratory distress, one should consider using the Venturi mask, which allows for delivery of a fixed concentration of oxygen. For example, at a 2 L/min oxygen flow rate, the oxygen concentration is 24% with a blue dilutor cap in place (Baxter Airlife Percento Mask). Using various caps and flow rates, oxygen concentration can be increased stepwise by 4% to 5% increments up to an inspired oxygen concentration of 50%. The proper method for using this device is to initiate the flow at the 24% oxygen concentration setting and then to observe the patient closely. If respiratory depression is not present, one may elect to increase the oxygen concentration to 28% and repeat the observation,

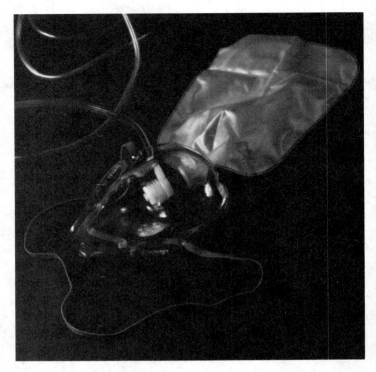

FIGURE 4-11. Nonrebreather mask.

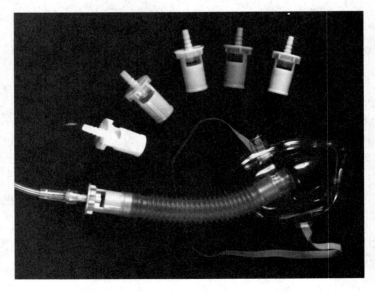

FIGURE 4-12. Venturi mask and oxygen regulator caps.

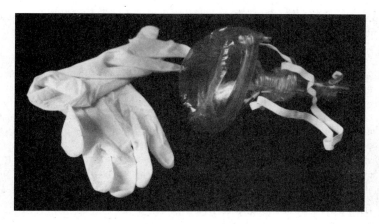

FIGURE 4-13. Resuscitation mask.

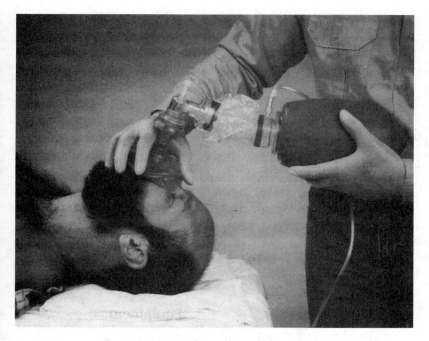

FIGURE 4-14. Bag-valve-mask device.

continuing to increase the oxygen concentration as long as the patient tolerates the previously lower concentration well.

Resuscitation mask (Figure 4-13)

A resuscitation mask is used to perform mouth-to-mask artificial ventilations. In this way mouth-to-mouth contact is avoided. The mask fits snugly onto the victim's face, covering the nose and the mouth. The victim's head should be tilted back, using the chin lift or jaw thrust maneuver. The rescuer can then blow into the tube on top of the mask. If one adds supplemental oxygen and regulates the oxygen flow at 10 L/min, a delivered oxygen concentration of about 50% is achieved. A one-way valve diverts the victim's exhaled air, protecting the rescuer from exposure to infectious diseases. Masks are available in a variety of sizes and configurations.

Bag-valve-mask (Figure 4-14)

The bag-valve-mask unit includes a self-inflating bag, a nonrebreathing valve, and a face mask. It can deliver 21% oxygen (room air) to a victim. By adding a supplemental oxygen source of 12 L/min, one can achieve an oxygen concentration of 40%. By adding a reservoir with an open end, one can obtain about a 90% oxygen concentration.

The mask of the bag-valve-mask unit is applied in the same way as the resuscitation mask, obtaining a tight seal around the nose and the mouth. One-person ventilations using the bag-valve-mask device are less effective than two-person techniques in which both hands are used to get a seal (Figure 4-15). It is

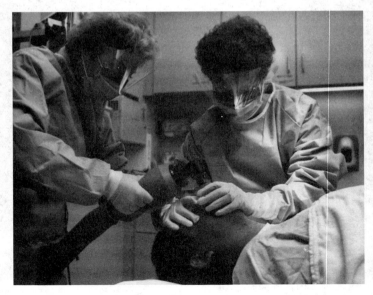

FIGURE 4-15. Use of bag-valve-mask device with oxygen reservoir.

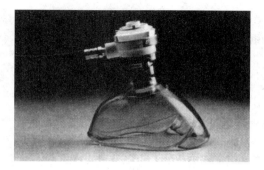

FIGURE 4-16. Oxygen-powered breathing device.

appropriate to use an oropharyngeal or nasopharyngeal airway in conjunction with the bag-valve-mask device. Without the mask, the bag can be used to perform ventilations via an endotracheal tube. Bags are available in adult and child sizes.

Although there are many brands of bag-valve-mask devices on the market, a transparent mask is recommended so that one may observe and intervene rapidly should emesis occur.

Oxygen-powered devices (Figure 4-16)

Oxygen-powered devices can deliver 100% oxygen at a rate of 100 L/min to a resuscitation mask, an attached mask, an endotracheal tube, or a transtracheal catheter insufflation device. Timing and length of oxygen delivery are left up to the operator. This device should *not* be used in children under 12 years of age. The rescuer must be trained in its proper use.

Text continues on p. 84

CARDIAC DYSRHYTHMIAS

When the normal rhythm from the sinus node fails or its conduction is disturbed, a dysrhythmia occurs. On the basis of current knowledge, there are two categories of dysrhythmias:

Abnormalities of conduction that are caused by conduction block, reentry, or reflection.

Abnormalities of impulse initiation caused by altered automaticity or triggered activity.

The reader is referred to cardiac textbooks for explanation of these phenomena.

Dysrhythmias Originating in the Sinus Node
Normal sinus rhythm

Rate	60 to 100 beats/minute
Rhythm	Regular
P waves	Present
QRS complex	Present; normal duration
P/QRS relationship	P wave preceding each QRS complex
PR interval	Normal

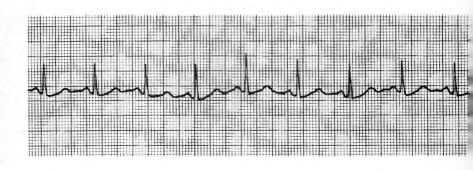

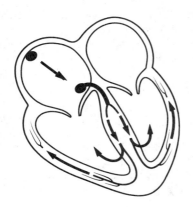

Impulse travels from SA to AV node through His Bundle to Purkinje fibers

■ **SIGNIFICANCE**

The SA node is the normal pacemaker of the heart; it is influenced both by the parasympathetic and the sympathetic branches of the autonomic nervous system.

■ **THERAPEUTIC INTERVENTION**

None required.

Sinus tachycardia

Rate	100 to 180 beats/minute
Rhythm	Regular
P waves	Present, may merge with T wave
QRS complexes	Present, normal duration
P/QRS relationship	P wave preceding each QRS complex
PR interval	Normal

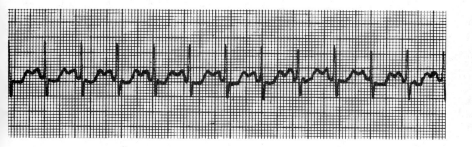

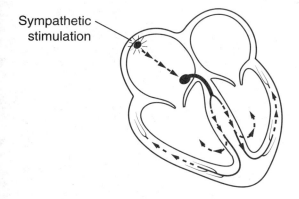

Sympathetic stimulation

SA node originates impulses at regular rate of greater than 100 / minute

■ **SIGNIFICANCE**

The normal pacemaker of the heart is firing at an increased rate because of anxiety, fever, pain, exercise, nicotine, caffeine, hyperthyroidism, heart failure, volume loss, or other reasons that may cause increased tissue oxygen demands. This condition may also be caused by decreased vagal tone (parasympathetic decrease), which allows the sinus node to increase its rate.

■ **THERAPEUTIC INTERVENTION**

Treat the cause. There is no specific drug given for sinus tachycardia except that with increased sympathetic discharge in a myocardial infarction a beta-blocker may be used. If sinus tachycardia is the dysrhythmia seen following cardiopulmonary arrest, a Swan-Ganz catheter should be placed, and the wedge pressure should be maintained at 15 to 18 mm Hg.

Sinus bradycardia

Rate	<60 beats/minute
Rhythm	Regular
P waves	Present
QRS complexes	Present; normal duration
P/QRS relationship	P wave preceding each QRS complex
PR interval	Normal

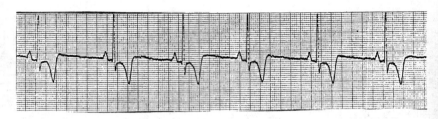

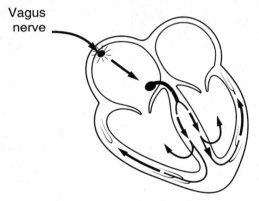

Vagus nerve

SA node originates impulses at a regular rate of less than 60 / minute

■ **SIGNIFICANCE**

The normal pacemaker, the SA node, is slowed by increased vagal tone (parasympathetic stimulation). Causes include sleep, a normal athletic heart, anoxia, hypothyroidism, increased intracranial pressure, acute myocardial infarction, and vagal stimulation (such as vomiting, straining at stool, carotid sinus massage, or ocular pressure). It may also be caused by beta-blocker and digitalis medications or may occur after cardioversion.

■ **THERAPEUTIC INTERVENTION**

Observe the patient for symptoms such as a decrease in blood pressure, decreasing level of consciousness, syncope, shock, or acidosis.

1. Hold digitalis or beta blocker medication.
2. Administer oxygen.
3. Keep patient supine if symptomatic.
4. Treat with atropine or a transcutaneous pacemaker if the patient develops symptoms (e.g., severe hypotension, syncope).
5. Administer IV infusion of dopamine or epinephrine if severe symptoms.

(See Figure 4-27.)

Sinus arrhythmia

Rate	60 to 100 beats usually; may increase with inspiration and decrease with expiration
Rhythm	Irregular
P waves	Present
QRS complexes	Present; normal duration
P/QRS relationship	P wave preceding each QRS complex
PR interval	Normal

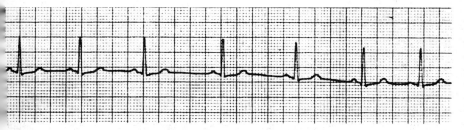

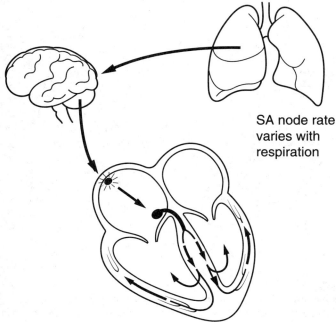

SA node rate
varies with
respiration

■ **SIGNIFICANCE**

This dysrhythmia is a normal finding in children and young adults due to parasympathetic influence. It often varies with the respiratory cycle, but this is not always true. For this variance to be considered a dysrhythmia, the variation must exceed 0.12 seconds between the longest and shortest cycles.

■ **THERAPEUTIC INTERVENTION**

None required.

Dysrhythmias Originating in the Atria

Premature atrial complex (PAC)

Rate	Usually 60 to 100 beats/minute
Rhythm	Irregular due to early beats
P waves	Present, but premature P wave may appear different in configuration (because it did not originate in the SA node)
QRS complexes	Present; normal duration; noncompensatory pause
P/QRS relationship	P wave preceding each QRS complex, though if it appears quite early, QRS may not follow
PR interval	Usually normal

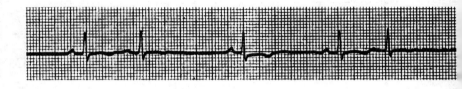

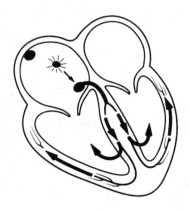

Atrial origin of
abnormal impulse

■ **SIGNIFICANCE**

PACs are the result of an irritable ectopic focus that may be caused by emotions, fatigue, alcohol, caffeine, nicotine, digitalis toxicity, congestive heart failure, electrolyte imbalance, hypoxia, or ischemia; sometimes the etiology is unknown. They may be a prelude to atrial fibrillation, atrial flutter, atrial tachycardia, or paroxysmal supraventricular tachycardia (PVST).

■ **THERAPEUTIC INTERVENTION**

Treatment is usually unnecessary but should be given if the patient is symptomatic. Drugs that could be used are quinidine, procainamide, and digitalis. If alcohol, caffeine, or nicotine is the cause, advise the patient to eliminate it.

Atrial flutter

Rate	Atrial rate of 230 to 350 beats/minute, ventricular rate usually 150 to 170 beats/minute
Rhythm	Regular or irregular
P waves	Sawtoothed pattern of flutter waves
QRS complexes	Present; normal duration
P/QRS relationship	Because of rapid atrial rate, there may be two or more flutter waves for every QRS; it may be regular or irregular
PR interval	Flutter to R wave interval may be fixed or variable

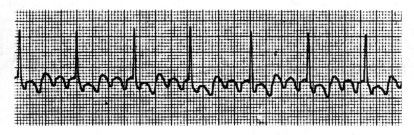

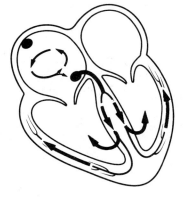

Reentry circuit in
right atrium; block
present in AV node

■ **SIGNIFICANCE**

A single reentry circuit within the right atrium is thought to be responsible for this dysrhythmia. The atrium fires at such a rapid rate that there is a block at the AV node, so that only every second, every third, or every fourth impulse reaches the ventricles. The ventricular response may be regular or irregular. Atrial flutter is a dangerous dysrhythmia in that ineffective atrial contraction may cause mural clots to form in the atria and consequently break loose, forming pulmonary or cerebral emboli. Atrial flutter may be seen in coronary artery disease, rheumatic heart disease, and pulmonary embolism.

■ **THERAPEUTIC INTERVENTION**

Reduce the ventricular rate with digitalis, verapamil, or propranolol. Then administer quinidine or procainamide to convert or prevent the arrhythmia. (See Figure 4-29.) If the patient is symptomatic, use synchronous cardioversion. (See Figure 4-28.)

Atrial fibrillation

Rate	Atrial rate 400 to 800 beats/minute; ventricular rate varies
Rhythm	Ventricular rhythm *always* irregularly irregular
P waves	Irregular, rapid; "fib waves" replace P waves
QRS complexes	Present, normal duration usually
P/QRS relationship	Indistinguishable P waves; irregular ventricular response
PR interval	Indistinguishable

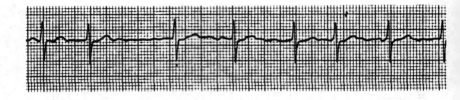

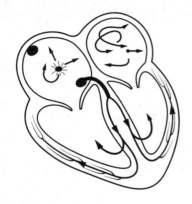

Random reentry circuits
within atria; variable degree
of block in AV node

■ **SIGNIFICANCE**

Multiple atrial pacemakers fire chaotically in rapid succession. The atria quiver and never firmly contract. The ventricles react in a sporadic fashion. Because of poor atrial emptying there is danger of mural clot formation and embolism. Cardiac output drops 15% to 20% because of lack of atrial kick. Atrial fibrillation is said to be uncontrolled if the ventricular rate is faster than 100 beats/minute. This dysrhythmia is frequently seen in the presence of coronary artery disease, pericarditis, congestive heart failure, rheumatic heart disease, hypertension, pulmonary embolus, hyperthyroidism, and digitalis toxicity.

■ **THERAPEUTIC INTERVENTION**

Check the ventricular response, both on the monitor and by checking apical pulse. Check the patient's blood pressure. If the patient is severely symptomatic (syncope, altered level of consciousness, deteriorating vital signs, and chest pain), administer synchronous cardioversion. (See Figure 4-28.) If the patient has been on digitalis therapy, obtain a serum digoxin level before cardioversion.

If the patient has not been on digitalis therapy before the onset of this dysrhythmia, he or she may be treated with digitalis or quinidine following a successful synchronous cardioversion. If the patient is stable with atrial fibrillation, rate control is achieved with digitalis, beta-blockers, and calcium channel blockers. Chemical conversion can be accomplished with quinidine, procainamide, and verapamil, or with newer agents such as flecainide, propafenone, sotalol, or amiodarone. Warfarin is used to prevent systemic thromboembolism. A new surgical technique called the Maze procedure is being used to abolish atrial fibrillation. (See Figure 4-29.)

Dysrhythmias Originating in the AV Junction

Junctional rhythm

Rate	Usually 40 to 60 beats/minute
Rhythm	Regular
P waves	May appear inverted or may not be present
QRS complexes	Present; normal duration
P/QRS relationship	P wave may appear inverted before or after the QRS complex or may be hidden in QRS
PR interval	Less than 0.12 second when P wave is present preceding QRS

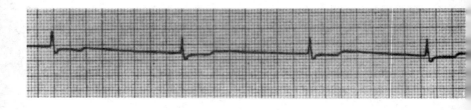

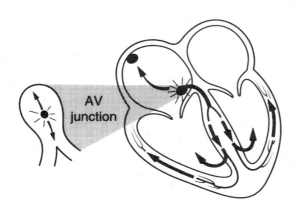

Impulse originates in AV junction

■ **SIGNIFICANCE**

Usually when higher pacemakers fail, the AV junction takes over as the pacemaker of the heart.

■ **THERAPEUTIC INTERVENTION**

If the patient has been on digitalis therapy, withhold digitalis and obtain a serum digoxin level to check for digitalis toxicity. There is no specific therapy for this dysrhythmia. If the patient becomes symptomatic (syncope, altered level of consciousness, and chest pain) as a result of the slow heart rate, give atropine sulfate. If the atropine is unsuccessful, transcutaneous pacing is indicated. (See Figure 4-27.)

Premature junctional complex (PJC)

Rate	Usually normal or bradycardic
Rhythm	Irregular due to early beats
P waves	May appear inverted or may not be present
QRS complexes	Present; normal duration
P/QRS relationship	P waves may appear inverted before or after the QRS complex or may be hidden in QRS; entire P/QRS complex is early
PR interval	Less than 0.12 second when P wave is seen in premature beat

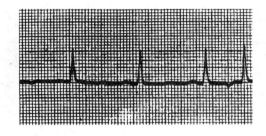

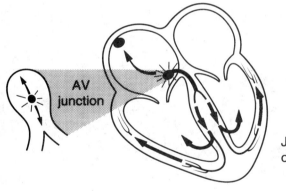

Junctional origin
of abnormal impulse

■ **SIGNIFICANCE**
The AV junction is the pacemaker. The dysrhythmia is usually seen in digitalis toxicity, ischemia, hypoxia, electrolyte imbalances, and congestive heart failure.

■ **THERAPEUTIC INTERVENTION**
If the patient is on digitalis therapy, withhold digitalis and obtain a serum digoxin level. Observe closely. Pharmacologic therapy may include quinidine or procainamide if the patient is symptomatic. Alcohol, caffeine, and nicotine should be withheld from the patient's daily routine.

Junctional tachycardia

Rate	60 to 180 beats/minute; 60 to 100 beats/minute is often called accelerated junctional rhythm
Rhythm	Regular
P waves	May appear inverted or may not be present
QRS complexes	Present; normal duration
P/QRS relationship	P waves may appear inverted before or after the QRS complex or may be hidden in QRS
PR interval	Less than 0.12 second when P wave is present

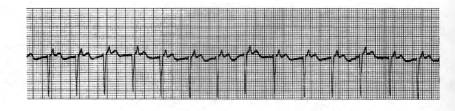

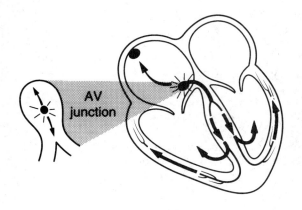

Ectopic focus in AV juncti-
beats regularly at rate of
60 -180 / minute

- ■ **SIGNIFICANCE**

  A junctional focus takes over as the heart's pacemaker. Junctional tachycardia has the same causes as PJCs.

- ■ **THERAPEUTIC INTERVENTION**

  Check vital signs. If the patient is on digitalis therapy, withhold digitalis and obtain a serum digoxin level. In the presence of hemodynamic instability, digitalis binding antibody may be administered. Usually no other treatment is necessary.

Wandering pacemaker

Rate	Usually 50 to 100 beats/minute
Rhythm	Usually regular or slightly irregular
P waves	Present; configuration varies
QRS complexes	Present; normal duration
P/QRS relationship	P wave proceeds most QRSs, though it may disappear
PR interval	Normal

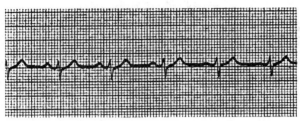

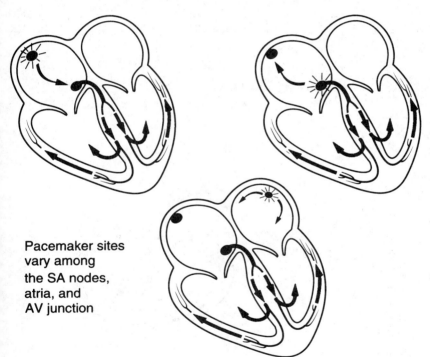

Pacemaker sites
vary among
the SA nodes,
atria, and
AV junction

■ SIGNIFICANCE

There is competition between two or more supraventricular foci in the SA node, atria, or AV junction, for control of the rhythm. Either the SA node is suppressed or other lower foci become excited and take over the pacemaker function of the heart.

■ **THERAPEUTIC INTERVENTION**

Treatment is usually unnecessary. If the patient is receiving digitalis, it may be wise to withhold the digitalis and obtain a serum digoxin level.

Paroxysmal supraventricular tachycardia (PSVT, reentry tachycardia)

Rate	100 to 280 beats/minute
Rhythm	Regular; sudden start and stop
P wave	Often buried in or distorting QRS; may be before QRS
QRS complexes	Present; usually normal duration though may be wide
P/QRS relationship	P wave for each QRS, or none seen
PR interval	Short or none

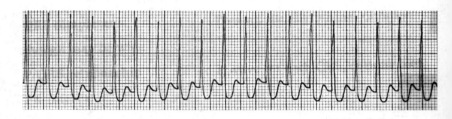

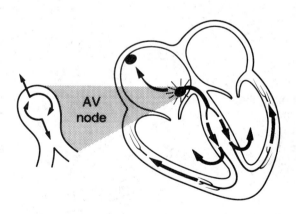

AV junction or atrium originates impulse

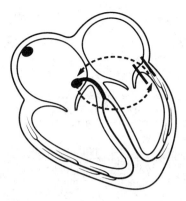

Circus movement between
AV node and accessory pathway

■ **SIGNIFICANCE**

Most frequently the rhythm is a reentry tachycardia occurring within the AV node. PSVT can also be due to circus movement between the AV node and an accessory pathway. Least frequently, the tachycardia originates within the atria. PSVT can occur in a normal heart, or in association with hypoxia, ischemia, electrolyte imbalances, stretch of the myocardium as in congestive heart failure, rheumatic heart disease, acute pericarditis, myocardial infarction, mitral valve prolapse, or with preexcitation such as Wolff-Parkinson-White syndrome. Non-paroxysmal atrial tachycardia is caused by digitalis toxicity. Physical signs in the patient are dyspnea, angina, diaphoresis, fatigue, anxiety, dizziness, and polyuria.

■ **THERAPEUTIC INTERVENTION**

Record the rhythm in multiple leads before treatment so that the mechanism of the arrhythmia can be determined. AV nodal reentry tachycardia is usually benign and self-limiting or easily terminated with vagal maneuvers, e.g., carotid sinus pressure, gagging, Valsalva maneuver, facial immersion in cold water, or coughing. Since this arrhythmia is usually initiated with a PAC, advise the patient to avoid excess caffeine, nicotine, and stress. If the patient is symptomatic with the PSVT, vagal maneuvers or drugs such as adenosine (first line), verapamil, and procainamide IV are used. If this is unsuccessful, cardiovert. (See Figures 4-28 and 4-29.)

If the patient is digitalis toxic, discontinue the digitalis preparation and correct any hypokalemia. Antiarrhythmic medications used in this case are phenytoin, lidocaine, and magnesium IV. If the patient is hemodynamically compromised, administer digitalis binding antibody.

Newer approaches being used are permanent ablation of the AV node by radiofrequency current, and surgical interruption of the accessory pathway.

Atrioventricular Blocks

First-degree AV block

Rate	Usually 60 to 100 beats/minute
Rhythm	Usually regular
P waves	Present
QRS complexes	Present; normal duration
P/QRS relationship	P wave preceding each QRS complex
PR interval	Greater than 0.20 seconds, consistent

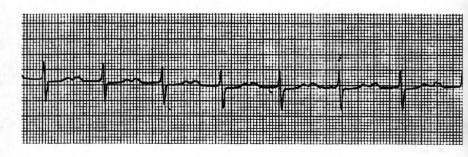

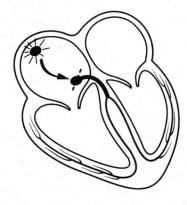

SA node originates impulse;
conduction delay at AV node

■ **SIGNIFICANCE**

The SA node initiates an impulse that is delayed through the AV node. This may be caused by anoxia, ischemia of the myocardium, AV node malfunction, edema following open heart surgery, myocarditis, thyrotoxicosis, rheumatic fever, and certain drugs, including digitalis, clonidine, and tricyclic antidepressants.

■ **THERAPEUTIC INTERVENTION**

Treat the underlying cause. If the patient is on digitalis therapy, withhold digitalis and obtain a serum digoxin level. Observe the patient for a higher degree of block. If the patient becomes symptomatic (syncope, altered level of consciousness, chest pain), administer atropine. If atropine administration is unsuccessful, prepare for pacemaker placement.

Second-degree AV block—type I
(Mobitz, type I or Wenckebach phenomenon)

Rate	Usually normal
Rhythm	Grouped beats
P waves	One preceding each QRS complex except for regular dropped ventricular complex at intervals
QRS complexes	Cyclic missed conduction; when QRS complex is present, it is of normal duration
P/QRS relationship	P wave before each QRS complex except for regular dropped ventricular complex at intervals
PR interval	Lengthens with each cycle until one QRS complex is dropped, then repeats

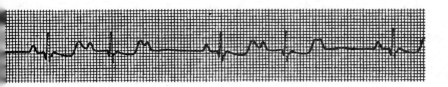

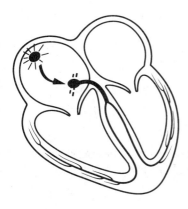

SA node originates impulse;
progressive conduction delay
at AV node

■ **SIGNIFICANCE**

Each atrial impulse takes longer to travel through the AV node, until a beat is finally dropped, and the entire cycle repeats itself. Although its cause is not well understood, this dysrhythmia is transient and commonly seen following inferior wall myocardial infarction or any other disorder that affects conduction through the AV node or the bundle of His, such as digitalis intoxication, myocarditis, or open heart surgery.

■ **THERAPEUTIC INTERVENTION**

If the patient is on digitalis therapy, withhold digitalis and obtain a serum digoxin level. Observe for progression of the AV block. If perfusion is impaired or serious dysrhythmias result from bradycardia, consider atropine and then a transcutaneous pacemaker. (See Figure 4-27.)

Second-degree AV block—type II (Mobitz, type II)

Rate	Atrial rate usually 60 to 100 beats/minute; ventricular rate usually slow
Rhythm	Regular
P waves	Two or more for every QRS complex
QRS complexes	Normal or prolonged duration when present
P/QRS relationship	Two or more nonconducted impulses appearing as P waves without QRS complexes following
PR interval	Normal or delayed on the conducted beat, but remains the same throughout the dysrhythmia

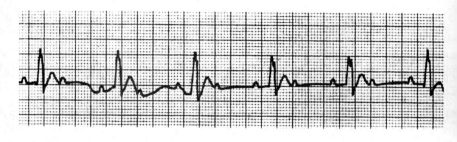

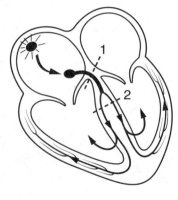

Partial intermittent block in
bundle of His or bundle branches

■ **SIGNIFICANCE**

One or more atrial impulses are not conducted through the AV node to the ventricles. This is usually the result of an inferior or anterior wall myocardial infarction, but may also be caused by anoxia, digitalis toxicity, edema following open heart surgery, or hyperkalemia.

■ **THERAPEUTIC INTERVENTION**

If the QRS is of normal duration, administer atropine. When this is ineffective or the QRS is wide, pacing is the treatment of choice. If the patient is on digitalis therapy, withhold digitalis and obtain a serum digoxin level. If hyperkalemia is the cause of the dysrhythmia, administer sodium polystrene sulfonate (Kayexalate) enema. Always administer supplemental oxygen. (See Figure 4-27.)

Complete AV block—third-degree heart block

Rate	Atrial rate 60 to 100 beats/minute; ventricular rate usually less than 60 beats/minute
Rhythm	Regular
P waves	Occur regularly
QRS complexes	Slow; narrow or wide (>0.12 second)
P/QRS relationship	Completely independent of each other
PR interval	Inconsistent

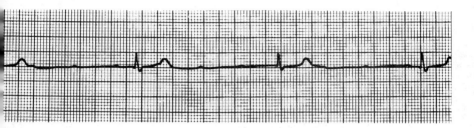

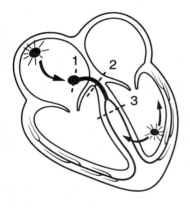

Complete block at AV node, bundle of His, or bundle branches; may have junctional or ventricular independent pacemaker

■ **SIGNIFICANCE**

In this dysrhythmia there is no conduction of the SA node impulse through the AV node. The AV junction or ventricle begins to initiate its own impulse; the atria and ventricles beat independently of each other. Causes may include digitalis toxicity, diaphragmatic or anterior myocardial infarction, myocarditis, or accidental injury during open heart surgery.

■ **THERAPEUTIC INTERVENTION**

If the patient is on digitalis therapy, withhold digitalis and obtain a digoxin level. Observe the ventricular rate closely. If the ventricular rate is slow, the patient will most likely be symptomatic (syncope, altered level of consciousness, and chest pain), and cardiac failure may soon result. Therapeutic intervention is the placement of a pacemaker. Be prepared to perform both basic and advanced life support. (See Figure 4-27.)

AV dissociation

Rate	May or may not be normal
Rhythm	P waves regular; QRS complexes regular
P waves	Vary; may be sinus, atrial, or junctional
QRS complexes	Normal duration or wide
P/QRS relationship	Varies; usually no relationship
PR interval	Inconsistent

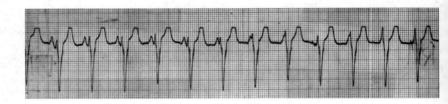

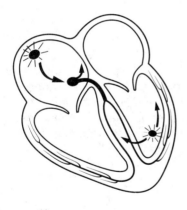

Junctional or ventricular focus
beating faster than sinus node

■ **SIGNIFICANCE**
The AV junction pacemaker accelerates to a rate exceeding that of the underlying sinus rate. There is independent beating of the atria and ventricles, but no heart block is present. This dysrhythmia is seen in acute inferior myocardial infarction and digitalis toxicity.

■ **THERAPEUTIC INTERVENTION**
Most often the patient is asymptomatic, and pacemaker therapy is not warranted. Direct therapy at the underlying cause.

Dysrhythmias Originating in the Ventricles

Premature ventricular complex (premature ectopic beat or extrasystole, PVC, PVB, VPD)

Rate	Usually 60 to 100 beats/minute
Rhythm	Irregular due to early beats
P waves	Present with each sinus beat; do not precede PVCs
QRS complexes	Sinus-initiated QRS complex normal; QRS of PVC wide and bizarre, greater than 0.12 second; full compensatory pause; usually has T wave of opposite polarity
P/QRS relationship	P wave before each QRS complex in normal sinus beats; no P wave preceding PVC
PR interval	Normal in sinus beat; none in PVC

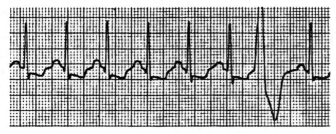

Single PVC

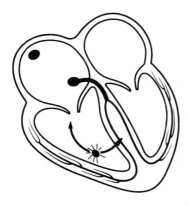

Ventricular origin of
abnormal impulse

■ **SIGNIFICANCE**

PVCs are indicative of an irritable ventricle. PVCs come from an impulse initiated by a ventricular cell. They may occur as a result of hypoxia, hypovolemia, ischemia, infarction, hypertrophy, hypokalemia, acidosis or the use of alcohol, nicotine, caffeine, or many other drugs. PVCs may originate from the same focus (unifocal PVCs) or from various foci (multifocal PVCs). Multifocal PVCs are of different configurations. PVCs may occur in repetitious patterns. If they occur every other beat, the condition is called bigeminy. If they occur every third beat, it is called trigeminy. If they occur in a pair, they are called a couplet. If three occur together, they are called a triplet. A series of three or more consecutive PVCs is commonly known as ventricular tachycardia.

■ **THERAPEUTIC INTERVENTION**

If the cause of the PVCs is known, treat the cause. If the patient is hypoxic, administer oxygen. If the patient is hypokalemic, give potassium. If the patient is hypovolemic, initiate volume replacement. Usually isolated PVCs are not treated except for the first 4 hours after a myocardial infarction. There is little conclusive evidence that PVCs adversely affect survival and that treatment enhances survival. Treatment is lidocaine in the form of an IV bolus followed by additional boluses and an IV drip. Other drugs that may be administered are atropine (if the PVCs are related to a slow heart rate), procainamide, quinidine, phenytoin, bretylium, or propranolol.

Ventricular tachycardia (V tach or VT)

Rate	100 to 250 beats/minute
Rhythm	Regular
P waves	Not seen
QRS complexes	Wide and bizarre
P/QRS relationship	None
PR interval	None

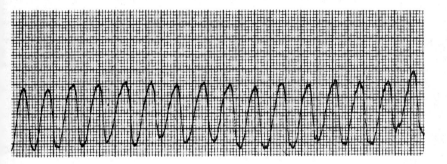

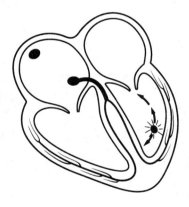

One ventricular pacemaker
fires rapidly

■ **SIGNIFICANCE**

This rhythm is actually several consecutive PVCs. It is rare in patients without underlying heart disease. The patient's hemodynamic response is based on the lack of atrial kick and the ventricular rate. Craney found that cardiac patients with a VT rate of 130 to 270 became dizzy, and loss of consciousness occurred beginning at a VT rate of 200.[3] Nonsustained VT (lasting less than 30 seconds) may not be treated unless the person is symptomatic or has underlying heart disease. Sustained VT is more often seen in those with prior myocardial infarction, chronic coronary artery disease, or dilated cardiomyopathy. Polymorphic VT (torsades de pointes) is often seen with drugs that prolong the QT interval, such as quinidine. If fast VT does not dissipate itself, it will deteriorate to ventricular fibrillation.

■ **THERAPEUTIC INTERVENTION**

Monomorphic VT at a rate faster than 150 beats per minute is treated in an emergency with synchronized cardioversion at 100, 200, 300, then 360 joules (J). Pulseless VT is treated as ventricular fibrillation. If the patient is stable, antiarrhythmic IV drugs such as lidocaine, procainamide, and bretylium are used. Polymorphic VT is treated by stopping the offending drug and giving IV potassium or IV magnesium. If this is not successful, use overdrive pacing or an IV isoproterenol drip. Oral antiarrhythmic drugs include quinidine, procainamide, flecainide, mexiletine, and amiodarone. An automatic implantable cardioverter defibrillator may be used when VT has resulted in cardiac arrest. If the site of the VT can be determined during electrophysiologic study, ablation or surgical subendocardial resection may be performed. (See Figures 4-24, 4-28, and 4-29.)

Ventricular fibrillation (VF)

Rate	Rapid, disorganized
Rhythm	Irregular
P waves	Not seen
QRS complexes	Extremely bizarre, wide patterns, appearing like baseline oscillations
P/QRS relationship	None
PR interval	None

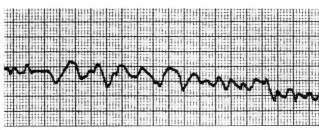

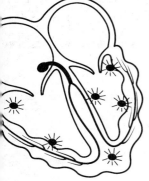

Ventricular ectopic
sites firing so fast
that quivering results

■ **SIGNIFICANCE**

This rhythm produces essentially no cardiac output; death will result if it is allowed to persist for more than 4 to 6 minutes. It is often initiated by ventricular tachycardia. Its most frequent cause is coronary artery disease.

■ **THERAPEUTIC INTERVENTION**

Begin basic and advanced cardiac life support immediately. The sooner defibrillation is performed, the greater the chance of success. Defibrillate three times at 200, 200 to 300 and 360 J, respectively. Administer 100% oxygen under positive pressure; administer epinephrine IV and repeat every 3 to 5 minutes. Allow the drug to circulate for 30 to 60 seconds and then reevaluate the patient's rhythm. If fibrillation continues, defibrillate at 360 J. If this is unsuccessful, the following treatments may be tried: (1) lidocaine, (2) bretylium, (3) magnesium sulfate, (4) procainamide, and in some cases (5) sodium bicarbonate. After each dose of medication, defibrillate with 360 J. If resuscitation is successful, the underlying cause of the arrest must be corrected. (See Figure 4-24.) Patients who survive at least one episode of cardiac arrest may receive an automatic implantable cardioverter defibrillator.

Idioventricular rhythm

Rate	20 to 40 beats/minute
Rhythm	Regular or irregular
P waves	None
QRS complexes	Wide and bizarre
P/QRS relationship	None
PR interval	None

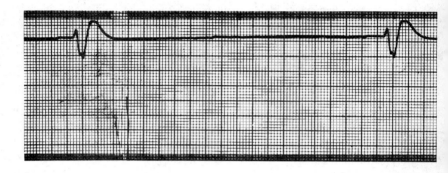

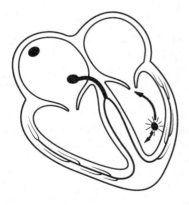

Ventricular focus originates
beat at very slow rate

■ **SIGNIFICANCE**

This dysrhythmia is associated with a poor prognosis; it probably indicates a large myocardial infarction with concurrent loss of a large amount of ventricular mass.

■ **THERAPEUTIC INTERVENTION**

Begin basic and advanced cardiac life support immediately. Intubate and give 100% oxygen under positive pressure. Administer epinephrine and atropine. (See Figure 4-25.)

Accelerated idioventricular rhythm

Rate	40 to 120 beats/minute
Rhythm	Regular
P waves	None
QRS complexes	Wide and bizarre
P/QRS relationship	None
PR interval	None

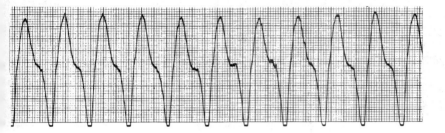

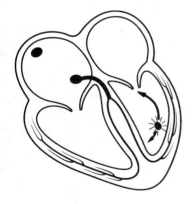

Ventricular focus originates beat
at rate of 40-120 / minute

- ■ **SIGNIFICANCE**
  This arrhythmia is seen during reperfusion with thrombolytic therapy for coronary occlusion. It can also reflect myocardial necrosis.
- ■ **THERAPEUTIC INTERVENTION**
  Often no drug intervention is needed. Keep the patient flat in bed and provide fluids until the arrhythmia disappears.

Asystole (ventricular standstill)

Rate	None
Rhythm	None
P waves	May or may not appear
P/QRS relationship	None
PR interval	None

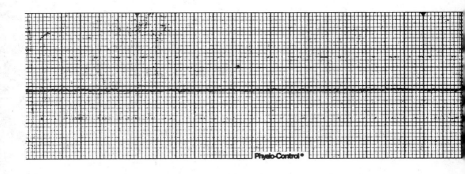

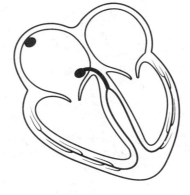

No impulses
from the heart

■ **SIGNIFICANCE**

Asystole often implies that the patient has been in cardiopulmonary arrest for a prolonged period; mortality is high (greater than 95%).

■ **THERAPEUTIC INTERVENTION**

Begin basic and advanced life support immediately. Intubate and give 100% oxygen under positive pressure. Administer epinephrine and atropine. Consider sodium bicarbonate administration. Confirm asystole by switching to another lead because occasionally ventricular fibrillation may appear as a flat line. Shocking asystole may eliminate return of spontaneous heart beats. Transcutaneous pacing may be effective only if asystole is of short duration. Consider termination of resuscitation efforts since this is a "terminal" rhythm. (See Figure 4-26.)

Pulseless electrical activity (PEA)

Pulseless electrical activity is a phenomenon in which some type of electrical activity other than VT or VF is present but there is not a palpable pulse. This group of dysrhythmias includes:

Electromechanical dissociation (EMD)
Pseudo-EMD
Idioventricular rhythms
Ventricular escape rhythms
Bradyasystolic rhythms
Post-defibrillation idioventricular rhythms

■ **SIGNIFICANCE**

Cardiac output is so low or nonexistent that the patient is essentially in cardiac arrest. Death almost always follows PEA, although there is survival from certain causes if recognized and treated early in the process. Causes include:

Hypovolemia
Hypoxia
Cardiac tamponade
Tension pneumothorax
Hypothermia
Massive pulmonary embolism
Drug overdoses, such as tricyclics, digitalis, beta-blockers, calcium channel blockers
Hyperkalemia
Acidosis
Massive acute myocardial infarction

■ **THERAPEUTIC INTERVENTION**

Initiate CPR, intubate, and administer positive pressure breathing right away. Identify the cause and apply specific interventions. For example, give volume expanders in hypovolemia. With suspected cardiac tamponade, perform pericardiocentesis. In tension pneumothorax, apply needle decompression. Proper airway management and aggressive hyperventilation should be pursued since hypoventilation and hypoxemia are frequent causes of PEA. Medications used in PEA include epinephrine IV every 3 to 5 minutes and atropine. Sodium bicarbonate may be useful in hyperkalemia, acidosis, and with tricyclic antidepressant overdose. (See Figure 4-25.)

ADVANCED LIFE SUPPORT TECHNIQUES

Administration of Medications in Cardiac Arrest

The ideal route for drug administration during cardiopulmonary resuscitation is IV through a central vein located above the diaphragm. But often it is easier to place a peripheral IV line, and CPR does not have to be stopped to do so. When drugs are given peripherally compared to the central route, peak drug levels are lower and circulation time is increased. To speed up drug delivery to the central circulation, peripheral catheters should be large bore and placed proximally, (e.g., antecubital). Any medication administered through a peripheral catheter should be given rapidly and flushed afterward with 20 to 30 ml of solution. Then elevate the extremity.

If insertion of an IV line is delayed, one may wish to consider administering medication via the endotracheal route. This route is particularly beneficial for children, in whom much time may be consumed attempting to find an IV route.

The lungs absorb medication rapidly, and the entire cardiac circulation passes through them, making the absorption of medication by the cardiovascular system rapid. It is interesting to note that the onset of action of atropine, epinephrine, and lidocaine given intratracheally to animals in cardiopulmonary arrest was 70% to 80% more rapid than the onset with IV drugs.

The following medications are readily absorbed via the intratracheal route:

Atropine	Isoproterenol
Bretylium	Lidocaine
Diazepam	Naloxone (Narcan)
Epinephrine (Adrenalin)	

The following medications should *not* be given via the intratracheal route:
Sodium bicarbonate; because of alkalinity and volume
Norepinephrine (Levophed); causes tissue necrosis and sloughing
Calcium chloride; causes tissue necrosis and sloughing

■ **PROCEDURE FOR INTRATRACHEAL ADMINISTRATION OF MEDICATIONS**
1. Advance a long, small-bore catheter beyond the end of the endotracheal tube.
2. Stop chest compressions.
3. Administer through the catheter 2 to 2½ times the recommended adult IV dose of the medication mixed with 10 ml of distilled water or normal saline.
4. Give four or five ventilations with the bag-valve device to distribute the medication.
5. Resume chest compressions.

The intraosseous route is an excellent alternative when IV access is not readily available, particularly in the pediatric patient. Although the intraosseous dose would be the same as the IV dose, some evidence suggests that higher intraosseous doses might be necessary, especially when epinephrine is administered.

Medication drips should be mixed in normal saline rather than D_5W. Hyperglycemia may lead to a worse neurologic outcome and increased mortality in the arrest victim. Supplemental administration of glucose should be reserved for documented hypoglycemia.

Carotid Sinus Massage

Carotid sinus massage is the procedure usually chosen before pharmacologic or electric therapies for cardioversion of PSVT. The procedure is performed to place pressure on the carotid bodies located in the carotid arteries. This pressure activates the autonomic nervous system, causing vagal nerve stimulation. As a result, conduction is slowed and the reentry circuit is interrupted, stopping the tachycardia.

■ **PROCEDURE**

1. Place the patient in a supine or Trendelenburg position with the neck extended.
2. Administer oxygen via nasal cannula at 4 to 6 L/min.
3. Initiate IV D_5W TKO.
4. Monitor the patient's ECG continuously.
5. Auscultate the carotids for the presence of bruits (murmurs); do not perform the massage if bruits are present.
6. Turn the patient's head to the left side. On the patient's right side, locate the carotid sinus by palpating the carotid artery just below the angle of the jaw (Figure 4-17).
7. Press the carotid artery between the fingers and the lateral processes of the vertebrae.
8. Apply pressure firmly in a small, circular motion, backward and medially.
9. Pressure should last no more than 5 seconds (less if a rhythm change is seen).
10. Carotid sinus massage may be repeated if it is unsuccessful the first time.

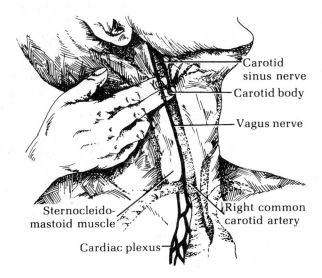

FIGURE 4-17. Location of the carotid sinus body.

(From Conover MB: *Understanding electrocardiography—arrhythmias and the 12 lead EKG.* St Louis,

■ **SPECIAL NOTES**

Warn the patient that the procedure is uncomfortable.

Have a crash cart and transcutaneous pacemaker standing by during the procedure.

Stop the procedure if there is a rhythm change.

Never massage both sides at once.

Successful conversion is often preceded by short periods of asystole, followed by a few PVCs before normal sinus rhythm resumes.

If the procedure is successful, continue to monitor the patient.

■ **COMPLICATIONS**

Dysrhythmias (ventricular tachycardia, ventricular fibrillation, asystole)

Cerebral occlusion (CVA)

Transient ischemia attack

■ **OTHER VAGAL MANEUVERS**

Valsalva maneuver

Facial immersion in cold water

Digital rectal massage

Gagging

Coughing

Precordial Thump ("Thumpversion")

Although the precordial thump may occasionally convert a patient out of VT or VF, the maneuver appears more likely to have no effect, or to exacerbate the rhythm (i.e., precipitate a pulseless rhythm or asystole). This is because the emergency rescuer has no control over when in the cardiac cycle the low-energy wave (approximately 4 J) will be delivered with the thump. Aggravation of the rhythm is likely if the thump is delivered during the vulnerable period (T wave).

Grauer and Cavallaro[4] recommend that the thump be used in "no-lose" situations. They generally reserve use of the thump for treatment of rhythms without a pulse (pulseless VT or VF), since there is nothing to lose from treatment of such rhythms. But in VT with a pulse, where there is "too much to lose," it is better to use synchronized countershock. It is also acceptable to avoid use of the thump in pulseless VT or VF when a defibrillator is close by. (See Figure 4-24.)

In acute onset asystole, rhythmic precordial thumps can produce a QRS complex and associated myocardial contraction until pacing is initiated.

■ **PROCEDURE** (Figure 4-18)

1. Locate the mid portion of the sternum, halfway between the suprasternal notch and the costal angle.
2. Make a fist with the dominant hand.
3. Deliver one blow with the fleshy part of the fist to the mid-sternum from 18 to 12 inches above the chest.
4. Check for return of pulse and continue with resuscitation as needed.

Remember to never deliver more than one precordial thump, and do not delay other resuscitation techniques for the thump. The precordial thump is not used with children.

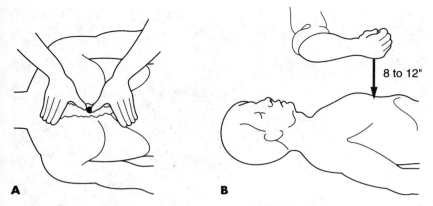

A   **B**

FIGURE 4-18. **A**, Finding correct location. **B**, Performance of precordial thump.

(From Persons CB: *Critical care procedures and protocols.* Philadelphia, 1987, Lippincott, p. 20.)

Defibrillation

The sooner defibrillation is delivered to a patient with pulseless ventricular tachycardia or ventricular fibrillation, the greater the chance of recovery. Without this intervention, death will ensue. Defibrillation depolarizes a critical mass of the myocardium so that the SA node or other intrinsic pacemaker can regain control.

On discovering a patient in pulseless ventricular tachycardia or ventricular fibrillation, the rescuer should defibrillate immediately three times if necessary. If unsuccessful, it is essential to begin basic and advanced life support techniques and medications before further defibrillation attempts. (See Figure 4-24.)

In addition to the manual mode, defibrillators are now available in automatic and semi-automatic designs, so rescuers can be more easily trained to defibrillate. It is essential to know how to operate the defibrillators in your work setting quickly and efficiently. Users should follow checklists each shift to ascertain that there is no malfunction of defibrillators. A more thorough evaluation by biomedical personnel is warranted every 3 to 6 months.

External defibrillation can be performed with the usual hand-held paddles or the newer ''hands-off'' disposable electrodes. Paddles and electrodes are available in adult and pediatric sizes. As soon as the adult paddles/electrodes fit onto a child's chest with good skin contact (usually over 1 year of age or 10 kg), they should be used, because transthoracic impedance is less and defibrillation more successful. Anterior-lateral paddle/electrode placement is commonly used (Figure 4-19), though anterior-posterior placement is an acceptable alternative (Figure 4-20). Paddles/electrodes should be placed 5 inches away from an internal pacemaker generator and never over nitroglycerin ointment/patches or EKG electrodes/wires. If the patient has an automatic implantable cardioverter defibrillator (ICD), the internal pads on the epicardium may deflect the energy when

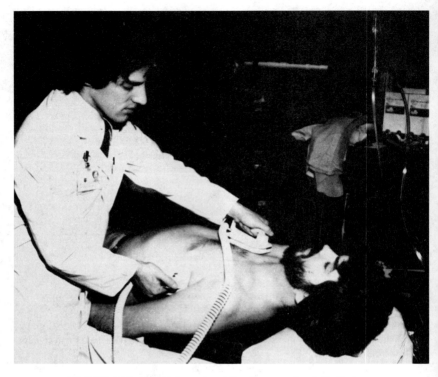

FIGURE 4-19. Anterior-lateral paddle placement for defibrillation.

the paddles are in their usual location. Side-to-side location of the paddles/electrodes may be successful in this circumstance.

Remember that transthoracic impedance is lower with rapid, successive shocks, so initial shocks in the adult are stacked: 200, then 200 to 300, and finally 360 J without pulse checks in between. Initially, 2 J/kg are used with children followed by 4 J/kg.

Disposable defibrillation electrodes are pregelled with conductive medium. When using paddles, always apply a conductive medium to them, even in an emergency. This conductive medium decreases transthoracic impedance and prevents skin burns. Commercially available paste or disposable pregelled pads may be used with the paddles. *Never* use alcohol-soaked pads because alcohol will ignite. Make sure that the paste is not smeared between the paddles on the chest, or arcing of the current may occur. There should be enough paste on the paddles to cover them completely, but never so much that the paste slides down onto the rescuer's hand, creating an electrical hazard.

Before defibrillation remove temporary transvenous pacing wires from the generator so its internal circuitry is not damaged. Always check permanent pacemaker function after defibrillation. Do not delay CPR or external defibrillation when an ICD is in place; proceed with the usual emergency protocols. If

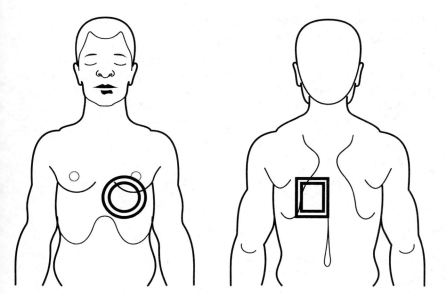

FIGURE 4-20. Anterior-posterior disposable defibrillation electrode placement.
(From Zoll PD: *1200 pacemaker/defibrillator operator's guide.* Woburn, Mass, Zoll Medical Corporation, 1992, p. 35.)

the ICD discharges when the caregiver's hands are on the patient, a small amount of current may be felt, but it is not dangerous.

■ **EXTERNAL DEFIBRILLATION PROCEDURE**

1. Verify loss of consciousness and absence of pulse and respirations.
2. Turn the machine on.
3. Check that the "synchronous/defibrillate" switch is in the defibrillate mode.
4. Select the desired energy level.
5. If paddles are used, apply a conductive medium to their surfaces.
6. Apply the disposable electrodes or hard paddles to the patient's unclothed chest in the desired location.
7. Confirm the dysrhythmia of ventricular tachycardia or fibrillation on the monitor scope.
8. If paddles are used, apply 25 pounds of pressure to them to decrease transthoracic impedance.
9. Charge the machine.
10. Observe closely and state aloud, "All clear." This means no person should be touching the patient, the bed, or any equipment attached to the patient.
11. Discharge the defibrillator by pressing the discharge buttons simultaneously.
12. Quickly interpret the rhythm on the monitor scope and proceed with the second shock if needed.

Emergency Thoracotomy/Open Chest Massage/ Internal Defibrillation

Thoracotomy and open chest massage (direct cardiac massage) or cross-clamping of the aorta may be required in cases of penetrating wounds to the heart, repeat pericardial tamponade not relieved by pericardiocentesis, tension pneumothorax, crush injuries to the chest, or any other incident for which ready access to the intrathoracic cavity is needed. Other examples include patients in arrest with chest wall deformities such as those found in patients with COPD and barrel chest.

■ **EQUIPMENT**

Gloves, masks, goggle, gowns	Sterile towels or drapes
Scalpel and blade	Suture material
Rib retractor	Vascular clamps
Forceps needle holder	Good lighting
Scissors	Povidone-iodine
Suction	
Defibrillator with internal paddles	
4 × 4 inch gauze soaked in saline	

■ **PROCEDURE (PERFORMED BY A PHYSICIAN)**
1. Place patient in supine position.
2. Ensure that patient is being ventilated.
3. Ensure placement of two large-bore IV lines.
4. Cleanse skin rapidly with povidone-iodine.
5. Apply simple skin draping.
6. Make a curvilinear incision 2 to 3 cm lateral to the left sternal border, extending to the midaxillary line in the fourth or fifth intercostal space. (See Figure 4-21.)
7. Spread the ribs and retract the lungs.
8. Introduce a gloved hand into the chest cavity.
9. Open the pericardial sac if necessary.
10. Massage the heart gently.
11. Perform internal defibrillation if needed (see below).
12. Determine if there is volume in the heart.
13. Determine if cross-clamping of the aorta is required.
14. Determine if there is an injury and repair it if possible.
15. It may be necessary to cross-clamp the aorta if bleeding is massive.
16. Once the procedure has been accomplished, transport the patient to the operating suite for irrigation, repair, closure, and chest tube placement.

Thoracotomy is of limited usefulness in medically caused cardiopulmonary arrest. Studies have shown improved survival when the chest is opened early during resuscitation efforts. Thoracotomy should only be performed by a trained physician.

■ **INTERNAL DEFIBRILLATION PROCEDURE**
1. Replace the external paddles of the defibrillator with internal paddles.
2. Turn the machine on.

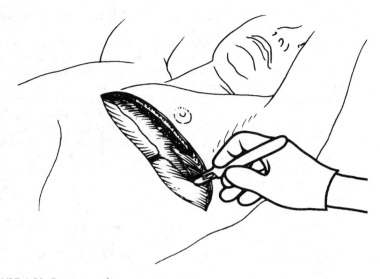

FIGURE 4-21. Emergency thoracotomy incision.
(From Wasserberger J, Ordog GJ, Dang C, Schlater TL: Emergency department thoracotomy, *Emer Med Clin North Am* 7(1):104, 1989.

3. Ensure that the ''synchronous/defibrillate'' switch is in the defibrillate mode.
4. Use sterile saline-soaked sponges as conductive medium; place them on the surfaces of the electrodes.
5. Select the dosage level (usually 10 to 20 J in an adult).
6. Place one paddle over the apex of the left ventricle and the other over the base of the right ventricle.
7. Charge the machine.
8. Ensure that all personnel are standing clear of the victim, the bed, and the electrical equipment.
9. Press the discharge buttons and discharge the current.
10. Quickly interpret the rhythm and assess pulses and breathing status; if these are not acceptable, resume internal massage and continue ventilation.

Cardioversion (Synchronous Electrical Countershock)

Synchronous cardioversion is the delivery of a countershock to the chest wall timed to coincide with the QRS. In this way, the shock is not delivered on the T wave, when it could initiate ventricular fibrillation. Synchronized cardioversion is used when a fast tachycardia is accompanied by signs and symptoms of intolerance. These dysrhythmias include ventricular tachycardia, paroxysmal supraventricular tachycardia, atrial fibrillation, and atrial flutter. If a patient has a wide-complex tachycardia of unknown etiology with hemodynamic instability, it should be treated as if it is ventricular tachycardia. Synchronized cardioversion is immediately indicated. (See Figures 4-28 and 4-29.)

Synchronized cardioversion can be an elective procedure for the conversion of atrial fibrillation and flutter when pharmacologic means have not worked. In the presence of digitalis toxicity, cardioversion should not be performed.

The patient in ventricular tachycardia who is pulseless, unconscious, hypotensive, or in pulmonary edema should receive unsynchronized shocks. This avoids any delay when attempting synchronization, since defibrillators may have difficulty differentiating the QRS from a T wave at a very fast rate.

This procedure should only be undertaken by adequately trained personnel who will not only be able to perform the procedure, but who will be able to manage any emergency situation that may result from the cardioversion.

■ NONEMERGENCY PROCEDURE

1. Explain the procedure to the patient.
2. Obtain written consent from the patient.
3. Give anticoagulation therapy for several weeks before the procedure.
4. Withhold digitalis for 24 to 72 hours before the procedure; a safe digitalis level in atrial fibrillation may be a toxic level in normal sinus rhythm.
5. Give the patient nothing by mouth (NPO) for 12 hours before the procedure to prevent emesis and aspiration.
6. Determine the serum potassium level; hypokalemia predisposes the patient to ventricular fibrillation.
7. Ask the patient to void.
9. If the patient wears dentures, remove them.
10. Continue at No. 4 of emergency procedure.

■ EMERGENCY PROCEDURE

1. Give a brief explanation of the procedure to the patient and/or the family.
2. Obtain consent from the patient or family if possible.
3. If the patient wears dentures, remove them.
4. Keep the room very quiet and dim (usually less sedation will be required).
5. Have a crash cart, transcutaneous pacemaker, and inhalation equipment standing by.
6. Give D_5W IV TKO with an 18-gauge or larger cannula.
7. Have midazolam (Versed) or diazepam (Valium) ready in bolus form; administer it slowly by IV push at small increments until the patient is no longer awake and alert.
8. Ensure that the patient is disconnected from all other electric equipment and oxygen.
9. Turn on the defibrillator unit.
10. Apply ECG electrodes to the patient away from the defibrillator paddle sites. Select a lead with a tall R wave.
11. Obtain a precardioversion 12-lead ECG and have it read by a physician; mark the strip with name, date, and time.
12. Turn on "synchronous" button and verify sensing of the QRS.
13. Set the energy level to 100 J.
14. Run an ECG strip throughout the procedure.

15. If hard paddles are used, cover the surfaces with conductive medium. (*Never* use alcohol-soaked pads—they will explode!)
16. Place the paddles or disposable defibrillation electrodes just to the right of the sternum in the second or third intercostal space and in the fifth intercostal space at the anterior axillary line.
17. Charge the machine.
18. Push down on the paddles with 25 pounds of pressure.
19. Quickly double-check the room to ensure that all personnel are standing clear of the patient, bed, and equipment. Announce, "All clear."
20. Press the discharge buttons simultaneously and hold them until the shock is delivered.
21. Observe the patient closely for respiratory rate and observe the ECG for the resulting rhythm.
22. If the procedure is unsuccessful, repeat it using 200, 300, then 360 J.
23. If the procedure is successful, run a postcardioversion ECG and mark the strip with date, name, and time.

■ **CARE OF PATIENT AFTER CARDIOVERSION**
1. Check the vital signs every 15 minutes for 1 hour, then every 30 minutes for 2 hours, then every 2 hours.
2. Monitor the cardiac rhythm and document any dysrhythmias.
3. Tend to burns that may have been produced by paddles.
4. Keep the patient under observation for 24 hours.
5. If there are no problems, the patient may be discharged.

■ **EARLY COMPLICATIONS**

Asystole	Ventricular tachycardia or fibrillation
Junctional rhythm	Embolization
Premature ventricular contractions	

■ **LATE COMPLICATIONS**
Reversion to atrial fibrillation or atrial flutter
Embolization

Pacemakers

A pacemaker is a technical system for providing low-energy electrical stimulation to the myocardium, which will result in depolarization of the heart. Temporary pacing is instituted in patients with hemodynamically unstable bradycardia (i.e., those with hypotension, change in mental status, myocardial ischemia, or pulmonary edema). Pacing is also used in bradycardic situations accompanied by PVCs if pharmacologic means have not increased the heart rate and eliminated these PVCs. The danger here is that the PVCs, if untreated, may lead to ventricular tachycardia or ventricular fibrillation. (See Figure 4-27.) In asystole, pacing is not usually successful if a long period of hypoperfusion has existed because the heart is then unable to respond to the pacing stimuli. If pacing is to be used successfully in the cardiac arrest victim, it should be started early. (See Figure 4-26.) Finally, pacing may be used to "overdrive" atrial and ventricular tachyarrhythmias. If the pacing is instituted for a few seconds at a rate faster than the tachycardia and then abruptly stopped, the heart's normal (and slower) pacemaker may take over. This overdrive pacing technique should be done only by skilled practitioners with a defibrillator nearby since it may accelerate the rate or trigger ventricular fibrillation.

Standby temporary pacing may be used in the following circumstances:
Stable bradycardias, when it is suspected that the patient may become unstable in the near future
Acute myocardial infarction
Symptomatic sinus node dysfunction
Second-degree heart block, type II
Third-degree heart block
Newly acquired left bundle branch block, right bundle branch block, alternating bundle branch block, or bifascicular block

Components of a Pacemaker System

■ **GENERATOR**
The generator houses the electronic circuitry that directs the pacing rate, current released, sensing of the patient's own underlying beats, and timing. In addition the power source or battery is contained therein.

■ **ELECTRODES**
The contact point with the myocardium (or chest wall) from which the energy is discharged is called the electrode.

■ **LEAD WIRE**
The insulated lead wire connects the generator to the electrodes. It carries the electrical stimulus to the heart and relays information about the patient's own beats back to the generator.

Mode of pacing—demand versus fixed rate

Many pacemakers are set to the demand mode, in which they fire when needed. A sensing circuit looks for the patient's own underlying beats. If the patient's rate falls below a preset rate, the pacemaker fires. Occasionally pacemakers may be set to fire at a fixed rate no matter what the patient's own heart is doing. The problem with this mode of pacing is that the paced beats may compete with the patient's own beats. There is a remote possibility that the pacemaker may fire on the patient's own T wave, causing ventricular tachycardia or fibrillation. In asystole, the fastest way to initiate temporary pacing may be in the fixed rate mode.

Types of pacemaker systems
Temporary transcutaneous (external)

Many of the newer defibrillators also have the ability to perform transcutaneous pacing. Disposable electrodes are placed anterior and posterior on the chest. The caregiver dials the appropriate settings and initiates pacing through the chest wall. See the procedure below. Because the skeletal muscle contraction is painful to the patient, IV sedation or analgesia is given. Electrical capture is usually obtained at 40 to 100 mA. Patients who require greater amounts of energy to capture the ventricle are those with large hearts, increased anterior-posterior chest size, large chest muscle mass, large pleural effusion, and pericardial tamponade. This system is used in emergencies until the patient is stabilized, and then consideration is given to placement of a temporary transvenous catheter when the personnel and equipment are available. It is also used when pacing is needed for only a short duration, such as a bradycardia resulting from a medication side effect or overdose.

■ **PROCEDURE FOR TRANSCUTANEOUS PACING**

1. Administer an IV analgesic/sedative medication.
2. Prepare the patient's skin for electrode application. The skin should be clean and dry. Clip the hair to promote electrode adherence, though shaving may be necessary in an emergency.
3. Attach the pacing electrodes to the pacing cable. Affix the pacing electrodes to the patient so that they "sandwich the heart." The anterior electrode is located at a left V2 or V3 position and the posterior electrode under the scapula to the left of the spine.
4. Attach the ECG electrodes to the ECG cable and apply to the patient's skin in the designated locations. These ECG electrodes must always be in place if demand pacing is used, so that the patient's own beats can be sensed.
5. Turn on the defibrillator/external pacing unit.
6. Select the pacing mode (usually demand) and the pacing rate (usually 60 to 100 beats per minute).
7. Ensure that the machine is sensing the patient's own ECG complexes.
8. If the patient is awake, activate the pacemaker at the lowest current setting. Increase the mA until ventricular electrical capture occurs. Electrical capture is verified by a pacing spike followed by a wide QRS and a tall broad T wave in the opposite direction. (See Figure 4-22.)
9. Increase the mA by 5% to 10% to ensure consistent capture.
10. If the patient is unconscious, initiate pacing with the mA up to maximum. Confirm electrical capture and decrease the mA until only that which is necessary for capture is used.

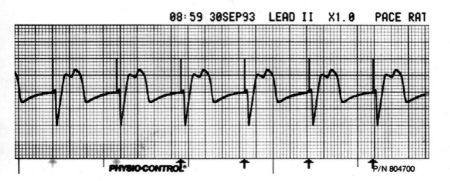

FIGURE 4-22. Ventricular capture with a transcutaneous pacemaker.

11. Verify mechanical capture by checking for a pulse and blood pressure.
    Caution: Assess the pulse in the right femoral artery, for a carotid artery pulse may be difficult to detect due to the muscle contraction with pacing. Measure blood pressure in the right arm because falsely elevated pressures are found in the left arm during transcutaneous pacing.

■ **PROBLEMS ENCOUNTERED WITH TRANSCUTANEOUS PACING**
   Patient discomfort
   Tell the patient in advance that he will feel a "thumping" sensation in his chest.
   Give the patient adequate IV analgesia/sedation before initiating pacing.
   Do not place the pacing electrodes over the nipple, cuts or abrasions, ECG electrodes, nitroglycerin patches or ointment, alcohol or acetone skin prep.
   Place the pacing electrode under the breast of the female patient rather than over breast tissue.
   Use only the amount of current necessary to capture the ventricle.
   Change the pacing electrodes every 24 hours.
   Lack of electrical capture
   Increase the mA.
   Check for adequate adherence to the patient's skin. The posterior electrode may have slid out of position due to diaphoresis.
   Check that all the cable connections are intact.
   Change position of the pacing electrodes. Alternate positions are side-to side and anterior-lateral.
   Correct any underlying acidosis and hypoxia that could be keeping the myocardium from responding to the electrical stimulus.
   Inability to sense the patient's underlying rhythm
   Increase the size of the ECG pattern on the monitor.
   Select a different lead.
   Check for adherence of the ECG electrodes.
   Change the position of the ECG electrodes to achieve different leads.

■ **ADVANTAGES**
   It can be done with minimal training by a variety of caregivers.
   It is quickly and simply initiated.
   The procedure is noninvasive and thus low risk.
   It is especially useful in patients with bleeding disorders, a compromised immune system, or who are receiving thrombolytic therapy.
   It allows more controlled insertion of a transvenous wire.
   It is less costly than other types of pacing.

■ **DISADVANTAGES**
   It is uncomfortable for the patient.

Temporary transvenous

In the transvenous approach a pacing catheter is threaded through a major vein such as the brachial, internal jugular, subclavian, or femoral, so that the electrodes are in contact with the endocardium of the right ventricle at the apex.

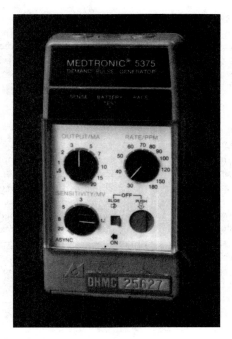

FIGURE 4-23. A temporary transvenous pacemaker generator.

The catheter may have a small balloon at its tip to help float it into position. Its location is then tracked by ECG recordings taken from the end of the pacing wire. The catheter may also be a stiffer type that is inserted under the guidance of fluoroscopy. This pacing wire is then connected to an external generator. Dials on the face of this generator are manipulated by the caregiver to control pacing rate, energy output, and sensing of the patient's own heart beats. (See Figure 4-23.) If pacing wires are placed in the atria and ventricles (dual chamber pacing), the AV interval is also set on the generator.

■ **ADVANTAGES**

It performs reliably once in place.

The patient experiences minimal discomfort during use.

■ **DISADVANTAGES**

It must be inserted by a physician.

Placement is time-consuming.

CPR must be interrupted during placement.

Fluoroscopy is sometimes required.

20% develop complications (e.g., pneumothorax, pericardial tamponade, infection, bleeding, thrombus formation).

The amount of energy it takes to capture the ventricle increases over time.

Its direct pathway to the heart presents a microshock hazard to the patient.

Temporary transthoracic

This emergency method of passing a needle directly through the chest wall until contact is made with the myocardium has been abandoned recently. Problems with this technique were a high risk of complications (e.g., pneumothorax, hemothorax, hemopericardium), delay in chest compressions, and poor reliability of pacing.

Permanent

In a permanent pacing system all the components are placed internally during an elective surgical procedure. Electrodes are put in contact with the endocardium of the right ventricle and/or atrium via a transvenous approach, or rarely the electrodes are screwed into the epicardium. The generator is usually located subclavicular, though it may be in the abdominal area. Settings are changed in the generator by placing a hand held programmer over the chest wall. Most patients are now followed in a pacemaker clinic in which their ECG is sent via telephone from their home to a technician or nurse who checks the function of their pacemaker. Permanent pacemakers are now being incorporated into automatic implantable cardioverter defibrillators to pace patients out of their tachyarrhythmias or to provide back-up pacing when asystole or bradycardia occurs after defibrillation.

Text continued on p. 110

TABLE 4-2   Advanced Cardiac Life Support: Drugs, Indications, and Adult Dosages

DRUGS: MOST COMMONLY AVAILABLE ADULT PREPARATION	INDICATIONS/PRECAUTIONS	DOSAGE (ADULTS)
Adenosine 3 mg/ml in 2-ml vial (total = 6 mg)	• First drug for narrow-complex PSVT • May be used diagnostically (after lidocaine) in wide-complex tachycardias of uncertain type *Precautions:* Transient side effects include flushing, chest pain or tightness, brief periods of asystole or bradycardia, ventricular ectopy. Less effective in patients taking theophyllines; avoid in patients on dypyridamole.	*IV rapid push:* Place patient in mild reverse Trendelenburg position before administration. Initial bolus of 6 mg given **rapidly** over 1-3 sec followed by NS bolus of 20 ml; then elevate the extremity. • Repeat dose of 12 mg in 1-2 min if needed. • A third dose of 12 mg may be given in 1-2 min if needed.
Aminophylline 25 mg/ml in 10-ml vial (total = 250 mg) 50 mg/ml in 10-ml vial (total = 500 mg)	• Third-line agent for acute pulmonary edema. *Precautions:* May cause VT. Avoid in PSVT and ischemic heart disease. Do not mix with other drugs.	*IV rapid loading dose:* 5 mg/kg give over 30-45 min • Never exceed 500 mg loading dose. • Follow with infusion of 0.5-0.7 mg/kg/hr.
Amrinone 5 mg/ml in 20-ml vial (total = 100 mg) Mix in 0.45% NS to maximum of 3 mg/ml (750 mg/250 ml)	• Severe CHF refractory to diuretics, vasodilators, and conventional inotropic agents *Precautions:* Causes tachyarrhythmias, hypotension, and thrombocytopenia. Can increase myocardial ischemia. Avoid extravasation.	*IV infusion:* 0.75 mg/kg given over 10-15 min • Follow by infusion of 5-15 μg/kg per min titrated to clinical effect. Optimal use requires hemodynamic monitoring.

Continued

(From American Heart Association: *Advanced cardiac life support algorithms and drugs, a 1993 handbook for adult and pediatric providers.* Dallas, 1993, American Heart Association.)
*Not yet FDA-approved

TABLE 4-2 Advanced Cardiac Life Support: Drugs, Indications, and Adult Dosages–cont'd

DRUGS: MOST COMMONLY AVAILABLE ADULT PREPARATION	INDICATIONS/PRECAUTIONS	DOSAGE (ADULTS)
Atropine Sulfate 0.1 mg/ml in 10-ml preloaded syringe (total = 1 mg) Can be given ET	• First drug for symptomatic bradycardia (Class IIa) • Second drug (after epinephrine) for asystole or bradycardic PEA (Class IIb) *Precautions:* Use with caution in presence of myocardial ischemia and hypoxia. Increases myocardial oxygen demand. Avoid in hypothermia. • Use with caution in infranodal (type II) AV block and new third-degree block with wide QRS complexes (Class IIb). Be prepared to pace or give catecholamines.	*Asystole or PEA:* 1 mg IV push • Repeat every 3-5 min (if asystole persists) to maximum dose of 0.03-0.04 mg/kg. *Bradycardia:* 0.5-1.0 mg IV every 3-5 min as needed; not to exceed total dose of 0.03-0.04 mg/kg • Use shorter dosing interval (3 min) and higher doses (0.04 mg/kg) in severe clinical conditions. *ET:* 1-2 mg diluted in 10 ml NS
β-Blockers *Metoprolol:* 1 mg/ml in 5-ml vial (total = 5 mg) *Atenolol:* 0.5 mg/ml in 10-ml ampule (total = 5 mg) *Propranolol:* 4 mg/ml in 5-ml vial (total = 20 mg)	• Supraventricular tachyarrhythmias (PSVT, atrial fibrillation/flutter) unconverted after adenosine or digoxin, or if ventricular response remains too fast • To reduce myocardial ischemia and damage in AMI patients with elevated heart rates, BP, or both *Precautions:* Do not give soon after calcium channel blocking agents like verapamil or diltiazem; can cause arrhythmias and hypotension. Avoid in bronchospastic diseases. Administer with monitoring of cardiac and pulmonary status.	*Metoprolol:* 5 mg slow IV at 5-min intervals to a total of 15 mg *Atenolol:* 5 mg slow IV (over 5 min). Wait 10 min, then give second dose of 5 mg slow IV (over 5 min). In 10 min, if tolerated well, may start 50 mg PO, then give 50 mg PO BID. *Propranolol:* 1-3 mg slow IV. Do not exceed 1 mg/min. Repeat a second dose after 2 min, if necessary.
Bretylium 50 mg/ml in 10-ml prefilled syringe (total = 500 mg) 50 mg/ml in 10-ml vial (total = 500 mg)	• Cardiac arrest from VF/pulseless VT after shock, epinephrine, lidocaine (Class IIa) • Refractory/recurrent VT after full doses of lidocaine (Class IIa)	*Cardiac arrest:* 5 mg/kg IV bolus. Repeat at 10 mg/kg in 5 min.

Precautions: Side effects include postural hypotension, nausea, and vomiting.

Calcium chloride

100 mg/ml in 10-ml vial (total = 1 g; a 10% solution)

- Known or suspected hyperkalemia (eg, renal failure)
- Hypocalcemia (eg, after multiple blood transfusions)
- As an antidote for toxicity (hypotensions and arrhythmias) from calcium channel blocker overdose
- Used prophylactically before IV calcium channel blockers to prevent hypotension

Precautions: Do not use routinely in cardiac arrest; do not mix with sodium bicarbonate.

Diltiazem

5 mg/ml in 5- or 10-ml vial (total = 25 or 50 mg)

- To control ventricular rate in atrial fibrillation and atrial flutter
- After adenosine to terminate refractory PSVT with narrow QRS complex and adequate BP. Alternatively use verapamil.

Precautions:
- Do not use calcium channel blockers for wide-QRS tachycardias of uncertain origin.
- Avoid calcium channel blockers in patients with WPW syndrome plus rapid atrial fibrillation/flutter and in patients with sick sinus syndrome or AV block without pacemaker.
- Expect BP drop due to peripheral vasodilation (more BP drop with verapamil than diltiazem). IV calcium can restore BP; consider prophylactic calcium before giving calcium channel blockers.
- Do not use with IV β-blockers.
- Avoid in patients on oral β-blockers.

Stable VT:
- 5-10 mg/kg over 8-10 min. Wait 10-30 min before next dose.
- Maximum total 30 mg/kg over 24 hours
- 5-10 ml IV for hyperkalemia and calcium channel blocker overdose
- 2 ml for prophylactic pretreatment before IV calcium channel blockers

- 15-20 mg (0.25 mg/kg) IV over 2 min
- May repeat in 15 min at 20-25 mg (0.35 mg/kg) over 2 min

Maintenance infusion:
5-15 mg/hr titrated to heart rate

Continued

(From American Heart Association: *Advanced cardiac life support algorithms and drugs, a 1993 handbook for adult and pediatric providers.* Dallas, 1993, American Heart Association.)
*Not yet FDA-approved

TABLE 4-2 Advanced Cardiac Life Support: Drugs, Indications, and Adult Dosages—cont'd

DRUGS: MOST COMMONLY AVAILABLE ADULT PREPARATION	INDICATIONS/PRECAUTIONS	DOSAGE (ADULTS)
Dobutamine 12.5 mg/ml in 20-ml vial (total = 250 mg) *IV infusion only:* Dilute 500-1000 mg (40-80 ml) in 250 ml NS or D₅W	• Use for pump problems (CHF, pulmonary congestion) with systolic BP 90-100 mg Hg and no signs of shock. *Precautions:* Avoid when systolic BP <90-100 mm Hg. May cause tachyarrhythmias, fluctuations in BP, headache, and nausea.	• Usual infusion rate is 2-20 μg/kg/min. • Titrate so heartrate does not increase greater than 10% of baseline. • Hemodynamic monitoring is required for optimal use.
Dopamine 40 mg/ml in 5-ml ampule (total = 200 mg) or 160 mg/ml (total = 800 mg) *IV infusion:* Mix 400-800 mg in 250 ml NS, LR, or D₅W	• Second drug for symptomatic bradycardia (after atropine) • Use for significant hypotension (systolic BP 70-100 mm Hg) and signs and symptoms of shock. May use in patients with hypovolemia but only after volume replacement. Use with caution in cardiogenic shock and CHF. *Precautions:* Do not mix with sodium bicarbonate. May cause tachyarrhythmias, excessive vasoconstriction.	*Low dose:* 1-5 μg/kg/min infusion rate ("renal doses") *Moderate dose:* 5-10 μg/kg/min ("cardiac doses") *High dose:* 10-20 μg/kg/min ("vasopressor doses")
Epinephrine Preloaded 10-ml syringe: 1 mg/10 ml Glass 1-ml ampule: 1 mg/ml Multi-dose 30-ml vial: 1 mg/ml Can be given ET	• *Cardiac arrest:* VF, pulseless VT, asystole, PEA • *Symptomatic bradycardia* after atropine and transcutaneous pacing (Class IIb)	*Cardiac arrest:* First dose: 1 mg IV push, may repeat every 3-5 min. *Alternative regimens for second dose of epinephrine (Class IIb):* • Intermediate: 2-5 mg IV push, every 3-5 min • Escalating: 1 mg-3 mg-5 mg IV push, 3 min apart • High: 0.1 mg/kg IV push, every 3-5 min *Endotracheal:* 2.0-2.5 mg diluted in 10 ml NS *Profound bradycardia:* 2-10 μg/min (add 1 mg to 500 ml NS; run at 1-5 ml/min)

Furosemide

10 mg/ml in ampules, vials, syringes of 2 ml, 4 ml, 10 ml

- For adjunctive therapy of acute pulmonary edema in patients with systolic BP >90-100 mm Hg; hypertensive emergencies.

Precautions: Dehydration, hypotension, electrolyte imbalance

IV push:

0.5-1.0 mg/kg given over 1-2 min. If no response, double the dose to 2 mg/kg IV, slowly over 1-2 min.

Isoproterenol

1 mg/ml in 1-ml vial

IV infusion:
Mix 1 mg in 250 ml NS, LR, or D_5W

- **Do not use for cardiac arrest patients.**
- Refractory torsades de pointes (but only after magnesium sulfate)
- *Temporary* control of bradycardia in heart transplant patients

Precautions: Increases myocardial oxygen requirements, which may increase myocardial ischemia. Do not give with epinephrine; can cause VF/VT.

- Infuse at 2-10 µg/min.
- Titrate to adequate heart rate.
- In torsades, titrate to heart rate that results in suppression of the VT.

Lidocaine

Preloaded 20 mg/ml in 5-ml syringe (total = 100 mg)

Also in 10 mg/ml in 5-ml vial (total = 50 mg)

Can be given ET

- Cadiac arrest from VF/pulseless VT (Class IIa)
- Stable VT, wide-complex tachycardias of uncertain type, wide-complex PSVT (Class I)

Precautions:

- *Prophylactic* use in AMI patients not recommended.
- Reduce maintenance dose (not loading dose) in patients with impaired liver function, left ventricular dysfunction.

Cardiac arrest from VF/VT:

- Initial dose: 1.0-1.5 mg/kg IV push
- For refractory VF may repeat at 1.0-1.5 mg/kg in 3-5 min; maximum total of 3 mg/kg.
- A single dose of 1.5 mg/kg in cardiac arrest is acceptable.

Nonarrested patient:

Stable VT, wide-complex tachycardia of uncertain type, significant ectopy:

- 1.0-1.5 mg/kg IV push. Repeat at 0.5-0.75 mg/kg every 5-10 min, maximum total 3 mg/kg.

Maintenance infusion:

2-4 mg/min (30-50 µg/kg per min)

Continued

(From American Heart Association: *Advanced cardiac life support algorithms and drugs, a 1993 handbook for adult and pediatric providers.* Dallas, 1993, American Heart Association.)
*Not yet FDA-approved

TABLE 4-2 Advanced Cardiac Life Support: Drugs, Indications, and Adult Dosages–cont'd

DRUGS: MOST COMMONLY AVAILABLE ADULT PREPARATION	INDICATIONS/PRECAUTIONS	DOSAGE (ADULTS)
Magnesium sulfate 10-ml ampule of 50% $MgSO_4$ = 5 g of magnesium 2-ml ampule (total = 1 g/2 ml) 10-ml preloaded syringe (total = 5 g/10 ml)	• Cardiac arrest associated with torsades de pointes, or suspected hypomagnesemic state • Refractory VF (after lidocaine and bretylium) • Perfusing torsades de pointes • Consider prophylactic administration in hospitalized patients with AMI (Class IIa). • Life-threatening ventricular arrhythmias due to digitalis toxicity, tricyclic overdose *Precautions:* Occasional fall in BP with rapid administration. Use caution with renal failure.	***Cardiac arrest:*** 1-2 g IV (2-4 ml of a 50% solution), diluted in 10 ml of D_5W, given over 1-2 min ***Acute myocardial infarction:*** Loading dose of 1-2 g (8-16 mEq), mixed in 50-100 ml of D_5W, over 5-60 min. Follow with 0.5-1.0 g (4-8 mEq) per hour for up to 24 hours. ***Torsades de pointes:*** Loading dose of 1-2 g (8-16 mEq), mixed in 50-100 ml of D_5W, over 5-60 min. Follow with 1-4 g/h (sufficient to control the torsades).
Morphine sulfate 2-5 mg/ml in 1-ml syringe	• Chest pain and anxiety associated with AMI, or cardiac ischemia • Acute cardiogenic pulmonary edema (if BP adequate) *Precautions:* • May compromise respiration; therefore use with caution in the compromised respiratory state of acute pulmonary edema. • Reverse with naloxone (0.4-0.8 mg IV). Administer slowly and titrate to effect. • Causes hypotension in volume-depleted patients.	• 1-3 mg slow IV (over 1-5 min) every 5-30 min
Nitroglycerin **SL tablets:** 0.3, 0.4 mg **Inhaler:** 0.4 mg/dose *IV infusion:* Ampules: Vials: 5 mg in 10 ml 25 mg in 5 ml 8 mg in 10 ml 50 mg in 10 ml 10 mg in 10 ml 100 mg in 10 ml	• Chest pain of suspected cardiac origin • Unstable angina • Complications of AMI, including CHF, left ventricular failure • Hypertensive crisis/urgency with chest pain *Precautions:* With evidence of AMI limit systolic BP drop to 10% if patient is normotensive, 30% if hypertensive, and avoid below 90 mm Hg. Patient should sit or lie down when receiving this medication.	***IV infusion:*** Route of choice for emergencies. Use IV sets provided by manufacturers. Infuse at 10-20 µg/min. Titrate to effect. Do not mix with other drugs. ***Sublingual:*** 0.3-0.4 mg, repeat every 5 min. ***Inhaler:*** Spray for 0.5-1 at 5-min intervals.

Nitroprusside

(*Light sensitive*)
10 mg/ml in 5-ml vial (total = 50 mg)
Mix 50 or 100 mg in 250 ml D_5 W or NS.

Cover drug with opaque material.

- Hypertensive crisis
- To reduce afterload in heart failure and acute pulmonary edema
- To reduce afterload in acute mitral or aortic regurgitation

Precautions: Wrap drug reservoir in aluminum foil. Hypotension, thiocyanate toxicity, and CO_2 retention. Other complaints include headaches, nausea, vomiting, and abdominal cramps.

IV infusion:
Begin at 0.1 µg/kg/min and titrate upward every 3-5 min to desired effect (up to 5 µg/kg/min).
- Use an infusion pump. Action occurs within 1-2 min.

Norepinephrine

1 mg/ml in 4-ml ampule
Mix 4 mg in 250 ml D_5W or D_5NS. Avoid dilution in NS alone.

For severe cardiogenic shock and hemodynamically significant hypotension (systolic BP <70 mm Hg). This is an agent of last resort for management of ischemic heart disease and shock.

Precautions: Increases myocardial oxygen requirements as it raises BP. May induce arrhythmias. Use caution in patients with acute ischemia; monitor cardiac output. Extravasation causes tissue necrosis.

IV drip only:
0.5-1.0 µg/min titrated to effect up to 30 µg/min

Procainamide

100 mg/ml in 10-ml vial (total = 1 g)
500 mg/ml in 2-ml vial (total = 1 g)

- Recurrent VT not controlled by lidocaine
- Refractory PSVT
- Refractory VF/pulseless VT
- Stable wide-complex tachycardia of unknown origin
- AF with rapid rate in WPW

Precautions:
- Patients with cardiac or renal dysfunction: reduce loading dose to 12 mg/kg and maintenance infusion to 1-2 mg/min
- Proarrhythmic, especially in setting of AMI, hypokalemia, or hypomagnesemia

Cardiac arrest:
30 mg/min (maximum total 17 mg/kg)
Other indications:
20-30 mg/min until one of following:
- Arrhythmia suppression
- Hypotension
- QRS widens >50%
- Total of 17 mg/kg given
Maintenance infusion:
1-4 mg/min

Continued

(From American Heart Association: *Advanced cardiac life support algorithms and drugs, a 1993 handbook for adult and pediatric providers.* Dallas, 1993, American Heart Association.)
*Not yet FDA-approved

TABLE 4-2 Advanced Cardiac Life Support: Drugs, Indications, and Adult Dosages—cont'd

DRUGS: MOST COMMONLY AVAILABLE ADULT PREPARATION	INDICATIONS/PRECAUTIONS	DOSAGE (ADULTS)
Sodium bicarbonate 50-ml preloaded syringe 8.4% sodium bicarbonate at 50 mEq/50 ml)	• Not recommended for routine use in cardiac arrest patients • Adequate ventilation and CPR are the major "buffer agents" in cardiac arrest. *Precautions:* There are specific indications for bicarbonate use: • Class I if patient has known preexisting hyperkalemia • Class IIa if known preexisting bicarbonate-responsive acidosis (e.g., diabetic ketoacidosis); tricyclic antidepressant overdose; to alkalinize urine in aspirin overdose • Class IIb if intubated and continued long arrest interval; upon return of spontaneous circulation after long arrest interval • Class III (harmful): hypoxic lactic acidosis (e.g., cardiac arrest and CPR without intubation)	• 1 mEq/kg IV bolus • Repeat half this dose every 10 min thereafter. • If rapidly available, use blood gas analyses to guide bicarbonate therapy (calculated base deficits or bicarbonate concentration).
Thrombolytic agents	ST segment elevation of 1 mm in 2 or more contiguous leads in context of signs and symptoms of AMI	Several dosing regimens are possible for thrombolytic therapy.

Alteplase:
Reconstitute to 1 mg/ml

Precautions: Usual exclusion criteria: active, internal bleeding; history of cerebral vascular event (stroke, AV malformation, neoplasm, head trauma, recent surgery, or trauma in last 14 days); aortic dissection; severe uncontrolled hypertension; bleeding diatheses; prolonged CPR with evidence of thoracic trauma; central lines, difficult intubation

Adjunctive therapy:
• 160-325 mg aspirin chewed as soon as possible
• Heparin should begin immediately and continue for 48 hours if alteplase is used.

Anistreplase:
Reconstitute 30 U in 50 ml sterile water or D$_5$W
Streptokinase:
Reconstitute to 1 mg/ml

• Common approach is two peripheral IV lines, *one exclusively for thrombolytic administration.*

Alteplase:
Standard regimen:
• Give 60 mg IV in first hour (of which 6-10 mg is given initially IV push)
• Then 20 mg/h for 2 additional hours
• Total dose ≤100 mg
Front-loaded regimen*:
• Give 15-mg bolus
• Then 0.75 mg/kg over next 30 min (not to exceed 50 mg)
• Then 0.50 mg/kg over next 60 min (not to exceed 35 mg)
• Total dose ≤100 mg

Anistreplase:
30 U IV over 2-5 min

Streptokinase:
1.5 million U in a 1-hour infusion*

Continued

(From American Heart Association: *Advanced cardiac life support algorithms and drugs, a 1993 handbook for adult and pediatric providers.* Dallas, 1993, American Heart Association.)
*Not yet FDA-approved

TABLE 4-2 Advanced Cardiac Life Support: Drugs, Indications, and Adult Dosages—cont'd

DRUGS: MOST COMMONLY AVAILABLE ADULT PREPARATION	INDICATIONS/PRECAUTIONS	DOSAGE (ADULTS)
Verapamil 2.5 mg/ml in 2-, 4-, and 5-ml vials (totals = 5, 10, and 12.5 mg)	• Drug of second choice (after adenosine) to terminate PSVT with narrow QRS complex and adequate BP **Precautions:** • Do not use calcium channel blockers, such as verapamil, for wide-QRS tachycardias of uncertain origin. • Avoid calcium channel blockers in patients with WPW syndrome and atrial fibrillation, sick sinus syndrome, or AV block without pacemaker. • Expect BP drop due to peripheral vasodilation. IV calcium can restore BP, and some experts recommend prophylactic calcium before giving calcium channel blockers. • Do not use with IV β-blockers. • Use extreme caution with oral β-blockers.	• 2.5-5.0 mg IV bolus over 1-2 min. Repeat 5-10 mg, if needed, in 15-30 min. Maximum dose: 30 mg. • Alternative: 5-mg bolus every 15 min to total of 30 mg • Older patients: administer over 3 min.

(From American Heart Association: *Advanced cardiac life support algorithms and drugs, a 1993 handbook for adult and pediatric providers.* Dallas, 1993, American Heart Association.)
*Not yet FDA-approved

TABLE 4-3   Drugs Used in Pediatric Advanced Life Support

DRUGS	DOSAGE (PEDIATRIC)	REMARKS
Adenosine	0.1-0.2 mg/kg Maximum single dose: 12 mg	Rapid IV bolus
Atropine sulfate	0.02 mg/kg	Minimum dose: 0.1 mg Maximum single dose: 0.5 mg in child, 1.0 mg in adolescent
Bretylium	5 mg/kg; may be increased to 10 mg/kg	Rapid IV
Calcium chloride 10%	20 mg/kg	Give slowly.
Dopamine hydrochloride	2-20 μg/kg per min	α-Adrenergic action dominates at ≥15-20 μg/kg per min.
Dobutamine hydrochloride	2-20 μg/kg per min	Titrate to desired effect.
Epinephrine for bradycardia	IV/IO: 0.01 mg/kg (1:10,000, 0.1 ml/kg) ET: 0.1 mg/kg (1:1000, 0.1 ml/kg)	Be aware of total dose of preservative administered (if preservatives are present in epinephrine preparation) when high doses are used.
Epinephrine for asystolic or pulseless arrest	*First dose:* IV/IO: 0.01 mg/kg (1:10,000, 0.1 ml/kg ET: 0.1 mg/kg (1:1000, 0.1 ml/kg IV/IO doses as high as 0.2 mg/kg of 1:1000 may be effective. *Subsequent doses:* IV/IO/ET: 0.1 mg/kg (1:1000, 0.1 ml/kg) • Repeat every 3-5 min. IV/IO doses as high as 0.2 mg/kg of 1:1000 may be effective.	Be aware of total dose of preservative administered (if preservatives are present in epinephrine preparation) when high doses are used.
Epinephrine infusion	Initial at 0.1 μg/kg per min Higher infusion dose used if asystole present	Titrate to desired effect (0.1-1.0 μg/kg per min).
Lidocaine	1 mg/kg	
Lidocaine infusion	20-50 μg/kg per min	
Sodium bicarbonate	1 mEq/kg per dose or 0.3 × kg × base deficit	Infuse slowly and only if ventilation is adequate.

(From American Heart Association: *Advanced cardiac life support algorithms and drugs, a 1993 handbook for adult and pediatric providers.* Dallas, 1993, American Heart Association.)

ADVANCED LIFE SUPPORT ALGORITHMS FOR ADULTS

The American Heart Association released new advanced cardiac life support algorithms in November, 1992.[1] It is suggested that these algorithms be used as educational tools rather than as dictums of emergency care. They are designed to provide a basic plan of care and are not meant to be followed blindly. Some patients may require care not outlined in or varied from that in the algorithms. When clinically appropriate, flexibility is accepted and encouraged. Also, they emphasize: Treat the patient, not the monitor. Adequate airway, ventilation, oxygenation, chest compressions, and defibrillation are more important than administration of medications and take precedence over initiating an intravenous line or injecting agents.

Therapeutic interventions in the algorithms are classified as follows:

CLASS	THERAPEUTIC INTERVENTION
I	Usually indicated and always acceptable; considered safe and effective.
IIa	Available evidence suggests it is probably useful and effective.
IIb	May be helpful and is probably not harmful, but not well established by evidence.
III	Inappropriate, without supporting data, and possibly harmful.

Within the flow diagrams themselves are the Class I recommendations. The footnotes present Class IIa, IIb, and III recommendations (Figures 4-24 to 4-29). See Tables 4-2 and 4-3 for adult and pediatric medications recommended for use when delivering advanced life support.

FIGURE 4-24. Algorithm for ventricular fibrillation and pulseless ventricular tachycardia (VF/VT).

(From American Heart Association: Guidelines for cardiopulmonary resuscitation and emergency cardiac care, JAMA 268:2217, 1992.)

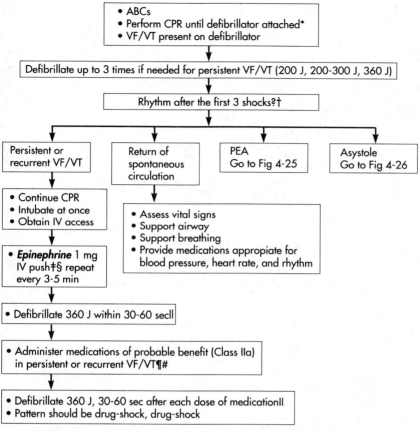

- ABCs
- Perform CPR until defibrillator attached*
- VF/VT present on defibrillator

↓

Defibrillate up to 3 times if needed for persistent VF/VT (200 J, 200-300 J, 360 J)

↓

Rhythm after the first 3 shocks?†

| Persistent or recurrent VF/VT | Return of spontaneous circulation | PEA Go to Fig 4-25 | Asystole Go to Fig 4-26 |

Persistent or recurrent VF/VT:

- Continue CPR
- Intubate at once
- Obtain IV access

↓

- **Epinephrine** 1 mg IV push‡§ repeat every 3-5 min

Return of spontaneous circulation:

- Assess vital signs
- Support airway
- Support breathing
- Provide medications appropiate for blood pressure, heart rate, and rhythm

↓

- Defibrillate 360 J within 30-60 sec‖

↓

- Administer medications of probable benefit (Class IIa) in persistent or recurrent VF/VT¶#

↓

- Defibrillate 360 J, 30-60 sec after each dose of medication‖
- Pattern should be drug-shock, drug-shock

* Precordial thump is a Class IIb action in witnessed arrest, no pulse, and no defibrillator immediately available.
† Hypothermic cardiac arrest is treated differently after this point.
‡ The recommended dose of **epinephrine** is 1 mg IV push every 3-5 min. If this approach fails, several Class IIb dosing regimens can be considered:
  - Intermediate: **epinephrine** 2-5 mg IV push, every 3-5 min
  - Escalating: **epinephrine** 1 mg-3 mg-5 mg IV push (3 min apart)
  - High: **epinephrine** 0.1 mg/kg IV push, every 3-5 min
§ **Sodium bicarbonate** (1 mEq/kg) is Class I if patient has known preexisting hyperkalemia
‖ Multiple sequenced shocks (200J, 200-300J, 360 J) are acceptable here (Class I), especially when medications are delayed
¶ • **Lidocaine** 1.5 mg/kg IV push. Repeat in 3-5 min to total loading dose of 3 mg/kg; then use
  - **Bretylium** 5 mg/kg IV push. Repeat in 5 min at 10 mg/kg
  - **Magnesium sulfate** 1-2 g IV in torsades de pointes or suspected hypomagnesemic state or severe refractory VF
  - **Procainamide** 30 mg/min in refractory VF (maximum total 17 mg/kg)
• **Sodium bicarbonate** (1 mEq/kg IV):
Class IIa
  - if known preexisting bicarbonate-responsive acidosis
  - if overdose with tricyclic antidepressants
  - to alkalinize the urine in drug overdoses
Class IIb
  - if intubated and continued long arrest interval
  - upon return of spontaneous circulation after long arrest interval
Class III
  - hypoxic lactic acidosis

> - Continue CPR
> - Intubate at once
> - Obtain IV access
> - Assess blood flow using Doppler ultrasound

↓

> Consider possible causes
> (Parentheses=possible therapies and treatments)
> - Hypovolemia (volume infusion)
> - Hypoxia (ventilation)
> - Cardiac tamponade (pericardiocentesis)
> - Tension pneumothorax (needle decompression)
> - Hypothermia
> - Massive pulmonary embolism (surgery, **thrombolytics**)
> - Drug overdoses such as tricyclics, digitalis, β-blockers, calcium channel blockers
> - Hyperkalemia*
> - Acidosis†
> - Massive acute myocardial infarction

↓

> - **Epinephrine** 1 mg IV push, *‡ repeat every 3-5 min

↓

> - If absolute bradycardia (<60 beats/min) or relative bradycardia, give **atropine** 1 mg IV
> - Repeat every 3-5 min up to a total of 0.04 mg/kg§

* **Sodium bicarbonate** 1 mEq/kg is Class I if patient has known preexisting hyperkalemia.
† **Sodium bicarbonate** 1 mEq/kg:
  Class IIa
  - if known preexisting bicarbonate-responsive acidosis
  - if overdose with tricyclic antidepressants
  - to alkalinize the urine in drug overdoses
  Class IIb
  - if intubated and long arrest interval
  - upon return of spontaneous circulation after long arrest interval
  Class III
  - hypoxic lactic acidosis
‡ The recommended dose of **epinephrine** is 1 mg IV push every 3-5 min.
  If this approach fails, several Class IIb dosing regimens can be considered.
  - Intermediate: **epinephrine** 2-5 mg IV push, every 3-5 min
  - Escalating: **epinephrine** 1 mg-3 mg-5 mg IV push (3 min apart)
  - High: **epinephrine** 0.1 mg/kg IV push, every 3-5 min
§ Shorter **atropine** dosing intervals are possibly helpful in cardiac arrest (Class IIb)

FIGURE 4-25. Algorithm for pulseless electrical activity (PEA) (electromechanical dissociation or EMD).

(From American Heart Association: Guidelines for cardiopulmonary resuscitation and emergency cardiac care, *JAMA* 268:2219, 1992.)

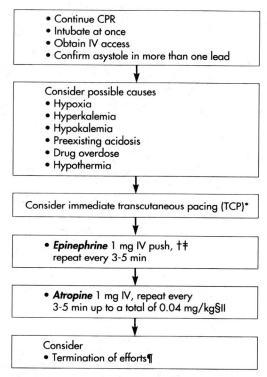

- Continue CPR
- Intubate at once
- Obtain IV access
- Confirm asystole in more than one lead

Consider possible causes
- Hypoxia
- Hyperkalemia
- Hypokalemia
- Preexisting acidosis
- Drug overdose
- Hypothermia

Consider immediate transcutaneous pacing (TCP)*

- *Epinephrine* 1 mg IV push, †‡
  repeat every 3-5 min

- *Atropine* 1 mg IV, repeat every
  3-5 min up to a total of 0.04 mg/kg§‖

Consider
- Termination of efforts¶

* TCP is a Class IIb intervention. Lack of success may be due to delays in pacing. To be effective TCP must be performed early, simultaneously with drugs. Evidence does not support routine use of TCP for asystole.

† The recommended dose of *epinephrine* is 1 mg IV push every 3-5 min. If this approach fails, several Class IIb dosing regimens can be considered:
- Intermediate: *epinephrine* 2-5 mg IV push, every 3-5 min
- Escalating: *epinephrine* 1 mg-3 mg-5 mg IV push (3 min apart)
- High: *epinephrine* 0.1 mg/kg IV push, every 3-5 min

‡ *Sodium bicarbonate* 1 mEq/kg is Class I if patient has known preexisting hyperkalemia.

§ Shorter *atropine* dosing intervals are Class IIb in asystolic arrest.

‖ *Sodium bicarbonate* 1 mEq/kg:
  Class IIa
  - if known preexisting bicarbonate-responsive acidosis
  - if overdose with tricyclic antidepressants
  - to alkalinize the urine in drug overdoses
  Class IIb
  - if intubated and continued long arrest interval
  - upon return of spontaneous circulation after long arrest interval
  Class III
  - hypoxic lactic acidosis

¶ If patient remains in asystole or other agonal rhythms after successful intubation and initial medications and no reversible causes are identified, consider termination of resuscitative efforts by a physician. Consider interval since arrest.

FIGURE 4-26. Asystole treatment algorithm.

(From American Heart Association: Guidelines for cardiopulmonary resuscitation and emergency cardiac care, *JAMA* 268:2220, 1992.)

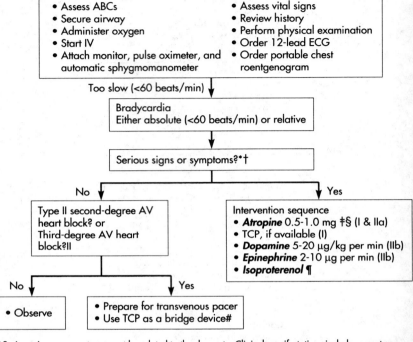

- Assess ABCs
- Secure airway
- Administer oxygen
- Start IV
- Attach monitor, pulse oximeter, and automatic sphygmomanometer

- Assess vital signs
- Review history
- Perform physical examination
- Order 12-lead ECG
- Order portable chest roentgenogram

Too slow (<60 beats/min)

Bradycardia
Either absolute (<60 beats/min) or relative

Serious signs or symptoms?*†

No

Type II second-degree AV heart block? or
Third-degree AV heart block?‖

Yes

Intervention sequence
- *Atropine* 0.5-1.0 mg ‡§ (I & IIa)
- TCP, if available (I)
- *Dopamine* 5-20 µg/kg per min (IIb)
- *Epinephrine* 2-10 µg per min (IIb)
- *Isoproterenol* ¶

No

- Observe

Yes

- Prepare for transvenous pacer
- Use TCP as a bridge device#

* Serious signs or symptoms must be related to the slow rate. Clinical manifestations include: *symptoms* (chest pain, shortness of breath, decreased level of conciousness) and *signs* (low BP, shock, pulmonary congestion, CHF, acute MI).
† Do not delay TCP while awaiting IV access or for *atropine* to take effect if patient is symptomatic.
‡ Denervated transplanted hearts will not respond to *atropine*. Go at once to pacing, *catecholamine* infusion, or both.
§ *Atropine* should be given in repeat doses in 3-5 min up to total of 0.04 mg/kg. Consider shorter dosing intervals in severe clinical conditions. It has been suggested that atropine should be used with caution in atrioventricular (AV) block at the His-Purkinje level (type II AV block and new third-degree block with wide QRS complexes) (Class IIb).
‖ Never treat third-degree heart block plus ventricular escape beats with *lidocaine*.
¶ *Isoproterenol* should be used, if at all, with extreme caution. At low doses it is Class IIb (possibly helpful); at higher doses it is Class III (harmful).
# Verify patient tolerance and mechanical capture. Use analgesia and sedation as needed.

FIGURE 4-27. Bradycardia algorithm (with the patient not in cardiac arrest).

(From American Heart Association: Guidelines for cardiopulmonary resuscitation and emergency cardiac care, *JAMA* 268:2221, 1992.)

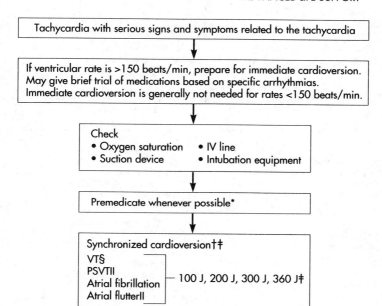

* Effective regimens have included a sedative (eg, *diazepam, midazolam, barbiturates, etomidate, ketamine, methohexital*) with or without an analgesic agent (eg, *fentanyl, morphine, meperidine*). Many experts recommend anesthesia if service is readily available.
† Note possible need to resynchronize after each cardioversion.
‡ If delays in synchronization occur and clinical conditions are critical, go to immediate unsynchronized shocks.
§ Treat polymorphic VT (irregular form and rate) like VF: 200 J, 200-300 J, 360 J.
|| PSVT and atrial flutter often respond to lower energy levels (start with 50 J).

FIGURE 4-28. Electrical cardioversion algorithm (with the patient not in cardiac arrest).
(From American Heart Association: Guidelines for cardiopulmonary resuscitation and emergency cardiac care, *JAMA* 268:2224, 1992.)

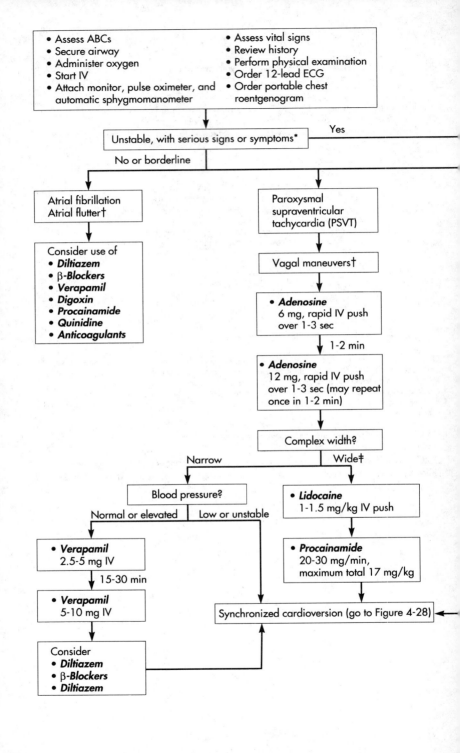

- Assess ABCs
- Secure airway
- Administer oxygen
- Start IV
- Attach monitor, pulse oximeter, and automatic sphygmomanometer

- Assess vital signs
- Review history
- Perform physical examination
- Order 12-lead ECG
- Order portable chest roentgenogram

Unstable, with serious signs or symptoms*   Yes

No or borderline

Atrial fibrillation
Atrial flutter†

Consider use of
- *Diltiazem*
- β-*Blockers*
- *Verapamil*
- *Digoxin*
- *Procainamide*
- *Quinidine*
- *Anticoagulants*

Paroxysmal supraventricular tachycardia (PSVT)

Vagal maneuvers†

- *Adenosine*
  6 mg, rapid IV push over 1-3 sec

1-2 min

- *Adenosine*
  12 mg, rapid IV push over 1-3 sec (may repeat once in 1-2 min)

Complex width?

Narrow   Wide‡

Blood pressure?

Normal or elevated   Low or unstable

- *Lidocaine*
  1-1.5 mg/kg IV push

- *Verapamil*
  2.5-5 mg IV

15-30 min

- *Verapamil*
  5-10 mg IV

Consider
- *Diltiazem*
- β-*Blockers*
- *Diltiazem*

- *Procainamide*
  20-30 mg/min, maximum total 17 mg/kg

Synchronized cardioversion (go to Figure 4-28)

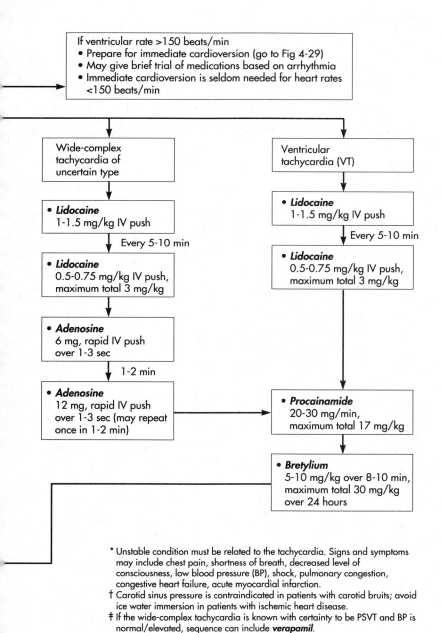

If ventricular rate >150 beats/min
- Prepare for immediate cardioversion (go to Fig 4-29)
- May give brief trial of medications based on arrhythmia
- Immediate cardioversion is seldom needed for heart rates <150 beats/min

Wide-complex tachycardia of uncertain type

Ventricular tachycardia (VT)

- *Lidocaine* 1-1.5 mg/kg IV push

  Every 5-10 min

- *Lidocaine* 0.5-0.75 mg/kg IV push, maximum total 3 mg/kg

- *Lidocaine* 1-1.5 mg/kg IV push

  Every 5-10 min

- *Lidocaine* 0.5-0.75 mg/kg IV push, maximum total 3 mg/kg

- *Adenosine* 6 mg, rapid IV push over 1-3 sec

  1-2 min

- *Adenosine* 12 mg, rapid IV push over 1-3 sec (may repeat once in 1-2 min)

- *Procainamide* 20-30 mg/min, maximum total 17 mg/kg

- *Bretylium* 5-10 mg/kg over 8-10 min, maximum total 30 mg/kg over 24 hours

* Unstable condition must be related to the tachycardia. Signs and symptoms may include chest pain, shortness of breath, decreased level of consciousness, low blood pressure (BP), shock, pulmonary congestion, congestive heart failure, acute myocardial infarction.
† Carotid sinus pressure is contraindicated in patients with carotid bruits; avoid ice water immersion in patients with ischemic heart disease.
‡ If the wide-complex tachycardia is known with certainty to be PSVT and BP is normal/elevated, sequence can include **verapamil**.

FIGURE 4-29. Tachycardia algorithm.
(From American Heart Association: Guidelines for cardiopulmonary resuscitation and emergency cardiac care, *JAMA* 268:2223, 1992.)

REFERENCES

1. American Heart Association: Guidelines for cardiopulmonary resuscitation and emergency cardiac care, *JAMA* 268:2171, 1992.
2. Benumof JL: Management of the difficult adult airway, *Anesthesiology* 75:1087, 1991.
3. Craney J, Stones R, Horowitz L, Gottlieb C: What is the relationship between ventricular tachycardia rate and hemodynamic compromise? Presented at the American Association of Critical Care Nurses National Critical Care Nursing Research Conference, May 12, 1991, Boston, Mass.
4. Grauer K, Cavallaro D: *ACLS certification preparation.* St Louis, 1993, Mosby Lifeline.

SUGGESTED READINGS

American Heart Association: *Advanced cardiac life support algorithms and drugs.* Dallas, 1993, the Association.

American Heart Association: Improving survival from sudden cardiac arrest: the "chain of survival" concept, *Circulation* 83:1832, 1991.

Automated external defibrillation. In American Heart Association: *Textbook of advanced cardiac life support.* Dallas, 1990, American Heart Association.

Barbiere CC, Libertore K: Automated external defibrillators: An update of additions to the ACLS algorithms, *Crit Care Nurs* 12(5):17, 1992.

Bennett B, Singh S: Management of ventricular arrhythmias: then and now, *Am J Crit Care* 3:107, 1992.

Blazing MA, Morris JJ: Atrial fibrillation: conventional wisdom reappraised, *Heart Disease and Stroke* March/April:78, 1992.

Bolgiano CS, Bunting K, Shoenberger MM: Administering oxygen therapy: what you need to know, *Nursing* 20(6):47, 90.

Brain AIJ: The Intavent laryngeal mask instruction manual. Berkshire, UK, 1992, Brain Medical Ltd.

Chronister C: Clinical management of supraventricular tachycardia with adenosine, *Am J Crit Care* 2:41, 1993.

Conover MB: *Understanding electrocardiography—arrhythmias and the 12 lead EKG.* St Louis, 1992, Mosby.

Cummins RO: From concept to standard-of-care? Review of the clinical experience with automated external defibrillators, *Ann Emerg Med* 18:1269, 1989.

Crockett P, McHugh LG: *Noninvasive pacing: what you should know.* Redmond, Wash, 1988, Physio-Control.

Crockett PJ, Droppert BM, Higgins SE: *Defibrillation: What you should know.* Redmond, Wash, 1991, Physio-Control.

deLuna AB, Coumel P, Leclercq JF: Ambulatory sudden cardiac death: mechanisms of production of fatal arrhythmia on the basis of data from 157 cases, *Am Heart J* 117: 151, 1989.

Emerman CL, Pinchak AC, Hancock D, Hagin JF: The effect of bolus injection on circulation times during cardiac arrest, *Am J Emerg Med* 8:190, 1990.

Fabius DB: Diagnosing and treating ventricular tachycardia, *J Cardiovasc Nurs* 7(3):8, 1993.

Feeney-Stewart F: The sodium bicarbonate controversy, *Dimensions of Crit Care Nurs* 9(1):22, 1990.

Gibbs W, Eisenberg M, Damon SK: Dangers of defibrillation: injuries to emergency personnel during patient resuscitation, *Am J Emerg Med* 8:101, 1990.

Gonzalez ER: Pharmacologic controversies in CPR, *Ann Emerg Med* 22(2, part 2):317, 1993.

Jaffe AS: The use of antiarrhythmics in advanced cardiac life support, *Ann Emerg Med* 22(2, part 2):307, 1993.

Kater KM, Kubrik NS, Kubrik M: Corralling atrial fibrillation with "Maze" surgery, *Am J Nurs* 92(7):34, 1992.

Kerber RE: Electrical treatment of cardiac arrhythmias: defibrillation and cardioversion, *Ann Emerg Med* 22(part 2):296, 1993.

Kinney MR, Packa DR, Andreoli KG, Zipes DP, eds: *Comprehensive cardiac care.* St Louis, 1991, Mosby.

Lounsbury P, Frye SJ: *Cardiac rhythm disorders.* St Louis, 1992, Mosby.

Lubliner C: When to expect heart block, *RN* 53(1):28, 1990.

Moser SA, Crawford D, Thomas A: Updated care guidelines for patients with automatic implantable cardioverter defibrillators, *Crit Care Nurs* 13(2):62, 1993.

Niemann JT: Cardiopulmonary resuscitation, *N Engl J Med* 327:1075, 1992.

Panacek EA, Munger MA, Rutherford WF, Gardner SF: Report of Nitropatch explosions complicating defibrillation, *Am J Emerg Med* 10:128, 1992.

Paradis NA: Epinephrine in cardiac arrest: a critical review, *Ann Emerg Med* 19:1288, 1990.

Paul SC: New agents for emergency management of supraventricular tachydysrhythmias, *Crit Care Nurs Q* 16(2): 35, 1993.

Roberts J, Hedges J: *Clinical procedures in emergency medicine.* Philadelphia, 1991, Saunders.

Somerson SJ, Sicilia MR: Emergency oxygen administration and airway management, *Crit Care Nurs* 12(4):23, 1992.

Stewart RD: Manual translaryngeal jet ventilation, *Emerg Med Clin North Am* 7(1):155, 1989.

Teplitz L: Transcutaneous pacemakers, *J Cardiovasc Nurs* 5(3):44, 1991.

Wasserberger J, Ordog GJ, Dang C, Schlater TL: Emergency department thoracotomy, *Emerg Med Clin North Am* 7(1):103, 1989.

CHAPTER 5

Intravenous Therapy and Laboratory Specimens

INTRAVENOUS LINES

An intravenous (IV) line is initiated so that fluids, medications, blood, and blood products can be placed into the vascular circulation. To initiate an IV line, one should have general familiarity with the peripheral vasculature of the limb of the access site. When determining where to start the line, consider the urgency of the situation—urgency may take priority over the best long-term site location. In the emergency situation, where IV access is critical, the IV is often started in the most accessible site.

Cannula and Needle Sizes for Fluid and Medication Administration

Blood and blood products—18-gauge or larger
Colloids (plasma or albumin)—20-gauge or larger
Crystalloids—21-gauge or larger
To give large volumes of fluid, use at least a 16-gauge or larger needle.

Types of cannulas used in intravenous therapy

hollow needle   A sharpened stainless steel or aluminum cannula.
winged needle   Also known as a ''scalp vein'' or a ''butterfly''; a stainless steel needle with two winglike plastic projections mounted where the needle meets the catheter to facilitate placement and anchoring.
indwelling catheter   Made of polyethylene, polyvinyl chloride, Silastic, or Teflon; better than a metal cannula for long-term use.
plain plastic catheter   Made without a needle tip; used when a cutdown is performed.
catheter-over-needle   A tapered catheter fitted over a needle; the needle is used to puncture the skin and the vein; the catheter is advanced over the needle; the needle is removed from the patient.

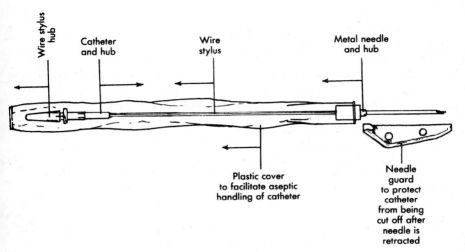

FIGURE 5-1. Intracath catheter inside needle.

catheter-inside-needle (Figure 5-1)   A sharp, hollow needle with a catheter inside the lumen; the needle punctures the skin and the vein; the catheter is advanced through the needle; the needle is removed from the patient but remains outside, over the end of the catheter, secured by an outer plastic clip. This type of device is often used for placement of a central venous pressure line, most often a subclavian line.

Site preparation

1. Apply a proximal tourniquet to sites in extremities to distend the vein. Use rubber tubing, a wide (commercially available) tourniquet, or a blood pressure cuff (most comfortable and most effective).
2. Keep the tourniquet in place for no more than 5 minutes or just until the vein dilates; if the vein does not dilate enough for cannulation:
   Rub the vein.
   Tap the vein.
   Hold the limb in a dependent position.
   Apply heat with a hot pack or warm towel.
   Have the patient open and close his fist.
3. Apply a 10% povidone iodine (Betadine) solution.
4. Make a wheal with 2% lidocaine over the puncture site if a large-bore needle is to be used.

Peripheral venipuncture technique

1. Stabilize the vein.
2. Use the smallest angle possible between the needle and the vein.
3. Puncture the skin and the vein with the bevel of the needle facing upward.

4. Advance the needle slowly.
5. Check for a blood return ("flashback").
6. Remove the tourniquet.
7. Slowly advance the needle as far as possible; it is often helpful to have the IV solution running while doing this to help float the catheter in and dilate the vein.
8. Place a small dab of antibiotic ointment at the puncture site.
9. Cover the site with sterile 2 × 2 inch gauze.
10. Secure the cannula with tape.
11. Make a loop with the IV tubing and secure it.
12. Label the IV site (type, gauge, time, date, initials).
13. Mark the drip rate and note if any medications have been added on the solution container.

Heparin lock

A heparin lock is a peripheral IV cannula without IV tubing attached. The distal end of the cannula is plugged. The purpose of this lock is to have ready access to a vein should the need arise or to have brief access to a vein should an intravenous medication be given. The cannula should be filled with a heparin solution so that it will not clot while it is not in use. It can be used if the patient does not require massive volume replacement and medications do not have to be diluted in large amounts of solution.

COMPLICATIONS OF INTRAVENOUS THERAPY

Hematoma
Fluid extravasation outside the vein and into the tissues
Phlebitis
Clot embolism
Catheter fragment embolism
Cellulitis
Sepsis
Fluid overload

PERIPHERAL INTRAVENOUS SITES IN THE ADULT

The most common sites for the initiation of IV lines in the adult patient are in the upper extremities. The choice of an IV site depends on:
Condition of the vein
Length of time the IV will be in place
Clinical condition of the patient
Age of the patient
Size of the patient
Purpose of the IV line

The following superficial veins of the upper extremities are appropriate for IV use.

The Digital Veins

These are located on the dorsal portions of the fingers. They can be cannulated with a scalp vein needle and should only be used in an absolute emergency when no other IV site is attainable. Large volumes of fluid cannot be given via these sites.

The Metacarpal Veins

Three metacarpal veins are formed by the junction of the digital veins; these are good IV sites because they are located between the metacarpal bones of the hand, which form natural splints. They are especially useful if long-term IV therapy is indicated, because future IVs can be initiated above the site. These should be avoided in the elderly, however tempting it may be, because the skin of elderly people is very thin and blood may extravasate into the hand.

The Cephalic Veins

These are located in the radial aspect of the dorsal venous network. They are formed by the union of the metacarpal veins on the radial aspect of the forearm. They are large, in a good location, and can accommodate a large-bore cannula. Their location provides natural splints.

The Accessory Cephalic Vein

This vein originates from the union of the dorsal veins and joins the cephalic vein below the elbow. It can accommodate a large-bore cannula and is a good vein to use for the administration of blood.

The Basilic Vein

This vein originates from the union of the dorsal veins on the ulnar aspect of the arm. It has a large capacity, but is often not chosen as an IV site because it is not readily accessible. This vein can be visualized by flexing the arm at the elbow and elevating it.

The Median Veins

The median antebrachial vein

This vein originates from the union of many veins on the palm of the hand. It ascends along the ulnar aspect of the arm and can sometimes be difficult to find.

The median cephalic/median basilic vein

This vein is located in the antecubital fossa. It is large and is frequently used to withdraw blood for laboratory specimens. It is also frequently used as an IV site in extreme emergency situations, such as cardiopulmonary arrest or multiple trauma, because access is usually very easy and the vein can accommodate a very large-bore cannula. It is important to remember that the brachial artery lies just behind this vein.

The following peripheral vein of the lower extremities is appropriate for IV use.

The Saphenous Vein

The small saphenous vein terminates at the deep popliteal vein, which enters the great saphenous vein, which terminates at the femoral vein. It is important to be aware that there is great danger of embolism when an IV is initiated at this site—it should only be used in cases of extreme emergency. If an IV is initiated at this site and the PASG is applied, a pressure bag must be placed over the IV bag, and the pressure must exceed that of the PASG to run.

The following peripheral vein of the neck is appropriate for IV use.

The External Jugular Vein

This vein is often overlooked. It is very large and easy to cannulate. It should be considered as an IV site in cardiopulmonary arrest and multiple trauma, especially for cases in which large amounts of fluids are to be administered over a short period of time. This vein can accommodate a very large-bore cannula.

PERIPHERAL INTRAVENOUS SITES IN INFANTS AND CHILDREN

The IV sites of choice in an infant or small child are the dorsum of the hand, the dorsum of the foot, and the scalp (in an infant). In the newborn, the umbilical vein should not be overlooked. **Be sure to anchor an IV extra securely in an infant or a small child because movement may dislodge it.** Gauze and tape wrapped around a tongue blade makes an excellent armboard.

INTEROSSEOUS INFUSIONS

An interosseous infusion is the administration of IV fluids and drugs directly into the bone marrow. It is best performed on children under the age of 2 when they are in:
- Cardiopulmonary arrest
- Hypovolemic shock
- Status epilepticus

It may also be performed in any other condition where the administration of fluid or medication is critical to the child's survival and the establishment of an IV is difficult.

Locate the anterior medial surface of the tibia, 2 cm below the tibial tuberosity (Figure 5-2). Other sites that may be used are the distal anterior femur, the medial malleolus, and the iliac crest.

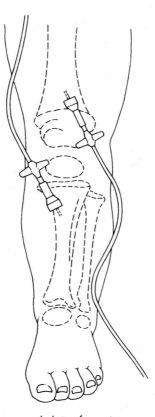

FIGURE 5-2. Recommended sites for an intraosseous infusion.

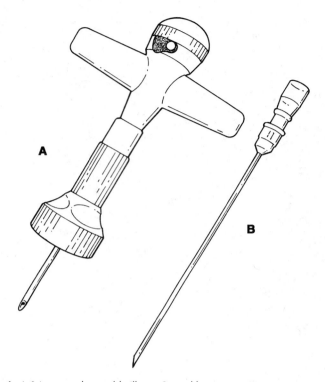

FIGURE 5-3. **A,** A 16-gauge disposable Illinois Sternal bone marrow aspiration needle. **B,** A 3-inch, 18-gauge B-D spinal needle.
(®Becton, Dickinson and Co., Rutherford, NJ)

Prepare the area with Betadine. Using a metal biopsy needle, such as an Illinois Sternal Bone Marrow Needle (Figure 5-3) or a Jamsheedy needle), advance the needle through the skin, fascia, and bony cortex with a back-and-forth boring motion. It is apparent that the needle is in the bone marrow when there is a popping sensation followed by a sudden absence of resistance, when the needle can stand upright without manual support, and when fluid flows freely through the needle. Aspirate, using a syringe. If bone marrow is returned, the needle has been placed correctly.

Once the needle is in place, tape it and infuse solutions and/or medications.

Venous Cutdown

A venous cutdown is a minor surgical procedure that is used if a peripheral IV site cannot be located or if a large volume of fluid is to be administered over a short period of time. A cutdown is usually done on the basilic vein (just above the elbow) or the saphenous vein (above the ankle). The saphenous vein is usually chosen when a cutdown is performed on a child (Figure 5-4, *A, B*).

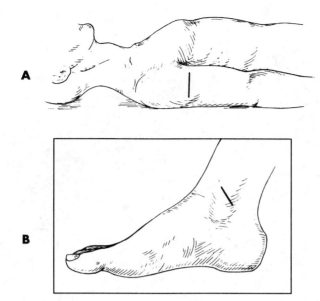

FIGURE 5-4. Common sites of venous cutdown. **A**, Cephalic vein. **B**, Saphenous vein.

■ **EQUIPMENT**
  Surgical gloves
  Surgical mask
  Scalpel handle and blades (11- or 15-gauge)
  Vascular scissors
  Suture scissors
  Lidocaine (1% or 2%)
  Suture material
  Forceps
  4 × 4-inch gauze squares
  Sterile towels
  Catheter (may use infant-feeding tube or IV connecting tubing)
  Antiseptic solution
  Hemostats
  Syringe and needle (25-gauge)
  Antibiotic ointment
  IV setup
  Tape
  Small vein retractor
■ **PROCEDURE (USUALLY PERFORMED BY A PHYSICIAN)** (FIGURE 5-5, A, B, C)
  1. Prepare the extremity with antiseptic solution.
  2. Drape the limb.
  3. Apply a local anesthetic.
  4. Make a transverse incision.

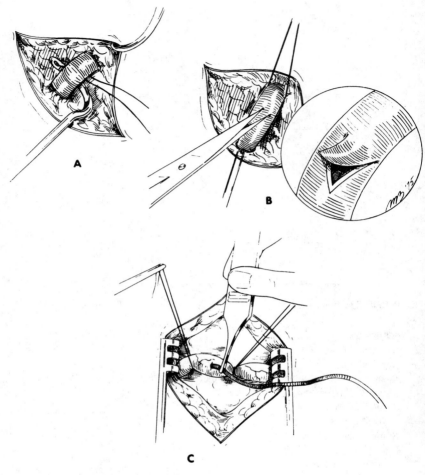

FIGURE 5-5. Venous cutdown. **A,** Isolating the vein. **B,** Cutting the vein. **C,** Inserting the cannula.

5. Dissect the tissue down to the vein.
6. Lift the vein.
7. Nick the vein with a scalpel.
8. Insert the cannula.
9. Secure the cannula with a suture.
10. Suture the wound around the cannula.
11. Apply antibiotic ointment.
12. Tape the cannula in place.
13. Label the IV site (gauge and type of cannula, date, time, caregiver's initials).

Central Vein Cannulation

Catheterization of the subclavian vein (Figure 5-6) is used to provide volume and to enable measurement of the central venous pressure. Catheterization of the internal jugular vein is used to provide large volumes over a short period of time. It should be remembered that catheterizing these sites carries a risk of pneumothorax. They should only be used in urgent situations.

Subclavian vein

This vein is located in the neck between the median and middle thirds of the clavicle and the sternal notch.

1. Place the patient in Trendelenburg's position to increase the size of the vein and decrease the possibility of air embolism.
2. Place a rolled towel between the patient's shoulder blades to provide a better angle.

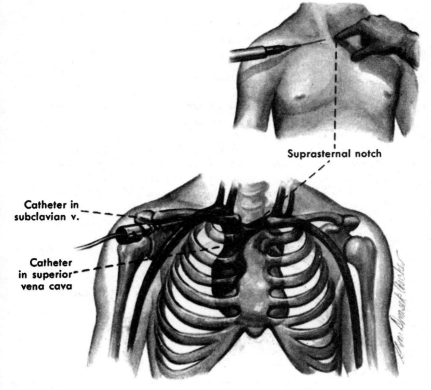

Suprasternal notch

Catheter in subclavian v.

Catheter in superior vena cava

FIGURE 5-6. Technique of percutaneous intraclavicular subclavian catheterization. Needle, inserted under midclavicle and aimed in three dimensions at top of posterior aspect of sternal manubrium (indicated by fingertip in suprasternal notch), lies in a plane parallel with frontal plane of patient and will enter anterior wall of subclavian vein.
(From Needle and cannula techniques, Chicago, 1971, Abbott Laboratories.)

3. Prepare the neck and upper chest with an antiseptic solution.
4. Anesthetize the area with 1% lidocaine at the inferior edge of the clavicle where the medial and middle thirds join.
5. Insert a 14-gauge or larger cannula (with a syringe on the end to avoid air embolism), aiming toward the suprasternal notch and keeping the cannula just under the clavicle.
6. Aspirate as the needle is advancing; if nonpulsating blood is drawn, the vein has been cannulated.
7. Advance the catheter through the needle; do not pull back on the catheter because it may be sheared off.
8. When the catheter is in place, withdraw the needle.
9. Clip on the catheter guard so that the needle will not shear off the catheter.
10. Suture the catheter and guard in place.
11. Apply antibiotic ointment to the puncture site.
12. Apply a dry sterile dressing.
13. Apply a waterproof dressing.
14. Label the cannulation site.

Internal jugular vein

1. Place the patient in Trendelenburg's position to increase the size of the vein and decrease the possibility of air embolism.
2. Place a rolled towel between the shoulder blades to provide a better angle.
3. Prepare the neck and upper chest with an antiseptic solution.
4. Drape the neck and upper chest area.
5. Anesthetize the area with 1% lidocaine at the junction of the middle and lower thirds of the anterior border of the sternocleidomastoid muscle.
6. Insert a 14-gauge or larger cannula (with a syringe on the end to avoid air embolism) close behind the sternocleidomastoid muscle, aiming toward the space formed by the clavicular and sternal heads.
7. Aspirate as the needle is advancing; if nonpulsating blood is drawn, the vein has been cannulated.
8. Advance the catheter through the needle; do not pull back on the catheter because it may be sheared off.
9. When the catheter is in place, withdraw the needle carefully.
10. Clip the catheter guard so that the needle will not shear off the catheter.
11. Suture the catheter and guard in place.
12. Apply antibiotic ointment to the puncture site.
13. Apply a dry sterile dressing.
14. Apply a waterproof dressing.
15. Label the cannulation site.

CENTRAL VENOUS PRESSURE

The central venous pressure (CVP) is a measurement of the right-sided pressures of the heart, blood volume, effectiveness of the heart as a pump, and vascular tone.

■ **PROCEDURE USING A SUBCLAVIAN INTRAVENOUS LINE**
1. Place the patient in a supine (flat) position.
2. Measure at the midaxillary line (5 cm from the top of the chest) in the fourth intercostal space at the level of the right atrium.
3. Place the manometer zero-reading at this point.
4. Fill the manometer from the attached IV solution (do not let it overflow).
5. Turn the stopcock on the IV line open to the patient and the manometer. The fluid level will fall and fluctuate (decreasing on inspiration and increasing on expiration).
6. When the fluid level appears stable, note where the top of the fluid column reaches.
7. Record this reading as the CVP.
8. Adjust the stopcock to close the manometer and open the IV line to the patient (make sure to readjust the IV solution drip rate).

The normal range of CVP is 4 to 10 cm of water pressure. A value greater than 10 cm may indicate tamponade, right heart failure, fluid overload, pulmonary edema, tension pneumothorax, or hemothorax. A value below 4 cm may indicate hypovolemia, vasodilation, dehydration, septic shock, or drug-induced shock.

PULMONARY ARTERY WEDGE PRESSURE

Pulmonary artery wedge pressure (PAWP) is a reflection of left ventricular pressure. It is measured with a Swan-Ganz catheter (Figure 5-7), which may be placed by a percutaneous or cutdown approach. A normal PAWP value is 6 to 12 cm of water.

■ **PROCEDURE**
1. Insert the catheter into the superior vena cava.
2. Inflate the balloon with air to let blood flow carry it through the right atrium and right ventricle into the pulmonary artery.
3. Once the catheter arrives at the pulmonary artery, deflate the balloon.
4. Advance the catheter a few centimeters more into a small branch of the artery.
5. When the balloon is once again inflated, it occludes the artery, and the tip of the catheter transmits a pressure that reflects left ventricular pressure (Figure 5-8).

VENOUS ACCESS DEVICES

During the last decade, the tremendous use of IV drugs and fluids has increased the need for reliable venous access. Venous access devices (VADs) can dependably provide such access and are essential in the medical management of patients requiring prolonged IV therapy such as those with cancer, Crohn's disease (requiring TPN), AIDS, sickle cell anemia, and cystic fibrosis. They are also extremely useful in blood drawing.

Because of the widespread and growing use of VADs throughout the country, it is imperative that the emergency department nurse be knowledgeable and

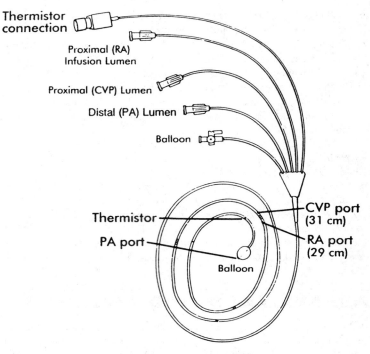

FIGURE 5-7. Swan-Ganz catheter.

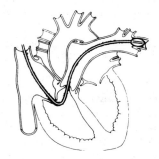

FIGURE 5-8. The tip of the catheter transmits a pressure that reflects left ventricular pressure.

skilled in the care and accessing of these devices that are a virtual lifeline for many people.

VADs are inserted under sterile conditions, most often into a major vein in the upper chest such as the subclavian, jugular, or cephalic. The device consists of a single-lumen or multi-lumen catheter with one, two or three noncommunicating internal lumens, each with a corresponding hub. Multi-lumen catheters allow separate infusion of IV drugs and solutions, blood sampling, and hemodynamic monitoring. One lumen may be used continuously, whereas others may be accessed intermittently.

CATHETER TYPES

VADs are classified as non-tunneled, tunneled, or implanted. All can be inserted either peripherally or in the larger central veins.

Non-tunneled Catheters

A non-tunneled venous catheter is inserted by venipuncture directly through the skin into the selected vessel. These are also known as ''percutaneous catheters.'' Peripheral catheters are often inserted by a physician or specially trained nurse, while central catheters are always inserted by a physician.

Non-tunneled VADs have the smallest internal lumen of all three types, but are quite versatile and can be used over long periods of time (weeks or months) for administration of medications, fluids, or blood products. They can also be used to obtain blood samples.

Non-tunneled catheters have high care requirements such as dressing changes and daily flushing and restrictions on activities such as swimming. A dressing must cover the exit site (the antecubital space or the neck) and may negatively impact patient self-image.

Tunneled Catheters

This type of catheter is available in many brands (Hickman, RAAF, Corcath, Groshong). It is inserted into a central vein by percutaneous venipuncture or surgical cutdown. These catheters are thick walled, large bore, and are available in single-lumen, double-lumen, and triple-lumen form. A portion of the catheter is tunneled through the subcutaneous space and exits the skin at the convenient site, usually on the chest. A Dacron cuff is located about 2 cm above the exit site. Fibrotic tissue grows around the cuff and acts as a barrier against ascending microorganisms and also prevents catheter dislodgement.

Tunneled catheters are the most versatile of all types of catheter. Because of their large bore it is usually easy to obtain blood samples while a double or triple lumen allows for multiple infusions. Also, tunneled catheters can often be repaired if damaged distal to the exit site.

Disadvantages of tunneled catheters include daily high care requirements such as dressing changes and flushes. Tunneled catheters are usually only inserted in those patients who have the mental and physical ability to care for them.

Venous Access Ports

A venous access port or implanted venous access device consists of a catheter attached to a portal body. The portal may be constructed of plastic, stainless steel, or titanium and contains a dense silicone septum overlying a reservoir. The septum can withstand 1000 to 2000 needle sticks. A specially designed needle called a Huber needle must be used to access this port. The Huber needle has a deflective noncoring point that tears rather than cores the septum.

Ports are not as versatile as tunneled catheters because incompatible solutions cannot be infused simultaneously into a single lumen device. For this reason, more and more double-lumen ports are being placed. Ports can be accessed for blood sampling as well as bolus and continuous infusions. There are little or no care requirements for the patient since the entire system is enclosed under the skin. The patient should be consulted as to whether he or she prefers a small wheal of lidocaine before access, because access necessitates a needle stick.

ACCESSING VENOUS ACCESS DEVICES

Various procedures in accessing VADs are used throughout the country; however, it can be reasonably assumed that the fundamental requirement for successful VAD maintenance is strict adherence to established protocols. Below are basic steps utilized during accessing for blood sampling.

Non-tunneled and Tunneled Catheters

1. Good hand washing and aseptic technique are essential in preparing to access the device.
2. Sterile gloves should always be worn.
3. Gather needed equipment before access.
      Laboratory tubes/test requisition
      Heparinized saline (10 U/ml)
      Alcohol wipes
      Two 10 cc syringes, one filled with saline
      18-gauge needles
      Syringes large enough to draw required amount of blood
      Sterile Luer lock caps
4. Prepare sterile barrier/place equipment on barrier.
5. Turn off any infusions/dual or triple lumen; clamp catheters that will not be used for blood sampling.
6. Clamp catheter to be used and remove Luer-Lock cap from catheter hub.
7. Attach 10-cc syringe to hub; withdraw 6 ml of blood for discard/clamp catheter.
8. Attach syringe large enough to accommodate blood needed for samples and withdraw that amount. Remember to draw samples for blood cultures first.

Blood needed for clotting studies should not be drawn from heparinized catheters.

9. Clamp catheter, remove collection syringe, inject blood samples into appropriate laboratory tubes.
10. Flush catheter with 10 cc N/S, then reattach to infusion. If dual-lumen or triple-lumen catheter, unclamp other catheters and restart those infusions.
11. If catheter is to be capped, flush with heparinized saline (10 U/ml), wipe hub with alcohol wipe, then cap with sterile Luer-Lock cap and tape for added security.

    NOTE: Groshong catheters do *not* require heparin flush.
12. Label blood sample tubes and send to laboratory.

ACCESSING AND DRAWING BLOOD SAMPLES FROM IMPLANTED PORTS

1. Have the patient lie supine or in semi-Fowlers position.
2. Wash hands thoroughly.
3. Palpate site to locate the port and septum; examine the site for signs and symptoms of infection.
4. Cleanse the site with povidone/iodine swabs; start at center and cleanse outward in a circular motion.
5. Make a small wheal above injection site with 1% lidocaine if patient desires.
6. Place needed equipment on sterile barrier.
    10-cc syringe filled with N/S
    18-gauge needle
    90 degree Huber needle
    Sterile gloves
7. Prime Huber needle with N/S.
8. Cannulate the port with the Huber needle; push the needle through the skin and septum until the bottom of the port is felt.
9. Check for correct placement by flushing with remaining saline in syringe; a correctly accessed port will flush easily with pain or swelling (infiltration).
10. Apply antimicrobial ointment to site.
11. Stabilize needle by placing 2 × 2 inch gauze pads under wings of needle and tape.
12. Clamp tubing and remove syringe.
13. Hook up to infusion tubing and tape connections. If no infusion is ordered, cap with sterile Luer-Lock cap after heparin flush.

Blood Sampling from Implanted Port:

1. If access is required, follow above procedure.
2. If access has been achieved, gather necessary equipment
    Alcohol wipes
    Two 10-cc syringes, one filled with saline
    One heparinized saline

Blood collection tubes/requisitions/labels

Syringe of appropriate size to draw required amount of blood

3. Wear sterile gloves.
4. Stop infusion and clamp the short extension tubing attached to the Huber needle hub.
5. If no infusion, ensure that tubing is clamped and remove Luer-Lock cap.
6. Attach 10-cc syringe, unclamp tubing, withdraw 6 cc of blood.
7. Clamp tubing, disconnect this syringe, and discard it.
8. Attach collection syringe, unclamp tubing, and slowly and steadily withdraw required amount of blood. Do not draw clotting studies from heparinized catheters.
9. Clamp tubing, disconnect syringe.
10. Flush Huber needle with 10 cc N/S and reconnect to infusion.
11. If no infusion, flush with heparinized saline (10 U/ml) then cap with sterile Luer-Lock cap.
12. Inject laboratory specimen tubes with blood, label and send to lab.

COMPLICATIONS INVOLVING VENOUS ACCESS DEVICES

1. **Infection** may occur at exit site, port pocket along catheter tunnel, or as septicemia.
2. **Obstruction**: Withdrawal occlusion—occurs when hospital personnel are unable to withdraw blood samples; fluid can still be infused unless there is intraluminal occlusion of the catheter.
   Intraluminal obstruction—occurs when blood cannot be withdrawn nor can fluids be infused.
   • Most commonly caused by clot formation or precipitation of drugs.
   • May require gentle instillation of thrombolytic agent (usually urokinase), always ordered by a physician.
3. **Extravasation:** Leakage from a vein or catheter into subcutaneous tissue. Symptoms are pain, swelling, erythema.
   Certain drugs can cause tissue necrosis.
   • Greatest risk is with implantable ports, usually secondary to dislodgment of Huber needle.
4. **Damaged catheters:** Only tunneled catheters can be repaired if damaged in the external portion.

INTRAARTERIAL LINES

Intraarterial lines may be established via a percutaneous puncture or cutdown. Before puncture of the artery, check collateral circulation. Check circulation in the forearm using the Allen test.

ALLEN TEST

To assess for the Allen sign (Figure 5-9, *A, B, C*), palpate both the radial and ulnar pulses. Occlude both arteries with firm pressure and raise the arm to

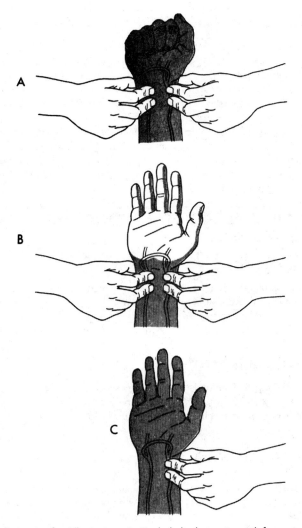

FIGURE 5-9. Assessing for Allen's sign. **A,** Occlude both arteries with firm pressure. **B,** Raise arm to blanch hand. **C,** Release ulnar artery for return of color to hand. (From Sheehy SB, Barber J: *Emergency nursing—principles and practice,* ed 2. St Louis, 1985, Mosby.)

blanch the hand. Release the ulnar artery and assess for return of color to the hand. If the hand does not perfuse (negative Allen sign), this indicates that the ulnar artery is not capable of maintaining circulation to the hand. Therefore, do not attempt a radial artery puncture in this wrist.

GENERAL PRINCIPLES OF IV THERAPY

- In emergency situations, look for a site that is easy to cannulate.
- The vein to be cannulated should be large enough to hold the cannula that will be introduced.
- If the purpose of the IV line is to provide a vehicle to administer large volumes of fluid over a short period of time, be sure to initiate the largest bore cannula possible.
- Whenever possible, try to initiate the IV in the patient's nondominant arm.
- Be sure to have all equipment ready ahead of time (including tape strips).
- If a patient is in shock, perfusion is decreased and medication absorption is erratic; IV administration of medications is much more reliable than other routes of administration.

DRAWING BLOOD FOR BLOOD GAS MEASUREMENT

Selection of Site

Choose the radial, brachial, or femoral artery (Figure 5-10, *A, B, C*).
Avoid limbs that demonstrate poor circulation.
Avoid limbs where hematomas are present.
If the radial artery is selected, check for the presence of a positive Allen test.

Suggested Equipment

Container of crushed ice (plastic bag or emesis basin is fine)
Rubber or cork stopper or commercial blood gas cap
5-ml glass syringe or specially treated plastic syringe
Two 22-gauge 1.5 inch needles
Two alcohol swabs
Sodium heparin, 0.5 ml (1000 U/ml)
One small dry gauze pad
Gummed label for syringe
Laboratory requisition slip with the following information: Concentration of oxygen patient is receiving and by what route (FiO_2) and patient's rectal temperature at the time the specimen is collected (both parameters affect calculation of values).

Drawing the Specimen

1. Explain the procedure to the patient.
2. Draw up 0.5 ml heparin into a *glass* or specially treated plastic syringe.
3. Flush the syringe with heparin (expel all air bubbles).
4. Replace the needle.

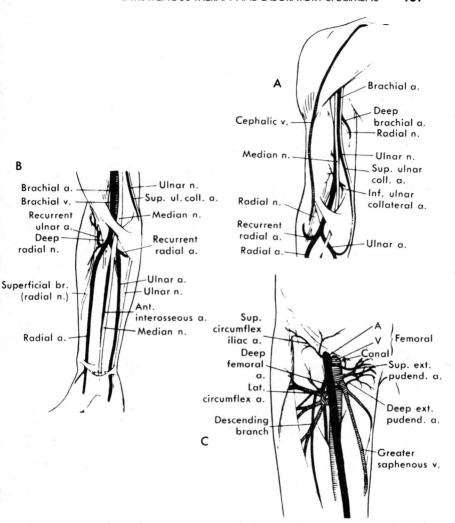

FIGURE 5-10. **A,** Brachial artery, a continuation of axillary artery. *Advantages:* Easy to locate, not much arterial spasm, and easy to immobilize. *Disadvantages:* Radial and medial nerves in close proximity and venous system in close proximity, making venous sampling possible. **B,** Radial artery extends from neck of radius to median side of styloid process. *Advantages:* No close proximity to veins; thus venous sampling is unlikely. *Disadvantages:* Puncture may produce spasm and artery is very small. **C,** Femoral artery branches from abdominal aorta and branches to superficial epigastric, superficial circumflex iliac, external pudendal, deep femoral, and descending genicular arteries. *Advantages:* Easily accessible. *Disadvantages:* May have large amount of interstitial bleeding before it is noticed. Close proximity to vein makes venous sampling possible.

(From Budassi SA: *JEN* 3(2):24, 1977.)

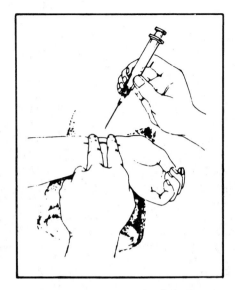

FIGURE 5-11. Puncture of radial artery.
(From Budassi SA: *JEN* 3(2):24, 1977.)

5. Select the puncture site.
6. Straighten the limb of the selected puncture site and position it on a firm surface.
7. Palpate the artery: assess the pulse and position of the artery.
8. Cleanse area over the puncture site with an alcohol swab (be sure to use plenty of friction and allow the alcohol to dry before the actual puncture).
9. Immobilize the artery between two fingers (be careful not to contaminate the puncture site).
10. Penetrate both the skin and the artery at a 45- to 90-degree angle, holding the syringe like a pencil (Figure 5-11).
11. If the syringe begins to fill and the plunger begins to move spontaneously, this is usually an indication that the needle is in the artery.
12. If the syringe does not begin to fill spontaneously, withdraw the needle slightly (it may have gone all the way through the artery).
13. If systolic blood pressure is less than 100 mm Hg, the syringe may not fill spontaneously, and it may be necessary to manually withdraw the plunger (e.g., during CPR).
14. If the blood sample is not bright red or is bluish in color, this may indicate that the specimen is venous—make another attempt at an arterial specimen.
15. Obtain 3 to 5 ml of arterial blood (some laboratories will accept less for analysis).
16. Withdraw the needle quickly.
17. Apply direct pressure with dry gauze.
18. Maintain pressure for 5 minutes (make certain to time it on your watch or the wall clock—it is difficult to estimate 5 minutes).

Care of the Specimen

1. Expel all air bubbles from the sample.
2. Stick the needle into a cork or rubber stopper or remove the needle and cap the syringe.
3. Place the gummed label (containing patient's name and hospital number) on the syringe.
4. Place the syringe into the container of ice.
5. Send the specimen to the laboratory immediately along with the completed laboratory request form. (If the specimen is being sent to a small laboratory, it frequently is helpful to call the laboratory before obtaining the arterial specimen so that the blood gas analyzer can be calibrated before the specimen arrives in the laboratory.)

Aftercare

Ensure that pressure is maintained over the puncture site for at least 5 minutes (sandbags will not do—use fingers!).

Do not use dressings or bandages that interfere with visualization of the puncture site. Patients with blood dyscrasias or those who are anticoagulated may require a longer period of pressure to ensure that bleeding has ceased.

Observe the puncture site for at least 1 minute following removal of manual pressure for formation of a hematoma.

Reassess pulse.

Interpretation of Arterial Blood Gas Values (Figure 5-12)

Notice the pH value: 7.35 to 7.45 = normal; above 7.45 = alkalosis; below 7.35 = acidosis.

Notice the bicarbonate level: 22 to 26 mEq = normal; above 26 mEq = metabolic alkalosis; below 22 mEq = metabolic acidosis.

Notice the Pco_2 value: 35 to 40 mm Hg = normal; above 45 mm Hg = respiratory acidosis; below 35 mm Hg = respiratory alkalosis.

Make an acid-base "diagnosis" on the basis of these criteria. Consider the effect of compensatory mechanisms on blood gas values. Even when the values are abnormal, they may not all fit the criteria. The variance is caused by the compensatory action—see the examples that follow.

DEFINITIONS

acid A hydrogen ion donor; carbonic acid (H_2CO_3) is an acid.

base A hydrogen ion acceptor; bicarbonate (HCO_3) is a base.

acidosis Increased acid concentration and/or decreased base concentration. A pH of less than 7.4 is considered acidosis. A pH less than 7.3 is considered within the "danger range." Severe acidosis is a central nervous system depressant. (Signs and symptoms: judgment errors, lethargy, disorientation.)

	pH	CARBONIC ACID	BICARBONATE
ACIDOSIS	Low	Increase	Decrease
ALKALOSIS	High	Decrease	Increase

Acid-base balance is normally maintained by three different body systems: the respiratory system, the renal system, and the buffer system.

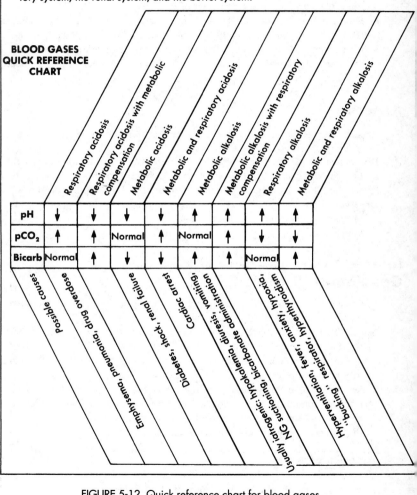

FIGURE 5-12. Quick reference chart for blood gases.
(From Budassi SA: *JEN* 3(2):24, 1977.)

alkalosis   Increased base concentration and/or decreased acid concentration. A pH greater than 7.4 is considered alkalosis. A pH greater than 7.6 is considered within the ''danger range.'' Severe alkalosis is a central nervous system excitant. (Signs and symptoms: tingling of fingertips, muscle spasms, seizures.)

pH   The hydrogen ion concentration of a solution; the relationship of carbonic acid (H_2CO_3) and bicarbonate (HCO_3) determines the pH of human serum. Acid-base balance is a function of the ratio of carbonic acid (H_2CO_3) to bicarbonate (HCO_3).

INTRAVENOUS SOLUTIONS

Dextrose (5%) in water (D_5W)

A hypotonic solution of dextrose in water containing 50 g dextrose monohydrate/liter.

■ **USE:**
TKO IV lines and nonelectrolyte fluid replacement, medical lines (emergency and other)

■ **CONTRAINDICATIONS:**
Head injuries; may increase intracranial pressure

Normal Saline

A crystalloid, isotonic solution containing:
9 g NaCl/L
145 mEq Na/L
145 mEq Cl/L

■ **USE:**
Restoration of water and salt loss in hypovolemic states; as irrigation solution

■ **CONTRAINDICATIONS:**
Congestive heart failure, pulmonary edema, renal impairment, edematous states with sodium retention

Dextrose (2.5%) and half normal saline

An isotonic solution containing:
25 g dextrose monohydrate/L
4.5 g NaCl/L

■ **USE:**
Maintenance fluid

■ **CONTRAINDICATIONS:**
Congestive heart failure, renal impairment, edema with sodium retention

Dextrose (5%) and Ringer's Lactate

A hypertonic solution containing:

50 g dextrose monohydrate	300 mg KCl/L
8.6 g NaCl/L	330 mg CaCl/L

- **USE:**
  To replace fluid and electrolyte loss
- **CONTRAINDICATIONS:**
  Congestive heart failure, renal impairment, edema with sodium retention

Ringer's Lactate

A crystalloid isotonic polyelectrolyte solution equaling the electrolyte concentration in human plasma and containing:

13 mEq Na/L	109 mEq Cl/L
4 mg K/L	2.8 mEq lactate/L

- **USE:**
  In hypovolemia for volume replacement
- **CONTRAINDICATIONS:**
  Congestive heart failure, renal impairment, edema with sodium retention, head injury, liver disease, respiratory alkalosis

Dextran 75

A colloid solution containing:
  6% Gentran in 0.7% NaCl
Should be administered through a blood filter.
- **USE:**
  Treatment of shock, hemorrhage, burns
- **CONTRAINDICATIONS:**
  Bleeding disorders, congestive heart failure, renal impairment

Plasma

A colloid solution and the liquid fraction of unclotted whole blood containing:

135 to 150 Na/L	98 to 106 Cl/L
3.5 to 5 K/L	22 to 30 HCl_3/L

Should be administered through a blood filter.
- **USE:**
  Volume replacement
- **CONTRAINDICATIONS:**
  Congestive heart failure, pulmonary edema

Plasmanate

A colloid and commercial IV solution containing:
Human albumin, 88%
Alpha globulin, 7%
Beta globulin, 5%
Polyelectrolyte solution
    100 mEq Na/L
    50 mEq Cl/L
Should be administered through a blood filter.
■ **USE:**
Blood volume expansion
■ **CONTRAINDICATIONS:**
Congestive heart failure, pulmonary edema

Salt-Poor Albumin

A colloid solution containing:
Normal human albumin, 25%
Alpha globulin, 7%
Protein, 12.5%
Should be administered through a blood filter.
■ **USE:**
Urgent fluid volume replacement because of trauma or burns; rarely used in trauma management today
■ **CONTRAINDICATIONS:**
Congestive heart failure, pulmonary edema

BLOOD AND BLOOD COMPONENTS

General Principles

If a patient is losing blood, he is losing *all* components.
Blood replacement with fresh whole blood cells is best, but it is usually difficult to obtain large amounts.
It requires 30 to 45 minutes to completely type and cross-match blood.
If the need is lifesaving, O negative blood may be given.
If the need is urgent, type-specific (A, B, AB, or O) unmatched blood can be given to decrease the hazard of reaction.

Complications

Mismatched blood
Hypothermia—banked blood is cold
Hypocalcemia—citrate in banked blood binds free calcium
Hyperkalemia—potassium levels increase in stored blood by 1 mEq/L/day

Acid-base problems—stored blood has a pH of 6.4 to 6.8; this causes an initial acidosis, but citrate causes conversion to bicarb and eventual alkalosis

Coagulation defects—especially disseminated intravascular coagulation (DIC)

Care of the Patient Receiving Volume Replacement

Check the airway frequently.
Auscultate the lungs.
Monitor the ECG.
Check urinary output.
Check temperature.
Check electrolytes.
Check hematocrit.

THE COLLECTION OF LABORATORY SPECIMENS

The Collection of Blood

Most patients have blood samples collected at some time during their emergency department visit. These blood values may be used to establish a baseline, identify trends, or diagnose a particular condition. Always explain to the patient that blood is going to be drawn for some test. If the patient asks the reason for the tests, try to explain. The patient should be lying or sitting while the specimen is being collected.

Selection of the site

Usually the median cephalic vein, located in the antecubital fossa, is used for the collection of blood. You may use any other peripheral site that is readily accessible. If an IV line must also be initiated, consider establishing the IV line and withdrawing a blood sample from that line before connecting the IV solution. This will save the patient an additional puncture and may save time.

Methods to find a vein

Apply a tourniquet and leave it in place for no longer than 5 minutes.
Lower the extremity, causing the site from which the specimen is to be collected to be dependent.
Apply warm soaks to the area.
Have the patient open and close his or her hand.
Use good direct lighting.
Feel for a vein with the fingers; sometimes good large veins are a bit deeper and cannot be visualized, but can be palpated.
In an absolute emergency situation, when a site for drawing blood cannot be located, the specimen may be drawn from the femoral vein. This site is not routinely recommended because of the increased incidence of infection and/or embolism.

Procedure

Once the site has been identified, cleanse it with an antiseptic solution such as alcohol or an iodine-based solution (be sure to check to see if the patient is allergic to any of these preparations). Avoid using alcohol if you are drawing an ethanol level.

Palpate the site above the proposed needle entry point; do not touch the actual site.

Have the patient open and close a fist to allow for venous filling.

Stabilize the vein with a thumb.

Draw the skin taut below the site to prevent the vein from moving during puncture.

Insert the needle at a 30-degree angle with the bevel facing up.

If using a Vacutainer, insert the laboratory tube at this point.

If using the needle-and-syringe technique, begin to pull back on the plunger of the syringe at this point.

Once the correct amount of blood has been collected, release the tourniquet.

Place a dry, sterile 2 × 2 inch gauze square over the needle insertion site and withdraw the needle.

Place a slight amount of pressure over the puncture site.

Place specimens into the correct laboratory tubes if the needle-and-syringe technique was used.

Do not force blood with pressure through the needle and into the laboratory tube.

Be sure to agitate carefully any tube that contains any type of preservative or chemical to allow for its dissemination.

Label all tubes carefully with the patient's name, hospital number, the date, and the caregiver's initials.

Do not have the patient bend the arm at the elbow to decrease bleeding; instead, have the patient elevate the arm.

LABORATORY ANALYSIS

The laboratory data base is an essential component in the assessment of patients in the emergency department. Expensive at best, laboratory tests should not be ordered indiscriminately, but should follow an interview and examination process that indicates the appropriate testing requirements for each patient.

A number of laboratory tests are frequently used within the emergency setting. In some departments it is a nursing responsibility to order routine tests when their need is established, whereas in other departments such orders are carried out by the physician on duty. In either case, a working knowledge of the common tests and the types of containers used to collect test specimens is necessary for the nurse involved (Table 5-1).

Specific Tests

Table 5-2 provides a quick overview of commonly ordered laboratory tests and corresponding normal lab values for each test.

TABLE 5-1   Tubes for Drawing Blood*

TUBE	PRESERVATIVE OR ANTICOAGULANT	TEST
Red top	None	Serologies, chemistry panels, routine chemistries
Lavender top	Ethylenediaminotetraacetate (EDTA)	Hematology, lipoprotein electrophoresis, acid phosphatase
Blue top	Sodium citrate (0.5 g)	Coagulation studies
Gray top	Sodium fluoride	Blood glucose, blood alcohol, drug screens and tests that will not be evaluated soon
Green top	Sodium heparin	Special procedures

*Adapted from Sheehy SB, Barber JM: *Emergency nursing: principles and practice,* ed 2. St Louis, 1985, Mosby.

Complete blood count

A complete blood count (CBC) is a routine hematologic screening test on serum; it includes hemoglobin, hematocrit, total red blood cell (RBC) count, white blood cell count and differential, and mean corpuscular cell volume (MCV), mean cell hemoglobin concentration (MCHC), and mean cell hemoglobin (MCH). Elements of this test may on occasion be ordered separately, which will lower the cost to the patient. Five milliliters of venous blood is generally required.

Urinalysis

A urinalysis should always be a clean-catch or catheter specimen collected in a sterile, dry container and examined within 30 minutes if unrefrigerated. The standard examination includes appearance, pH, specific gravity, glucose and ketones, protein semiquantitation, and microscopic examination of the sediment for casts, crystals, RBCs, and bacteria.

Blood glucose

Venous blood for glucose levels should be obtained as a clot specimen in a patient whom you suspect has an abnormality in glucose metabolism. Collect the specimen before starting intravenous solution infusions or administering dextrose. Two to three milliliters is necessary to perform the test. Record the conditions under which the blood was drawn—that is, whether the patient was fasting, approximate time of last meal, and so on.

Blood urea nitrogen

The blood urea nitrogen (BUN) test measures the amount of circulating urea in the blood, which is the end product of protein metabolism and is normally

TABLE 5-2   Normal Laboratory Values for Commonly Ordered Laboratory Tests

Serum chemistry
Bilirubin (Bili)

Total	03.–1.5 mg/dL
Direct	0–0.2 mg/dL

Creatinine (Creat)

Female	0.6–1.1 mg/dL
Male	0.8–1.3 mg/dL

Urea nitrogen (BUN) — 8–23 mg/dL
Glucose-fasting (Gluc) — 65–110 mg/dL
Electrolytes (Lytes)

Potassium (K^+)	3.8–5.0 mEq/L
Chlorides (Cl)	95–103 mEq/L
Carbon dioxide (CO_2)	24–30 mM
Sodium (Na)	136–142 mEq/L

Arterial blood gases

pH	7.35–7.45
Po_2	80–105 mm Hg
Pco_2	35–45 mm Hg

Serum enzymes

Amylase	15–90 U/L
Creatinine phosphokinase (CPK)	25–145 mU/ml
Lactic dehydrogenase (LDH)	110–250 mU/ml
Alanine amino transaminase (SGPT)	5–35 mU/L
Aspartate amino transaminase (SGOT)	10–40 mU/ml

Hematology
Coagulation

Bleeding time	< 8 minutes
Partial thromboplatin time (PTT)	24–36 seconds
Prothrombin time (PT)	70%–100%
Thrombin time	11.9–18.5 seconds

Hematocrit

Female	37%–47%
Male	42%–52%

Hemoglobin

Female	12.0–16.0 g/dL
Male	14.0–18.0 g/dL

Erythrocytes

Female	$4.2–5.4 \times 10^6$ cu mm
Male	$4.6–6.2 \times 10^6$ cu mm

Sedimentation rate

Female	up to 20 mm/hr
Male	up to 9 mm/hr

Leukocytes — $4.8–10.8 \times 10^3$ cu mm
Platelets — $150–400 \times 10^3$ cu mm
Urinalysis

Color	yellow
pH	4.6–8
Specific gravity	1.001–1.035
Glucose	$\emptyset$

excreted in the urine. An elevation of the BUN may indicate renal failure, renal hypoperfusion, or obstructive uropathy. A 1-ml amount of venous blood is required to perform the test.

Serum electrolytes

The venous specimen should be withdrawn from a vein and collected in a specimen container in as atraumatic a procedure as possible to avoid hemolysis, which results in a false elevation of the serum potassium. Electrolytes include potassium, chlorides, and carbon dioxide content. Although each of these elements can be tested individually, the implications of the result may change depending on the values of the other electrolytes in concert with one another.

Serum creatinine

The serum creatinine test evaluates renal functions by measuring creatinine, a waste product that is found in skeletal muscle and is usually filtered by the renal glomerulus. The serum creatinine may be elevated in acute renal failure. A 3-ml amount of venous blood is needed to perform the test.

Cardiac enzymes

Tests for cardiac enzymes include creatinine phosphokinase (CPK), lactic dehydrogenase (LDH), and serum glutamic-oxaloacetic transaminase (SGOT). Levels may be elevated in cardiac muscle infarction, as well as in patients with acute muscle injury or multiple injections. Therefore, cardiac isoenzymes are usually evaluated also, specifically those that elevate in cardiac muscle infarction (LDH fraction 1 and CPK-MB). A 5 ml volume of venous blood is required for this test.

Toxic screen

A toxic screen may be ordered specific to a certain drug or as a screen for sedatives, hypnotics, and narcotics. It measures the exact amount of circulating drug per volume of plasma. This is a very expensive test and takes a long time to run. Most facilities send the specimen out to a bioanalysis laboratory, but this delays receipt of the results because of transit time. A 5-ml amount of venous blood is required to perform this test.

Serum drug level

A serum drug level is generally ordered specific to a drug such as digoxin. It measures the concentration of drug in the blood at the time the level is drawn. The test requires 2 to 5 ml of venous blood.

Serum amylase

Serum amylase is generally evaluated in patients with upper abdominal pain. The test measures the amount of circulating amylase, which is a digestive enzyme for carbohydrates and is elevated most notably in acute pancreatitis. This test requires 3 ml of venous blood.

Arterial blood gases

Arterial blood gases are analyzed from arterial specimens collected in heparinized tubes or syringes. Elements include serum pH, PCO_2, PO_2, and bicarbonate levels. Results help determine the acid-base status of the internal environment and the degree of oxygenation of the tissues. Most test results include the percentage of oxygen saturation of the red blood cells. The minimal specimen required is 3 ml, which is collected under aseptic conditions.

White blood count and differential

A white blood count (WBC) and differential may be ordered instead of a CBC when an infection is suspected. However, both these elements must be ordered and evaluated together, since the WBC may not be elevated even in severe infections, whereas the differential will. Mild to moderate leukocytosis may indicate an infectious process that is bacterial in origin. The differential is an evaluation of the different types of leukocytes that are found in the serum: neutrophils (56% of the total), eosinophils (2.7%), basophils (0.3%), and lymphocytes (34%). Neutrophils are also called ''polys,'' or polymorphonucleocytes, and ''segs,'' or segmented cells. Monocytes are nongranular leukocytes and may be seen in chronic inflammatory conditions in small numbers. Bands are new neutrophils that are formed in response to overwhelming bacterial invasion that taxes the older neutrophil population. Such a condition is referred to as a **shift to the left**. The WBC and differential are collected in a clot tube devoid of preservatives or anticoagulants. To perform the test, 3 to 5 ml venous blood is needed.

Coagulation studies

Various elements of the coagulation series evaluate the different stages of clotting. The studies include protime, partial thromboplastin time, platelet count, Lee white clotting time, and prothrombin consumption time.

Prothrombin time

This test identifies defects in stage 3 of coagulation. A calcium-binding anticoagulant is added to the patient's serum, and the time between addition of this element and the formation of a fibrin clot is measured.

Partial thromboplastin time

This test identifies defects in stage 2 of coagulation. It measures factors XII, XI, X, IX, VIII, V, II, and I. The test measures the clotting time of plasma when elements of the clotting process are added to calcium-free and platelet-poor plasma in a predetermined sequence.

Prothrombin consumption time (PCT)

This test measures prothrombin utilization time. It identifies defects in stage 1 and 2 of coagulation and is also used to elevate coagulation of blood.

Platelet count

This test identifies the number of platelets in a peripheral smear and confirms defects in stage 1 of coagulation.

Lee white clotting time

This test measures the time it takes for a fibrin clot to form in venous blood and identifies defects in stage 4 of coagulation.

BLOOD SAMPLING IN PEDIATRIC PATIENTS

Specimens may be obtained by finger-stick, heel-stick, or regular venipuncture technique, depending on the amount of the specimen required. If using conventional venipuncture technique, the appropriate size needle for collection would be between 19 or 23 gauge. Pediatric-size vacuum tubes are available in 3- and 5-ml sizes.

Finger-Stick/Heel-Stick Technique

Cleanse the site.
Apply a small sterile dressing at the completion of the procedure.

BLOOD FOR BLOOD CULTURES

Particular care must be taken when obtaining specimens for blood culture.
1. Separate containers are required for specimens for aerobic, anaerobic, and fungal cultures.
2. The stopper of a culture medium container must be cleansed using betadine followed by dry wiping or air drying.
3. It is recommended that the caregiver wear sterile gloves when obtaining the specimen to avoid contamination of the puncture site.
4. The site must also be prepared in the same way as the culture medium stopper.
5. The needle must be changed each time a culture medium is inoculated.
6. The ratio of blood to medium should be 1:10.
7. The laboratory slip is labeled with the patient's name, hospital number, date, time, and body temperature, and any antibiotics the patient is taking are listed.
8. The culture medium container is labeled with the patient's name, the hospital number, date, time, and caregiver's initials; also include the patient's hospital/emergency department number.

SPINAL FLUID

Usually three to five specimens are sent to the laboratory following a spinal tap.
1. Number the tubes serially during collection.
2. If only one tube is collected, this tube should be sent to the microbiology

section of the laboratory for division of the specimen under aseptic conditions following examination for necessary cultures.

3. Transport specimens to the laboratory immediately following collection; do not allow these specimens to sit in the department for prolonged periods.

URINE SPECIMENS

All urine specimens collected in the emergency department should be obtained by at least a midstream clean catch. On occasion it will be necessary to obtain a urine specimen by catheterization of the bladder.

1. Use sterile containers.
2. If the physician orders a urinalysis, split the urine and save a specimen (refrigerated) in case a culture and sensitivity test is ordered later.
3. Do not allow specimens to remain at room temperature for more than 30 minutes.

PERCUTANEOUS FLUID OR WOUND DRAINAGE SPECIMENS

Fluids from body cavities or wounds should be collected in a sterile syringe and then transferred to a sterile test tube or bottle. Be sure that specimens collected for anaerobic testing are free of air bubbles before being sent to the lab. If the patient is taking any medication, be sure to indicate what it is on the laboratory slip.

EMESIS AND GASTRIC LAVAGE MATERIAL

If the specimen is to be collected from gastric lavage, be sure to send the sample from the initial aspirate. If it is known or suspected what the ingested substance is or if there is an unusual smell about the patient, be sure to indicate this on the laboratory slip—it may aid in identification of toxic material.

STOOL SPECIMENS

If stool is to be sent to the laboratory for culture, it should be warm and newly evacuated. It should be sent to the laboratory in a sterile container. If the specimen is obtained by rectal swabbing, be sure that there is particulate matter on the swab. *Do not add saline or any other liquid to the specimen because this may destroy certain parasites.*

THROAT SWABS AND SPUTUM SPECIMENS

A throat culture is usually obtained via the oropharyngeal route using a long, sterile, cotton-tipped swab. The swab should then be placed in a sterile culture tube and transported to the laboratory as soon as possible.

Sputum can be collected directly into a dry, sterile container. The specimen should come from deep within the tracheobronchial tree. Saliva is not an acceptable sputum specimen. The specimen should be taken to the laboratory immediately. If the patient cannot cough or is unconscious, it may be necessary to obtain a specimen by suctioning the tracheobronchial tree.

SUGGESTED READINGS

Camp-Sorrell, D: Implantable ports: everything you always wanted to know, *J Intrav Nurs* 15:262, 1992.

Sheehy SB, Barber JM: *Emergency nursing: principles and practice,* ed 2. St Louis, 1985, Mosby.

Sheehy SB, Marvin JA, Jimmerson CL: *Clinical trauma care: the first hour,* St Louis, 1989, Mosby.

Wickham, R: Long-term venous access devices. In Kitt S, Kaiser J, eds: *Emergency nursing: a physiologic and clinical perspective.* Philadelphia, 1990, Saunders.

CHAPTER 6

Shock and Hemodynamic Monitoring

Shock is a complex syndrome that develops due to inadequate or inappropriate tissue perfusion leading to cellular hypoxia and a buildup of toxic metabolites. Three main components responsible for supplying the cells with nutrients and oxygen are the:

Heart, which functions as a pump

Blood, fluid which serves as the transporter

Vascular system, which provides the transportation network

If radical changes occur in any of these areas, shock may rapidly ensue.

CLASSIFICATION OF SHOCK

Hypovolemic

Decreased intravascular volume loss that may be caused by trauma; hemorrhage from other causes (GI bleeding or a ruptured ectopic pregnancy); severe burns; or dehydration resulting from diarrhea, polyuria, profuse diaphoresis, emesis, or excessive nasogastric suctioning.

Cardiogenic

Inefficiency of the heart as a pump; occurs in myocardial infarction, cardiac tamponade, pulmonary embolus, myocarditis, or cardiomyopathies.

Distributive

Maldistribution of blood volume due to changes in vascular resistance and permeability.

1. *Septic*   An overwhelming infection that causes an endotoxin release that results in vasodilation and decreased tissue perfusion.
2. *Anaphylactic*   A severe allergic reaction that results in histamine release, increased capillary permeability, and dilation of the arterioles and venules.
3. *Neurogenic*   Dilation of arterioles and venules caused by loss of sympathetic tone.

Obstructive

Obstruction to the outflow of blood from the heart caused by massive pulmonary embolism, pericardial tamponade, tension pneumothorax, or severe aortic stenosis.

The first hour of therapeutic intervention for shock is usually the most important. Management can be difficult, and the mortality rate is high. To choose the appropriate therapeutic intervention, it is vital to determine if the cause is a volume deficit problem, a pump failure problem, or a vascular dilation problem.

Despite the initiating etiology of shock, the final common pathway for all categories of shock is inadequate oxygen delivery at the cellular level. The immediate end-points of therapy for all categories of shock are to restore and maintain adequate delivery of oxygen and nutrients by preventing or reversing anaerobic metabolism.

It is, however, important to note that the most important factor in the success of early treatment is the experience of the medical and nursing staff,[1] for early recognition of decreased oxygen delivery and prompt initiation of therapy to restore tissue perfusion and oxygenation is critical to improving patient outcome.

PATHOPHYSIOLOGY OF SHOCK

Understanding the basic pathophysiology of shock is an essential component toward further appreciation of the clinical presentation and progression seen with each category of shock.

Regardless of the etiologic event, the primary pathophysiologic outcome in shock consists of hypoperfusion, which results in tissue hypoxia, acidosis, and end organ dysfunction.[2]

Rice[3] describes the shock state as having the potential for progressing through four stages:

Initial stage
Compensatory stage
Progressive stage
Refractory stage

Speed of progression and clinical manifestations seen with each stage will vary with each patient. The following pathophysiologic mechanisms are described according to each stage of shock:

Initial Stage

- Decrease in cardiac output
- Decrease in tissue perfusion
- Decrease in aerobic metabolism
- Increase in anaerobic metabolism
- Increase in lactic acid production

Compensatory Stage

- Decrease in cardiac output
- Activation of compensatory mechanisms

Compensatory mechanisms in shock

The activation of compensatory mechanisms occurs in an attempt to preserve vital organ function. The four most prominent mechanisms are discussed below.

■ **SYMPATHETIC NERVOUS SYSTEM**
When the sympathetic nervous system is activated following trauma, epinephrine is released. Epinephrine causes an increase in heart rate. Cardiac output and blood pressure increase, resulting in peripheral vasoconstriction.

■ **RENIN-ANGIOTENSIN MECHANISM**
When renal perfusion is decreased, the renin-angiotensin mechanism is activated. When renin is released, it causes the release of angiotensin I and angiotensin II. This effect causes the release of aldosterone into the system. Aldosterone causes increased sodium reabsorption at the renal tubule level. As sodium is reabsorbed, fluid is also reabsorbed. This fluid is then shunted into the venous system, resulting in increased intravascular volume, increased blood return to the right side of the heart, increased cardiac output, and increased blood pressure. Aldosterone may be a factor in decreased urinary output.

■ **RELEASE OF ANTIDIURETIC HORMONE**
In hypovolemic states, the anterior pituitary gland releases antidiuretic hormone (ADH). ADH causes the reabsorption of water at the renal collecting duct level. The water is shunted into the venous system, where it causes an increased intravascular volume, increased blood return to the right side of the heart, increased cardiac output, decreased urine output, and increased blood pressure. Like aldosterone, ADH release may also be a factor in decreased urinary output.

■ **INTRACELLULAR FLUID SHIFT**
Fluid shifts from intracellular spaces to intravascular spaces, causing increased vascular volume, increased blood return to the right side of the heart, increased cardiac output, and increased blood pressure. Because of the ''cellular dehydration,'' the patient, if awake, will complain of being thirsty.

Progressive Stage

- Decrease in compensatory mechanisms
- Hypoperfusion of vital organs
- Decrease in cardiac output

- Decrease in blood pressure
- Decrease in myocardial oxygen supply
- Decrease in myocardial function

Refractory Stage (irreversible)

- Multiple system organ failure
- Profound hypotension
- Severe hypoxemia
- Renal shutdown
- Intractable circulatory failure

Throughout the four stages of shock, five main organ systems are affected.

EFFECT OF SHOCK ON THE FIVE VITAL ORGANS

Heart

Decreased coronary artery perfusion causes decreased function of the heart muscle as a pump; stroke volume and blood pressure decrease.

Brain

If oxygen and nutrient supplies are inadequate, brain function diminishes and unconsciousness ensues.

Lungs

As the partial pressure of oxygen decreases because of decreased blood volume or blood pressure, gas exchange does not take place at the capillary membrane level.

Liver

Glycogen stores are depleted by an excess of circulating epinephrine; metabolic acids that are normally detoxified in the liver cause acidosis.

Kidneys

A drop in cardiac output causes a decrease in blood flow through the kidneys; decreased urinary output and renal failure result.

TYPES OF SHOCK

Hypovolemic Shock

Hypovolemic shock is the most frequent category of shock, resulting from a loss of blood, plasma, or fluid and electrolytes. The most common cause of hypovolemic shock is trauma that produces ruptured internal organs, lacerations, disrupted vasculature, long bone fractures, or pelvic fractures. Hypovolemic shock may also result from other conditions that result in fluid volume loss, such as a massive crush injury, severe burn injury, gastrointestinal bleed, ruptured aortic aneurysm, aortic dissection, ruptured ectopic pregnancy, peritonitis, intestinal obstruction, severe diarrhea, severe nausea and vomiting, or severe diaphoresis.

In general, the easiest way to discuss hypovolemic shock is in terms of blood loss resulting from trauma. The degree of shock depends on the following:

- Amount of blood lost
- Rate of blood loss
- Age of the patient
- Patient's overall physical condition
- Patient's ability to mobilize compensatory mechanisms

The blood volume of an adult (expressed in milliliters) is equal to 70% or 80% of *ideal* body weight in kilograms. A child contains 80 to 90 ml/kg of body weight.[4] The diagnosis of hypovolemic shock is made by clinical observation, physical examination, laboratory analysis, arterial pressure, central venous pressure (CVP), and pulmonary capillary occlusive pressure (PaOP) measurements. The initial goal in the treatment of hypovolemic shock is identifying and treating the cause while restoring volume by rapid infusion of fluids.

Classification of hypovolemic shock

Four classes of hypovolemic shock have been described[4]:

Class I: Less than 15% blood loss

■ **SIGNS AND SYMPTOMS**
- Mild tachycardia

■ **THERAPEUTIC INTERVENTIONS**
- Control bleeding
- Replace primary fluid losses

Class II: 15% to 30% blood loss

■ **SIGNS AND SYMPTOMS**
- Tachycardia
- Mild decrease in pulse pressure
- Mild increase in diastolic pressure
- Mild increase in respiratory rate
- Mildly cool skin

■ **THERAPEUTIC INTERVENTIONS**
- Manage airway.
- Administer oxygen.
- Administer IV fluids.
- Control bleeding if possible.
- Consider surgery.

Class III: 30% to 40% blood loss

■ **SIGNS AND SYMPTOMS**
- Airway difficulties possible
- Tachypnea
- Tachycardia
- Hypotension
- Restlessness, anxiety, or decreased level of consciousness
- Cool, clammy skin
- Cool extremities
- Delayed capillary refill
- Decreased urinary output
- Decreased CVP and PaOP

■ **THERAPEUTIC INTERVENTIONS**
- Manage airway.
- Administer oxygen.
- Administer IV fluids.
- Administer crystalloids and blood products.
  NOTE: Replace blood loss with crystalloids at a rate of 3 L of crystalloids to 1 L of blood loss.
- Consider autotransfusion.
- Control bleeding, if possible.
- Prepare patient for diagnostic studies and/or surgery.

Class IV: Greater than 40% blood loss

■ **SIGNS AND SYMPTOMS**
- Decreased level of consciousness
- Tachycardia
- Hypotension
- Narrowed pulse pressure
- Tachypnea
- Cool, clammy skin
- Delayed capillary refill
- Decreased urinary output
- CVP less than 5 mm H_2O
- PaOP less than 4 mm H_2O

■ **THERAPEUTIC INTERVENTIONS**
- Manage airway.
- Administer oxygen.
- Administer IV fluids.
- Give blood products as soon as possible.
- Control bleeding, if possible.
- Consider emergency surgical intervention.

Distributive Shock

Distributive shock occurs when there is an abnormal distribution of intravascular volume due to a decrease in vascular resistance. Categories of distributive shock include septic, anaphylactic, and neurogenic shock.

Septic shock

Septic shock is usually caused by an overwhelming gram-negative infection that results in vasodilation and decreased tissue perfusion. It may also be caused by immune system suppression, invasion of organs by toxic substances, or the failure of the immune system to react to bacteria. It is important to remember that blood volume in septic shock is essentially normal. The infection may come from a source such as an indwelling urinary catheter or a severe burn injury, or it may occur as a postpartum complication. Mortality from septic shock is high—30% to 50%.[5] Death from septic shock is more common in the very young and the very old.

The usual cause of the infection is a gram-negative bacillus such as *Escherichia coli, Pseudomonas, Staphylococcus, Proteus, Salmonella,* or *Bacteroides.* It is occasionally caused by gram-positive cocci or, on rare occasions, fungi, viruses, or yeast. Bacteria enter the vascular system and cause the release of endotoxins into the circulation. This causes fluid leaks into the interstitial spaces, increased vascular permeability and vasodilation, and hypotension.

■ **SIGNS AND SYMPTOMS**
- Decreased blood pressure or normal blood pressure with widened pulse pressure
- Decreased cardiac output
- Tachycardia
- Hyperventilation
- Hypocapnia
- Hyperpyrexia
- Chills/tremors/rigors
- Pink, warm, dry skin
- Petechiae
- Decreased level of consciousness
- Metabolic acidosis
- Nausea and vomiting
- Diarrhea
- Positive cultures

Initially, the presentation of septic shock is that of a hypodynamic state.[6] The initial response is arterial and venous vasodilation that results in decreased preload and decreased systemic vascular resistance ultimately causing hypotension. Shock may later progress to a hypodynamic state. In hypodynamic shock the cardiac output falls as a consequence of decreased intravascular volume and myocardial depression leading to decreased cellular perfusion. This causes a stagnation of blood and resultant anaerobic metabolism and acidosis.

■ **THERAPEUTIC INTERVENTIONS**
- High-flow oxygen
- IV fluids

- Antibiotics (be sure to obtain cultures first)
- Inotropic agents and vasodilators for alpha-adrenergic effects
- Dopamine (Intropin)
- Dobutamine (Dobutrex)
- Naloxone (Narcan): considered investigational
- Corticosteroids (controversial)
- Heparin (controversial)
- Surgical intervention

Anaphylactic shock

Anaphylactic shock is an antigen/antibody reaction that occurs when a sensitized person is exposed to an antigen that is characterized by acute changes in vascular permeability and bronchial hyperactivity. It develops rapidly (usually within 20 minutes following exposure)[6] and may be caused by medications (e.g., antibiotics, such as penicillin), contrast media, sera, insect bites and stings, or ingestion of foodstuffs. When the antigen/antibody reaction occurs, a histamine release causes arterioles, venules, and capillaries to dilate. When the capillaries dilate, capillary permeability increases and intravascular fluid leaks into the interstitial spaces. This causes a form of relative hypovolemia and shock.

■ **SIGNS AND SYMPTOMS**
- Respiratory difficulty:
   Stridor
   Airway obstruction
   Bronchospasm
   Wheezing
- Hypotension
- Tachycardia
- Dysrhythmias
- Urticaria/angioneurotic edema
- Pruritus
- Warm skin
- Cardiopulmonary arrest

■ **THERAPEUTIC INTERVENTIONS**
- ABCs
- High-flow oxygen
- IV fluids
- Epinephrine 0.1 to 0.5 ml of a 1:10,000 solution by slow IV push (may be repeated in 5 to 15 minutes if necessary). Propranolol (Inderal) should be available in the event persistent hypertension and tachycardia occur.
- Aminophylline for bronchospasm
- Beta-agonist aerosol (e.g., metaproterenol) for bronchospasm
- Antihistamines: (e.g., diphenhydramine) to decrease circulating histamines
- Steroids to reduce inflammatory response

Neurogenic shock

Neurogenic shock is caused by a decrease of sympathetic tone. This results in a dilation of arterioles and venules, which causes relative hypotension. Neurogenic shock may result from deep general anesthesia, spinal anesthesia, spinal cord injury, or severe brainstem injury at the level of the medulla. It is usually a diagnosis of exclusion when all other causes of shock are ruled out.

■ **SIGNS AND SYMPTOMS**
- Decreased blood pressure
- Rapid, shallow respirations or no respirations
- Tachycardia
- Paraplegia or quadriplegia
- Cool, clammy skin above the level of the lesion
- Priapism
- History of recent spinal anesthesia
- History of recent head trauma

■ **THERAPEUTIC INTERVENTIONS**
- ABCs
- Supine position
- IV fluids with crystalloids
- IV vasopressors for alpha-agonist effects
- Dopamine
- Phenylephrine
- Cervical spine protection

Cardiogenic Shock

Cardiogenic shock (seen with a 35% to 70% destruction of the left ventricular myocardium) is defined as a low cardiac output state with hypotension and signs of inadequate tissue perfusion.[7] Characterized as primary cardiac pump failure, it may be seen in the setting of acute myocardial infarction, myocardial contusion, myocardial rupture, myocarditis, cardiomyopathies, dysrhythmias, or pericardial tamponade. Pump failure is the inability of the heart to produce an adequate cardiac output. When myocardial infarction occurs, part of the myocardium becomes dysfunctional. If the infarct is large (usually involving more than 40% of the ventricle),[8] cardiac output decreases. When cardiac output decreases, blood pressure also decreases and tissue perfusion becomes inadequate, causing shock.

Therapeutic interventions are aimed at improving cardiac output, increasing tissue perfusion, and limiting myocardial damage. Cardiogenic shock occurs in 15% to 20% of myocardial infarction patients. Mortality is 75% to 95%.

■ **SIGNS AND SYMPTOMS**
- Signs of myocardial infarction (chest pain, nausea and vomiting, syncope)
- ECG changes indicative of myocardial infarction
- Cardiac dysrhythmias
- Elevated cardiac isoenzymes
- Shallow, rapid respirations
- Hypoxemia
- Decreased peripheral pulses
- Decreased blood pressure (if blood pressure increases, it does so at the expense of myocardial ischemia)

- Decreased cardiac output/cardiac index
- Elevated pulmonary artery occlusive pressure (greater than 18 mm Hg)
- Decreased level of consciousness (or anxiety or restlessness)
- Pale, cool, clammy skin
- Oliguria (less than 0.5 to 1 ml/kg/hour)
- Metabolic acidosis

■ **THERAPEUTIC INTERVENTIONS**

Aimed at optimizing preload, afterload, and contractility (See section on hemo-dynamic monitoring.)

- Correcting preload
  Low preload:
    Decreased CVP
    Decreased PaOP
    Decreased PAD
      Administer fluids
  High preload:
    Elevated CVP
    Elevated PAOP
    Elevated PAD
      Administer diuretics, venodilation (nitroglycerin)
- Correcting afterload
  Low afterload:
    Decreased blood pressure
    Decreased SVR
      Administer dopamine
  High afterload:
    Increased blood pressure
    Elevated SVR
      Administer sodium nitroprusside, dobutamine
- Correcting contractility (inotropy):
  Low cardiac output
    Administer dobutamine, epinephrine, and dopamine (if afterload within normal limits)
- Intraaortic Balloon Pump (IABP) to increase cardiac output, oxygen delivery, and blood flow to the coronary arteries and to decrease myocardial oxygen consumption
- High-flow oxygen and/or therapeutic intubation
- Antiarrhythmic agents

Obstructive Shock

Obstructive shock occurs as a result of an obstruction to the outflow of blood from the heart or from an increased resistance to ventricular filling (diastole). Massive pulmonary contusion, coarctation of the aorta, or aortic stenosis may cause an obstruction of outflow of blood, whereas pericardial tamponade or tension pneumothorax may result in increased resistance to ventricular filling.[9]

Regardless of the causes, the end result is a decrease in cardiac output and inadequate tissue perfusion.

■ **SIGNS AND SYMPTOMS (will vary according to cause)**

Pulmonary embolism
- Dyspnea
- Tachypnea
- Chest pain
- Anxiety
- Hypoxemia

Coarctation of aorta
- Systemic hypertension (upper extremities)
- Lower blood pressure in lower extremities

Aortic stenosis
- Chest pain
- Dyspnea
- Cyanosis
- Syncope
- Hypoxemia
- Cough
- Mental status changes

Pericardial tamponade
- Elevated CVP
- Cyanosis
- Distended neck veins
- Decreased CO
- Decreased blood pressure
- Muffled heart sounds

Tension pneumothorax
- Decreased CVP
- Decreased CO
- Decreased blood pressure
- Hypoxemia
- Severe shortness of breath
- Jugular vein distension
- Tracheal deviation
- Mediastinal shift

■ **THERAPEUTIC INTERVENTIONS (vary according to cause)**

Pulmonary embolism
- Oxygen
- System anticoagulation
- IV access

Coarctation of the aorta
- IV access
- Oxygen
- Prepare patient for cardiac catheterization, aortogram and/or operating room

Aortic stenosis
- IV access
- Supportive treatment of symptoms
- Prepare patient for cardiac catheterization or operating room (valve replacement)
- Oxygen

Pericardial tamponade
- IV access
- Oxygen
- Pericardiocentesis/pericardial window

Tension pneumothorax
- IV access
- Oxygen
- Needle thoracostomy
- Chest tube placement

FLUID REPLACEMENT

One of the most important therapeutic interventions for a patient in shock is to gain vascular access so that fluids and blood products can be administered to replace volume and to increase preload and cardiac output to improve oxygen delivery. The number of intravenous accesses required depends on the severity of shock.

Sites

Choose sites that can accommodate large-bore cannulas for rapid fluid volume replacement. In the emergency setting, when time is critical, choose sites that are easily accessible and easy to cannulate.

Peripheral

External jugular vein
Antecubital (fossa) vein
Saphenous vein
Femoral vein

Central

Internal jugular vein
Subclavian vein

CAUTION: Caution should be exercised in using subclavian or jugular veins for treatment of hypovolemic shock, since the great veins are usually collapsed, increasing the possibility of complications such as hemothorax or pneumothorax.[10]

Surgical cutdown

Brachial vein
Femoral vein
Saphenous vein

Intraosseous

Intraosseous infusion is a temporary method to obtain intravascular access in children when other vascular sites are not readily available. A rigid needle is placed through the bone cortex into the medullary cavity. The anterior medial aspect of the tibia is the preferred site. Positioning the needle 1 to 3 cm below the proximal tibial tuberosity is preferred, although any site along the tibia may be used. The midanterior distal one-third of the femur, iliac crest, humerus, and sternum are other sites that may be considered (depending on the patient's age). Intraosseous access should be replaced with conventional intravenous access as soon as possible.

Size of Cannula

Use the largest-gauge, shortest-length cannula possible. Whenever possible, in the adult patient, use a 16-gauge or larger cannula, so that both IV fluids and blood products can be infused. If a surgical cutdown is performed, attempt to cannulate the vein with a No. 8 (or larger) feeding tube.

Type of Tubing

Use standard *macrodrip* tubing (do not use *microdrip*) or other larger commercially available tubing. Inline manual pumping devices may be used to facilitate rapid fluid flow. Avoid IV extension tubing and standard stopcocks whenever possible during the resuscitation phase of fluid replacement. The increased length of tubing causes an increase in the coefficient of friction and slows the flow rate and delivery rate of the fluid. The inner diameter of standard stopcocks will slow flow rate.

CAUTION: Use only high-flow stopcocks.

IV Adjuncts

A rapid infusion device or pressure cuff used on an IV bag significantly increases the rate of fluid delivery.
If warming devices are used, be sure that the product chosen does not slow fluid flow rate.

Temperature of Fluids

Ideally, fluids should be warmed to 104° F. Rapidly infused fluids that are room temperature or colder may cause hypothermia. Commercially available fluid warmers may be used to warm fluids and blood. IV fluids may also be warmed by placing bags of IV fluids near the defrosting unit in prehospital vehicles, placing chemical heat packs on IV bags, coiling IV tubing through basins of warm water, and heating IV bags in a microwave. Whichever method is chosen, fluid temperatures must never exceed 104° F.

CAUTION: *Remember, blood and blood products cannot and should not be microwaved.*

Types of Fluids

The choice of replacement fluid for resuscitation of shock depends on the type and severity of shock. Crystalloid solutions are usually the solutions of choice in mild shock and in the early resuscitation phases of trauma. There continues to be considerable controversy in selecting the correct fluid to resuscitate patients in moderate to severe shock. At this time, there is evidence to support the opinion that crystalloids and colloids probably have equal effects, if the amount administered yields the same hemodynamic end points.[10] The American College of Surgeons Committee on Trauma (ACSCOT) recommends the following fluid replacement schedule:[4]

15% to 30% blood loss—crystalloid solutions

>30% to 40% blood loss—crystalloid solutions and blood products

When administering crystalloids, remember that they should replace blood volume loss on a 3:1 ratio.

Crystalloids

Crystalloid solutions used to increase intravascular volume in shock contain electrolytes in isotonic or hypertonic concentrations. Crystalloids are readily available and relatively inexpensive options for volume replacement.

■ ISOTONIC SOLUTIONS

Isotonic solutions have a concentration that is similar to the normal concentration of extracellular fluid.

- 0.9% sodium chloride
- Lactated Ringer's injection
- Ringer's solution

CAUTION: Administration of large amounts of normal saline may cause hyperchloremia, hypernatremia, and acidosis.

CAUTION: Administration of large amounts of lactated Ringer's solution may elevate lactate level in patients who may be in lactic acidosis.

■ HYPERTONIC SOLUTIONS

Hypertonic solutions have a concentration greater than extracellular fluid. Administration of hypertonic solutions draws interstitial and intracellular fluid into the intravascular space.

- 3% sodium chloride
- 5% sodium chloride
- 7.5% sodium chloride

Hypertonic solutions are being used experimentally in prehospital care and in some institutions.

CAUTION: **May lead to hypernatremia and hyperosmolarity.**

NOTE: Consider administering hypertonic solutions via infusion pump.
The most frequently recommended crystalloid solutions are Ringer's lactate solution and 0.9% sodium chloride solution.

Colloids

Colloids are volume expanders that do not diffuse easily across normal capillary membranes and increase plasma oncotic pressure.

Blood/blood components

In major hypovolemic situations consider the administration of whole blood or packed cells. The amount of blood to request for type and cross-match depends on local protocol. In general, in instances of major trauma, blood should be typed and cross-matched for at least four units, with instructions to the blood bank to keep two units ahead of demand.

If a patient has received 3 to 4 L of crystalloid solution without improvement and/or stabilization of vital signs, the need for blood products becomes evident.

Fresh whole blood. This is the ideal solution; it contains red blood cells (and hemoglobin), plasma, and clotting factors. Potential complications associated with administration of fresh whole blood include volume overload, infusion of excess potassium and sodium, and infusion of anticoagulant.

Packed red blood cells. This is whole blood in which plasma has been extracted. Because plasma contains factors that may cause transfusion reactions and transmit infectious diseases, the risks of these are greatly reduced when using packed cells. In addition to reducing these risks, the amount of citrate, phosphate, free potassium, and debris is less than that contained in whole blood. Packed red blood cells improve the oxygen carrying capacity of the blood while preventing fluid overload.

Problems inherent with the administration of large amounts of packed cells involve bleeding disorders, as a result of platelets and clotting factors that are minimally functional. The patient must be observed very closely for abnormal bleeding.

O negative packed red blood cells. When blood is required immediately without time for type and cross-match for type-specific matching, O negative packed cells should be given. O negative type blood can be universally accepted. When large amounts of O negative blood have been administered, there may be a reaction later when type-specific or type and cross-matched blood is given.

Type-specific, uncross-matched red blood cells. Type-specific uncross-matched cells may be given, if one can wait 15 to 20 minutes for the processing of type-specific, uncross-matched blood. Type-specific blood is preferable to O negative blood.

Type-specific and cross-matched red blood cells. Processing of type-specific and cross-matched red cells may take 30 minutes to 1 hour. Type-specific and cross-matched red blood cells are the most preferable type because risk of transfusion reactions are lower. However, in the resuscitation phase of shock, one may not have the luxury of waiting an hour for type and cross-matched red blood cells.

Albumin

Human serum albumin (5%) is a volume expander derived from the plasma utilized to increase or maintain oncotic pressure. Human serum albumin does not contain blood group antibodies. The shelflife of albumin is 3 to 5 years.

CAUTION: Albumin and Plasmanate are not recommended for use in trauma resuscitation, as they may increase bleeding from raw, abraded surfaces, they infuse slowly, they may cause an error in the type and cross-match process for blood, and they are relatively expensive.

■ **STROMA-FREE HEMOGLOBIN**

This material is hemoglobin that has been extracted from current or outdated red blood cells. The advantages are that it has no incompatibility factors and a great affinity for oxygen. The disadvantages are its 2-hour to 4-hour half-life and the fact that its affinity for oxygen is so great that oxygen does not release easily. There are also indications that stroma-free hemoglobin causes increased coagulation problems. At the present time, stroma-free hemoglobin is under clinical investigation.

Plasma substitutes

Currently available plasma substitutes include hetastarch, low-molecular-weight dextran, and high-molecular-weight dextran. Advantages of plasma substitutes include the following: readily available, can be administered without delay associated with typing and cross-matching blood, and do not transmit hepatitis or HIV. Plasma substitutes do not contain plasma proteins, clotting factors, or improve oxygen transport.

■ **DEXTRAN**

Dextran is a polysaccharide prepared from sucrose. Low-molecular-weight (dextran 40) and high-molecular-weight (dextran 70) dextrans are volume expander alternatives that improve intravascular volume for approximately 24 hours.[10] When administered in large doses, dextran can alter coagulation and result in prolongation of bleeding times and impair platelet function.

■ **HETASTARCH**

Hetastarch is a synthetic compound with an indefinite shelf-life. Hetastarch has similar volume expansion characteristics as 5% albumin, but Hetastarch may last up to 36 hours, and is less expensive than 5% albumin.

■ **PERFLUOROCARBON (FLUOROCARBON)**

Perfluorocarbon is a synthetic product that is known to effectively load and unload oxygen. The question of long-term effects still remains. Perfluorocarbon is currently under investigation and not generally available for clinical use.

CAUTION: In many shock states the capillary membranes may allow diffusion of colloids from the intravascular space into the interstitium.[11]

Massive Transfusion Considerations

If a patient has received more than 50% of his or her blood volume over a 3-hour period, observe the patient for the following conditions.

Hypothermia

Unwarmed blood may lead to hypothermia. Hypothermic conditions shift the oxyhemoglobin curve to the left. Cold blood products have a higher viscosity and therefore a slower flow rate.

Hyperkalemia

When red blood cells hemolyze, potassium is released. As some red blood cell hemolysis is inevitable, one must carefully monitor the patient's serum electrolytes, especially potassium, and treat resulting findings appropriately. If hyperkalemia does occur, it is usually transient, and as the patient stabilizes, this condition usually corrects itself.

Hypocalcemia

Banked blood contains citrate. Citrate binds free calcium. If citrated whole blood is administered at greater than 100 ml/min, give 10 ml of a 10% solution of calcium chloride with each 10 U of whole blood.[4]

Acidosis

Banked blood has a pH of 7.1. Multiple transfusions of banked blood may lead to acidosis. Monitor arterial blood gases for acidosis and EKG for dysrhythmias that are induced by acidosis.

Alkalosis

Although initially acidosis is a concern, eventually the citrate contained in banked blood is converted to bicarbonate in the liver. Monitor the patient's arterial blood gases for alkalosis.

Clotting disorders

Loss of clotting factors in most banked blood results in prolonged coagulation times and coagulation disorders. One should carefully monitor the patient's prothrombin time, partial thromboplastin time, and watch for any excessive bleeding. Administer 1 U of fresh frozen plasma for 10 U of whole blood given.

Debris

Banked blood often contains debris. Although it is not known if this debris is harmful, it is recommended that a 160-mm micropore filter be used during massive transfusions.[4]

Autotransfusion

Autotransfusion is a procedure in which blood is collected, filtered, anticoagulated, and then reperfused into the same patient. Autotransfusion is most commonly used as a therapy for hypovolemic shock.

When there is a massive blood loss into the thoracic cavity and banked blood is not readily available, autotransfusion should be considered. In the emergency setting, autotransfusion should be used in patients who have suffered chest trauma with accompanying hypotension or in patients requiring an open thoracotomy where blood loss is expected to be 500 cc or more. Blood from sources other than the thorax are considered contaminated and should not be used.

Most autotransfusion systems (ATS) use a closed-chest drainage system designed with access to the collection chamber for retransfusion. Blood that has been drained into the collection chamber to be used for autotransfusion should be retransfused within 6 hours of initiating collection.[12]

The use of anticoagulant in autotransfusion continues to be controversial. It has been recommended that addition of anticoagulant may be more appropriate in patients with large volume blood loss than in patients whose blood loss is slow and gradual.[13]

Advantages

- Readily available
- No time delay for lab type and cross-match
- No risk of transfusion reaction
- Fresh whole blood, intact clotting factors, platelets, red blood cells
- No risk of communicable disease transmission

Disadvantages

- Increase in free plasma hemoglobin as a consequence of hemolysis
- Potential for coagulopathies
- Potential for air embolism
- Potential for microembolization of fat and/or microaggregates

Contraindications

- Blood greater than 4 hours old
- Large clots
- Known coagulopathy
- Enteric contamination
- Malignant neoplasms
- Pericardial, mediastinal, or systemic infections
- Poor liver or renal function

Consider obtaining the following baseline lab values prior to initiating autotransfusion:

Complete blood count (CBC)	Split products of fibrinogen
Hemoglobin	BUN and creatinine
Hematocrit	Serum potassium
PT and PTT	Serum calcium
Platelets	Arterial blood gases
Thrombin time	Urinalysis
Plasma fibrinogen	

Procedure: Collection using the Atrium Autotransfusion System (Figure 6-1)

1. Fill water seal to 2 cm.
2. Fill suction control chamber to ordered suction pressure.
3. Assure ATS access line is clamped.
4. Connect patient.
5. Apply regulated suction until gentle bubbling occurs.
6. Closely monitor blood volume outputs in collection chamber.
7. When 500 cc of blood volume has drained into the collection chamber, clamp the ATS blood bag clamp.
8. Remove spike port cap.
9. Insert ATS bag spike into ATS access line using a firm twisting motion.
10. Place bag below closed chest drainage system.
11. Open ATS access line and blood bag clamps.
12. Gently bend ATS bag upward where indicated to initiate blood transfer.
13. Once blood evacuation is complete, clamp ATS access line and blood bag clamps.
14. Disconnect blood bag from ATS access line.

Reinfusion

1. Prime a microemboli blood filter and IV blood tubing with 0.9% sodium chloride solution.
2. Spike ATS blood bag with primed microemboli filter and blood tubing.
3. Hang ATS blood bag.
4. Open filtered air vent on top of ATS blood bag.
5. Open IV clamp to complete priming and assure all air has been evacuated.
6. Attach to patient IV access.
7. Begin infusion.

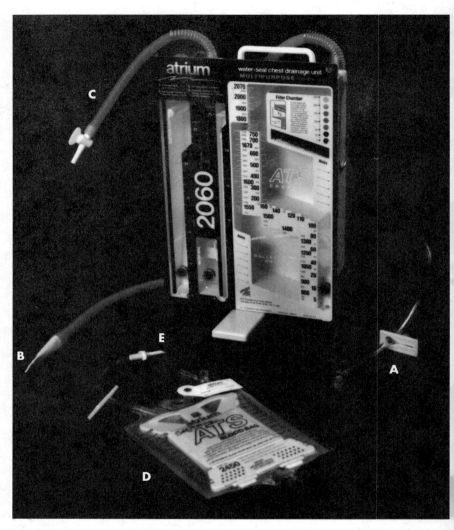

FIGURE 6-1. Atrium Autotransfusion System (ATS) (closed chest drainage). **A**, ATS access line. **B**, Patient tube connector. **C**, Suction line. **D**, ATS blood bag. **E**, ATS blood bag spike. (From Atrium Medical Corp., Hollis, New Hampshire.)

CAUTION: If using a pressure infusor, close the filtered air vent.

Maximum infusor pressure is 150 mm Hg.
Do not infuse entire blood volume in ATS blood bag through blood filter and IV tubing—air emboli can result.
Record chest drainage.
Record amount of autotransfused blood.
Document type and amount of anticoagulant used.
Observe the patient for:
    Excessive bleeding
    Hypothermia
    Air embolism
    Fat embolism

HEMODYNAMIC MONITORING

Successful management of shock, regardless of the classification, may be optimized by the use of hemodynamic monitoring. Hemodynamic status can be assessed through noninvasive methods (noninvasive BP, orthostatic vital signs, urine output, and evaluation of mental status) or with the use of invasive methods (pulmonary artery catheters and arterial pressure monitoring).

Invasive hemodynamic monitoring provides continuous physiologic data about the cardiovascular system. The information provided by this technology is a valuable adjunct to other assessment data.

Controversies currently exist surrounding the use of invasive hemodynamic monitoring.

Evidence suggests that data alone obtained from invasive hemodynamic monitoring cannot predict outcome and/or improve survival. Intelligent use of the data can guide the practitioner toward successful use of volume and pharmacological agents for patients in shock.[14]

Types of Monitoring

Noninvasive monitoring

- Blood pressure
- Postural vital signs
■ **POSTURAL VITAL SIGNS**
Postural vital signs should be assessed in all patients with (1) evidence of significant fluid loss through bleeding, vomiting, diarrhea, perspiration, or wound drainage; (2) unexplained tachycardia; (3) hypotension without tachycardia; (4) history or suspicion of chronic or concealed bleeding; or (5) blunt abdominal or chest trauma.

Contraindications Postural vital signs are not indicated if other injuries or the patient's general condition preclude safe administration of the test.

Rationale for the test When a patient assumes a vertical position, gravity tends to cause sequestration (pooling) of blood in the capacitance vessels of the legs and trunk. Normally, individuals adapt readily to this postural change through rapid vasoconstriction of the vessels in which the blood tends to pool. This adjustment is not possible for the volume-depleted patient whose vasoconstrictor potential has already been maximally used.

Interpreting results Postural changes (from lying to sitting or standing) that result in a *decrease* of 20 mm Hg or more in the systolic or diastolic blood pressure or an *increase* of 20 beats or more per minute in the pulse rate is a *positive* test result. The patient should be considered *hypovolemic* until proved otherwise.

CAUTION! The patient may experience weakness, dizziness, visual disturbances, or fainting during the test. These symptoms are promptly eliminated in most instances when the patient lies down again. Be certain to protect the patient during the assessment of postural vital signs to prevent injuries.

Procedure

1. With the patient supine, take and record the blood pressure and pulse as a baseline against which changes of both measures taken after position changes can be evaluated.
2. Have the patient sit up to a 90-degree position, and again record the blood pressure and pulse.
3. Have the patient stand, if possible, and again record the blood pressure and pulse. If significant changes occur, or if the patient's symptoms become acute during the sitting portion of the test, eliminate the third step and consider the results of the sitting portion positive.

Correct charting of the results is done in the following manner (Figure 6-2):

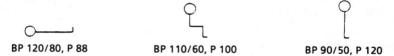

BP 120/80, P 88   BP 110/60, P 100   BP 90/50, P 120

FIGURE 6-2. Charting postural vital signs.
(From Bookman LB, Simoneau JK: *JEN* 3:43, 1977.)

Invasive Monitoring

- Arterial pressure
- Central venous pressure (CVP)
- Pulmonary artery pressure (systolic [PAS] and diastolic [PAD])
- Pulmonary artery occlusive pressure ("wedge pressure" PaOP)
- Cardiac output/index (C0/C1)
- Systemic vascular resistance (SVR)

Definitions

The following terms are commonly used while caring for the patient requiring hemodynamic monitoring:

preload The volume of blood filling the ventricles during diastole. Central venous pressure (CVP) reflects right ventricular (RV) preload. Pulmonary artery diastolic (PAD) and pulmonary artery occlusive/wedge (PaOP) reflect left ventricular preload.[15]

afterload The resistance the ventricles must work against during systole to eject its volume. Pulmonary vascular resistance (PVR) reflects RV afterload. Systemic vascular resistance (SVR) reflects left ventricular (LV) afterload.

contractility The force with which the heart muscle contracts.

Arterial pressure monitoring

Invasive arterial pressure monitoring provides direct measurement of arterial systolic and diastolic blood pressure. In addition, the presence of an arterial catheter allows for blood sampling for determination of arterial blood gas values and other laboratory studies.

Arterial pressure monitoring is achieved through cannulation of an artery either percutaneously or via surgical cutdown. The arterial vessels most commonly used are the radial and femoral arteries. The brachial artery may be used for short-term monitoring. The artery is cannulated using sterile technique and the cannula is attached to a pressurized system that provides a continuous infusion (3 cc/hr) of heparinized saline to maintain patency of the system.

Patient preparation

Before insertion of the arterial catheter, an Allen's test should be performed. An Allen's test assesses the ability of the ulnar artery to maintain perfusion if the radial artery is cannulated (Figure 6-3).

Equipment needed:

Sterile drapes	Pressure bag
Sterile gloves	Transducer holder
Betadine solution/ointment	Benzoin
1% lidocaine for infiltration	Tape
TB or 3-cc syringe	Bandages
20 gauge 1½ inch Intracath	2 × 2s
Heparinized saline (1000 U/500 cc N/S)	
Pressure tubing/transducer	
Monitor with pressure measurement capability	

Interpreting Results

■ WAVEFORM ANALYSIS

The arterial pressure consists of two phases: systole and diastole. Arterial systole signifies opening of the aortic valve with subsequent rapid ejection of blood into the aorta. Following this ejection, there is runoff of blood from the proximal aorta to the peripheral arteries. On the arterial waveform (Figure 6-4), this event is displayed as a sharp rise in pressure followed by a fall in pressure. As the pressure decreases, the aortic valve quickly closes, resulting in a small elevation in arterial pressure on the downslope. This is termed the **dicrotic notch**.

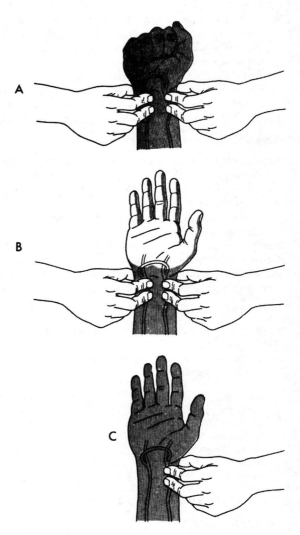

FIGURE 6-3. Assessing for Allen's Signs. **A**, Occlude both arteries with firm pressure. **B**, Raise arm to blanch hand. **C**, Release ulnar artery for return of color to hand.
(From Sheehy SB: *Emergency nursing: principles and practice,* ed 3. St Louis, 1985, Mosby.)

Diastole occurs following closure of the aortic valve and continues until the next systole.[16]

Mean arterial pressure (MAP) is the average arterial pressure during systole and diastole. MAP is influenced by cardiac output or the volume of blood in the arterial system and the elasticity or resistance of the arteries (SVR).[17]

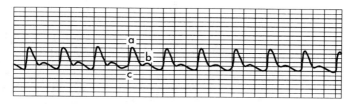

FIGURE 6-4. Arterial waveform. **A**, Systole. **B**, Dicrotic notch. **C**, Diastole.

The formula for calculating MAP is:

$$Pd + \frac{Ps - Pd}{3}$$

where
  Pd = diastolic pressure
  Ps = systolic pressure.

Normal values

Systolic pressure (SBP) = 110 to 120 mm Hg
Diastolic pressure (DBP) = 70 to 80 mm Hg
Mean arterial pressure (MAP) = 70 to 105 mm Hg[18]

Potential complications

An invasive monitoring device has potential complications inherent in its use.
Complications seen with invasive arterial monitoring may include:
  • Thrombosis/emboli
  • Infection/sepsis
  • Neurovascular compromise/distal ischemia
  • Bleeding
  • Coagulopathy (secondary to heparin)

■ **THERAPEUTIC INTERVENTIONS**
  • Frequent neurovascular assessments of extremity
  • Meticulous site care
  • Immobilization of extremity
  • Frequent assessment for site bleeding/oozing

Central Venous Pressure Monitoring

Central venous pressure (CVP) monitoring provides information about:
  • Pressure in the great veins
  • Blood volume
  • Right ventricular function
  • Central venous return[19]
Catheter placement for pressure measurement can be performed percutaneously
or via surgical cutdown. Veins commonly used for cannulation include internal

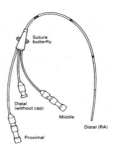

FIGURE 6-5. Central venous catheter.
(From Abbott Laboratories, Mountain View, Cal.)

and external jugular and subclavian veins and, less frequently, the antecubital veins.

Central venous catheters are manufactured with single, double, or triple lumens. CVP can also be measured via a pulmonary artery catheter. (See Figure 6-5.)

The decision to place a single-lumen or multilumen central line is determined by the actual or anticipated venous access needs of the patient. Considerations to help make the decision include:

- Need for CVP monitoring
- Need for frequent blood sampling
- Amount and frequency of medication administration
- Need for blood/blood product administration
- Need for maintenance fluid
- Patient's current vascular access

Recommendations exist regarding the use of the various ports of multilumen catheters:

The distal port (16-gauge/brown*) should be used for pressure monitoring, administration of blood products, and general access, since it is within close proximity to the right atrium.

The middle port (18-gauge/blue*) may be used for general access.

The proximal port (18-gauge/white*) is recommended for blood sampling and general access.

All ports of these catheters should be flushed with 2.5 mg of heparin (100 U/ml) following intermittent use.[14]

CVP can be measured using pressurized systems and a transducer (*see* Arterial Pressure Monitoring) or a water manometer.

Central pressures obtained from pressurized systems are measured in mm Hg. Those values obtained from a water manometer are measured in cm H_2O.

Normal values:

2 to 6 mm Hg

2 to 8 cm H_2O

*Color and gauge may vary with manufacturer.

To convert mm Hg to cm H_2O, multiply mm Hg $\times$ 1.36.[17] All central venous pressure measurements are mean pressures.

Patient preparation and equipment: *See* Pulmonary Artery Pressure Monitoring.

Interpreting results: Central venous pressure waveform analysis

The CVP waveform consists of three positive waves: **a**, **c**, and **v** followed by **x**, **x₁**, and **y** descent or negative waves. The **a** wave signifies atrial systole and is immediately followed by the **x** descent, which reflects atrial relaxation. The **c** wave signifies closure of the tricuspid value and may have a distinct appearance, may appear as a notch on the **a** wave, or may be absent. The **v** wave signifies right atrial filling, which occurs concomitantly during right ventricular (RV) systole. During RV systole, the closed leaflets of the tricuspid valve bulge into the right atrium. The **y** descent following the **v** wave represents opening of the tricuspid valve and RV filling (Figure 6-6).[16]

Central veins are influenced by the intrathoracic pressure changes that occur during the respiratory cycle. During spontaneous respiration (inspiration), negative pressure within the intrathoracic space causes the CVP to drop. Pressures rise during spontaneous expiration. The opposite phenomenon occurs with mechanically delivered breaths.

The pressure that is delivered with mechanically controlled breaths results in positive pressure within the intrathoracic space during both the inspiratory and expiratory phases of controlled ventilation.[20] During inspiration and to a lesser degree during expiration, the CVP will rise.

To minimize the influence that these changing pressures have on the waveform, CVP should be measured at end expiration, whether the patient is breathing spontaneously or with mechanical ventilation.[16] Intrathoracic pressures at end expiration are relatively constant and allow for a more stable pressure waveform (Figures 6-7 and 6-8).[21]

Potential complications

- Pneumothorax (related to insertion)
- Hemothorax (related to insertion)

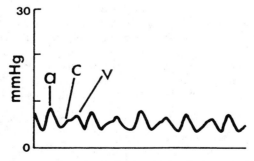

FIGURE 6-6. Central venous pressure waveform with identified **a**, **c**, and **v** waves.
(From Abbott Laboratories, Mountain View, Cal.)

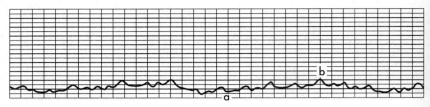

FIGURE 6-7. Central venous pressure waveform during spontaneous respirations. **A**, Inspiration, **B**, End expiration.

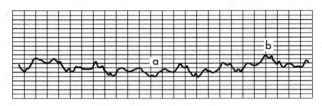

FIGURE 6-8. Central venous pressure waveform during mechanical ventilation. **A**, Inspiration. **B**, End expiration.

- Vessel thrombosis/occlusion
- Bleeding
- Infection/sepsis
- Air embolus
- Neurovascular compromise (at an antecubital site)

■ **THERAPEUTIC INTERVENTIONS**

Frequent neurovascular assessment of extremity (if indicated)
Meticulous site care
Maintenance of a closed system

Pulmonary Artery Pressure Monitoring

Pulmonary artery (PA) pressure monitoring provides direct measurement of pressure within the pulmonary artery. Monitoring is achieved through percutaneous cannulation of a central vein. Central veins commonly used include internal and external jugular and subclavian veins. Femoral and antecubital veins may be used if necessary. Use of a PA catheter allows for direct monitoring of PA pressures (systolic, diastolic, and mean) and central venous pressure and indirect measurement of left ventricular function (PA occlusive/wedge pressure [PaOP]) (Figure 6-9). Other hemodynamic values that may be obtained using the PA catheter include:

- Cardiac output/index
- Systemic vascular resistance
- SvO_2 (mixed venous oxygen saturation)*

*Using a fiberoptic pulmonary catheter.

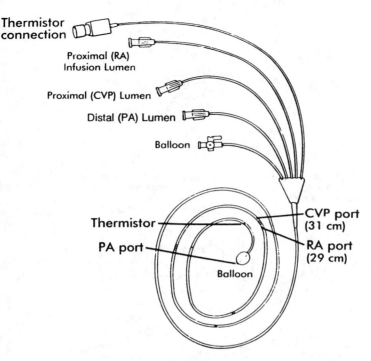

Thermistor connection

Proximal (RA) Infusion Lumen

Proximal (CVP) Lumen

Distal (PA) Lumen

Balloon

Thermistor

PA port

CVP port (31 cm)

RA port (29 cm)

Balloon

FIGURE 6-9. Pulmonary artery thermodilution catheter.

Patient preparation

The patient is prepared for any central vein catheterization using aseptic technique. The patient is placed in the Trendelenburg position to allow for venous distension. The skin is prepped with povidone/iodone solution, and the area is draped with sterile towels. The site is infiltrated with 1% lidocaine before cannulation to provide local anesthesia. A percutaneous sheath introducer is inserted first; this allows for immediate vascular access via the side port. Before the PA catheter insertion, the nurse connects and primes all ports of the catheter with a heparinized flush solution. If a fiberoptic catheter is used, the nurse should perform a preinsertion calibration via the oximetric computer/monitor. The PA catheter is advanced into position via the diaphragm of the introducer. It is advanced into the right atrium (RA), right ventricle (RV), and then the PA (Figure 6-10). Continuous cardiac monitoring is required during and after the procedure. During placement of the PA catheter, the role of the nurse may include:

- Observing for cardiac dysrhythmias (PVCs, V-tach)
- Administering lidocaine IVP if indicated (1 mg/kg)
- Observing waveforms and recording pressures (RA, RV, PA systolic and diastolic, PaOP)
- Inflating and deflating the catheter balloon according to physician direction

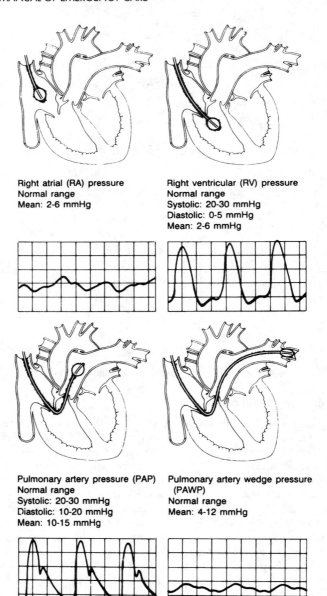

Right atrial (RA) pressure
Normal range
Mean: 2-6 mmHg

Right ventricular (RV) pressure
Normal range
Systolic: 20-30 mmHg
Diastolic: 0-5 mmHg
Mean: 2-6 mmHg

Pulmonary artery pressure (PAP)
Normal range
Systolic: 20-30 mmHg
Diastolic: 10-20 mmHg
Mean: 10-15 mmHg

Pulmonary artery wedge pressure
 (PAWP)
Normal range
Mean: 4-12 mmHg

FIGURE 6-10. Flow directed balloon-tipped catheter as it passes through the right side of the heart, wedging in a distal pulmonary artery with corresponding pressure waveforms and normal values.

(From Alspach JG: *AACN core curriculum for critical care nursing,* ed 4. Philadelphia, 1991, Saunders.

After the catheter is successfully inserted, a portable chest x-ray is taken to confirm catheter placement and to check for pneumothorax.

PaOP measurements should not be performed by nursing staff until chest x-ray film confirmation and physician approval are obtained. Pulmonary infarction may occur if the catheter tip is too far advanced into the pulmonary vasculature.

Equipment needed

Sterile drapes	Percutaneous sheath
Sterile gloves	Introducer kit (8.5 FR)*
Povidone/iodone solution/ointment	Pulmonary artery catheter (#7 French)*
1% lidocaine for infiltration	Monitor/computer for SvO_2†
3 cc syringe	Lidocaine (100 mg Bristojet)
Heparinized saline solution (1000 U/500 cc	Pressure bag
normal saline)	Transducer holder
Pressure tubing/transducers	Benzoin
Pressure monitor	Tape
Cardiac output computer*	2 × 2s

Interpreting results

■ PULMONARY ARTERY WAVEFORM ANALYSIS

PA pressure consists of two phases: systole and diastole. Systole signifies opening of the pulmonic valve with subsequent rapid ejection of blood into the PA. On the PA waveform, this event is displayed as a sharp rise in pressure followed by a fall in pressure as the volume decreases. When pressures within the right ventricle become less than pressures within the PA, the pulmonic valve abruptly closes. This abrupt closure of the pulmonic valve produces a small notch on the downslope called the **dicrotic notch**. Diastole follows closure of the pulmonic valve. During diastole, the pulmonary system receives runoff blood flow. Further blood flow from the right ventricle does not occur until the next systole. Provided that there is no pulmonary or mitral valve disease, the PA diastolic value (end-diastolic pressure) corresponds closely to the left ventricular end-diastolic pressure (LVEDP).[15]

> *Normal PA systolic pressure (same as RV systolic):*   20 to 30 mm Hg
> *Normal PA end-diastolic pressure:*   8 to 12 mm Hg

See Figure 6-11. *See* Interpreting Results, Central Venous Pressure Monitoring.

■ PULMONARY ARTERY OCCLUSIVE/WEDGE PRESSURE WAVEFORM ANALYSIS

PaOP is obtained following balloon inflation of the PA catheter. When the PA catheter is positioned in a small branch of the pulmonary artery and balloon inflation takes place, the flow of blood to that segment of the vessel is occluded. PaOP reflects left atrial pressure and has a similar appearance to right atrial pressure (presence of **a**, **c**, and **v** waves). The **a** wave represents left atrial sys-

---

*Not required for CVP catheter placement.
†Only if fiberoptic PA catheter is used.

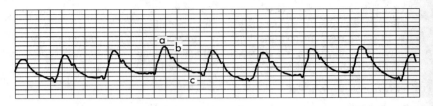

FIGURE 6-11. Pulmonary artery waveform. **A**, Systole, **B**, Dicrotic notch, **C**, Diastolic.

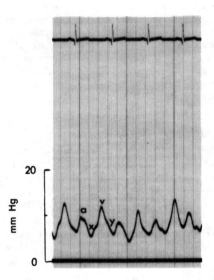

FIGURE 6-12. Normal pulmonary artery wedge (PAW) pressure waveform showing *a* and *v* waves and *x* and *y* descents. The mean of this PAW pressure is about 8 mm Hg.
(From Daily EK, Schroeder JS: *Techniques in bedside hemodynamic monitoring,* ed 4. St Louis, 1989, Mosby.)

tole, the **c** wave, often difficult to observe, signifies closure of the mitral valve, and the **v** wave represents filling of the left atrium.[16]

Similar to a CVP reading, a PaOP pressure is recorded as a mean value (Figure 6-12).

Normal PaOP = 4 to 12 mm Hg[16]

Potential complications

Potential complications seen with pulmonary artery pressure monitoring include:
- Thrombosis/emboli
- Infection/sepsis
- Bleeding
- Coagulopathy (secondary to heparin)

- Pneumothorax
- Hemothorax
- Pulmonary infarction
- Air embolus
- Ventricular dysrhythmias
- Ventricular perforation
- Distal neurovascular compromise*

■ **THERAPEUTIC INTERVENTIONS**
- Meticulous site care
- Maintenance of a closed system
- Performing wedge pressures only when indicated
- Ongoing assessment of PA waveform
- Continuous cardiac monitoring
- Assuring that balloon is deflated after each wedge pressure is obtained
- Routine documentation of catheter position (in cm)

Cardiac Output Determination

Cardiac output (CO) is the amount of blood ejected from the left ventricle per minute. CO is a product of stroke volume and heart rate. Stroke volume (SV) equals the amount of blood ejected by the left ventricle with each contraction.

$$CO = SV \times HR$$

where HR = heart rate.[17]

Using the PA catheter, cardiac output is measured via the thermodilution method. The thermodilution method is based on the theory of temperature change as an indicator of circulating blood volume. The thermistor port of the PA catheter, when attached to a cardiac output computer, provides an accurate measurement of blood temperature (core temp).

The nurse quickly injects a predetermined amount of room temperature† D_5W (5 or 10 ml) through the proximal lumen of the PA catheter. This procedure is repeated three times. An average of the three values is obtained provided they are within an acceptable range of each other. Studies have shown an expected variance of 4% to 10% to occur between sequential measurements.[21]

The thermistor senses the temperature of the blood in the PA: the cardiac output computer calculates the cardiac output in liters per minute:

$$Normal\ CO = 4\ to\ 8\ L/min^{[15]}$$

Cardiac index (CI) or the corrected CO according to body size and based on body surface area (BSA) is determined by:

$$CI = CO/BSA$$
$$Normal\ CI = 2.5\ to\ 4.0\ L/min^{[17]}$$

---

*Seen with femoral or peripheral sites.
†Iced injectate may be indicated in the hypothermic patient to allow for an adequate temperature difference.

Physiologic changes that may influence CO/CI include:
- Any changes in heart rate (affects diastolic filling time)
- Changes in preload (increased preload, increased CO; decreased preload, decreased CO)
- Extreme changes in afterload (decrease in CO)
- Venous constriction (increase in CO)
- Venous dilation (decrease in CO)
- Hypothermia (decreases in CO)

Systemic Vascular Resistance

Systemic vascular resistance represents the average resistance to blood flow within all vascular beds of the systemic circulation. SVR is a calculated value rather than a direct value. Pressure differences from either end of the circulatory system and measurements of blood flow determine SVR.[19]

$$SVR = \frac{MAP - CVP}{CO} \times 80$$

Normal values $= 770$ to 1500 dyne sec/cm

Any change in MAP, CVP, or CO will influence SVR.
Conditions resulting in a decreased SVR:
- Neurogenic shock
- Hyperthermia
- Cardiogenic shock (uncompensated)
- Hypovolemia (uncompensated)

Conditions resulting in an elevated SVR:
- Hypothermia
- Hypovolemia (compensated)
- Low cardiac output (compensated)

Accuracy of Data

To assure accuracy and reliability of the data obtained from any pressurized hemodynamic monitoring system, the following steps should take place prior to data collection:

1. Zero-calibrate the system to atmospheric air.
2. Level transducer to phlebostatic axis or midchest (Figures 6-13 and 6-14).
3. Check all connections for tightness and proper alignment.
4. Check catheter for proper position.
5. Check extremity for proper position and alignment.
6. Determine dynamic response by performing a square wave test (Figure 6-15).

The dynamic response represents a function of the entire monitoring system, which includes any component of the fluid path between the transducer and the catheter tip. This response measures the ability of the fluid-filled system to accurately reproduce pressure changes that occur in the cardiovascular system (waveforms). A good dynamic response reflects:

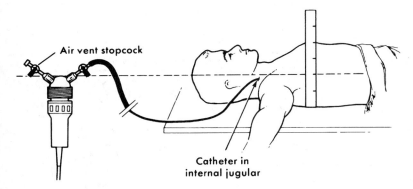

FIGURE 6-13. The patient's midchest position is measured, marked, and used as an anatomic reference point for placement of the transducer.
(From Daily EK, Schroeder JS: *Techniques in bedside hemodynamic monitoring,* ed 4. St Louis, 1989, Mosby.)

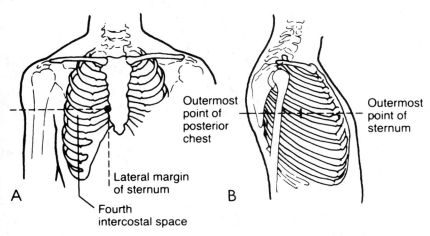

FIGURE 6-14. The phlebostatic axis. The crossing of two imaginary lines defines the assumed position of the monitoring catheter tip within the body, i.e., right atrial levels. **A,** A line that passes from the fourth intercostal space at the lateral margin of the sternum down the side of the body beneath the axilla. **B,** A line that runs horizontally at a part midway between the outermost position of the anterior and posterior surfaces of the chest.
(From Darovic G: *Hemodynamic monitoring, invasive and noninvasive clinical application.* Philadelphia, 1987, Saunders.)

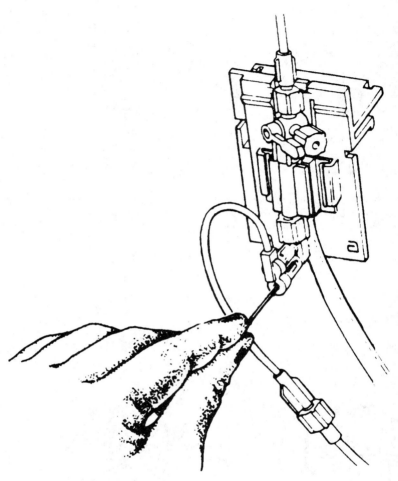

FIGURE 6-15. Method for performing a square wave test
(From Abbott Laboratories, Mountain View, Cal.)

- Accurate representation by the transducer due to a high natural frequency of the monitoring system
- The pressures within the patient's blood vessels
- Pressures within the heart chambers[22]

The square wave test determines the dynamic response of a hemodynamic system. This test is performed by activating the fast flush mechanism. The portion of the wave that is square is produced by the fast flush. Closure of the fast flush system produces the wave or oscillation after the square wave[22] (Figure 6-16).

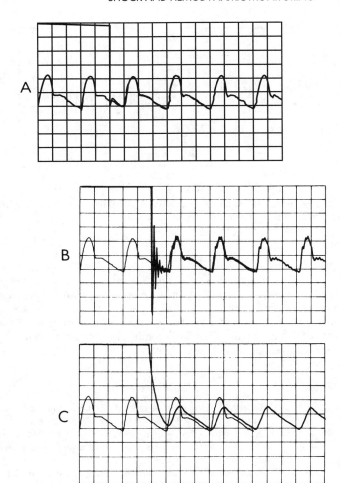

FIGURE 6-16. Assessing dynamic response. **A,** Optimally damped. The fast flush trace ends with small undershoot followed by an even smaller overshoot. **B,** Acceptable. The fast flush trace ending in rapid oscillations that subside prior to the next patient waveform indicates a high natural frequency system. Patient waveform distortion will be minimal despite underdamping. **C,** Overdamped. The fast flush trace slowly returns toward the next patient waveform without any sign of oscillation.

Continued.

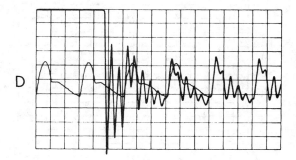

D

FIGURE 6-16, cont'd. D, Highly underdamped. The fast flush trace ends in a series of oscillations that persist into the next patient waveform.
(From Abbott Laboratories, Mountain View, Cal.)

The clinical presentation of shock can occur for a variety of reasons. The common thread in all shock states is a reduction in tissue perfusion with a resultant imbalance of cellular oxygen supply and demand. Measures to optimize CO and improve tissue perfusion remain the hallmarks of treatment. Prompt diagnosis and treatment remain essential contributing factors in reducing the overall morbidity and mortality in shock states.

REFERENCES

1. Herckes R, Bihari DJ: Management of shock. In Tinker J, Zapol W, eds: *Care of the critically ill patient.* New York, 1992, Springer-Verlag, pp 259-84.
2. Mouchawar A, Rosenthal M: A pathophysiological approach to the patient in shock. In Rosenthal M, ed: *Recent advances in critical care medicine: international anesthesiology clinics.* Boston, 1993, Little, Brown, pp 1-20.
3. Rice V: Shock a clinical syndrome: an update. Part 2, The stages of shock, *Crit Care Nurs* 11(5):74, 1991.
4. American College of Duraglan's Committee on Trauma; *Advanced trauma life support instructor manual.* Chicago, 1993, the Committee.
5. Sheehy SB, Barber JM: *Emergency nursing,* ed 3. St. Louis, 1992, Mosby.
6. Summers G: The clinical and hemodynamic presentation of the shock patient, *Crit Care Nurs Clin North Am* 2(2):161, 1990.
7. Houston M: Pathophysiology of shock, *Crit Care Nurs Clin North Am* 2(2):143, 1990.
8. Franaszek JB: Cardiogenic shock. In Rosen P et al, eds: *Emergency: emergency medicine,* ed 2. St Louis, 1988, Mosby.
9. Boyd J, Stanford G, Chernow B: The pathophysiology of shock. In Tinker J, Zapol W, eds: *Care of the critically ill patient.* New York, 1992, Springer-Verlag, pp 243-57.
10. Trunkey DD, Salber PR, Mills J: Shock. In Saunders CE, Ho MT, eds: *Current emergency diagnosis and treatment.* Norwalk, Conn, 1992, Appleton and Lange, pp 51-67.
11. Kuhn MM: Colloids versus crystalloids, *Critical Care Nurse* 11(5):37, 1991.

12. American Association of Blood Banks: *Standards for blood banks and transfusion services manual,* ed 14. Bethesda, Md, 1991, the Association.

13. Blansfield J: Emergency autotransfusion in hypovolemia, *Crit Care Nurs Clin North Am* 2(2):195, 1990.

14. Holder C, Alexander J: A new and improved guide to IV therapy, *AJN* 43, 1990.

15. Palmer D: Advanced hemodynamic assessment, *Dimens Crit Care Nurs* 1(3):139, 1982.

16. Daily E, Schroeder T: *Techniques in bedside hemodynamic monitoring,* ed 4. St Louis, 1989, Mosby.

17. Alspach J, ed: *American Association of Critical Care Nurses, core curriculum for critical care nursing,* ed 4. Philadelphia, 1991, Saunders.

18. Swearingen PL: *Manual of critical care: applying nursing diagnoses to adult critical illness.* St Louis, 1988, Mosby.

19. Darovic G: *Hemodynamic monitoring: invasive and noninvasive clinical application.* Philadelphia, 1987, Saunders.

20. Thielen J: Air Emboli: a potentially lethal complication of central venous lines, *Focus* 17(5):374, 1990.

21. Quaal S: Hemodynamic monitoring: a review of the literature, *Appl Nurs Res* 1(2):58, 1988.

22. Abbott Critical Care Systems: *Hemodynamic monitoring learning program.* Chicago, 1989, Abbott Laboratories, Hospital Product Division.

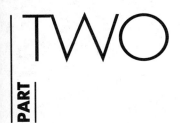

PART TWO

Medical Emergencies

Cardiac Emergencies

Chest pain can be the chief patient complaint in a variety of different but serious cardiac emergencies. Anytime the heart is in jeopardy the caregiver must ascertain the problem and begin treating it without the luxury of lengthy assessments or in-depth history taking. This chapter presents the essential elements of cardiac assessment in the emergency setting. It then outlines, by point of origination, various cardiac conditions that can produce chest pain and the corresponding emergency treatments. Common noncardiac conditions that produce chest pain are also listed. Finally, congestive heart failure, a common cardiac emergency, is discussed. This chapter is not designed to be a definitive course in cardiac care, but rather provides rapid detection methods and initial treatment options for suspected cardiac problems.

ASSESSMENT OF CHEST PAIN

Determine vital signs, skin vital signs (color, temperature, and moistness), pulse oximetry or arterial blood gas (ABG).

Examine a rhythm strip (lead II or MCL) for the presence of dysrhythmias.

Further examine the chief complaint and obtain a brief history.

Use the PQRST mnemonic to assist in gathering facts about the pain.

P = Provokes

What provokes the pain? What makes it better? What makes it worse?

Q = Quality

What does it feel like? Is it sharp? Dull? Burning? Stabbing? Crushing? (Try to let the patient describe it before offering choices.)

R = Radiates

Where does the pain radiate? Is it in one place? Does it go to any other place?

S = Severity

How severe is the pain? On a scale of 1 to 10, with 1 being the least pain and 10 being the worst, what rating would you give the pain? (Watch for nonverbal clues with this question. A patient may be writhing in pain and tell you the pain is a 2, or a patient may sit there very calmly and quietly and tell you the pain is a 10.)

T = Time

When did it start? How long did it last?
Other useful data to collect
   Find out if the patient has a history (or a family history) of heart disease, lung disease, stroke, or hypertension.
   Ask if the patient is taking any medications. (Use words such as "heart pills" or "water pills" if necessary.)
   Ask if it hurts to take a deep breath.
   Find out what the patient was doing when the pain began.
   Ask if the patient has ever had this pain before.
   Ask if it is different this time.
   Check the patient for level of consciousness.
   Check the patient's pupils for equality, reaction to light, and accommodation. (Remember that 10% of the population has unequal pupils.)
   Examine the neck veins for distension.
   Check the trachea to see that it is in a midline position.
   Inquire as to a recent history of trauma.
In these early phases of myocardial infarction, it is essential to pay particular attention to the relief of pain and the prevention of dysrhythmias.

ELECTROCARDIOGRAPH MONITORING

Monitoring on a four-lead monitoring system (with an automatic lead switch button) is shown in Figure 7-1, *A, B, C.*

When monitoring on a three-lead ECG monitor (without an automatic lead switch button), the best lead placement to use is Lead II or MCL_1. Leads II and MCL_1 are the best leads to monitor for dysrhythmias.

Standard 12-Lead Electrocardiograph

The standard 12-lead ECG (Figures 7-2 and 7-3) takes 12 views of the heart's electrical activity and records it on a wax-coated, standardized ECG paper.
   Before beginning:
   1. Check to be sure that all leads are placed correctly.
      a. "Green and white on the right, Christmas trees (red and green) below the knees" is a helpful memory aid.
      b. Ensure that there is a conduction medium between the electrodes and the patient.
      c. Avoid placing the electrodes over large muscle masses.

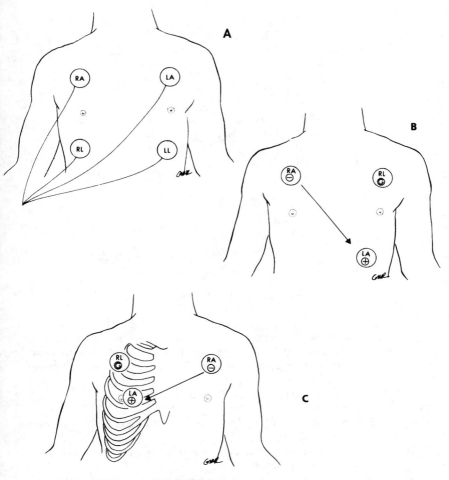

FIGURE 7-1. Lead placement for four-lead monitoring system (with automatic lead switch button), **A,** Monitoring on three-lead system (without automatic lead switch button). **B,** Lead II. **C,** Lead MCL$_1$.

2. Ensure that lead wires are not touching anything metal (this will cause 60-cycle interference).
3. Explain to the patient what you are doing.

When beginning:

1. Standardize the machine at the beginning of each lead.
2. Record at least four complexes in each lead.
3. If 60-cycle interference occurs, check for the following:
   a. Loose leads
   b. Leads and wires against metal
   c. Other electrical machines that could be unplugged

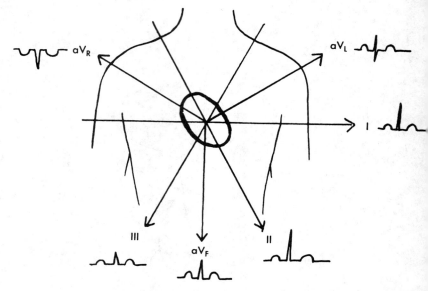

FIGURE 7-2. The six limb leads.

4. If the patient will be transferred to a coronary care or intensive care unit where an ECG will be done each day, mark their chest where the chest leads are placed to ensure that the leads will have the same placement each time the ECG is recorded.

5. Attempt to maintain the patient's modesty.

At the conclusion:

1. End the ECG with at least 15 seconds of lead II recording (used for dysrhythmia detection).

2. Record the patient's name, the date, and the time the ECG was taken directly on the ECG strip.

3. Interpret the strip or relay it to the appropriate individual for interpretation.

Interpretation

When current flows toward a lead (arrowheads, positive electrode), an upward ECG deflection occurs. When current flows away from a lead (arrowhead, positive electrode), a downward deflection of the ECG occurs. When current flows perpendicular to a lead (arrowhead, positive electrode), diphasic deflection of the ECG occurs.

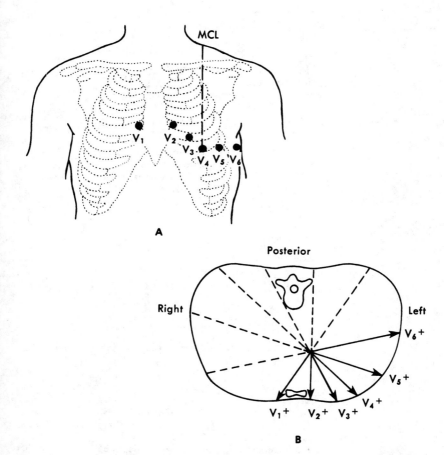

FIGURE 7-3. Electrode positions of the precordial leads. **A,** V_1, fourth intercostal space at right sternal border; V_2, fourth intercostal space at left sternal border; V_3, halfway between V_2 and V_4; V_4, fifth intercostal space at midclavicular line; V_5, anterior axillary line directly lateral to V_4; V_6, midaxillary line directly lateral to V_5. **B,** Precordial reference figure. Leads V_1 and V_2 are called right-sided precordial leads; leads V_3 and V_4, midprecordial leads; and leads V_5 and V_6, left-sided precordial leads.

(Adapted from Andreoli K et al: *Comprehensive cardiac care: a text for nurses, physicians, and other health practitioners*, ed 6. St Louis, 1987, Mosby.)

When examining a 12-lead ECG, examine each of the 12 leads individually and note any of the following:

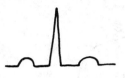

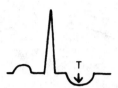

Normal

Ischemia
Decreased blood supply
T wave inversion
May indicate ischemia
without myocardial infarction

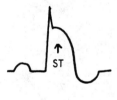

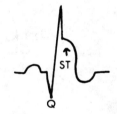

Injury
Acute or
recent; the
more elevated
the ST segment,
the more recent
the injury

Infarct
Significant Q wave
greater than 1 mm
wide and half the
height + depth of
the entire complex
Indicates myocardial
necrosis

The leads directly recording the area of infarct will demonstrate changes. An anterior wall myocardial infarction appears in leads V_1, V_2, and V_3.

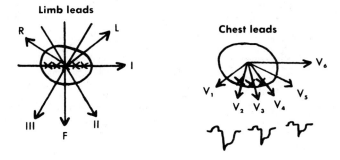

An inferior wall myocardial infarction appears in leads II, III, and V_F.

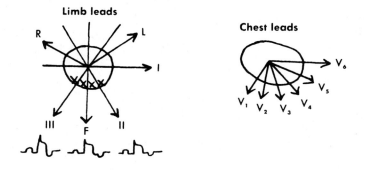

A lateral wall myocardial appears in leads I, aV_L, V_5, and V_6.

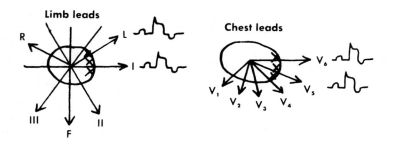

A posterior wall myocardial infarction appears in leads V_1 and V_2. The first r wave is tall, there is a depressed ST segment, and there is an elevated t wave.

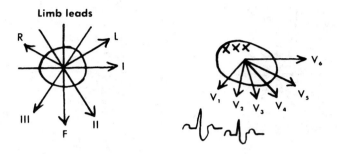

Plotting a simple axis

An axis is a graphic representation of the main vector in the heart.

■ **EQUIPMENT**
12-lead ECG
Graph paper
Ruler
Writing instrument

■ **PROCEDURE**
1. Draw leads I and aV_F lines on graph paper.

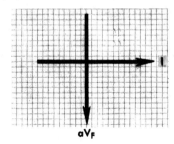

2. Examine lead I of the ECG.
   a. Determine if it is positive or negative.
   b. Determine by how much.

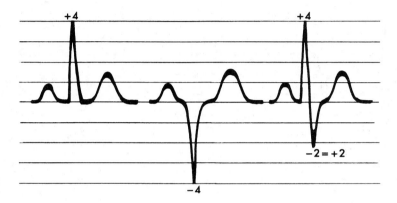

3. Plot the positive inflection or negative deflection on the graph paper by drawing a perpendicular line.
   a. Positive goes *toward* the lead.
   b. Negative goes *away from* the lead.

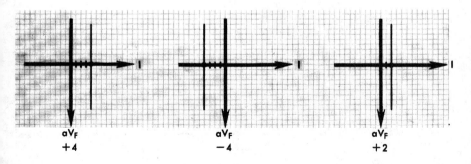

4. Examine lead aV$_F$ of the ECG.
   a. Determine if it is positive or negative.
   b. Determine by how much.

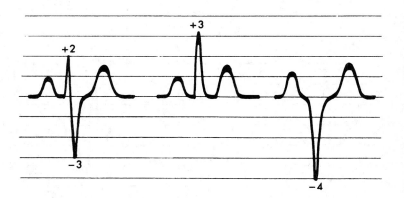

5. Plot the positive inflection or negative deflection on the graph paper by drawing a perpendicular line.
   a. Positive goes *toward* the lead.
   b. Negative goes *away from* the lead.

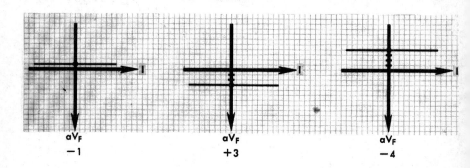

6. The intersection of the plots of leads I and aV$_F$ is the axis.

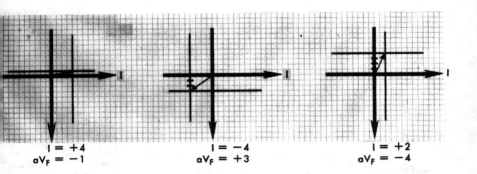

I = +4
aV$_F$ = −1

I = −4
aV$_F$ = +3

I = +2
aV$_F$ = −4

7. Superimpose a protractor compass over the graph paper to determine the exact degree of axis or estimate the degree of axis by quadrants.

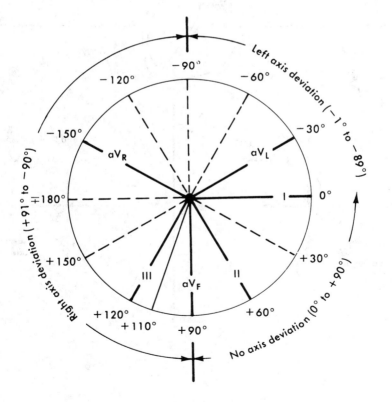

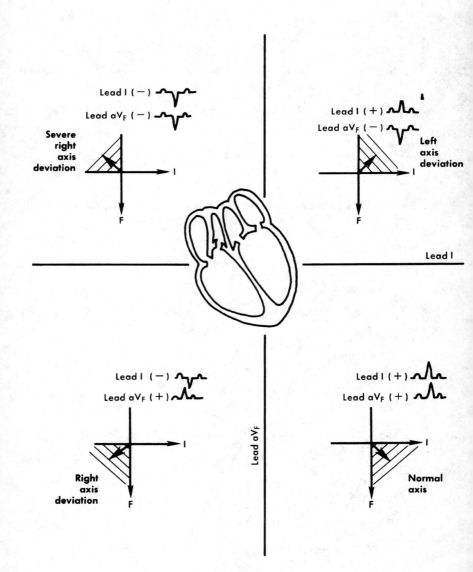

CHEST PAIN CAUSED BY REDUCED CORONARY ARTERY BLOOD FLOW

Angina Pectoris

When the myocardium becomes anoxic, a condition known as angina pectoris occurs.

Described as retrosternal discomfort, it usually occurs as a result of increased cardiac output and increased oxygen demand with an underlying diseased coronary artery system.

Most angina is caused by a partial occlusion of the coronary arteries, usually because of atherosclerosis.

It can also be caused by arterial spasms, emboli, or a dissecting aortic aneurysm.

Is not usually sharply localized.

Refer to Table 7-1 for a differential diagnosis of angina.

stable (typical) The pain that occurs is predictable and follows events such as exercise, heavy work, or strain.

unstable (preinfarction) Attacks are prolonged and more severe and occur more frequently.

Prinzmetal's (variant) The pain occurs while the patient is at rest and usually at the same time each day; during the attack the ST segment may be elevated. The prognosis is poor, with a 50% mortality the first year. In the early stages of the disease, if coronary catheterization indicates it, coronary artery bypass surgery is usually recommended.

TABLE 7-1   Differential Diagnosis of Angina

	STABLE ANGINA	UNSTABLE ("PREINFARCTION") ANGINA
Location of pain	Substernal; may radiate to jaws and neck and down arms and back	Substernal; may radiate to jaws and neck and down arms and back
Duration of pain	1 to 15 minutes	5 minutes, occurring more frequently
Characteristic of pain	Ache, squeezing, choking, heavy; burning	Same as stable angina, but more intense
Other symptoms	None, usually	Diaphoresis; weakness
Pain worsened by	Exercise; activity; eating; cold weather; reclining	Exercise; activity; eating; cold weather, reclining
Pain relieved by	Rest; nitroglycerin; isosorbide (Isordil)	Nitroglycerin, Isordil may only give partial relief
ECG findings	Transient ST depression; disappears with pain relief	ST segment depression; often T-wave inversion; but ECG may be normal

Myocardial Infarction

Myocardial infarction (MI) is a localized ischemic necrosis of an area of the myocardium caused by a narrowing of one or more of the coronary arteries. The narrowing may be caused by a thrombus, spasm, or hemorrhage. The size and location of the infarction depend on the location of the block in the coronary artery.

Clinical findings in myocardial infarction

Pain of sudden onset that lasts from several minutes to several days. It is usually localized in the substernal area and radiates up into the jaw or down into the arm. It also may have an atypical presentation, such as a toothache or other painful sensation.

Frequently described as crushing, sharp, or burning, or as a pressure, tightness, or choking.

Nausea and vomiting.

Blood pressure is usually decreased.

Increased pulse.

Edema caused by decreased cardiac output and increased venous pressure.

Heart sounds will vary depending on the physiologic status of the myocardium.

■ **THERAPEUTIC INTERVENTIONS**

Medications

■ **NITROGLYCERIN**
   Sublingual
   Administer an initial dose of nitroglycerin 0.4 mg or 1/150 g.

   Monitor blood pressure before and after nitroglycerin administration.

   Do not administer nitroglycerin unless systolic blood pressure is above 100 mm Hg.

   If the initial dose is not effective, administer an additional tablet (again, ensuring that the patient's systolic pressure is greater than 100 mm Hg). A third dose can be given if needed and tolerated.

   The contents of a 10-mg capsule of nifedipine can also be squirted under the patient's tongue if coronary spasm is suspected.

   Intravenous. Administer 5 to 10 µg/min and increase by 10 µg/min every 5 to 10 minutes until pain is relieved, systolic blood pressure drops to between 90 and 100 mm Hg, or the patient becomes symptomatic. Maximum IV dose is between 100 and 200 µg/min.

■ **TRANSDERMAL NITROPASTE**
Transdermal nitropaste is an alternative to nitroglycerin tablets. It is applied to the chest wall, usually over the left side of the chest, in a ½ inch to 1 inch area. The onset of action with nitropaste is slower than with tablets but the duration of action is longer than with tablets. If the patient develops an adverse reaction, this too will be longer in duration.

   Both nitroglycerin and nitropaste can lose potency over time. If the patient has taken several nitroglycerin tablets or has applied nitropaste without effect, you may choose to administer nitroglycerin from a fresh supply to ensure potency.

■ **MORPHINE SULFATE**

Morphine sulfate is the drug of choice for chest pain of myocardial origin. Besides relieving pain as a narcotic-analgesic, morphine sulfate reduces preload and decreases myocardial oxygen demand.

Administer slowly intravenously at a dosage of 2 to 10 mg, titrated to effect.

Do not give if systolic blood pressure is below 90 mm Hg.

If hypotension should occur, elevate the patient's legs to facilitate venous return to the central circulation, as for nitroglycerin-induced hypotension.

If there is respiratory depression, administer naloxone hydrochloride (Narcan) 0.8 mg IV. Naloxone acts rapidly and reverses the effects of morphine sulfate.

The presence of chronic obstructive pulmonary disease is a relative contraindication to the use of morphine sulfate.

■ **LIDOCAINE**

The prophylactic use of lidocaine in the treatment of suspected MIs has come under question due to its proarrhythmic potential. Although lidocaine is widely administered, some argue that it should be used only if ectopy develops. Prophylactic lidocaine is given by bolus-bolus method or bolus-IV drip method.

Bolus-bolus method

When given by bolus-bolus method, the initial dose should be 1 to 2 mg/kg given slowly over 1 to 2 minutes.

If lidocaine is given too rapidly, seizures may occur.

The initial bolus is followed 5 minutes later by an additional bolus of 50 mg.

Repeat the 50-mg bolus every 10 minutes up to a total dosage of 325 mg.

This method of administration should be considered, especially in the prehospital setting, because it is difficult to control an IV drip rate in a moving rescue vehicle.

Bolus-IV drip method

Lidocaine can also be given by slowly administering an initial bolus of 1 to 2 mg/kg IV, followed by a *drip* of 2 g lidocaine in 500 ml of D_5W running at a rate of 1 to 4 mg/min to maintain a constant blood level.

Do not administer lidocaine without an initial loading-dose bolus.

If an IV drip is started before a loading-dose bolus is given, an effective blood level of lidocaine may take a long time to reach or may never be attained.

Thrombolytic therapy

Pharmacologic agent is administered to dissolve thrombi that typically form at the site of athersosclerotic lesion. Can be a stand-alone treatment or used in conjunction with percutaneous transluminal coronary angioplasty (PTCA) or percutaneous directional coronary angioplasty (PDCA).

■ **GOALS**

Prevention of myocardial necrosis
Reduction of myocardial ischemia
Limitation of myocardial infarct size
Improvement of left ventricular function

■ **INDICATIONS**

Acute chest pain indicative of MI

TABLE 7-2 Coronary Arteries in Myocardial Infarction

RIGHT CORONARY ARTERY

LEFT CORONARY ARTERY

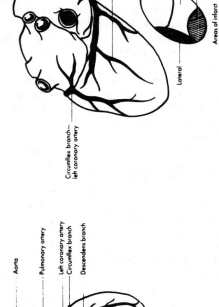

Supplies:

Right atrium

Right ventricle

Posterior surface of left ventricle

50% to 60% of SA node

Bundle of His

Block causes:

Infarction of posterior wall of left ventricle

Infarction of posterior half of interventricular septum

In inferior myocardial infarction (leads II, III, aV_F) anticipate second-degree heart block, Mobitz type I block, Wenckebach block

Left circumflex branch

Supplies:

Left atrium

Free wall of left ventricle

40% to 50% of SA node

8% to 10% of AV node

Bundle of His

Right bundle

Block causes:

Lateral wall infarction

Posterior wall infarction (near base)

Left anterior descending branch

Supplies

Interventricular septum

Block causes:

Infarction of anterior wall of left ventricle

Effect on papillary muscle (which attaches to mitral valve)

Infarction of anterior wall of septum

In anterior myocardial infarction (leads V_1, V_2, V_3) anticipate second-degree heart block, Mobitz type II block

ECG changes indicating acute myocardial ischemia

Lack of relief with nitroglycerin

Treatment can be initiated within 6 hours of onset of pain

Types of agents

Streptokinase and tissue plasminogen activator (tPA)

Method of administration: intravenous

NOTE: Heparin therapy is usually initiated concurrently to prevent rethrombus

Streptokinase:

1,500,000 IV administered via constant infusion over 60 minutes

tPA:

10 mg IV push bolus over 1 to 2 minutes followed immediately by a 50-mg infusion over 1 hour. Then 20-mg is administered over 1 hour followed by another 20-mg dose over 1 hour. A total of 100 mg is administered.

■ **COMPLICATIONS**

Bleeding

Reocclusion

Reinfarction

Allergic reaction

Reprofusion dysrhythmias

Hematoma at insertion site

Percutaneous Transluminal Coronary Angioplasty/ Percutaneous Directional Coronary Athrectomy

Nonsurgical methods of revascularizing myocardial tissue. Under sterile conditions in a catheterization lab, a steerable catheter is threaded into the coronary artery through a femoral artery sheath and positioned at the site of the coronary stenosis. The plaque is either flattened against the artery wall (PTCA) or cut away and removed altogether (PDCA).

■ **GOALS**

Prevention of myocardial necrosis

Reduction of myocardial ischemia

Limitation of myocardial infarct size

Improvement of left ventricular function

CHEST PAIN ORIGINATING FROM THE PERICARDIUM

Acute Pericarditis

Acute pericarditis is an inflammation of the pericardial sac and can occur as a result of the following conditions:

Idiopathic—following viral or febrile illness. Etiology may not be able to be established.

Infection—viral, bacterial, or fungal in origin

Connective tissue disease

Malignancy—breast, lung, and other tumors can metastasize to the pericardium

Uremia

Drug induced

Post-myocardial infarction (Dressler's syndrome)

Postpericardiotomy

■ **SIGNS AND SYMPTOMS**

Severe chest pain that increases with respirations or activity

Fever and chills

Diaphoresis

Dyspnea

Tachycardia or other dysrhythmias

Pericardial friction rub (increased when patient leans forward)

Malaise

ST segment elevation of 1 to 3 mm in all ECG leads except aV_R and V_1

Decreased blood pressure (if effusion has occurred)

■ **THERAPEUTIC INTERVENTIONS**

Treatment of underlying etiology

Chest x-ray film—may assist in establishing etiology

Oxygen

Sedation

Rest

Antibiotics

Analgesia (salicylates)

Nonsteroidal antiinflammatories

Corticosteroids

Much reassurance

Cardiac Tamponade

Cardiac tamponade is a condition in which blood leaks into the pericardial sac. It may be caused by:

Infection

Neoplasm

Open heart surgery

Cardiac catheterization

Dissecting aortic aneurysm

Trauma—most common cause

The compression of the heart caused by the increased fluid in the pericardial sac prevents adequate venous return from the systemic circulation. This produces a critical decrease in cardiac output.

■ **SIGNS AND SYMPTOMS**

The speed and severity in which signs and symptoms develop depend on the rate of fluid accumulation, pericardial compliance, and intravascular volume. An initial but temporary hypertensive state can exist as decreased cardiac output causes a compensatory vasoconstriction and an increase in peripheral vascular resistance. The patient may develop profound shock with as little as 150 to 200 ml of blood into the pericardial sac. Other signs and symptoms include:

Tachycardia
Elevated CVP (greater than 15 mm Hg)
Decreased blood pressure*
Distended neck veins* } Beck's Triad
Distant heart sounds*
Decreased arterial pressure
Decreased systolic blood pressure
Narrow pulse pressure
Weak, thready pulse
Cyanosis
Increased respiratory rate
Dyspnea
Paradoxical pulse (see below)
Restlessness
Loss of apical cardiac impulse
Shock
Widening cardiac silhouette on chest x-ray film

Paradoxical pulse

Paradoxical pulse is found in one third of patients experiencing acute pericardial tamponade. It will be noted by an abnormal fall in systolic blood pressure during inspiration.

■ **PROCEDURE**
1. Apply a blood pressure cuff to the patient's arm.
2. Inflate the cuff to a level above systolic pressure.
3. Deflate the cuff slowly until the first systolic sound is heard. During normal inspiration the systolic sound will disappear.
4. Deflate the cuff until all systolic sounds can be heard during both inspiration and expiration.
5. Note the point at which all systolic sounds can be heard.
6. The difference in millimeters of mercury between the pressure at which the systolic sound disappears during inspiration and the pressure at which all systolic sounds can be heard is called a paradox.

NOTE: A paradox of more than 10 mm Hg indicates a paradoxical pulse.

■ **THERAPEUTIC INTERVENTIONS**
CVP monitoring
Oxygen
PASG to increase venous return to the right side of the heart and correct hypovolemia
Volume expansion using normal saline
Pericardiocentesis (see below)

Pericardiocentesis (Figure 7-4)

■ **EQUIPMENT**
16- to 18-gauge needle
50-ml syringe
Fluoroscopy (PROCEDURE should ideally be done in cardiac catheterization lab)

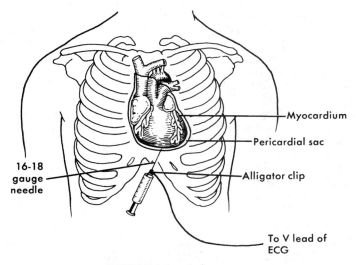

FIGURE 7-4. Pericardiocentesis.

Alligator clips (sterile)
Kelly clamp
3-channel ECG machine
Defibrillator
Three-way stopcock (metal)
Local anesthetic agent
Antiseptic solution
Gloves
Sterile drapes

■ **PROCEDURE**

1. Prepare the patient's chest at the left inferior costal margin and the xyphoid.
2. Administer a local anesthetic to the area.
3. Attach the limb leads to the patient's extremities and to the V5 and V6 precordial leads.
4. Attach one end of an alligator clip to the hub of the 16-gauge needle and the other end of the clip to the V lead of the ECG machine.
5. Attach the needle to the syringe via the three-way stopcock.
6. Run the ECG machine on the V-lead setting.
7. Advance the needle in a subxyphoid approach between the left inferior costal margin and the xyphoid at a 30- to 45-degree angle to the body, advancing toward the tip of the right scapula.
8. Gently aspirate the syringe as the needle is advanced; if blood returns and there is no ST-segment elevation on the ECG, the needle has probably entered the pericardial sac. If an ST-segment elevation appears on the ECG,

the needle has pierced the epicardium. If this occurs, withdraw the needle slowly until the ST segment returns to normal. If the needle has gone all the way through to the myocardium, a pulsation will be felt up through the needle and the syringe.

9. Once blood is being withdrawn from the pericardial sac, attach a Kelly clamp to the needle at the level of the skin to avoid accidental advancement of the needle.

NOTE: Blood withdrawn from the pericardial sac should not clot because it has been defibrinated in the sac. Also, samples should be placed in sterile tubes for lab analysis.

■ **COMPLICATIONS**
Laceration of a coronary artery
Laceration of the lung
Laceration of the ventricle
Cardiac dysrhythmias
Increased tamponade

CHEST PAIN OF AORTIC ORIGIN

Aortic Dissection (Figure 7-5)

Aortic dissection occurs primarily in men. It is frequently seen in conjunction with arteriosclerotic heart disease and hypertension. Other causes of dissection are trauma and Marfan's syndrome, which occur primarily in the young.

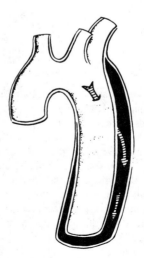

FIGURE 7-5. A dissecting aortic aneurysm.

An aortic dissection is a tear in the intimal layer of the aorta that allows blood to leak between the intimal and medial layers. There are three types of aortic dissection.

Type I

Dissection of the descending aorta to and beyond the aortic arch (occurs in two thirds of cases).

Type II

Dissection of the ascending aorta alone.

Type III

Dissection from beyond the left subclavian artery.

Dissection may cause occlusion of major vessels that branch off from the aorta, such as the myocardial, cerebral, mesenteric, and renal vessels. Rupture of the dissection may have two results: (1) rupture into the pericardial sac causing pericardial tamponade and (2) rupture into the chest cavity causing exsanguination.

■ **SIGNS AND SYMPTOMS**

Chest pain—described as excruciating or tearing; anteroposterior in nature (may be confused with myocardial infarction, back pain, pericarditis, or peptic ulcer)
Dyspnea
Orthopnea
Diaphoresis
Pallor
Apprehension
Syncope
Tachycardia
Absence of major arterial pulses *unilaterally*
Blood pressure differences between arms (in a thoracic aortic dissection)
Hypertension
Pulse at the sternoclavicular joint
Murmur of aortic insufficiency (in type II)
Hemiplegia or paraplegia
Shock
Widened mediastinum

■ **THERAPEUTIC INTERVENTIONS**

High Fowler's position
Oxygen
IV D_5W TKO
Nitroprusside
Propranolol
Much support and reassurance
Preparation for surgery
PASG if dissection is ruptured and patient is in shock

CHEST PAIN OF OTHER ORIGINS

Hyperventilation

Hyperventilation is one of the most common conditions. It may occur as a result of anxiety, or it may be caused by a disease process such as salicylate overdose, myocardial infarction, or intracerebral bleeding. Pay close attention to associated signs and symptoms that may lead to the discovery of an underlying disorder. Avoid "tunnel vision" and keep your mind open to all possibilities for the cause. Hyperventilation may be a response to a disease process that, when treated with the traditional breathing into a paper bag, could cause serious complications. *Medical illness must be ruled out* before assuming that the hyperventilation is caused by anxiety or an hysterical response.

■ **CAUSES**

Anxiety	Pulmonary hypertension
Pregnancy	Pulmonary edema
Fever from any cause	Smoke inhalation
Trauma	Anemia
Pain	Intracerebral bleeding and increased intracranial pressure
Liver disease	Central nervous system lesion
Pulmonary embolus	Fibrosis of lung tissue
Stress	Exercise
Diabetic ketoacidosis	Fatigue
High altitude	
Thyrotoxicosis	

No matter what the cause of hyperventilation, it is accompanied by a fall in PCO_2 (hypocapnia), which causes constriction of cerebral vasculature, respiratory alkalosis, and symptoms of tetany. PCO_2 may drop to as low as 15 mm Hg.

■ **SIGNS AND SYMPTOMS**

Anxiety or panicky appearance
Shortness of breath
Tingling of fingers and toes
Periorbital numbness
Carpopedal spasm
Syncope
Confusion

■ **THERAPEUTIC INTERVENTIONS**

Therapeutic intervention for hyperventilation syndrome should only be undertaken after medical disease and trauma have been ruled out as the cause of the hyperventilation.

Speak with the patient; make the patient aware of what is going on.
Have the patient talk. (It is difficult to hyperventilate while talking.)
Act in a calm, reassuring manner; never be demanding or demeaning.
Demonstrate proper breathing for the patient and say, "Breathe like I am breathing."
Once the patient seems to be aware of what is going on, have the patient watch a clock with a second hand and breathe once every 5 seconds.

If none of these seems to be working, have the patient rebreathe into a paper bag (carbon dioxide rebreathing).

Always remember to look for underlying causes of hyperventilation other than anxiety or hysteria.

OTHER CAUSES OF CHEST PAIN

See Table 7-3 for differential diagnosis.

Hiatal hernia
Gastric or peptic ulcer
Pancreatitis
Esophageal spasm
Mallory-Weiss syndrome
Borhave's syndrome
Trauma
Degenerative disk disease
Xyphoidalgia
Costochondritis
Mondor's disease
Postherpetic syndrome

CONGESTIVE HEART FAILURE

Congestive heart failure (CHF) is a symptom complex in which the heart can no longer produce sufficient cardiac output, at normal filling pressure, to meet metabolic demands. CHF may be seen as an individual entity or in conjunction with pulmonary edema, angina, or MI.

Onset of symptoms may be sudden (acute pulmonary edema) or gradual (chronic CHF). Causes of congestive heart failure include

Hypertension—systemic or pulmonary
Fluid overload
Increased intracranial pressure
Myocardial infarction with failure (most common of CHF)
Valvular heart disease
Coronary artery disease
Cardiomyopathy
Dysrhythmias
Tachycardia (more than 180 beats/minute)
Bradycardia (less than 30 beats/minute)
Fever from any cause
Hyperthyroidism
Post-pneumothorax
Adult respiratory distress syndrome (ARDS)
Oxygen toxicity
Uremic pneumonia
Intracranial tumors
Drugs such as methotrexate, busulfan, hexamethonium, and nitrofurantoin

TABLE 7-3 Differential Diagnosis of Chest Pain

CAUSE	ONSET OF PAIN	CHARACTERISTIC OF PAIN	LOCATION OF PAIN
Acute myocardial infarction	Sudden onset; lasts more than 30 minutes to 1 hour	Pressure, burning, aching, tightness, choking	Across chest; may radiate to jaws and neck and down arms and back
Angina	Sudden onset; lasts only few minutes	Aches, squeezing, choking, heaviness, burning	Substernal; may radiate to jaws and neck and down arms and back
Dissecting aortic aneurysm	Sudden onset	Excruciating, tearing	Center of chest; radiates into back; may radiate to abdomen
Pericarditis	Sudden onset or may be variable	Sharp, knifelike	Retrosternal; may radiate up neck and down left arm
Pneumothorax	Sudden onset	Tearing, pleuritic	Lateral side of chest
Pulmonary embolus	Sudden onset	Crushing (but not always)	Lateral side of chest
Hiatal hernia	Sudden onset	Sharp, severe	Lower chest; upper abdomen
Gastrointestinal disturbance or cholecystitis	Sudden onset	Gripping, burning	Lower substernal area, upper abdomen
Degenerative disk (cervical or thoracic spine) disease	Sudden onset	Sharp, severe	Substernal; may radiate to neck, jaw, arms, and shoulders
Degenerative or inflammatory lesions of shoulder, ribs, scalenus anterior	Sudden onset	Sharp, severe	Substernal; radiates to shoulder
Hyperventilation	Sudden onset	Vague	Vague

TABLE 7-3   Differential Diagnosis of Chest Pain—Cont'd

HISTORY	PAIN WORSENED BY	PAIN RELIEVED BY	OTHER
Age 40 to 70 years; may or may not have history of angina	Movement, anxiety	Nothing; no movement, stillness, position, or breath holding; only relieved by medication (morphine sulfate)	Shortness of breath, diaphoresis, weakness, anxiety
May have history of angina; circumstances precipitating; pain characteristic; response to nitroglycerin	Lying down, eating, effort, cold weather, smoking, stress, anger, worry, hunger	Rest, nitroglycerin	Unstable angina appears even at rest
Nothing specific, except that pain is usually worse at onset		Nothing	Blood pressure difference between right and left arms, murmur of aortic regurgitation
Short history of upper respiratory infection or fever	Deep breathing, trunk movement, maybe swallowing	Sitting up, leaning forward	Friction rub, paradoxic pulse over 10 mm Hg.
None	Breathing	Nothing	Dyspnea, increased pulse, decreased breath sounds, deviated trachea
Sometimes phlebitis	Breathing	Not breathing	Cyanosis, dyspnea, cough with hemoptysis
May have none	Heavy meal, bending, lying down	Bland diet, walking, antacids, semi-Fowler's position	
May have none	Eating, lying down	Antacids	
May have none	Movement of neck or spine, lifting, straining	Rest, decreased movement	Pain usually on outer aspect of arm, thumb, or index finger
May have none	Movement of arm or shoulder	Elevation and arm support to shoulder postural exercises	
Hyperventilation, anxiety, stress, emotional upset	Increased respiratory rate	Slowing of respiratory rate	Be *sure* hyperventilation is from nonmedical cause!

Anemia
Pericardial disease
Pulmonary embolus

■ **SIGNS AND SYMPTOMS**

Shortness of breath
Dyspnea
Weakness
Dependent edema
Distended neck veins
Hepatomegaly
Bilateral rales
Increased circulation time
Weight gain

■ **MONITORING PARAMETERS**

ABCs
Vital signs
Cardiac monitor
Auscultation of the lungs
Auscultation of the heart
Observation of neck veins
Observation for peripheral edema
Obtaining a history and performing a brief physical examination
Pulse oximetry/arterial blood gas
Chest x-ray film
CBC, lytes, BUN, CR
Cardiac enzymes

■ **THERAPEUTIC INTERVENTIONS**

Acute

High flow oxygen—may require intubation
Morphine sulfate—venous dilation decreases preload; sedation relieves anxiety and depression of respiratory center reduces hyperventilation
Diuretics—reduces preload. Rapid-acting loop diuretics; if no clinical response within 15 to 30 minutes, repeat dose
Aminophylline—used if bronchospasm present not relieved by oxygen, morphine, and diuretics
Dopamine or dobutamine
Rotating tourniquets
IV D_5W at TKO
Digoxin—may have adverse affects in setting of acute MI with CHF. Is also a weaker inotropic compared to dopamine or dobutamine. In an acute crisis should be used to control atrial arrhythmias and not for management of pump failure.

Chronic

Bedrest in high Fowler's position
Oxygen therapy
Digitalis therapy—used in presence of reduced left ventricular ejection fraction

Diuretics
Low-sodium diet
Angiotensin-Converting Enzyme (ACE) Inhibitors—systemic vasodilation
reduces afterload:
Captopril
Enalapril
Lisinopril

SUGGESTED READINGS

Dolan J: *Critical care nursing—clinical management through the nursing process.* Philadelphia, 1991, FA Davis.

Proehl J: *Adult emergency nursing procedures.* Boston, London, 1993, Bartlett Publishers.

Hartshom J, Lamborn M, Moll ML: *Introduction to critical care nursing.* Philadelphia, 1993, Saunders.

Heger JW, Roth JT, Niemann RF, Criley JM: *Cardiology—house officer series.* Baltimore, 1993, Williams & Wilkins.

CHAPTER 8

Pulmonary Emergencies

GENERAL ASSESSMENT

Severe dyspnea is a common chief complaint in the emergency setting. Questions to ask to assist with a diagnosis include:

- When did this begin?
- What brought it on? What were you doing when it started?
- Did it come on gradually or suddenly?
- Is it difficult to get air out?
- Has this ever happened before?
- Is it extremely difficult to breathe?
- Have you ever had lung disease? Heart disease? Asthma? High blood pressure?
- Do you smoke?
- Are you taking any medications? For your heart? For retained water?
- Do you have difficulty walking up stairs?

Other assessment parameters in the patient with a pulmonary disorder are:

Ensure ABCs.

Listen for noises (remember, noisy breathing is obstructed breathing.)

Check level of consciousness.

Check skin vital signs (color, temperature, and moistness).

Check character of respirations.

Check for use of accessory muscles.

Check for paradoxical chest movement.

PULMONARY EMBOLUS

Pulmonary embolus is one of the most difficult diagnoses to make because it is often confused with myocardial infarction, pneumothorax, and other conditions involving chest pain. It is not a disease, but rather a complication of a disease. Pulmonary embolus is caused by a free-flowing thrombus from the venous system of the legs, pelvis, or right side of the heart.

The thrombus lodges in a branch of the pulmonary artery, causing partial or total occlusion and sometimes infarction. An embolus may consist of clotted blood, fat, air, or amniotic fluid. Septic emboli from blood-borne bacteria and tumor emboli from intravascular metastases also occur.

■ **CAUSES**
Trauma
Long-bone fractures
Surgery (especially abdominal or pelvic)
Obesity
Decreased peripheral circulation
Congestive heart failure with myocardial infarction
Thrombophlebitis
Cardiac disease
Atrial fibrillation
Prolonged immobilization
Acute infections
Blood dyscrasias
Amniotic fluid emboli (in childbirth)
Air emboli (from scuba diving or poor IV technique)
Oral contraceptives
Neoplasms

■ **PREVENTION**
Frequent ambulation on long trips
Avoiding long periods of standing
Early postoperative ambulation
Elastic stockings for those on bed rest
Range of motion exercises for those on bed rest
Good IV technique
Careful management and movement of severely traumatized patients
Prophylactic anticoagulants for high-risk patients

■ **SIGNS AND SYMPTOMS**
There may be absolutely no prodromal signs or symptoms preceding a terminal event. When signs and symptoms do appear, they may be vague. The following is a list of some of the more common signs and symptoms:
Shortness of breath
Tachypnea
Tachycardia
Angina-like chest pain
Pallor or cyanosis
Anxiety
Occasionally decreased blood pressure
Possible wheezing
Right bundle branch block with right axis deviation, peaked T waves in limb leads, and depressed T waves in the right precordial leads (V_1, V_2, and V_3)

■ **THERAPEUTIC INTERVENTIONS**
ABCs
Oxygen at high flow rate
IV D_5W TKO

Analgesia (usually meperidine—avoid morphine)
Bronchodilators
Treatment of dysrhythmias
Heparin (5000 U bolus, then 1000 U per hour continuous infusion); monitor
    clotting times carefully
Thrombolytic therapy (TPA, urokinase)
Posteroanterior and lateral chest x-ray films
Ventilation/perfusion lung scan
Much reassurance
When 60% of the pulmonary vasculature is blocked, cardiac function is compromised. If a large pulmonary embolus lodges in the main, right, or left pulmonary artery, sudden death may occur.

SPONTANEOUS PNEUMOTHORAX

Spontaneous pneumothorax may occur in the absence of trauma. It occurs most often in young persons (16 to 26 years old) and is more commonly associated with males than females. The usual cause is a ruptured congenital bleb or a bulla that has developed from chronic obstructive pulmonary disease. Other causes of spontaneous pneumothorax include:

Too great mechanical ventilation pressures
Rupture of a cyst
Abscess
Fungal disease
Cancer
Tuberculosis
Trauma
Chest compression in cardiopulmonary resuscitation
Tracheostomy complication
Subclavian puncture complication

■ **SIGNS AND SYMPTOMS**

The signs and symptoms of spontaneous pneumothorax may be minimal. Classic signs and symptoms are usually associated with pneumothorax of 40% or greater.

Dyspnea
Tachypnea
Cyanosis
Sudden onset of pleuritic chest pain
Agitation
Decreased breath sounds

Severe signs and symptoms of tension pneumothorax include:

Decreased motion of chest wall
Mediastinal shift
Distended neck veins
Deviated trachea
Tympany on percussion
Shock

The absolute diagnosis of pneumothorax is made by chest x-ray examination. If symptoms are severe, however, do not delay therapeutic intervention until a chest x-ray film is available.

■ **THERAPEUTIC INTERVENTIONS**
Therapy is aimed toward reexpansion of the collapsed lung.
Oxygen
Analgesia
Needle placement in the anterior chest wall or chest tube
IV D_5W TKO
Bed rest in high Fowler's position
Much reassurance

PLEURAL EFFUSION

Abnormal collections of pleural fluid in the pleural space result in an effusion. Effusions take up space in the thoracic cavity, thus reducing lung volumes. Pleural effusions may be classified as transudative or exudative. Transudative effusions are caused by systemic factors, whereas exudative effusions are caused by disease of the pleura itself.

■ **CAUSES**

TRANSUDATIVE	EXUDATIVE
CHF	Infectious diseases
Cirrhosis	Neoplastic diseases
Pericardial disease	Collagen vascular diseases (systemic lupus erythematosus,
Pulmonary	rheumatoid pleuritis)
embolus	Postabdominal surgery
Peritoneal dialysis	Trauma

■ **SIGNS AND SYMPTOMS**
Dull, aching chest pain
Dullness to percussion (affected area)
Decreased breath sounds
Egophony (near top of fluid line)
Pleural friction rub
Dyspnea
Cough
Local or referred pleuritic pain
Signs and symptoms of congestive heart failure, infection, or pleural effusion
Chest x-ray film—two views: effusion will appear as a homogeneously dense opaque area. Fluid will often shift with change in body position.

■ **TREATMENT**
Thoracentesis
Oxygen
Analgesia
Subsequent treatment based on underlying cause

PNEUMONIA

Pneumonia results from a bacterial, viral, or fungal infection. The patient will often have a history of recent upper respiratory tract infection, otitis media, or conjunctivitis before the onset of pneumonia. However, the patient could have no known medical problems before pneumonia is manifest. It frequently appears in very young or very old persons who are debilitated in some way.

Pneumonia is classified according to the organism that causes it (pneumococcal, streptococcal, or viral) and according to its location (bronchial or lobar). Some of the more common causes of pneumonia are:

Debilitation
Underlying cardiovascular disorder
Underlying pulmonary disorder
Rapid environmental temperature changes
Smoking
Diabetes mellitus
Steroids
Immunosuppression
Aspiration (frequently seen in alcohol or drug abusers or persons with head injury)
Foreign body

■ SIGNS AND SYMPTOMS
  ### Bacterial pneumonia
  Dyspnea
  Sudden onset
  Chills
  Fever 39.4° to 40° C (103° to 104° F)
  Toxicity
  Productive cough and purulent sputum
  Chest pain (may be referred diaphragmatically and be mistaken for a gastrointestinal disorder)
  Diaphoresis
  Tachypnea
  Nausea and vomiting
  Cyanosis
  Rales
  Otitis media
  Conjunctivitis
  Apprehension
  Abdominal distension
  ### Nonbacterial pneumonia
Same symptoms as bacterial pneumonia
Insidious onset
Preceded by upper respiratory infection
Myalgia
Headache
May have seasonal pattern

■ **THERAPEUTIC INTERVENTIONS**

Oxygen

Bed rest in high Fowler's position

Pneumococcal—penicillin G (600,000 U every 12 hours)

Staphylococcal—methicillin nafcillin (1 to 2 g every 4 to 6 hours IV)

Gram-negative—Tobramycin or gentamicin (1 to 3 mg/kg every 8 hours often in conjunction with a cephalosporin)

Mycoplasmal—erythromycin, tetracycline, doxycycline

Aspiration—penicillin G (1,200,000 U every 6 hours)

■ **COMPLICATIONS**

Rupture of pneumatocele producing pneumothorax

Empyema

Therapeutic intervention for both of these complications is placement of a chest tube.

PULMONARY EDEMA

The key to survival in pulmonary edema is prompt recognition and rapid therapeutic intervention. Pulmonary failure is also known as backward failure or circulatory overload. It is most often a result of backward pressure into the left side of the heart and lungs. This transmits an increased pressure into the pulmonary capillaries and produces a leak of fluid from the capillaries into the alveoli. (See box below.) Normally the fluid content of the lungs is about 20% of their total volume. In acute pulmonary edema, the fluid content of the lungs can rise as high as 1000% of normal.

Pulmonary edema is a symptom complex, not a diagnosis. Several diseases may produce pulmonary edema:

Mechanism of Pulmonary Edema of Cardiac Origin

Myocardial infarction

↓

Left ventricular failure

↓

Increased pressure in left ventricle

↓

Increased pressure in pulmonary venous system

↓

Loss of plasma oncotic pressure

↓

Leak of fluid into interstitial tissue

↓

Reflex spasm of airways (cardiac asthma) and pulmonary alveoli

↓

Pulmonary edema and interference with gas exchange

↓

Decreased Po_2 and acidosis

Myocardial infarction (with left ventricular failure)
Aortic insufficiency
Aortic stenosis
Mitral stenosis
Myocarditis
Amyloidosis
Hypertension
Coronary artery disease
Dysrhythmias (tachycardias >180 beats per minute and bradycardias <30 beats per minute)
Hyperthermia
Hyperthyroidism
Exercise
Severe congestive heart failure
Adult respiratory distress syndrome
Heroin overdose
Inhalation of pulmonary irritants
Pulmonary embolism
High altitude
Neurogenic causes
Volume overload
Anemia
Uremia
Disseminated intravascular coagulation (DIC)
Near-drowning
Renal impairment
Lymphatic obstruction
Bacteremic sepsis
Beriberi
General anesthesia

■ **SIGNS AND SYMPTOMS**

Shortness of breath
Chest tightness
Cough
Cyanosis (central and peripheral)
Rales, rhonchi, wheezing
Distended neck veins
Pink, frothy sputum
Peripheral edema
Tachycardia
Paroxysmal nocturnal dyspnea (PND) or orthopnea
Cheyne-Stokes respirations
S_3 gallop and decreased heart sounds

■ **GOALS IN TREATMENT**

Decreased hypoxia
Improved ventilation

Decreased pulmonary capillary wedge pressure
Improved myocardial contractility
■ **MONITORING PARAMETERS**
Ensure ABCs.
Attempt to obtain a brief history.
Check vital signs.
Patient will usually be tachypneic, tachycardic, and hypertensive.
Monitor for dysrhythmias.
A dysrhythmia may have precipitated the pulmonary edema, or the dysrhythmia may have been caused by the hypoxic condition.
Auscultate the lungs.
Rales and rhonchi will be heard.
Wheezing is suggestive of cardiac asthma caused by a reflex spasm of the airways.
Auscultate the heart.
There will often be distant, muffled heart sounds of an S_3 caused by ventricular distension.
Observe external jugular (neck) veins.
The jugular vein reflects pressures found in the right atrium. Turn the patient's head to the right or left and observe the vein at the posterior border of the sternocleidomastoid muscle; the patient should be in semi-Fowler's position. Neck vein distension 2 inches above the sternal notch suggests right atrial congestion.
Observe for peripheral edema.
Pay particular attention to dependent parts, such as the arms, legs, feet, and sacral area.
■ **THERAPEUTIC INTERVENTIONS**
The following therapeutic interventions will alter circulatory and ventilatory dynamics but may not alter the underlying disease process. Once the patient is out of a life-threatening condition, status must be reevaluated to determine proper therapeutic intervention for the condition that caused the pulmonary edema.
Place the patient in high Fowler's position with legs dependent.
Administer high-flow oxygen to treat hypoxia.
Place patient on a cardiac monitor.
Initiate an IV line for the administration of medications.
Administer morphine sulfate 2 to 5 mg over 2 minutes, repeat at 15 minute intervals (up to 20 mg)
Nitroglycerin causes venous pooling and dilated vasculature that produces a decreased venous return to the right heart, provided that blood pressure is in an acceptable range. Start by giving 0.3- to 0.6-mg tablet sublingually while setting up a continuous intravenous infusion to be started at 5 to 10 μg/min. Increase by 10 μg every 2 to 5 minutes until dyspnea improves.
Give furosemide to produce diuresis and decrease intravascular volume.
Administer in a dose of 20 to 80 mg by IV push. The caregiver can

expect to see a response 5 to 15 minutes after Lasix administration. Use particular caution with the patient who has been digitalized or has been on previous diuretic therapy because hypokalemia-induced dysrhythmias or hypotensive states caused by excessive diuresis may result from furosemide administration.

Perform arterial blood gas analysis. The following blood gas values are desirable:

Po_2: 80 mm Hg; Pco_2: 30 to 40 mm Hg; pH: 7.45.

Place a Foley catheter if the patient is unable to control urination.

Give reassurance. These patients experience feelings of suffocation and doom. They need much verbal support and touch communication.

HIGH-ALTITUDE PULMONARY EDEMA

High-altitude pulmonary edema (HAPE) usually occurs in patients who have made a very rapid ascent to altitudes above 10,000 feet over sea level and have engaged in heavy physical activity for the first 3 days at that altitude. It can occur much sooner in patients with underlying pulmonary or cardiac disease. Symptoms may begin to occur from 6 to 36 hours after change of altitude. HAPE can also occur in patients who normally live at high altitudes but go to sea level for 2 or more weeks and then return to high altitude. It may be seen in patients with no history of cardiac or pulmonary disease who have marked hypertension. Therapeutic intervention is return to a lower altitude, oxygen therapy, and bed rest.

ASTHMA

Asthma is reversible airway disease where there is an obstruction of air flow caused by one or more of the following (''the three S's''):

Spasm
Swelling
Secretions

These produce bronchospasm, hypoxia, and anxiety. Asthma may occur at any age and may be the result of:

Bronchial-tree sensitivity to inhalants such as dust, pollen, mold, animal dander, gases, or insecticides
Ingestion of foods such as shellfish, milk, or chocolate
Stress and depression
Exercise
Smoking
Pulmonary emboli
Allergies
Cardiogenic causes
Nasal polyps
Hiatal hernia
Mechanical obstructions (such as tumors)

■ **SIGNS AND SYMPTOMS**
Wheezing (most commonly expiratory, but may also be inspiratory); *remember that in severe bronchospasm there may be no wheezing, as there may be no air movement.*
Dyspnea
Cough
Tachycardia
Hypertension
Mild cyanosis
Use of accessory muscles of respiration
Possible history of asthma
Usually a history of upper respiratory infection

■ **THERAPEUTIC INTERVENTIONS**
Bed rest in high Fowler's position
Epinephrine 0.1 to 0.3 ml of 1:1000 solution subcutaneously (adult dosage)
Oxygen
Bronchodilators—0.5 mg albuterol in 2.5 cc NS via nebulizer
IV NS at 100 to 200 cc/hr
Corticosteroids
Fluid and electrolyte replacement
Much verbal reassurance

STATUS ASTHMATICUS

Status asthmaticus is severe asthma that does not respond to epinephrine. The diagnosis is usually made through the patient's history.

■ **SIGNS AND SYMPTOMS**
Dyspnea (usually increases gradually over a few days)
Chest tightness
Tachycardia
Nonproductive cough
Wheezing on inspiration and expiration (if bronchospasm is severe there may be no wheezing because there may be no air movement)
Anxiety
Sitting forward, using accessory muscles of respiration
Mild cyanosis
Distended neck veins in expiration

■ **THERAPEUTIC INTERVENTIONS**
Arterial blood gas determinations
Humidified oxygen
Bronchodilators by inhalation
IV NS at 1000 cc/hr or greater
Epinephrine 0.4 ml of 1:1000 solution subcutaneously every half hour for three to five doses
Aminophylline 500 mg in 50 ml D_5W IV over 5 to 10 minutes (adult) followed by continuous infusion at 0.6 mg/kg/hr

Intubation if severe
Corticosteroids
Antacids
Expectorants
Accurate recording of intake and output

BRONCHITIS

Bronchitis is a syndrome in which there is a frequent and productive cough. The cause of bronchitis is believed to be chronic irritation of the bronchial mucosa by such things as smoking, air pollution, or chronic inhalation of irritant substances.

■ **SIGNS AND SYMPTOMS**
Dyspnea
Productive cough that worsens in the evenings or when there is damp weather

■ **THERAPEUTIC INTERVENTIONS**
Removing the cause (the source of the irritation)
Moving to a climate where there is warm, dry, dust-free air if possible
Rest
Relaxation
Bronchodilators
Expectorants
Antibiotics
Fluids (at least 4 liters per day by mouth)

CHRONIC OBSTRUCTIVE PULMONARY DISEASE

Chronic obstructive pulmonary disease (COPD) is a process in which there is a loss of elasticity in the lung tissue and destruction of the alveolar walls. The patient with COPD will have much difficulty exhaling and will have difficulty with gas exchange. The specific cause of COPD is not known, but smoking appears to contribute to it (90% of COPD patients have a history of heavy smoking—more than 1 pack per day). Other causative factors may include pollution, industrial inhalants such as silicon, and tuberculosis.

■ **SIGNS AND SYMPTOMS**
Patient states that he or she has emphysema
Severe dyspnea that increases over a number of days
Cyanosis (especially of the lips, nailbeds, and earlobes)
Clubbing of fingers
Faint breath sounds, wheezes, or rales
Prolonged expiratory phase of respiration
Use of accessory muscles of respiration
Subclavicular and tracheal drawing-in on inspiration
Productive cough
History of smoking
Barrel chest

■ **THERAPEUTIC INTERVENTIONS**

Bed rest in high Fowler's position

IV D_5W TKO

Bronchodilators, first line of defense is beta-agonists by inhalation (reduce standard nebulized dose 25 to 50% in patients with known cardiac disease)

Oxygen at 2 L/min; observe the patient carefully; do not hesitate to give oxygen if the patient is hypoxic; the most severe life-threatening problem for these patients is hypoxemia

Adequate hydration

SMOKE INHALATION

The inhalation of smoke and other noxious fumes usually occurs during a fire in an enclosed space. Severe pulmonary damage, such as chemical pneumonitis or asphyxia caused by increased levels of carboxyhemoglobin, may result. The burning of synthetic materials produces noxious chemicals that produce additional problems in the respiratory tract (Table 8-1).

When caring for the victim of smoke inhalation, ask a few questions:

- How long were you exposed?
- Were you in a confined space?
- What type of material burned?
- How much of the material burned?

The primary manifestation of smoke inhalation is pulmonary edema. This may not appear for 24 to 48 hours.

■ **SIGNS AND SYMPTOMS**

Mild irritation of the upper airways or burning pain in the throat or chest

Singed nasal hairs

Hypoxia

TABLE 8-1   Toxic Products of Combustion*

MATERIAL	USE	MAJOR TOXIC CHEMICAL PRODUCTS OF COMBUSTION†
Polyvinyl chloride	Wall and floor covering, telephone cable insulation	Hydrogen chloride (P), phosgene (P), carbon monoxide
Polyurethane foam	Upholstery	Isocyanates, (toluene-2,4-diisocyanate) (P), hydrogen cyanide
Lacquered wood veneer, wallpaper	Wall covering	Acetaldehyde (P), formaldehyde (P), oxides of nitrogen (P), acetic acid
Acrylic	Light diffusers	Acrolein (P)
Nylon	Carpet	Hydrogen cyanide, ammonia (P)
Acrilan	Carpet	Hydrogen cyanide, acrolein (P)
Polystyrene	Miscellaneous	Styrene, carbon monoxide

*From Genovesi MG, Tashkin DP, Chopra S, Morgan M, McElroy C: *Chest* 71:441, 1977.

†P indicates a pulmonary irritant.

Facial burns
Sputum that contains carbon
Rales
Rhonchi
Wheezes
Dyspnea
Restlessness or agitation
Cough
Hoarseness
Other signs of pulmonary edema (usually appear hours later)
■ **THERAPEUTIC INTERVENTIONS**
ABCs
Humidified oxygen
IV D₅W TKO
Arterial blood gas values and appropriate therapy
Carboxyhemoglobin levels
Coughing, chest physical therapy, suctioning
Admission and observation for 24 to 48 hours
Endotracheal intubation, cricothyrotomy, or tracheostomy if indicated
Bronchodilators
Nasogastric tube
Steroids

CARBON MONOXIDE POISONING

Carbon monoxide is a colorless, odorless gas formed by the burning of organic matter. Inhalation of CO can lead to tissue hypoxia. CO has a 200 to 250 times greater affinity for hemoglobin than does oxygen. In the bloodstream CO displaces oxygen from the hemoglobin molecule thus decreasing oxygen content. CO also shifts the oxyhemoglobin dissociation curve to the left. This impairs the ability of hemoglobin to release oxygen molecules and may cause tissue injury. The brain and heart are most sensitive to CO poisoning.
■ **SIGNS AND SYMPTOMS**
Carboxyhemoglobin levels 20% to 40%
Headache
Dizziness
Irritability and confusion
Nausea
Angina (with preexisting heart disease)
Levels greater than 40%
Arrhythmias
Seizures
Coma
■ **TREATMENT**
High-flow oxygen
Intubation
Hyperbaric oxygen therapy

ADULT RESPIRATORY DISTRESS SYNDROME

Adult respiratory distress syndrome (ARDS) (otherwise known as shock lung, Da Nang lung, pulmonary contusion, congestive atelectasis, posttraumatic lung, and traumatic wet lung) is a pulmonary insult caused by a sudden congestion and atelectasis with hyaline membrane formation resulting from loss of surfactant and build-up of mucus along the alveoli. It is a syndrome of acute progressive failure caused by a variety of insults, such as:

Cardiopulmonary bypass
Infection
Pulmonary edema
Inhaled toxins
Hemorrhagic shock
Massive transfusions
Lung contusion
Massive fat emboli
Aspiration
Overdose
Eclampsia
Disseminated intravascular coagulation

Initially the lungs appear normal. Then there is progressive atelectasis, increased interstitial and alveolar edema, and marked ventilation-perfusion abnormalities that result in progressive hypoxemia and difficulty in breathing as lung compliance decreases.

■ **SIGNS AND SYMPTOMS**

Dyspnea
Tachypnea
Cyanosis
Hypoxemia
Hypocapnea
Pulmonary hemorrhage
Hypotension

■ **THERAPEUTIC INTERVENTIONS**

ABCs
Intubation—endotracheal or tracheostomy
Ventilation with volume-cycled ventilator and positive-end expiratory pressure
    (PEEP)
Dehydration with diuretics and fluid restriction
Medication, possibly with steroids to enhance surfactant production; perhaps
    heparin
Suction

Benefits of PEEP

Prevents the collapse of alveoli.
Increases functional residual capacity.
Improves VQ relationship.
Combats pulmonary edema.
Enhances Fio_2

Dangers of PEEP

Oxygen toxicity

Fluid overload

Decreased cardiac output

Possible pneumothorax (especially in patients with chronic obstructive pulmonary disease)

Infection

If PEEP fails, hyperbaric oxygenation may be used if a chamber is readily available, or one may elect to use a bypass oxygenator as a last effort.

NEAR-DROWNING

Drowning is the second leading cause of accidental death in the United States. It is the fourth leading cause of death in children.

Drowning or near-drowning occurs when an individual cannot stay afloat because of fatigue, lack of skill as a swimmer, panic, an acute medical incident while in the water (e.g., a myocardial infarction or a seizure), being traumatized, or hyperventilating in preparation for a long-distance swim underwater. A near-drowning may also be a suicide attempt.

There are three categories of near-drowning and drowning:

dry drowning Asphyxiation caused by decreased oxygen as a result of laryngotracheal spasm (prevents entrance of water as well as oxygen into trachea), causing cerebral anoxia, edema, and unconsciousness.

wet drowning The victim makes a desperate respiratory effort, and the lungs fill with fluid rather than air.

secondary drowning The recurrence of respiratory distress (usually in the form of pulmonary edema or aspiration pneumonia) that occurs following successful resuscitation from the initial near-drowning incident. It can occur anywhere from 3 to 4 minutes to several days after the incident.

Seawater

Seawater is a hypertonic solution; fluid transverses into the alveoli because of an osmotic pull across the alveolar capillary membrane that results in pulmonary edema; it also causes hemoconcentration and hypovolemia.

Fresh water

Fresh water is a hypotonic solution; fluid transverses rapidly out of the alveoli into the blood by diffusion. Because the fresh water contains contaminants such as chlorine, algae, and mud, surfactant breakdown occurs and fluid begins to seep into the alveoli once again, resulting in pulmonary edema; it also causes hemodilution and hypervolemia.

■ **SIGNS AND SYMPTOMS**

History of immersion

Dyspnea that progresses

Wheezing

Rales

Rhonchi

Cough (sometimes with pink, frothy sputum)

Tachycardia
Cyanosis
Elevated temperature (but cold water may cause hypothermia)
Chest pain
Mental confusion
Seizure
Increased muscle tone
Unconsciousness
Respiratory or cardiac arrest

■ **THERAPEUTIC INTERVENTIONS**
ABCs
Protection of cervical spine
Warming
Fresh water—5% dextrose in water
Salt water—Ringer's lactate or normal saline
High-flow oxygen intubation if necessary
Intubation is necessary
PEEP
Frequent suctioning
Elevating head of bed if c-spine cleared
Correction of acid-base imbalances
Antibiotics
Steroids
Isoproterenol or epinephrine for bronchospasm
Bronchodilators
Nasogastric tube
Central venous pressure line, arterial pressure line, or pulmonary capillary
    wedge pressure line
Admission for a minimum of 24 hours of observation
NOTE: Do not attempt to drain fluid from the lungs at the time of the incident, as
this would waste time that could be used in the resuscitation effort.

This chapter reviews many of the common pulmonary conditions seen in the
emergency department. Patients with these conditions often exhibit signs of air
hunger and are usually extremely anxious. Rapid assessment, intervention, and
reasssurance are key to preventing life-threatening respiratory complications.
Airway or breathing problems are often components of other medical emergencies such as multiple trauma or myocardial infarction, which are discussed in
other chapters of this book.

SUGGESTED READINGS

Corre K, Rothstein RJ: Assessing severity of adult asthma and need for hospitalization,
    Ann Emerg Med 14:45, 1985.
George RB et al, eds: *Chest medicine: essentials of pulmonary and critical care medicine.*
    Baltimore, 1990, Williams & Wilkins.
Glankler DM: Caring for the victim of near drowning, *Crit Care Nurse* 13:25, 1993.
Goldstein RA, ed: Advances in the diagnosis and therapy of asthma, *Chest* 87 (suppl):15,
    1988.

Haponik EF, Munster AM: *Respiratory injury: smoke inhalation and burns.* New York, 1990, McGraw-Hill.

May HL: *Emergency medicine.* Boston, 1992, Little, Brown.

Rowe BH, Keller JL, Oxman AD: Effectiveness of steroid therapy in acute asthma, *Am J Emerg Med* 10:301, 1992.

Tintinalli JE: Non-traumatic pneumothorax. In Callaham ME: *Current concepts in emergency medicine.* Toronto, 1987, Decker.

Neurologic Emergencies

Several types of neurologic emergencies bring a patient to the emergency department. Some of the more common ones are presented in this chapter.

HEADACHE

The chief complaint of a headache is a symptom of some underlying disorder and is not a diagnosis in itself. The diagnosis of headache is based on the patient's history.

- Is this the first headache?
- When did it start?
- Was there any trauma?
- Is there nausea or vomiting?
- Is there meningismus?
- Have there been any personality changes since the onset?
- Has there been any memory loss?
- Have there been any recent infections?
- Have there been any recent vision problems? Diplopia? Photophobia?
- Have there been any recent neurologic problems?
- Has blood pressure been elevated? For how long?
- Have there been any emotional problems?
- Is the patient currently taking any medications?
- Has the patient ever had any seizures? Recently?

Using the PQRST mnemonic, assess the pain:

P = Provokes: What makes the pain better? What makes it worse? Has the patient taken any medications for it?

Q = Quality: What does the pain feel like? Describe it.

R = Radiates: Where is the pain? Where does it go?

S = Severity: How severe is the pain? (This is not a particularly good index item for assessing headache because it is very subjective.)

T = Time: When did it start? When did it end? How long did it last?

Some common causes of headache:

Stress

Systemic illness

Intracranial hemorrhage
Intracranial tumor
Intracranial inflammations
Vascular problems
Temporal arteritis
Trauma

Migraine Headache

■ **SIGNS AND SYMPTOMS**
Recurrent pain
Severe pain
Pulsatile pain
Motor and visual problems
Anorexia
Nausea and vomiting
Emotional irritability
Syncope
Diaphoresis
Photophobia/phonophobia
Gastrointestinal disturbances
May be preceded by ''aura''
Possible family history of migraines

Cluster Headaches *(a form of migraine headache)*

■ **SIGNS AND SYMPTOMS**
Unilateral pain
Severe pain
Pain usually on one side of face or in one eye
Nasal congestion
Lacrimation
Ptosis
Diaphoresis
■ **THERAPEUTIC INTERVENTION**
Pain relief
    Usually with dihydroergotamine or sumatriptan
    Possibly with a narcotic analgesic
Nausea and vomiting relief
    With antiemetics
Anxiety relief
    With a sedative

Tension Headaches

Tension headaches usually occur in times of emotional distress. Pain is believed to be caused by contraction of the scalp and the muscles of the cervical area.

■ **SIGNS AND SYMPTOMS**
Dull headache (a tight, constricting feeling)
Bilateral pain (frontal or occipital)
■ **THERAPEUTIC INTERVENTIONS**
Mild analgesics
Identifying the cause of the pain and treating it

Traumatic Headaches

Local tissue damage from trauma may result in a headache, probably caused by muscle contractions and tension on the extracranial vasculature. Concussions and contusions are frequently followed by headaches. Intracerebral bleeds are usually accompanied by the complaint of a severe headache if the patient is conscious. For further information on intracranial bleeds, see Chapter 18.

Extracranial Headaches

There are many causes of extracranial headaches. These may include:
Glaucoma
Toothaches
Ear problems
Sinus congestion
These headaches are treated in accordance with their cause.

Temporal Arteritis

Temporal arteritis is a condition in which there is severe headache in one temporal area. The pain may also involve the neck or jaw area or both.
■ **SIGNS AND SYMPTOMS**
Severe headache
Patient is usually over 50 years old
Pain when temporal area is touched
Visual disturbances
History of polymyalgia rheumatica
■ **THERAPEUTIC INTERVENTIONS**
Steroids
Biopsy for definite diagnosis

HYPERTENSION

Hypertension is a product of cardiac output multiplied by peripheral vascular resistance. It can be benign or malignant (Table 9-1). A patient with a blood pressure of 160/90 or higher should be considered hypertensive. A diastolic blood pressure of greater than 130 mm HG is considered a hypertensive crisis. If hypertension is present with any of the following, the situation is considered an absolute emergency:
Cerebrovascular accident

TABLE 9-1 Comparison of Benign and Malignant Hypertension

	BENIGN (GRADUAL PHASE)	MALIGNANT (ACCELERATED PHASE)
Duration	More than 10 years	Less than 2 years
Onset	Gradual; frequently asymptomatic	Sudden; symptomatic
Encephalopathy	Rarely	Often

Myocardial infarction
Grade III or IV retinopathy
Angina pectoris
Congestive heart failure
Renal insufficiency
Aortic dissection

The elevated blood pressure may be determined in the following ways:

On physical examination (especially with sustained abdominal bruit)
In accordance with family history
By age (if the patient is less than 25 years old and has hypertension, it is probably caused by renal vascular disease)
By laboratory examination (urinalysis, BUN, creatinine, electrolytes, uric acid, calcium, lipids, and glucose)
By chest x-ray examination
By ECG
By intravenous pyelogram

Some patients will have an elevated blood pressure but no evidence of end-organ damage. This may be because the blood pressure increase is secondary to some other problems, such as:

Drug withdrawal (especially clonidine or propranolol)
Drug interactions (such as the combination of monoamine oxidase inhibitors and Chianti wine)
Direct drug effects (such as from amphetamines, tricyclics, or phencyclidine)
Pheochromocytoma
Head trauma
Guillain-Barré syndrome

Therapeutic intervention focuses on the underlying cause. Essential hypertension usually originates from the kidneys, adrenal glands, nervous system, coarctation of the aorta, or toxemia.

■ **SIGNS AND SYMPTOMS**

Headache
Epistaxis
Tinnitus
Syncope

■ **COMPLICATIONS (Table 9-2)**

Minor

Coronary hypertrophy

TABLE 9-2 Complications of Hypertension

	I	II	III	IV
Fundi	Vascular spasms	Vascular sclerosis	Hemorrhage and/or exudates	Papilledema
Heart	Left ventricular hypertrophy	Congestive heart failure	Myocardial ischemia	Myocardial infarction
Vascular	Atherosclerosis	Aneurysm with or without rupture	Dissection of aneurysm	Rupture of aneurysm
Brain	Cerebrovascular insufficiency	Encephalopathy	Cerebral thrombosis	Intracranial or subarachnoid hemorrhage
Renal	Benign nephrosclerosis	Malignant nephrosclerosis	Impaired renal function; low specific gravity; proteinuria; hematuria	Elevated creatinine and BUN

Left ventricular hypertrophy
Grade III retinopathy
Abnormal ECG or dysrhythmias
Conduction disturbances
Major
Cerebrovascular accident
Aortic dissection
Congestive heart failure
Renal insufficiency
Encephalopathy
Grade IV retinopathy
Myocardial infarction
Cerebral thrombosis
Peripheral vascular insufficiency
Sudden death

Hypertensive Encephalopathy

■ **SIGNS AND SYMPTOMS**
Fluctuating levels of consciousness or coma
Headaches
Seizures
Grade IV retinopathy
■ **THERAPEUTIC INTERVENTIONS**
Administration of an antihypertensive agent (Table 9-3)
Treatment of underlying condition

TABLE 9-3 Commonly Used Antihypertensive Medications

DRUG	COMMON BRAND NAME	DOSE (DAILY)	MAJOR ACTION	COMMON SIDE EFFECTS	UNIQUE PROBLEMS
Thiazide diuretics	Diuril, Hydrodiuril, Esidrix, Zaroxolyn	0.5-2 g 25-50 mg 25-100 mg 5-10 mg	Renal sodium and water increase by inhibition of Na reabsorption in distal tubule	Hypokalemia, decreased glomerular filtration rate, increased uric acid	Further compromise of impaired renal or hepatic functions, severe hyperglycemia
Furosemide	Lasix	40-200 mg	Inhibits Na reabsorption in ascending limb of Henle's loop	Fluid and electrolyte imbalance, hyperuricemia	Eighth nerve damage (rare)
Alpha-methyldopa	Aldomet	1-2 g	Central effect most profound	Sedation, postural hypotension, retention of sodium and water, impotence common	Positive direct Coombs' test (20%), hemolytic anemia, reversible liver damage, drug fever
Propranolol	Inderal	80-160 mg (may be much higher)	Beta-adrenergic blockade	Exacerbates congestive heart failure, exacerbates asthma, many central nervous system side effects (e.g., depression, hallucinations)	Masks signs and symptoms of hypoglycemia
Clonidine	Catapres	0.4-2 g	Many actions both peripheral and central (most important); causes stimulation of central centers that inhibit sympathetics	Dry mouth, sedation	Hyperirritability, marked rebound of hypertension with acute withdrawal
Hydralazine	Apresoline	100-200 mg/day, rarely more than 400 mg/day	Direct relaxation of smooth muscles, arteries much more than veins	Numerous effects including headaches, palpitations, dizziness, nasal congestion, flushing, peripheral neuropathy, myocardial ischemia	Acute rheumatoid states (10%), lupus-like syndrome

Drug	Preparation	Dose	Mechanism	Side effects	Additional effects
Reserpine (rarely used)	Many preparations such as Serpasil	0.1-1.0 mg	Depletes catecholamine status leading to decreased peripheral resistance and cardiac output	Depression (do not use if patient is depressed), gastrointestinal upset	Extrapyramidal tract signs, gastrointestinal bleeding
Spironolactone	Aldactone	100 mg	Competitive antagonist of aldosterone in renal tubules	Hyperkalemia with or without other diuretics	Gynecomastia, masculinization, gastrointestinal upset
Triamterene	Dyrenium	200-300 mg	Direct action on tubular transport, not competitive antagonist of aldosterone	Hyperkalemia	Gastrointestinal symptoms, megaloblastic anemia (rare)
Prazosin	Minipress	3 mg to start, with first dose 1 mg only; may increase to 20 mg slowly	Alpha-adrenergic blocking agent at postsynaptic receptors	Postural hypotension; syncope, especially in salt-depleted patient (first dose phenomenon); palpitations, drowsiness, headache	Positive antinuclear factor ($\frac{1}{3}$ of patients)
Minoxidil	Loniten	10-40 mg	Vasodilation by direct relaxation of arteriolar smooth muscle	Fluid retention, reflex activation of sympathetic nervous system	Pericardial effusion
Guanethidine	Ismelin	25-50 mg	Inhibition of sympathetic nerves, inhibition of indirect activity of sympathetic amines (e.g., tyramine), presynaptic action caused by impaired release of neurotransmitter from peripheral adrenergic neurons	Postural hypotension (severe), weakness, fluid retention, precipitation of congestive heart failure	Hypertensive crisis (rare) with use in patients with pheochromocytoma or with sympathomimetics in "cold remedies"; in relation to tricyclics, guanethidine action is antagonized, and if tricyclics are withdrawn, profound hypotension may result if guanethidine is continued.

Continued

TABLE 9-3 Commonly Used Antihypertensive Medications—cont'd

DRUG	COMMON BRAND NAME	DOSE (DAILY)	MAJOR ACTION	COMMON SIDE EFFECTS	UNIQUE PROBLEMS
Labetalol	Normodyne	600 mg	Vasodilation by alpha, adreno-receptor blockade; also beta blockade	Fatigue, dizziness Postural hypotension (uncommon) Bradycardia (uncommon) Contraindications: Asthma Heart failure Heart block Severe tachycardia	Hypertensive crisis possible if used when pheochromocytoma is present
Captopril	Capoten	75-450 mg	Competitive inhibition of angiotensin-I converting enzyme	Proteinuria Hypotension, especially when CHF is present Elevated BUN	Agranulocytosis

From Rosen P et al: *Emergency medicine*, ed 2. St Louis, 1987, Mosby.

Hypertensive Cerebrovascular Syndromes (Transient Ischemic Attacks and Hemorrhages)

■ **SIGNS AND SYMPTOMS**
Headache
Decreased level of consciousness
■ **THERAPEUTIC INTERVENTIONS**
For intracerebral bleeding
Oxygen
Furosemide
Possible surgery
For cerebrovascular accident
Sodium nitroprusside

Toxemia

■ **SIGNS AND SYMPTOMS**
Elevated blood pressure
Peripheral edema
Proteinuria
Seizures
Decreased level of consciousness
■ **THERAPEUTIC INTERVENTIONS**
Immediate delivery (via induction of labor or cesarean section)
Diazoxide
Sodium nitroprusside
Magnesium sulfate for seizures

Left Ventricular Failure

■ **SIGNS AND SYMPTOMS**
Dyspnea
Pink, frothy sputum
Rales
Bronchospasm
■ **THERAPEUTIC INTERVENTIONS**
Oxygen
Antihypertensive agent

Aortic Dissection (See also Chapter 7)

■ **SIGNS AND SYMPTOMS**
Chest pain that radiates to back
Hypertension
Blood pressure discrepancies between arms
Pulse discrepancies between femoral areas

■ **THERAPEUTIC INTERVENTIONS**
Sodium nitroprusside
Beta blockade
Surgery

Drug Overdose

■ **THERAPEUTIC INTERVENTIONS**
Sodium nitroprusside

Drug Withdrawal

■ **THERAPEUTIC INTERVENTIONS**
Clonidine—alpha and beta blockade
Propranolol—bed rest, nitroglycerin

Pulmonary Edema

■ **SIGNS AND SYMPTOMS**
Shortness of breath
Possible chest tightness
Anxiety
Inability to lie flat
Rales, rhonchi, wheezes
Distended neck veins
Pink, frothy sputum
■ **THERAPEUTIC INTERVENTIONS**
Morphine sulfate
Nitroglycerin
Oxygen/positive pressure
Furosemide
Bed rest in high Fowler's position
Aminophylline
Monitor condition

MAO Inhibitors

■ **THERAPEUTIC INTERVENTIONS**
Phentolamine
Phenoxybenzamine

Glomerulonephritis

■ **THERAPEUTIC INTERVENTIONS**
Hydralazine
Diazoxide
Furosemide

Hyperthyroidism

■ **THERAPEUTIC INTERVENTIONS**
Alpha and beta blockade
Iodine
Propylthiouracil

SEIZURES

A seizure is a symptom, not a disease. It is a period of abnormal electrical activity in the brain. There are two classes of seizures:
   Generalized, which include tonic-clonic and absence
   Partial, which includes focal
Seizures may occur as a result of head trauma, tumor, vascular disorders, metabolic abnormalities, overdoses, or infections. It is important to obtain past history of seizures, information on what happened preceding the seizure, any history of recent trauma, and the patient's vital signs.

Generalized Seizures

Tonic-clonic (formerly Grand Mal)

In tonic-clonic seizure there is a sudden loss of organized muscle tone. This causes a severely decreased level of consciousness, extensor muscle spasms, apnea, and bilateral clonic movements. The patient fades into a postictal state in which there is muscle relaxation, deep breathing, and a depressed level of consciousness. The seizures may be idiopathic or may be caused by an easily identifiable condition, such as hypoxia.

■ **THERAPEUTIC INTERVENTIONS**
Protect airway patency, administer oxygen.
Protect patient from injury.
Administer naloxone 0.8 mg and dextrose 50% 50 ml IV if cause is unknown.
Give diazepam IV or lorazepam IV.

Absence (formerly Petit Mal)

Absence seizures are usually caused by a cortical lesion and generally occur in children between 4 and 12 years old. The child may appear confused and disinterested, have a glassy stare, blink, and make lip-smacking movements. During the seizure the patient may respond to verbal commands.

■ **THERAPEUTIC INTERVENTIONS**
Diazepam IV
Ethosuximide IV

Partial Seizures

Focal (Jacksonian) seizure

Focal or Jacksonian seizures usually occur unilaterally and are caused by a focal brain lesion such as a tumor, abscess, infarction, or eschar. This type of seizure is usually not life-threatening, but it does not respond well to anticonvulsant medications.

■ **THERAPEUTIC INTERVENTIONS**
Diazepam or phenobarbital (although they may not work)
Be sure to do a brief neurologic examination on all seizure patients once the postictal period has passed.

Status Epilepticus

Status epilepticus is a series of consecutive seizures or a continuous seizure that is not responsive to traditional therapeutic interventions.

■ **THERAPEUTIC INTERVENTIONS**
Try to determine the cause once the seizure is controlled.
Treat the cause if possible.
Clear the airway.
Provide oxygen (consider 100% oxygen and endotracheal intubation if seizure is prolonged).
Consider IV.
Consider naloxone.
Consider dextrose 50%—50 ml.
Consider thiamine 50 to 100 mg if possibility of alcoholism exists.
Consider diazepam 2.5 mg increments IV, ET, or per rectum (to 15 mg) adult dose.
Consider phenytoin 25 to 50 mg/min loading dose (to 1 g) adult dose; be sure to give phenytoin via *normal saline solution,* not D$_5$W. Patient should also be on a cardiac monitor.
Consider phenobarbital 130 mg every 10 to 15 minutes (to 1 g)—adult dose.
Consider paraldehyde 1 to 4 ml IV or 5 to 10 ml IM—adult dose.
Consider general anesthesia if status has not responded to any of these.

STROKE (CEREBROVASCULAR ACCIDENT)

Stroke is caused by the occlusion or rupture of a cerebral blood vessel by occlusion or hemorrhage.

Occlusion

Embolus—From the heart or large arteries, caused by atrial fibrillation, myocardial infarction, or surgery; sudden onset.
Thrombosis—Often the cause of a transient ischemic episode; gradual onset. It is often caused by hypertension, age, diabetes, smoking, or elevated lipids.

Hemorrhage

Intracerebral bleeding—sudden onset; usually resulting from hypertension.
Subarachnoid bleeding—sudden onset; there are no known risk factors.
Cerebellar bleeding—sudden onset; usually resulting from hypertension.

■ **SIGNS AND SYMPTOMS**

Headache
Vertigo
Ataxia
Nausea and vomiting
Sudden neurologic deficit
Unequal pupils
Hemiparesis
Aphasia/dysphasia
Dysphagia
Decerebrate posturing
Sleepiness
Coma
Decreased BP on left side (left subclavian artery occlusion)
Frequently occurs in early morning hours
Find out if the patient has a history of any of the following:

Hypertension	Subacute bacterial endocarditis
Hyperlipidemia	Prosthetic heart valve
Diabetes	Collagen disease
Smoking	Use of birth control pills
Heart problems	Recent neck trauma
Atrial fibrillation	

■ **THERAPEUTIC INTERVENTIONS**

Ensure ABCs.
Keep the patient lying flat. This causes loss of autoregulation and a decreased
  mean arterial pressure. (Remember, cerebral perfusion pressure is equal to
  mean arterial pressure minus intracranial pressure.)
Decrease blood pressure—usually with nitroprusside.
Correct dysrhythmias.
Consider anticoagulants.
Consider aspirin.
Consider surgery.
Consider osmotic diuretics to decrease cerebral edema.
Consider steroids.
Consider antipyretics.
Consider seizure prophylaxis.
NOTE: If diagnosis of stroke is certain, do not administer dextrose 50%.

Categories of Cerebrovascular Accident

Transient ischemic attack

A transient ischemic attack (TIA) is a neurologic deficit that lasts for less than
12 hours. Most last only about 5 to 30 minutes. There are two causes, thrombosis and embolus. A TIA may be a prodrome to a cerebrovascular accident.

Reversible ischemic neurologic deficit

Symptoms will occur over 24 hours and may last for weeks. The patient may have minimal, partial, or no permanent deficit.

Stroke in evolution

Symptoms last longer than 24 hours with an increasing neurologic deterioration, with residual deficits present.

Completed stroke

There will be permanent neurologic damage.

■ **THERAPEUTIC INTERVENTIONS**
Ensure ABCs.
Consider anticoagulants.
Consider surgery.

UNCONSCIOUSNESS

Unconsciousness is by definition the opposite of consciousness. It is the depression of consciousness or the lack of awareness of self or anything surrounding self. This condition continues despite attempts to provide a stimulus. There are two causes of coma—structural lesions and metabolic or toxic states.

Examine the patient to determine if the coma is focal or diffuse and if it seems to be organic (as it is 95% of the time) or functional. Ascertain whether the patient is improving or getting worse with each passing minute. Pay strict attention to the ABCs. Perform a brief neurologic examination.

■ **THERAPEUTIC INTERVENTIONS**
The main purpose of therapeutic intervention is to protect the patient from further deterioration and to try to isolate the cause of the unconsciousness.
ABCs
Naloxone 0.8 mg IV, to rule out narcotic overdose
Dextrose 50% 50 ml IV, to rule out hypoglycemia and to protect the brain from hypoglycemia
Thiamine 50 to 100 mg IV, if alcohol abuse is suspected, to prevent Wernicke Korsakoff syndrome
Flumazenil to rule out benzodiazepine overdose
Left lateral swimmer's position with head dependent to prevent aspiration
Cervical spine precautions, if trauma is a possibility
Hyperventilate with 100% oxygen if head trauma is suspected as the cause
Other treatment depends on findings.
The causes of unconsciousness can be remembered using a simple mnemonic:
A = Alcoholism
E = Epilepsy/environmental conditions
I = Insulin (too much or too little)
O = Overdose (or underdose)
U = Uremia (or other metabolic causes)
T = Trauma or tumors
I = Infection or ischemia

P = Psychiatric
S = Stroke (i.e., CVA or other neurologic or cardiovascular causes)
In the differential diagnosis process, be sure to assess the following:

Temperature	Presence of paralysis
Respirations	Occurrence of trauma
Blood pressure	Abdomen
Pulse	Extremities
Skin vital signs (color, temperature, moistness)	Presence of Babinski's reflex
Pupils	Presence of Battle's sign
Breath odor	Presence of hematotympanum
Presence of needle tracks	Presence of raccoon eyes
Presence of petechiae	Presence of Brudzinski's sign
Lung sounds	Presence of Kernig's sign
Deep tendon reflexes	Presence of incontinence
Presence of posturing	Presence of tongue lacerations

Consider the following laboratory tests to assist with diagnosis:

CBC	Urinalysis
Platelet count	Monitor:
Electrolyte levels	ECG
Glucose levels (serum and urine)	Cerebrospinal fluid pressure
BUN	X-ray examinations:
Creatinine levels	skull
Toxicology screen	face
Cholesterol level	chest
Magnesium level	abdomen
Calcium level	Scan:
Phosphorus level	head
Bilirubin level	lungs

BOTULISM

Botulism is caused by the ingestion of foods that have been improperly canned (high bacteria content before canning), especially those with low acid content, such as green beans. It can also occur in infants who have been fed unprocessed raw honey.

■ **SIGNS AND SYMPTOMS**

Usually develop 12 to 36 hours after ingestion of contaminated food, but may be delayed up to 4 days.

Dilated fixed pupils/limited eye movement
Dry mouth/sore throat
Diplopia
Urinary retention
Distended abdomen
Postural hypotension
Difficulty swallowing
Constipation
Headache

Decreased deep tendon reflexes
Difficulty chewing
Nasal tone to voice
Respiratory paralysis
Patient remains awake and alert throughout
NOTE: May mimic stroke, Guillain-Barré syndrome, myasthenia gravis, or arsenic intoxication.

■ **LABORATORY TEST**
Blood specimens for determination of presence of toxins

■ **THERAPEUTIC INTERVENTIONS**
ICU admission
ABCs (especially good respiratory support)—may require tracheostomy and
  ventilator assistance
Gastric lavage or emesis if ingestion is recent—then magnesium sulfate, as
  toxin is slowly absorbed
Antitoxin
Reporting to CDC in Atlanta

GUILLAIN-BARRÉ SYNDROME

Guillain-Barré syndrome is an acute paralytic disease that causes a decrease of
myelin in the nerve roots and the peripheral nerves.

■ **SIGNS AND SYMPTOMS**
Tingling sensation in the extremities (for hours to weeks)
Severely decreased deep tendon reflexes
Symmetrical paralysis, usually beginning in lower extremities and gradually
  ascending to respiratory muscles

■ **THERAPEUTIC INTERVENTIONS**
ABCs (consider endotracheal intubation and ventilator)
General supportive care

MYASTHENIA GRAVIS

Myasthenia gravis is a defect in neuromuscular transmission. It is most common
in persons in their twenties and thirties, and occurs more frequently in females
than males. Myasthenia gravis usually affects only the facial and neck muscles;
in a myasthenia crisis there is a sudden onset that may cause respiratory
paralysis.

■ **SIGNS AND SYMPTOMS**
Increasing fatigue
Delayed recovery of muscle strength
Weak eye muscles
Weak facial muscles
Weak jaw muscles
Weak pharyngeal muscles
Diplopia
Dysphagia

Inability to handle secretions
Possible aspiration
■ **THERAPEUTIC INTERVENTIONS**
ABCs (consider endotracheal intubation)
Neostigmine 1 mg IV in myasthenia crisis
Medications that precipitate myasthenia include:
Barbiturates
Opiates
Quinidine
Quinine
Any muscle relaxants
Andrenocorticotropic hormone (ACTH)
Steroids
Aminoglycosides
Certain antibiotics

PARALYTIC SHELLFISH POISONING

Saxitoxin is a toxin produced by marine protozoans that interferes with neuron membrane permeability to sodium ions. The toxin is consumed by shellfish such as oysters, clams, and sea snails that produce the phenomenon known as *red tide*. When these shellfish are consumed by humans, they cause paralytic shellfish poisoning.

■ **SIGNS AND SYMPTOMS**
Paresthesias (progressive)
Paresthesias of the mouth and head only
Dysphagia
Tremors
Vertigo
Flaccid quadriplegia
Dysarthria
Respiratory paralysis
■ **THERAPEUTIC INTERVENTIONS**
ABCs (consider endotracheal intubation and ventilator)
Good supportive care
The prognosis for paralytic shellfish poisoning is usually good after 24 hours.

As is obvious from the headings in this chapter, neurologic emergencies covers a wide variety of topics from the not-so-serious to the life-threatening. It is extremely important for emergency nurses to be familiar with all aspects of neurologic emergencies to be better able to intervene in the life-threatening events.

SUGGESTED READINGS

Abbott RO et al: Risk of stroke in male cigarette smokers, *N Engl J Med* 315:717, 1986.
Auer RV: Progressive review: hypoglycemic brain damage, *Stroke* 17:699, 1986.
Cherington M et al: Lightning strikes: nature of neurological damage in patients evaluated in hospital emergency departments, *Ann Emerg Med,* 21(5):575, 1992.

Frommer DA: Stroke. In Rosen P et al, eds: *Emergency medicine,* ed 2. St Louis, 1987, Mosby.

Gill JS et al: Stroke and alcohol consumption, *N Engl J Med* 315:1041, 1986.

Gillum RF et al: International diagnostic criteria for acute myocardial infarction and acute stroke, *Am Heart J* 108:150, 1984.

Henry GL: *Headache.* In Rosen P et al, eds: *Emergency medicine,* ed 2. St Louis, 1987, Mosby.

Huff JS: *Coma.* In Rosen P et al, eds: *Emergency medicine,* ed 2. St Louis, 1987, Mosby.

Joint National Committee on Detection, Evaluation, and Treatment of High Blood Pressure: The 1984 Report of the Joint National Committee on detection, evaluation, and treatment of high blood pressure, *Arch Intern Med* 144:1045, 1984.

Matthews J: *Hypertension.* In Rosen P et al, eds: *Emergency medicine,* ed 2. St Louis, 1987, Mosby.

Tomlanovich MC, and Yee AS: Seizure. In Rosen P et al, eds: *Emergency medicine,* ed 2. St Louis, 1987, Mosby Co.

Whisnanta JP: The decline of stroke, *Stroke* 15:160, 1984.

Abdominal Pain

Abdominal pain is a symptom, not a diagnosis. The fact that the patient is complaining of abdominal pain is indicative of something happening that is causing this symptom to appear. Some conditions change so quickly that approximately one half of presenting diagnoses are changed by the time patients receive appropriate treatment. There are three types of abdominal pain—visceral, parietal, and referred.

Visceral Pain

Visceral pain may be caused by the stretching of a viscus. The patient usually describes it as cramping or gas pains. It is pain that intensifies and then decreases and is usually centered around the midline of the abdomen. It is a diffuse pain that is difficult to localize on examination. In response to the pain, the patient may be diaphoretic and have nausea and vomiting, decreased blood pressure, tachycardia, and spasms of the abdominal wall muscles. Many inflammatory conditions begin with the signs and symptoms of visceral pain. Some of these more common conditions include:

Appendicitis
Cholecystitis
Pancreatitis
Intestinal obstruction

Parietal Pain

Parietal pain develops after visceral pain. It is a steady aching pain that is caused by inflammation. Parietal pain is stimulated by palpation or any tension in the peritoneal area. The pain is more localized. Parietal pain is associated with appendicitis.

Referred Pain

Referred pain is pain felt away from the original source of the pain. One theory is that this occurs as a result of fetal development and nerve growth or relocation.

PROBLEM AREA	PAIN REFERRED TO
Fluid collected under diaphragm	Top of shoulder
Ruptured peptic ulcer	Back
Pancreas	Midline back or directly through to back
Biliary tract	Around right side to scapula
Dissecting or ruptured aneurysm	Low back and thighs
Renal colic	Groin and external genitalia
Appendix	May be epigastric region
Uterine disease	Low back
Rectal disease	Low back

It is important for the caregiver to note that each individual reacts differently to pain. Someone whose condition would normally show a demonstration of severe pain may not demonstrate it. Someone whose condition would lead one to believe that the expression of pain should be minimal may complain of severe pain. Treat each patient individually, in accordance with the perceived expression of pain.

ASSESSMENT OF THE PATIENT WITH ABDOMINAL PAIN

There are three points to consider when examining a patient with abdominal pain:

Try to determine the possible diagnosis.

Try to determine if the patient requires hospital admission.

Try to determine if the patient requires surgery.

When assessing the patient with a complaint of abdominal pain, the caregiver should use a format that is easy to remember and one that will provide a complete assessment. A tool that could be used is the "PQRST" mnemonic:

- **P** = Provokes

  What provokes the pain?

  Is there anything that makes it better?

  Is there anything that makes it worse?

- **Q** = Quality

  Ask the patient to describe the pain. Do not make suggestions unless the patient is unable to describe the pain. If the patient needs some "help," suggest words such as "sharp," "dull," or "pressure." If the pain is caused by an event in the hollow viscus, the patient may describe the pain as "like being punched in the gut."

DESCRIPTION	POSSIBLE CAUSE
Severe, sharp	Infarction or rupture
Severe, controlled by medication	Pancreatitis, peritonitis, small bowel obstruction, renal colic, biliary colic
Dull	Inflammation, low-grade infection
Intermittent pain	Gastroenteritis, small bowel obstruction

- **R** = Radiates

  Ask the patient to point to the location of the pain. Ask if the pain radiates to any other place.

- **S** = Severity
  Ask the patient, "On a scale of 1 to 10, with 1 being the least and 10 being the worst, give the pain a number." This is a very subjective finding and will vary in accordance with how the patient tolerates pain.
- **T** = Time
  Ask the patient how long he or she has had the pain. Ask when it started and when it ended. Ask if this pain has ever been felt before. Pain of sudden onset is usually associated with rupture, tortion, strangulation, or vascular problems. Pain that is gradual in onset is usually caused by an inflammatory or obstructive process, such as pain that occurs with appendicitis or intestinal obstruction. Generally, the more acute the underlying process, the more acute the pain.

ASSOCIATED SIGNS AND SYMPTOMS

Nausea, Vomiting, and Anorexia

When nausea and vomiting appear to be the highlights of the clinical findings, the most likely causes are gastroenteritis, acute gastritis, pancreatitis, or an obstruction located high in the intestinal structure. If vomiting is intractible or feces are present in the vomitus, this suggests an intestinal obstruction in progress. If there is blood in the vomitus, this suggests gastritis or gastric ulcer. If pain precedes vomiting, this suggests appendicitis.

Diarrhea and Constipation

When there is abdominal involvement in an emergency situation, it is often accompanied by a change in bowel content.

DESCRIPTION	POSSIBLE CAUSE
Diarrhea	Inflammatory disease
Constipation (or no flatus)	Dehydration, paralytic ileus, intestinal obstruction
Clay-colored stool	Biliary obstruction
Melena (black tarry stool)	High intestinal bleeding
Bright red blood	Low intestinal bleeding
Bloody diarrhea	Amebic dysentery, Crohn's disease, ulcerative colitis

Fever and Chills

Repeated fever and chills indicate bacterial infection, pyelonephritis, or appendicitis. Intermittent fever and chills may indicate acute cholecystitis.

Urinary Tract Symptoms

SYMPTOM	MAY INDICATE
Burning on urination	Urinary tract infection
Pain on urination	Obstruction somewhere in urinary tract
Hematuria or dysuria	Urinary tract infection or renal colic

Gynecologic Symptoms

Most gynecologic symptoms indicate gynecologic problems, such as pelvic inflammatory disease, ruptured ectopic pregnancy, ruptured ovarian cyst, or ruptured corpus luteum. Vaginal bleeding may indicate miscarriage, ruptured ectopic pregnancy, or one of many other gynecologic disorders.

Gastrointestinal Upset

If a meal was consumed by several people but only one person complains of associated signs and symptoms, the caregiver should rule out the possibility of gastroenteritis. If many persons complain of GI problems, there is a possibility of food poisoning. If there is a history of ingestion of fatty foods followed by abdominal pain, this may indicate acute cholecystitis. If there is a history of alcohol abuse, the caregiver must be sure to rule out pancreatitis. If abdominal pain starts just before eating and eating causes relief of pain, the caregiver should assume that the problem may be caused by a gastric ulcer or associated gastric disorder.

Age-Related Factors

Intussusception is rarely seen in persons over age 2. Intestinal obstruction is rarely seen in persons under age 40. Appendicitis occurs most frequently in persons between the ages of 5 and 45.

Remember that if major blood loss and hypovolemia have occurred, the signs of abdominal pain may be obscured.

PAIN IN THE FOUR QUADRANTS OF THE ABDOMEN

Physical Examination and Laboratory Analysis

Sometimes the patient's physical appearance offers clues to the diagnosis.
• What position is the patient lying in?
• Vital signs
  Temperature will often be normal for a while and then elevate in the course of the disease process. Temperature will elevate if there is a rupture or peritonitis or when an infection is fulminant.
  Pulse will usually be evidenced as tachycardia.
  Respirations will be shallow, and there will be very little motion of the abdominal wall when there is peritonitis. Rapid respirations may indicate shock pancreatitis or peritonitis.
  Hypotension may indicate an acute condition that may require surgery.

Inspection
Observe the patient's abdomen.
Check for abdominal wall movement.

If the patient's hips are flexed and the knees drawn up toward the chest, this may be suggestive of appendicitis, a pelvic abscess, or a psoas abscess.

If peristaltic movements or abdominal distension are observed, this may be suggestive of intestinal obstruction.

Ascites may be indicative of liver disease.

An abdominal aneurysm may be evidenced by a visible or palpable abdominal mass.

Auscultation

Bowel sounds are difficult to assess in the emergency care setting because it takes a full 3 to 5 minutes of auscultation before the absence of bowel sounds can be established. Normally, there are 10 to 20 peristaltic sounds per minute (Figure 10-1).

Palpation

Palpate the abdomen as gently as possible. Check for spasms, tenderness, and any masses. Be sure to observe the patient's face during this examination, as this may be a clue to the patient's level of pain. Remember to palpate the area that hurts the most last so the examination can be completed without interruption.

Percussion

Percussion is probably the least useful of all examination tools because it is difficult to assess the findings. Areas that are normally dense will produce dull sounds.

Tympany

Tympany is a sign that gas is present. Conditions that sometimes present with this sign are appendicitis and sigmoid colon obstruction. Urinary retention offers the sign of dullness over the suprapubic area.

Ascites

Ascites (shifting dullness) is the presence of fluid where it normally should not be. Ascites could also suggest a tumor, congestive heart failure, or blood in the peritoneal cavity. If you suspect the patient to have ascites remember to measure the abdominal girth with a tape measure and mark the area. After percussion, proceed to palpation. Start the initial abdominal examination with auscultation first, then proceed to percussion.

Laboratory Tests and X-ray Examination

Perform the following laboratory tests on the patient with abdominal pain:

Serum electrolytes
Serum amylase
Urinalysis
Urine amylase
Complete blood count (including hematocrit and hemoglobin)
Blood urea nitrogen

Right Upper Quadrant

Cholecystis
Hepatitis
Hepatomegly
Biliary Colic
Pancreatitis
Perforated Duodenal Ulcer
Rightsided Nephrolithiosis
Myocardial Ischemia
Right Lung Pneumonia

Right Lower Quadrant

Appendicitis
Intestinal Obstruction
Crohn's Disease
Diverticulosis
Fecal Perforation
Ectopic Pregnancy
Ovarian Cyst
Salpingitis
Strangulated Hernia
Kidney or Ureteral Stone

The Four Quadrants of the Abdomen

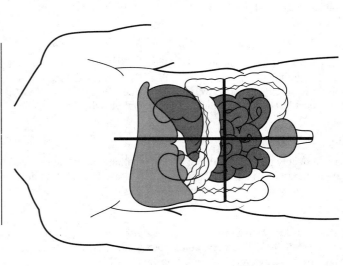

FIGURE 10-1. The four quadrants of the abomen.

Left Upper Quadrant

Pancreatitis
Gastric Ulcers
Gastritis
Splenic Rupture
Diverticulitis
Leftsided Nephrolithies
Myocardial Ischemia
Left Lung Pneumonia
Pulmonary Embolism
Pericarditis

Left Lower Quadrant

Early Appendicitis
Sigmoid Perforation
Sigmoid Diverticulitis
Colon Perforation
Ulcerative Colitis
Salpingitis
Ovarian Cyst
Ectopic Pregnancy
Strangulated Hernia
Kidney or Ureteral Stone

The following x-ray studies may be obtained:
   Upright chest
   Upright abdominal
   Left lateral decubitus
   Plain abdominal film
   Intravenous pyelogram (IVP)
   Intravenous cholangiogram
   Upper GI series
   Lower GI series
Conditions where surgery should be considered:

Appendicitis	Cholecystitis (may consider lithotripsy)
Bowel obstruction	Pancreatitis
Bowel infarction	Salpingitis
Ruptured ectopic pregnancy	Perforation of viscus
Ureteral stone	Ruptured intraabdominal aneurysm
Peritonitis	Massive GI bleed
Diverticulitis	

Chronic conditions where abdominal pain is a major symptom:

Ulcerative colitis	Irritable bowel syndrome
Crohn's disease	Regional enteritis
Reflux esophagitis	

Conditions outside the abdomen that may present with the symptom of abdominal pain:

Hepatitis	Empyema
Rheumatic fever	Pleurisy
Myocardial infarction	Hip joint disease
Pneumothorax	Spinal tumor
Pneumonia	

INFLAMMATORY CONDITIONS THAT CAUSE ABDOMINAL PAIN

Acute Appendicitis

■ **SIGNS AND SYMPTOMS**
   Anorexia
   Nausea and vomiting
   Pain in right lower quadrant, at McBurney's point
   Afebrile (unless ruptured)
   Guarding posture (fetal position, hips flexed and knees drawn up)
   Elevated white count
■ **THERAPEUTIC INTERVENTION**
   IV Ringer's lactate
   If ruptured:
      Nasogastric tube
      Rectal acetaminophen for fever control

Acute Pancreatitis

■ **SIGNS AND SYMPTOMS**
Severe epigastric pain following ingestion of alcohol or large amounts of food
Nausea and vomiting
Abdominal distension
Abdominal tenderness
Abdominal rigidity
■ **THERAPEUTIC INTERVENTION**
IV Ringer's lactate
Analgesia for pain management
Nasogastric tube
Antibiotics
Chest x-ray film (20% to 50% of patients with pancreatitis have associated pulmonary complications)

Ulcerative Colitis

■ **SIGNS AND SYMPTOMS**
Bloody diarrhea
Frequent stools (usually more than 20 per day)
Abdominal cramps
Weight loss
Weakness
If perforated:
  Fever
  Tachycardia
  Generalized signs of sepsis
■ **THERAPEUTIC INTERVENTION**
IV Ringer's lactate or normal saline
Antibiotics
Hospital admission

Toxic Megacolon

Toxic megacolon is a severe dilation of the colon associated with colitis.
■ **SIGNS AND SYMPTOMS**
Fever
Explosive diarrhea
A quiet abdomen
Prostration
Possible shock-like state
■ **THERAPEUTIC INTERVENTION**
IV Ringer's lactate
Hospital admission

Esophagitis

Esophagitis is an inflammation of the hiatal esophagus usually caused by the regurgitation of gastric acids. It is often accompanied by a hiatal hernia or gastric ulcer. It may also be caused by the ingestion of a caustic substance such as lye or another strong alkali or acid.

■ **SIGNS AND SYMPTOMS**
Steady, substernal pain that is increased by swallowing
Occasional vomiting
Weight loss
Obstruction
Bleeding
Foul breath

■ **THERAPEUTIC INTERVENTION**
Bland diet
Antacids
Surgery to correct anatomic defect
If caused by caustic ingestion:
    ABCs
    Dilation of the esophagus
    Antibiotics

Gastritis

Gastritis is an inflammation of the gastric mucosa. It can occur as a result of ingestion of a gastric irritant, hyperacidity, bile reflux, or shock.

■ **SIGNS AND SYMPTOMS**
Epigastric pain
Nausea and vomiting
Mucosal bleeding
Epigastric tenderness on palpation

■ **THERAPEUTIC INTERVENTION**
Antacids
Bland diet
Sedative (if nausea is severe)
Nasogastric tube
Fluid replacement
Anticholinergic medications

Peptic Ulcer

A peptic ulcer can occur in the stomach and the duodenum. It is usually caused by hyperacidity.

■ **SIGNS AND SYMPTOMS**
Burning pain in the epigastric region, usually occurring early in the morning
    and just before meals
Pain relieved by antacids, bland foods, or vomiting

Symptoms that occur during stressful periods when production of gastric acids
   is increased

■ **THERAPEUTIC INTERVENTION**
Antacids
Bland diet
Sedation
Nasogastric tube if severe vomiting
Fluid and electrolyte replacement

OBSTRUCTIVE CONDITIONS THAT CAUSE ABDOMINAL PAIN

Intestinal Obstruction

An intestinal obstruction may be caused by a large variety of syndromes. Intestinal obstruction may be caused by a hernia, fecal impaction, adhesions, tumors, paralytic ileus, intussusception, regional enteritis, volvulus, gallstones, abscesses, and hematomas. There may be a primary mechanical obstruction or a secondary obstruction caused by an inflammatory condition or a nervous system problem. The primary danger of an intestinal obstruction is dehydration. Other dangers include infarction and perforation of the bowel.

■ **SIGNS AND SYMPTOMS**
Nausea and vomiting
Abdominal pain
Constipation/obstipation
Abdominal distension

■ **THERAPEUTIC INTERVENTION**
IV Ringer's lactate or normal saline
Antibiotics
Nasogastric tube
Possible surgery

Cholecystitis

Cholecystitis is an inflammation of the gallbladder that may be exacerbated by the presence of gallstones.

■ **SIGNS AND SYMPTOMS**
Abdominal pain of sudden onset (especially following ingestion of fried or
   greasy foods) in the epigastric region, radiating to the right upper quadrant
Low-grade fever (100.4° F [38° C])
Nausea and vomiting
Local and rebound tenderness
Referred pain into the right subclavicular area
Slight jaundice
Usually overweight, over 40 years old, and female

■ **THERAPEUTIC INTERVENTION**
Nasogastric tube
IV Ringer's lactate or normal saline
Possible surgery

Esophageal Obstruction

Most of the time an esophageal obstruction is the result of a foreign body ingestion.

■ **SIGNS AND SYMPTOMS**
History of foreign body ingestion
Cervical subcutaneous emphysema (if there is a perforation)
Patient complains of "something stuck" in his throat

■ **THERAPEUTIC INTERVENTION**
If the object does not have sharp edges and can pass into the stomach, it can usually pass through the intestines without difficulty.
Retrieval of the object through esophagoscopy.

Incarcerated Hernia

An incarcerated hernia is a protrusion of bowel or other abdominal contents through the abdominal musculature but not through the skin. There is usually a good blood supply to the hernia unless it is incarcerated. Hernias are most commonly found in the inguinal, femoral, and umbilical areas.

■ **SIGNS AND SYMPTOMS**
The patient notices the herniation.
Pain in the abdominal wall following exertion.

■ **THERAPEUTIC INTERVENTION**
If the hernia is not incarcerated, manual attempt, by a surgeon, at replacement
If incarcerated, surgery

HEMORRHAGIC CONDITIONS THAT CAUSE ABDOMINAL PAIN

Upper GI Bleeding

There are several causes of upper GI bleeding, or bleeding proximal to the ligament of Treitz.

■ **SIGNS AND SYMPTOMS**
Hematemesis
Melena (blood and stomach acids mix with stool)
Possible shock
Possible history of chronic alcohol ingestion
Epigastric tenderness
Possible jaundice, an enlarged spleen, and an enlarged liver

Specific areas of upper GI bleeding
Bleeding peptic ulcer

Two thirds of all cases of upper GI bleeding are caused by peptic ulcers. The bleeding is caused by the granulation of the ulcer that erodes into a vessel during the healing process.

■ **THERAPEUTIC INTERVENTION**
ABCs
IV Ringer's lactate or normal saline
Bedrest
Oxygen
Iced-saline gastric lavage through a large (Ewald) tube
Surgery if bleeding is uncontrolled and the patient shows signs and symptoms of shock
Blood replacement

Bleeding Esophageal Varicies

Patients with liver disease have a high risk of developing esophageal varicies. Portal hypertension causes collateral vessels to develop between the stomach and the systemic veins of the lower esophagus. Rupture of these vessels can rapidly cause death. It is the cause of death in over one third of patients with cirrhosis of the liver.

■ **SIGNS AND SYMPTOMS**
Massive bleeding from the upper GI tract
History of chronic alcohol ingestion or portal hypertension

■ **THERAPEUTIC INTERVENTION**
ABCs
Balloon tamponade with a Sengstaaken-Blakemore tube (Figure 10-2)
Intraarterial vasopressin
Surgery

Mallory-Weiss Syndrome

This syndrome is usually caused by retching and vomiting that is not synchronized with gastric regurgitation. This causes bleeding at the cardioesophageal junction.

■ **SIGNS AND SYMPTOMS**
History of retching and vomiting with normal gastric content emptying, followed by hematemesis on subsequent vomiting episodes

■ **THERAPEUTIC INTERVENTION**
Whole blood transfusions
Balloon tamponade with a Sengstaaken-Blakemore tube (Figure 10-2)
Intraarterial vasopressin
Surgery

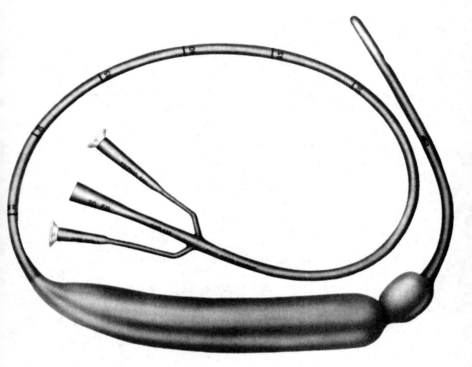

FIGURE 10-2. Blakemore tube.

Borhave's Syndrome

Borhave's syndrome is the term for small tears of the esophagus that are caused by vomiting following a large meal. It is thought to be caused by distension of the esophagus.

■ **SIGNS AND SYMPTOMS**

Bloody expectoration when the patient clears vomitus

Possible massive bleeding if tears are severe

Pain in the esophagus

■ **THERAPEUTIC INTERVENTION**

ABCs

Close observation

Surgery if bleeding is heavy and uncontrolled

Lower GI Bleeding

Bleeding from the large bowel and rectum is usually caused by ruptured diverticula, ulcerative colitis, tumors, cecal ulcers, ruptured hemorrhoids, or polyps.

■ **SIGNS AND SYMPTOMS**
Bright red blood from the rectum
■ **THERAPEUTIC INTERVENTION**
Control of bleeding (depends on the source)
Possible surgery

HOW TO INSERT A NASOGASTRIC TUBE

1. Measure the length of the tube required by measuring from the tip of the patient's earlobe to the tip of the nose and from the tip of the nose to the umbilicus; mark the tube at this point.
2. Explain the procedure to the patient.
3. Lubricate the tube at the tip and a few inches up from the distal end with a water-soluble lubricant.
4. Place the patient in high Fowler's position.
5. Have the patient place his or her head in a sniffing position.
6. Check the patient for a deviated septum.
7. Insert the tube via the nares, instructing the patient to swallow as the tube is being passed; using a small amount of water and having the patient sip and swallow during this process usually helps (unless water is contraindicated).
8. Continue to pass the tube until it is at the level previously marked; if the patient begins to choke or cough during the procedure, stop and allow the patient to rest; if coughing and choking continue, remove the tube and begin again, as the tube may have inadvertently passed into the trachea.
9. Check to be sure the tube is in the stomach (while air is being injected into the tube, auscultate the epigastric region for the sound of air movement or aspirate the tube for the presence of stomach contents.)
10. Secure the tube by taping it to the nose and the forehead.
11. Connect the distal end of the tube to intermittent suction if the tube is single lumen and to continuous suction if the tube is double lumen. (Single-lumen tubes are uncommon in current practice.)

HOW TO INSERT A SENGSTAAKEN-BLAKEMORE TUBE

1. Explain the procedure to the patient.
2. Check the tube balloons for patency.
3. The pharynx may be anesthetized.
4. Lubricate the tube with a water-soluble lubricant at the tip and several inches up from the distal end.
5. Insert the tube via the nares for approximately 50 cm.
6. Check to be sure the tube is in the stomach; while air is being injected into the tube, auscultate the epigastric region for the sound of air movement or aspirate the tube for the presence of stomach contents.
7. Fill the gastric balloon with 200 to 250 ml of radiopaque (Hypaque) dye and double-clamp it.

8. Apply gentle traction to check for placement and to wedge the balloon into the cardioesophageal junction.
9. Aspirate the stomach contents to check for continued bleeding; if bleeding is present, inflate the esophageal balloon to a pressure between 25 and 45 mm Hg by attaching the distal end of the balloon to a sphygmomanometer.
10. Double-clamp the tube.
11. Obtain an abdominal x-ray film to verify the tube's position.
12. A small nasogastric tube may be passed to the upper end of the gastric balloon to allow upper esophageal aspiration if required.
13. The esophageal balloon should be deflated every 8 hours to avoid necrosis.
14. Be sure to monitor the patient closely for airway obstruction and keep equipment close by in case the balloons must be deflated rapidly.

SUGGESTED READINGS

Burkhart C: Guidelines for rapid assessment of abdominal pain indicative of acute surgical abdomen, *Nurse Practitioner* 17(6):39, 1992.

DeVault K, Castell DO: The irritable stomach syndrome, *Am J Gastroenterol* 3:399, 1992.

Gallegos N, Hobsley M: Abdominal pain—parietal or visceral? *J Royal Soc Med* 85(7): 379, 1992.

Jess L: Acute abdominal pain, *Nursing* 23(9):34, 1993.

Malasanos L: *Health assessment,* ed 4. St Louis, 1990, Mosby.

O'Toole M: Advancement assessment of the abdomen and gastrointestinal problems, *Nurs Clin North Am* 25(12):771, 1990.

Weber FH, McCallum RW: Clinical approaches to irritable bowel syndrome, *Lancet* 340(12):1447, 1992.

Blood Disorders

There are several disorders of the blood, but only the three most common will be discussed here: sickle cell disease and crisis, hemophilia, and anemia.

SICKLE CELL DISEASE

Sickle cell disease is an inherited disorder that occurs in 7% of West Africans and African Americans. It is an autosomal recessive disease with an altered hemoglobin molecule. A person with sickle cell disease has two sickle cell genes and rarely lives past early adulthood. A person who has sickle cell *trait* has one sickle cell gene, and the disease remains clinically inactive.

SICKLE CELL CRISIS (VASO-OCCLUSIVE CRISIS)

Sickled cells carry a normal amount of hemoglobin, but the cells have a tendency to clump together because of their sickled shape. As these cells clump, obstruction becomes evident and oxygen and other nutrients do not reach capillaries distal to the blockage, resulting in ischemia.

This causes severe pain and leads to chronic and acute organ dysfunction and frequent infections.

Sickle cell crisis may be precipitated by cold, stress, infection, metabolic or respiratory acidosis, high altitude, or unknown factors. It usually occurs more frequently at night. If the ischemic state is not corrected, local tissue necrosis occurs.

Common sites of sickle cell crisis/pain in children are the hands, feet, and abdomen (mimicking appendicitis). In adults, pain commonly occurs in the long bones, large joints, and the spine.

■ **SIGNS AND SYMPTOMS**

Pain (episodic and in target areas)
History of sickle cell disease
Weakness
Pallor

■ **THERAPEUTIC INTERVENTIONS**
Analgesia
    Acetaminophen or codeine for mild-to-moderate pain
Ketorolac or morphine sulfate for moderate-to-severe pain
Oxygen
IV D5% in ½ normal saline or D_5W for hydration
Antibiotics for the infection
Local heat
Warm environment
Emotional support
■ **COMPLICATIONS**
Recurrent crisis
Chronic hemolytic anemia
Frequent infections
Transient aplastic crisis
Cholelithiasis and cholecystitis
Delayed sexual maturation
Priapism
Renal disease/failure
Bone disease (infarction leading to avascular necrosis of femoral heads)
High-output cardiac failure
Autosplenectomy
Pneumonia
Meningitis
Osteomyelitis
Pulmonary embolus
Cor pulmonale
Chronic skin ulcers
High incidence of spontaneous abortion, perinatal mortality,
    maternal mortality
Hepatomegaly
Hepatic infarction
Jaundice
Coma
Death

HEMOPHILIA

In its simplest expression, hemophilia can be viewed as a bleeding disorder
caused by the absence of a clotting factor. However, hemophilia is actually a
catch-all term for a number of bleeding disorders.

Hemophilia (factor VIII deficiency or factor IX deficiency) is an X chromo-
some, sex-linked disorder that occurs recessively in males and is transmitted by
females. The level of bleeding disorder can be quite variable. Factor VIII (anti-
hemophilia factor) deficiency occurs in 1 of 10,000 people. Factor IX deficiency
occurs in 1 of 40,000 people. Both are usually manifested by hemarthrosis of

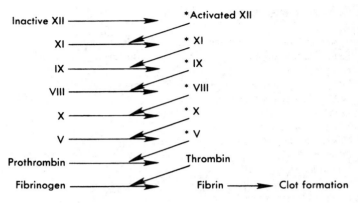

FIGURE 11-1. Clotting factors (intrinsic mechanisms).

the knees, elbows, and ankles, but bleeding can also occur in the central nervous system, the oral or nasal mucosa, the urinary tract, or the GI tract. It may first be seen in infancy when excessive bleeding occurs on circumcision, with bleeding gums, and/or epistaxis.

Figure 11-1 schematically depicts the primary clotting mechanism. Each factor is a protein or glycoprotein that circulates in the plasma. Clotting factors circulate in an inactive form. Initiation of clotting factors first requires factor activation. This occurs whenever a cut or bruise is sustained. The subsequent factors are activated in a domino-like fashion until fibrinogen becomes fibrin and a clot is formed. If any one of these factors is removed from the sequence or inactivated, clotting will not take place.

Hemophilia Type A (Factor VIII Disorder)

Hemophilia type A is a factor VIII disorder. In the majority of patients, factor VIII may be present but not functional, or is functioning at less than normal capacity. The actual severity of the disease depends on the functional activity of the factor in each patient.

In type A hemophilia, the functional level of factor VIII can be augmented by transfusion with fresh frozen plasma, fresh plasma, cryoprecipitate (from pooled plasma), or factor VIII concentrate. The amount of factor VIII in the plasma is small. Consequently, the patient may be at risk of fluid overload and infectious diseases. Cryoprecipitate and factor VIII concentrate are smaller in volume but carry a high risk of hepatitis and other infectious diseases. D-Desaminoarginine vasopressin (DDAVP) stimulates the release, but not the formation, of factor VIII and may be used for mild hemophilia bleeds.

Hemophilia Type B (Christmas Disease)

The less common form of hemophilia, known as type B hemophilia or Christmas disease, is the absence or functional defect of factor IX. Bleeding caused by factor IX deficiencies can be treated with fresh frozen or fresh plasma or factor IX concentrate. Cryoprecipitate cannot be used because it does not contain factor IX.

Episodes of hemarthrosis that result from type A or B hemophilia are usually self-limiting; the joint capsule can only distend to a certain point before the bleeding eventually is tamponaded. To treat, immobilize and elevate the joint and apply ice over a light pressure dressing. After administering therapeutic products that correct coagulation problems, aspirate the blood in the joint. Advise the patient to limit weight-bearing and recommend range of motion exercises. A hematologic and orthopedic follow-up should be performed.

A third type of bleeding disorder that is not really hemophilia is von Willebrand's disease. It is a decrease in von Willebrand factor, a plasma protein necessary for platelet function. It is usually evidenced by mucocutaneous bleeding, such as epistaxis or excessive vaginal bleeding during menstruation. Bleeding problems are treated with fresh frozen or fresh plasma, cryoprecipitate, or DDAVP.

Treatment for all hemophilia and von Willebrand's disorders is rapid factor replacement or other therapeutic intervention mentioned above and close observation for further bleeding.

ANEMIA

Anemia is defined as a hemoglobin less than 50% of normal value. Normal hematocrit at sea level in a male should range between 42% and 53%. Normal hematocrit at sea level in a female should range between 37% and 47%.

Identify the cause of the anemia and treat the cause. Remember, when an acute bleed occurs, hematocrit and hemoglobin will remain the same as normal until some rehydration occurs.

■ **TYPES OF ANEMIA**
Macrocytic hypochromic
Macrocytic
Normocytic normochromic

■ **SIGNS AND SYMPTOMS**
Weakness and fatigue
Syncope
Dyspnea on exertion
Palpitations
Possible CHF
Possible myocardial infarction
Possible shock

The diagnosis of anemia can be made on the basis of history as well as:
    Orthostatic vital signs
    Abnormalities in
        CBC
        Reticulocyte count
        Wright's stain

■ **THERAPEUTIC INTERVENTIONS**
Folate (oral)
Treat underlying condition
Three of the most common blood disorders have been briefly discussed. For a more in-depth evaluation, the reader is referred to the suggested reading list.

SUGGESTED READINGS

Lederman A: The last days of Helen Banks, *Nursing* 22(8):42, 1992.

Martinelli AM: Sickle cell disease—etiology, symptoms, patient care, AORN, 53(3):716, 1991.

Mills D: When blood won't clot, *RN* 55(11):28, 1992.

Pfaff JA, Geninatti M: Hemophilia, *Emerg Med Clin North Am* 11(2):337, 1993.

Rivers R, Williamson N: Sickle cell anemia complex disease, nursing challenge, *RN* 53(4):24, 1990.

Saunders DY, Severance HW, Pollack CV Jr: Sickle cell vaso-occlusive pain crisis in adults: alternative strategies for management in the emergency department, *Southern Med J* 85(8):808, 1992.

Turner T: A helping hand for haemophiliacs . . . paediatric haemophilia service, *Nurs Times* 84(49):26, 1988.

Metabolic Emergencies

ENDOCRINE EMERGENCIES

Overproduction or underproduction of certain hormones may result in endocrine emergencies. Often a stressful event triggers a crisis of the endocrine system.

DIABETES EMERGENCIES

Diabetes mellitus is a chronic condition in which the body is unable to metabolize glucose, the body's major source of energy, due to a lack of effective insulin. There are two major types of diabetes: type I (also called insulin-dependent diabetes mellitus or juvenile onset diabetes), characterized by insulin deficiency, and type II (also called noninsulin-dependent diabetes mellitus or adult onset diabetes), characterized by insulin resistance. The goal in treatment of diabetes is to balance food intake/energy output (exercise) and the use of insulin (which may be endogenous or exogenous) to maintain the blood glucose levels at or near the normal range. When that balance is not achieved, diabetes emergencies may occur.

Hypoglycemia

Hypoglycemia is the most common acute complication of diabetes and the most common side effect of insulin and oral hypoglycemic agents. As more and more individuals with diabetes follow intensive therapy regimens (three or more insulin injections per day or use of an insulin pump, as recommended by the American Diabetes Association based on the results of the Diabetes Control and Complications Trial),[1] it is likely that there will be an increase in the frequency of severe hypoglycemia seen in the Emergency Department. Severe hypoglycemia is defined as a condition in which assistance is needed to obtain treatment. Mild and moderate hypoglycemia are common self-treated conditions.

The normal blood glucose range is 80 to 120 mg/dl (4.4 to 6.6 mmol/L). Hypoglycemia, or low blood glucose, is defined as a blood glucose level below 50 mg/dl (2.8 mmol/L). In an individual whose blood glucose normally runs

281

very high, or with a very sudden drop in blood glucose, symptoms of hypoglycemia may be present at higher blood glucose levels (>50 mg/dl).

All those who take medication for their diabetes are at risk for hypoglycemia. An increased risk exists for those with type I diabetes practicing intensive therapy (three or more insulin injections a day or use of an insulin pump) and those with type II diabetes taking a long-acting oral hypoglycemic agent, such as chlorpropamide (Diabinese).

■ **CAUSES**
Too much insulin*
Too much exercise/activity
Too little food
Alcohol

■ **SIGNS AND SYMPTOMS**
Mild hypoglycemia. Characterized by adrenergic symptoms:†
Shaking
Sweating
Tachycardia
Hunger
Pallor
Tingling of lips
Anxiety
Palpitations
Restlessness
Moderate hypoglycemia. Characterized by neuroglycopenic symptoms:
Irritability
Inability to concentrate
Drowsiness
Confusion
Slurred speech
Staggered gait
Weakness
Blurred vision
Headache
Severe hypoglycemia. May result in:
Unconsciousness
Seizures
Rarely, death

■ **THERAPEUTIC INTERVENTIONS**
Treatment of hypoglycemia in the conscious patient
• Recognize symptoms.
• Confirm blood glucose level (a fingerstick, blood glucose test performed with a light-reflectance meter is adequate to begin treatment if the equip-

---

*Too much insulin may include accidental or intentional overdoses of insulin or oral hypoglycemic agents.

†These symptoms may be masked with long-standing diabetes, autonomic neuropathy (specifically, hypoglycemic unawareness), beta blockers or alcoholism.

Treatment of Hypoglycemia

Each of the following contain 15 g of carbohydrate
½ cup orange juice
⅓ cup apple juice
½ cup regular soda (not diet soda)
½ oz box raisins
10 jelly beans
3 tsp honey or syrup
3 glucose tablets
8 Lifesavers
8 small sugar cubes
4 tsp sugar
1 small tube cake frosting
1 small tube glucose gel

ment is functioning properly and the operator has been well-trained in the procedure).

- Obtain laboratory analysis of blood glucose for confirmation of the meter result.
- Administer 15 g of rapid-acting carbohydrate (see examples in the box above).
- If no improvement in 10 minutes, repeat adminstration of 15 g of carbohydrate.

Treatment of hypoglycemia in the semi-conscious or unconscious patient
- Confirm blood glucose level, as above.
- Administer 50% dextrose 25 to 50 ml IV.
- A continuous infusion of D_5W or $D_{10}W$ to maintain blood glucose in the normal range may be necessary.

  or

- Administer glucagon 1 mg IM (0.5 mg in children ages 3 to 5, 0.25 mg in children less than 3 years).
- If no improvement in 20 minutes, repeat the glucagon.
- Once the patient can swallow, give 20 g of carbohydrate by mouth to prevent a recurrence and to restock depleted glycogen stores.
- Vomiting is common following the administration of glucagon, so position the patient to avoid aspiration.
- Glucagon may not be effective if the liver glycogen stores have been depleted.
- Monitor blood glucose levels, vital signs and neurological status.

Following successful treatment of hypoglycemia, it is helpful for the patient to reflect on possible causes as an aid to prevention of hypoglycemia in the future. Recalling past insulin doses (see Table 12-1), time of injection, food intake, activity, and special circumstances may help to identify the cause of hypoglycemia. Frequent or prolonged hypoglycemia may result in permanent neurologic damage.[2] Early recognition of symptoms and prompt treatment is the key. Rec-

TABLE 12-1   Types of Insulin—Onset, Peak, and Duration of Action

TYPE	ONSET*	PEAK*	DURATION*
Short-acting			
Regular	½-1	2-4	6-8
Semilente	1-2	3-8	10-16
Intermediate-acting			
NPH	1-2	6-12	18-24
Lente	1-3	6-12	18-24
Long-acting			
Ultralente	4-6	8-20	24-28

*In hours following subcutaneous administration. These times are approximate and are based on biosynthetic human insulin. Animal insulins tend to have slightly longer action times. Individual variations in insulin absorption and action may be caused by many factors, including dose, injection technique, injection site, temperature of insulin, exercise following injection, and insulin antibodies.

ommend to the patient that identification, such as a Medic-Alert necklace or bracelet, be worn.

Reactive Hypoglycemia

Reactive, or postprandial, hypoglycemia is described as hypoglycemia that occurs in response to a meal, generally 1 to 2 hours after eating. This occurs in people who do not have diabetes.

■ **CAUSES**
Altered GI motility after gastric surgery
Fructose intolerance
Impaired glucose tolerance
Insulinoma
Idiopathic

■ **THERAPEUTIC INTERVENTIONS**
Administer oral glucose.
Refer for further work-up of etiology and treatment plan.

Hyperglycemic Emergencies
Diabetic ketoacidosis

Diabetic ketoacidosis (DKA) is the most common endocrine emergency and accounts for about 80% to 90% of hyperglycemic emergencies. This is an acute complication of diabetes and in some cases may be the initial presentation of new-onset diabetes. DKA is characterized by dehydration, electrolyte losses, ketonuria, and acidosis, resulting from an inadequate amount of available insulin. When insulin is unavailable for the transport of glucose into cells, fatty acids are metabolized into ketone bodies in the liver. An accumulation of ketones results in metabolic acidosis.

DKA usually occurs only in type I diabetes, but under conditions of extreme stress may be seen in type II diabetes. There is a 6% to 10% mortality rate associated with the precipitating cause, the DKA itself or complications of the treatment.

■ **CAUSES**
Omission of insulin injection(s)
Inadequate insulin dose
New-onset diabetes
Illness
Infection
Myocardial infarction
Cerebrovascular accident
Trauma
Surgery
Steroids
Pancreatitis
Pregnancy
Emotional stress
Unknown etiology

■ **SIGNS AND SYMPTOMS**
Nausea
Vomiting
Anorexia
Kussmaul respirations (rapid, deep breathing)
Acetone on the breath (fruity-smelling breath)
Abdominal pain
Drowsiness
Weakness
Thirst
Polyuria
Tachycardia
Orthostatic hypotension
Poor skin turgor
Dry mucous membranes
Hyperglycemia (>250 mg/dl)
pH <7.3
Serum bicarbonate <15 mEq/L
Ketonuria
Glucosuria
Mental status ranging from normal to coma

■ **DIFFERENTIAL DIAGNOSIS**
Alcoholic ketoacidosis
Hyperglycemic hyperosmolar nonketotic coma
Starvation ketosis
Uremia

Lactic acidosis

Toxin ingestion

■ **THERAPEUTIC INTERVENTIONS**

The goals of treatment are fluid and electrolyte replacement, reversal of ketone-mia and hyperglycemia, and determination and treatment of the precipitating cause. Correction that occurs too rapidly may result in cerebral edema, hypogly-cemia, or hypokalemia.

Laboratory evaluation

Obtain a blood glucose level. If unable to do so rapidly, give an unconscious patient 25 g of dextrose to rule out hypoglycemia, the most common cause of altered mental status in a person with diabetes. (This small amount of glucose would not be harmful to a person in DKA.)

Obtain urine ketones, serum glucose, electrolytes, ketones, BUN, creatinine levels.

Obtain arterial blood gases.

Additional studies may be needed to determine precipitating cause.

Fluid replacement

Administer normal saline at 1 L/hr for 1 to 2 hours, then 100 to 500 ml/hr.

Change to ½ normal saline when the patient is no longer hypovolemic.

The total fluid deficit generally averages 6 L.

Insulin

Administer insulin following the first liter of saline (see Table 12-1).

IV insulin is recommended, as IM or SC insulin is erratically absorbed in the presence of hypovolemia.

A bolus or 5 to 10 units of regular insulin may be given, or a continuous infusion may be started (remember to prime the tubing and discard the first 30 to 50 ml of the insulin/NS solution).

The rate of infusion should be titrated for a reduction in the patient's blood glucose of 100 mg/dl/hr.

Insulin therapy must be aggressive until ketogenesis stops.

When the blood glucose level falls to 250 mg/dl or below, the IV fluid should be changed to fluid containing 5% dextrose.

Subcutaneous insulin must be given 1 to 4 hours before discontinuing the insulin infusion.

Electrolyte replacement

Initially, the potassium level may be high.

Fluid resuscitation, insulin, and correction of acidosis all reduce extracel-lular potassium.

Replace potassium, after documented urine output, at 20 to 40 mEq/L.

Phosphate replacement may be necessary.

Sodium bicarbonate may be necessary if the arterial blood pH is ≤7.1.

Monitor electrolytes every 2 to 4 hours.

Follow-up

Determine the precipitating cause and plan treatment.

Patient and family education is needed if the cause was the omission of an insulin dose during illness.

Hospital admission is usually indicated. In mild cases of DKA the patient may be discharged home from the Emergency Department following treatment if the following conditions have been met:

Vital signs are normal.

Patient tolerates po fluids.

Blood glucose is <300 mg/dl.

There is a normal pH.

Bicarbonate is >15 mEq/L.

The precipitating cause has been determined and corrected.

Follow-up with the patient's private medical doctor has been arranged.

Hyperosmolar hyperglycemic nonketotic coma

Hyperosmolar hyperglycemic nonketotic coma (HHNC) accounts for about 10% to 20% of hyperglycemic emergencies. This is an acute complication of type II diabetes and is characterized by dehydration, extreme hyperglycemia, electrolyte imbalances, and altered mental status. Acidosis is not present in HHNC, in contrast to DKA (Table 12-2). This may represent the initial presentation of type II diabetes. The high mortality rate of 40% to 70% may be due to the existence of severe underlying conditions, the lack of aggressive treatment, or a delay in establishing the diagnosis. With an increase in the elderly population, it is likely that HHNC will be seen more frequently in the future. Potential complications of treatment include cerebral edema, systemic hypoperfusion, cerebral infarction, and hypokalemia.

■ **CAUSES**

Illnesses

Chronic renal insufficiency

Gram-negative pneumonia

Gram-negative urinary tract infection

GI bleed

Gram-negative sepsis

Myocardial infarction

Uremia

Vomiting

Acute viral illness

Pulmonary embolism

Subdural hematoma

Cerebrovascular accident

TABLE 12-2   Comparison of Diabetic Ketoacidosis (DKA) and Hyperosmolar Hyperglycemic Nonketotic Coma (HHNC)

	SERUM GLUCOSE	pH	SERUM KETONES	SERUM OSMOLALITY	URINE GLUCOSE	URINE KETONES
DKA	300-1500 mg/dl	<7.3	Present	Inconclusive	Present	Present
HHNC	600-2000 mg/d	WNL	Absent	350-475 mOsm/L	Present	Absent to trace

Pancreatitis
Burns
Heat stroke
Medications
Thiazide diuretics
Steroids
Phenytoin
Propranolol
Cimetidine
Immunosuppressive agents
■ **THERAPEUTIC INTERVENTIONS**
Hyperalimentation
Tube feeding without sufficient free water
Dialysis
Recent cardiac surgery
■ **SIGNS AND SYMPTOMS**
Dehydration
Hyperglycemia (>600 mg/dl)
Hyperosmolality (>300 mOsm/L)
Absent or minimal ketones
pH >7.3
Serum bicarbonate >20 mEq/L
Mental status ranges from drowsy to unresponsive
Seizures
■ **DIFFERENTIAL DIAGNOSIS**
DKA
Alcoholic ketoacidosis
Lactic acidosis
Other causes of altered mental status
■ **THERAPEUTIC INTERVENTIONS**
The goals of treatment are rehydration, correction of electrolyte imbalances, reduction of glucose, and determination and treatment of precipitating cause.

Laboratory evaluation
Blood sugar level
Serum glucose, electrolytes, BUN, creatinine
CBC
Urinalysis
Arterial blood gases
Other studies may be necessary to determine underlying cause
Serum osmolality may be calculated as follows:

$$\text{Osmolality (mmol/L)} = \text{serum sodium} \times 2 + \text{blood glucose}/18 + \text{BUN}/2.8$$

Fluid replacement
Begin fluid resuscitation with normal saline. Give 1 L over the first hour.
Change to ½ NS and reduce the rate when the patient's blood pressure responds and urine output is adequate.

When the blood glucose drops to 250 mg/dl or below the fluid should contain 5% dextrose.

The average fluid deficit is 9 to 12 L.

Electrolyte replacement

After urine output is documented and before insulin is given, begin potassium replacement, initially at 10 mEq/hr, then by adding 20 to 30 mEq/L IV fluid.

Check the potassium level every 2 hours until it is stable.

Insulin

The goal is to reduce the blood glucose level by 100 mg/dl/hr.

With acidosis, hyperkalemia, or renal failure, insulin is needed and should be given IV or IM until the blood glucose has dropped to 250 mg/dl or the osmolality has been reduced to 315 mmol/L.

In some cases insulin is not necessary because the fluid replacement is adequate to reduce the blood glucose levels.

Follow-up

Admission to an intensive care unit is indicated.

Determination and treatment of the precipitating cause is essential.

Diabetes insipidus

In diabetes insipidus the kidneys are unable to resorb water because the action of antidiuretic hormone (ADH) is not effective in increasing the permeability of the renal tubules. Thus the kidneys are unable to concentrate urine appropriately, and excessive amounts of dilute urine are excreted. The condition may be temporary or permanent, depending upon the amount of hypothalamic secretory tissue remaining.

Nephrogenic diabetes insipidus may occur, resulting in a lack of response of the renal tubules to appropriate levels of ADH. This situation may be caused by familial conditions, renal disease, electrolyte imbalances, or lithium carbonate. This condition does not respond to ADH replacement therapy, so it must be treated with dietary sodium and protein restrictions, thiazide diuretics, and nonsteroidal antiinflammatory drugs.

■ **CAUSES**

Tumors in the hypothalamus/pituitary region

Head trauma

Surgical trauma

Ischemia of the hypothalamus/pituitary gland

CNS infections

Phenytoin

■ **SIGNS AND SYMPTOMS**

Polyuria (3 to 15 L/day)

Polydipsia

Specific gravity <1.005

Urine osmolality <300 mOsm/L

Serum osmolality >295 mOsm/L

Serum sodium >145 mEq/L

Weight loss
Fatigue
- **THERAPEUTIC INTERVENTIONS**
Fluid replacement
Replacement of ADH
    Vasopressin tannate in oil
    Lysine vasopressin spray
    Desmopressin acetate (DDAVP)

SYNDROME OF INAPPROPRIATE ANTIDIURETIC HORMONE

Secretion of ADH is sustained and abnormal in the syndrome of inappropriate antidiuretic hormone (SIADH), resulting in water intoxication. This condition is characterized by hyponatremia and hypotonicity.
- **CAUSES**
Malignancies
Pulmonary disease
CNS disorders
Pain
Stress
General anesthesia
Oral hypoglycemic agents
Psychotropic drugs
Antineoplastic agents
Narcotics
More common in elderly
- **SIGNS AND SYMPTOMS**
Fatigue
Headache
Confusion
Decreased level of consciousness
Nausea and vomiting
Diminished tendon reflexes
Seizures
Weight gain without edema
Dilutional hyponatremia
Decreased plasma osmolality
Increased urine osmolality
Increased urine sodium
Increased specific gravity
- **THERAPEUTIC INTERVENTIONS**
Hypertonic saline and furosemide (check serum sodium every hour)
Fluid restriction
IV normal saline or oral salt supplements
Potassium replacement

THYROID EMERGENCIES

The thyroid hormone has an effect on nearly every organ system. Severe thyroid dysfunction, both hypothyroid and hyperthyroid, presents a significant medical emergency.

Thyroid Storm (Hyperthyroid Crisis)

Thyroid storm, a hyperthyroid crisis, may occur in a previously undiagnosed hyperthyroid patient who is under significant stress. If not promptly diagnosed and treated, this condition may progress to exhaustion, cardiac failure, and death. Death may occur within 2 hours if this condition goes untreated.[3] The mortality rate is 20% to 60%. Thyroid storm is four times more likely to occur in women than in men.

■ **CAUSES**

Stress
Infection
DKA
Embolism
Surgery
Trauma
Manipulation of the thyroid gland

■ **SIGNS AND SYMPTOMS**

Fever
Anxiety
Agitation
Tremors
Nausea, vomiting
Tachydysrhythmias
Tachypnea
Hypertension
Diaphoresis
Flushing
Abdominal pain
Muscle weakness
Exophthalmos
Decreased level of consciousness
Psychosis
Pulmonary edema
Cardiac failure
Hypercalcemia
Hyperglycemia
Metabolic acidosis

■ **THERAPEUTIC INTERVENTIONS**

The goals of treatment are to reduce the fever and prevent life-threatening arrhythmias.

Cooling blanket
Acetaminophen (not aspirin)
Cardiac monitor
Oxygen
Elevate head of bed
Corticosteroids
IV fluids containing dextrose
B vitamins
Propranolol
Propylthiouracil
Iodine—sodium iodide, potassium iodide, or Lugol's solution
Treatment of underlying illness

Myxedema Coma (Hypothyroid Coma)

Myxedema coma is the very rare, very serious crisis of hypothyroidism. Respiratory failure is the usual cause of death from myxedema coma. The mortality rate is 30% to 80%.

■ **CAUSES**
Infection
Congestive heart failure
General anesthesia
Surgery
Trauma
Sedatives
Narcotics
Antidepressants
Exposure to cold temperatures
Stress

■ **SIGNS AND SYMPTOMS**
Hypothermia without shivering
Bradycardia
Hypoventilation
Hypotension
Hyponatremia
Hypoglycemia
Dry skin
Respiratory or metabolic acidosis
Fatigue
Seizures
Lethargy
Stupor
Coma

■ **THERAPEUTIC INTERVENTIONS**
Oxygen
Thyroid hormone replacement
Glucocorticoids

Gentle hydration
Sodium replacement
Passive warming
Vigorous treatment of infection
Possible intubation and ventilation

Thyroiditis

Thyroiditis is usually characterized by anterior neck pain that comes on gradually or suddenly after an upper respiratory infection. It is most often caused by a bacteria.

■ **SIGNS AND SYMPTOMS**
Increased neck pain when the head is turned
Fever
Hoarse voice
Elevated pulse
Increased neck pain on swallowing
Firm or nodular thyroid

■ **THERAPEUTIC INTERVENTIONS**
Aspirin
Bedrest
Antibiotics
Propranolol
Glucocorticoids
Possible surgery

ADRENAL EMERGENCIES

The adrenal cortex produces corticosteroids, which control metabolism and fluid and electrolyte balance. The adrenal medulla produces epinephrine and norepinephrine, which affect the autonomic nervous system.

Acute Adrenal Insufficiency

Acute adrenal insufficiency, or Addison's disease, is a decreased secretion of cortisol and aldosterone. The onset of this condition is often triggered by an underlying illness or stress. Long-term steroid use causes adrenal atrophy; thus rapid discontinuation of steroids may result in acute adrenal insufficiency.

■ **SIGNS AND SYMPTOMS**
Nausea and vomiting
Abdominal cramping
Diarrhea
Headache
Fever
Hypotension
Weakness

Irritability
Fatigue
Lethargy
Dehydration
Tachycardia
Weight loss
Anorexia
Truncal obesity
Hyperpigmentation, particularly over knuckles, in creases of hands, in axilla, in the gums, and in recent scars
Moon face
Hyponatremia
Hyperkalemia
Hypercalcemia
Hypoglycemia
Hypochloremia
Azotemia
■ **THERAPEUTIC INTERVENTIONS**
Laboratory evaluation
   Cortisol
   ACTH
   Electrolytes
   Glucose
Fluid and electrolyte replacement
Administration of hydrocortisone
Cardiac monitoring
Determination and treatment of precipitating cause

Pheochromocytoma

Pheochromocytoma is a tumor of the adrenal gland that is usually benign. The tumor stimulates excessive secretion of catecholamines. The hallmark symptom of this condition is extreme hypertension, which may be persistent or paroxysmal.

■ **SIGNS AND SYMPTOMS**
Hypertension
Headache
Diaphoresis
Pallor
Tremor
Chest pain
Abdominal pain
Palpitations
Mental status changes
■ **THERAPEUTIC INTERVENTIONS**
Control the hypertensive crisis.
Maintain volume status.

Observe for cardiac arrhythmias.

Stabilize for surgery.

Disruptions in the production of endocrine hormones result in medical emergencies that require prompt assessment, diagnosis, and correction, along with determination and treatment of a precipitating cause.

ELECTROLYTE DISORDERS

Electrolytes, ions that conduct electrical current, are essential for properly functioning cells and maintenance of fluid balance and acid-base balance. An excess or deficit of any of the vital electrolytes may result in a life-threatening crisis.

CALCIUM PROBLEMS

Hypocalcemia

Hypocalcemia is an unusual diagnosis in the emergency setting. It is uncommon and usually a chronic condition. If there is a deficiency of parathyroid hormone (PTH) or if there is PTH impairment, serum calcium levels are reduced.

■ **SIGNS AND SYMPTOMS**

Laryngeal spasm with stridor

Numbness and tingling (circumorally and in distal extremities)

Tetany

Dysrhythmias

Seizures

Muscle cramps

Hyperactive reflexes

■ **THERAPEUTIC INTERVENTIONS**

Acute

Administer a calcium gluconate IV 10% solution over 10 to 15 minutes (rapid administration could cause hypotension). Calcium chloride may be substituted, but **be aware that local tissue necrosis may occur.**

Seizure precautions

Calcifediol

Chronic

Ergocalciferol

Vitamin D treatment

Increased dietary intake of calcium

Oral calcium

Hypercalcemia

Hypercalcemia is usually a complication of a malignancy, but may also be caused by hyperparathyroidism, thiazide diuretics, hypervitaminosis D, hyperthyroidism, or Addison's disease. It is usually not acute or life-threatening. The goals of treatment are to decrease the serum calcium level, which can usually be accomplished by rehydration, and to detect and treat the underlying cause.

■ **SIGNS AND SYMPTOMS**
Nausea and vomiting
Thirst
Dry nose
Dysrhythmias and shortened QT interval
Weakness
Itching
Dehydration from polyuria
Postural hypotension
Elevated BUN
Lethargy to coma
Confusion

■ **THERAPEUTIC INTERVENTIONS**
Administer an IV of normal saline at 200 ml/hr (or in accordance with CVP).
Furosemide may be given to prevent fluid overload.

MAGNESIUM PROBLEMS

Hypomagnesemia

Magnesium is contained primarily in green vegetables. It is absorbed at the small bowel level and is excreted by the kidneys. Many enzyme systems that control the permeability of cell membranes, muscle contractions, oxidative phosphorylation, fat and nucleic acid synthesis, and the stabilization of nuclear proteins are activated by magnesium.

Decreased magnesium is caused by poor dietary intake or when magnesium needs are increased, such as in pregnant women, nursing mothers, and growing children. It can also be caused by chronic alcohol use, malabsorption syndromes, nasogastric suctioning, vomiting, diarrhea, or by renal loss. Decreased magnesium can also occur as a result of hypoparathyroid or hyperparathyroid disease, hyperthyroidism, or during treatment of diabetic ketoacidosis. Hypomagnesemia should also be considered in patients who have received massive transfusions with citrated blood, those with acute pancreatitis, and those who have recently had a cardiopulmonary bypass.

■ **SIGNS AND SYMPTOMS**
Nausea, vomiting, and diarrhea
Anorexia
Decreased level of consciousness
Muscle fibrillation, tremors, hyperreflexia
Ataxia
Vertical nystagmus
Tetany
Psychosis
Hallucinations
Dysrhythmias
Paroxysmal supraventricular tachycardia
Ventricular tachycardia

Ventricular fibrillation
Apathy
Leg cramps
Insomnia
Confusion
- **THERAPEUTIC INTERVENTIONS**
Administer oral, IM, or IV magnesium

Hypermagnesemia

Hypermagnesemia is a life-threatening condition. Fortunately, it is uncommon.
Usually hypermagnesemia results from iatrogenic excessive administration of
magnesium-containing products such as antacids, enemas, dialysate solution, or
in patients with renal failure or overdoses of lithium. It may also be seen in
patients with diabetic ketoacidosis, Addison's disease, viral hepatitis, or hypothermia.

- **SIGNS AND SYMPTOMS**
  ### Mild (3 to 5 mEq/L)
  Bradycardia
  Nausea and vomiting
  Decreased deep tendon reflexes
  Hypotension
  Red, warm skin
  Diaphoresis
  Muscular weakness
  ### Moderate (5 to 10 mEq/L)
  Decreased level of consciousness
  Prolonged P-R interval, QRS complex, and QT interval
  Paralysis
  ### Severe (>15 mEq/L)
  Third-degree heart block
  Paralysis of respiratory muscles
  Asystole
- **THERAPEUTIC INTERVENTIONS**
ABCs
Decreased magnesium intake
Administer an IV of 0.45% normal saline and diuretics to enhance excretion (if
    normal renal function)
If greather than 5 mEq/L, give calcium chloride, 5 ml of a 10% solution over 30
    seconds (may be repeated)
Consider renal dialysis with magnesium-free dialysate

PHOSPHOROUS PROBLEMS

Hypophosphatemia

In humans 80% to 85% of phosphate is in bones and teeth and 15% to 20% is intracellular. The main source of phosphate is food products. It is important to cellular structure and function, serum calcium levels, and glycolysis and oxygen delivery. It is excreted by the kidneys. Hypophosphatemia is more common in diabetes, chronic alcohol use, and chronic bowel disease.

Signs and symptoms begin when serum phosphorous is less than 2 mg/100 ml and becomes life-threatening when levels are less than 1 mg/100 ml. Hypophosphatemia results from loss of the mineral through the intestines or kidneys or intracellular phosphate shifts caused by sepsis, respiratory alkalosis, epinephrine administration, or hepatic failure.

- **SIGNS AND SYMPTOMS**
  Moderate decrease
  Weakness
  Confusion
  Tremors
  Pain in bones
  Joint stiffness
  Chest pain
  Muscle pain
  Tingling of fingers and circumoral area
  Severe decrease
  Seizures
  Anisocoria (unequal pupils)
  Paralysis
  Coma to death
- **THERAPEUTIC INTERVENTIONS**
  Decrease intake of substances that cause decreased phosphorous, such as phosphorous-binding antacids.
  Replace with oral or (if severe) IV phosphorus.

Hyperphosphatemia

Hyperphosphatemia is considered present when serum phosphorous levels are above 4.5 mg/100 ml. It is most commonly caused by lack of phosphorous excretion at the renal level and can occasionally be caused by phosphorous moving from the intracellular to the extracellular spaces as a result of cellular tissue destruction.

- **SIGNS AND SYMPTOMS**
  Pruritis
  Tetany
  Calcium phosphate deposits in joints and blood vessels
  Nausea, vomiting, anorexia

Muscle weakness

Tachycardia

■ **THERAPEUTIC INTERVENTIONS**

Administer phosphate binding agents, such as aluminum, magnesium, or calcium antacids.

Decrease dietary intake of phosphorus.

If severe, dialysis may be necessary.

POTASSIUM PROBLEMS

Hypokalemia

Hypokalemia is defined as a serum potassium level below 3.5 mEq/L. It results from excess potassium excretion in urine that could be caused by use of diuretics, excess potassium excretion in feces resulting from diarrhea or malabsorption, metabolic alkalosis, intracellular shift of potassium, or a magnesium deficiency. Normal serum potassium levels are 3.5 to 5 mEq/L.

■ **SIGNS AND SYMPTOMS**

Muscle weakness

Fatigue

Leg cramps

Nausea, vomiting

CNS irritability

Paresthesias

Paralysis

Decreased reflexes

Paralytic ileus

Polydipsia

Dysrhythmias (PVCs, atrial tachycardia, nodal tachycardia, ventricular tachycardia, ventricular fibrillation)

Respiratory or cardiac arrest

■ **THERAPEUTIC INTERVENTIONS**

Replace potassium orally with potassium chloride.

IV infusion rate

    <10 to 20 mEq/hr

    Concentration <30 to 40 mEq/L

    May irritate vein

    Do not give as IV bolus.

Closely monitor for dysrhythmias.

Monitor serum potassium and other electrolytes.

Monitor hourly urine output.

Consider potassium-sparing diuretics.

Hyperkalemia

Hyperkalemia (serum potassium levels above 5 mEq/L) may be caused by major crush injuries, severe electrical burns, major thermal burns, severe acidosis (potassium increases by 0.6 mEq/L with each decrease of 0.1 U of pH), renal failure, potassium overdose, increased intake potassium, decreased urinary excretion, extracellular shift, overuse of salt substitutes, lupus, sickle cell disease, amyloidosis, or gastrointestinal disorders.

- **SIGNS AND SYMPTOMS**

Dysrhythmias
> Sinus bradycardia, sinus arrest, first degree heart block, junctional rhythms, idioventricular rhythms, ventricular tachycardia, ventricular fibrillation, asystole

Decreased reflexes
Paresthesias
Paralysis
Irritability
Anxiety
Abdominal cramping
Diarrhea
Weakness
Respiratory and/or cardiac arrest

- **THERAPEUTIC INTERVENTIONS**

Therapeutic intervention is aimed at increasing cellular uptake of potassium.
Administer calcium gluconate 10 to 20 ml of 10% solution IV slowly.
> Rapid acting; lasts 30 to 60 minutes.
> Antagonizes potassium at the cell membrane.
> Especially useful in dialysis patients, particularly in cardiac arrest situations resulting from hyperkalemia.
> Not recommended for use in patients who are on digitalis.
>> or:

Administer sodium bicarbonate 44 mEq (1 amp) IV slowly.
> Causes cells to absorb potassium immediately; lasts 1 to 2 hours.
>> or:

Administer insulin and glucose.
> D_{10} (500 ml) with 10 to 20 U regular insulin over ½ to 1 hour.
> Takes about 30 minutes to start working, but lasts 4 to 6 hours.
> Check serum glucose. Observe closely for hypoglycemia.
>> or:

Administer kayexelate (a cation exchange resin).
> 25 g retention enema (followed by 15 ml of 70% solution of sorbitol to promote diarrhea)
> Takes about 2 hours to start working
>> or:

Administer furosemide and saline
> 40 mg Lasix in normal saline at 100 ml/hr
> *Problem:* Has a slow onset and causes an excessive electrolyte excretion.

or:
Renal dialysis
    Efficient/effective

SODIUM PROBLEMS

Hyponatremia

Intracellular and extracellular fluids normally have the same osmolality. The electrolyte that controls the extracellular osmolality is sodium. A serum sodium level of less than 135 mEq/L is considered hyponatremia. This can occur when there is an actual decrease in the volume of extracellular sodium or an increase in the volume of extracellular fluid, resulting in dilutional hyponatremia. Excessive extracellular fluid may be caused by congestive heart failure, hepatic failure, or subnormal availability of antidiuretic hormone (ADH). Sodium loss can be caused by use of diuretics, vomiting, severe burns (third spacing), and lack of dietary sodium.

■ **SIGNS AND SYMPTOMS**

Severity of signs and symptoms depends on the level of serum sodium, affecting the amount of brain cell edema.

    Lethargy
    Postural hypotension
    Tremors
    Cool, clammy skin
    Headache
    Edema
    Confusion
    Seizures
    Coma

■ **THERAPEUTIC INTERVENTIONS**

Treat cautiously, overtreatment is dangerous.
Consider IV fluid and sodium replacement.
Replace other electrolyte losses.

Hypernatremia

Hypernatremia is defined as a serum sodium level above 145 mEq/L. It can result either from an increase in sodium or a decrease in fluid. Fluid decrease is the most common cause. Fluid loss may occur as a result of renal causes, fever, hyperventilation, or excessive perspiration.

An increase in extracellular sodium causes fluid to move from the intracellular spaces to the extracellular spaces in an attempt to achieve osmotic equilibrium. The resulting cellular "dehydration" causes CNS depression and possibly intracerebral hemorrhage.

■ **SIGNS AND SYMPTOMS**

Thirst
Fatigue

Lethargy
Confusion
Coma
■ **THERAPEUTIC INTERVENTIONS**
Treat the underlying cause and bring serum sodium levels to within normal
limit.
Ensure hypotonic replacement (gradually), usually with D_5W and/or 0.45% nor-
mal saline solution, in accordance with calculations, correct slowly to avoid
cerebral edema.
Consider hemodialysis.

ALCOHOL EMERGENCIES

Acute alcohol intoxication or other alcohol-induced problems may create a medical emergency. Acute intoxication or acute withdrawal from alcohol can be
life-threatening. It is essential to determine that there is no underlying cause of
illness or injury other than alcohol intoxication, such as head trauma, diabetic
ketoacidosis, or overdose.
Obtain a good history whenever possible:
• When was the patient's last drink?
• How much did the patient drink? (Remember that it is the *amount* of alco-
hol and not the type that affects the blood alcohol level.)
• How much does the patient usually drink each day? How much each
week?
• When was the last time the patient ate?
• Is the patient taking any medications?
• Has the patient taken any medications or drugs? (Specifically ask about
disulfiram [Antabuse] and metronidazole [Flagyl].)
• Does the patient have any other medical illness?

Acute Intoxication

Acute intoxication is caused by consumption of a large amount of alcohol over
a short period of time. Acute intoxication can occur at various levels, depending
on the patient's drinking frequency, the amount of food consumed with the
alcohol, and the physiologic tolerance of the drinker (Table 12-3).
■ **SIGNS AND SYMPTOMS**
Hypothermia or hyperthermia
Tachycardia
Hypotension
Hypovolemia
Arrhythmias
Respiratory depression
Aspiration (common)
Nausea/vomiting
Abdominal pain
Hypoglycemia

TABLE 12-3 Blood Alcohol Levels and Associated Signs and Symptoms

BLOOD ALCOHOL PERCENTAGE IN 70 KG PERSON	SIGNS AND SYMPTOMS
0.05%	Very few
0.10% (legally intoxicated in most states)	Giddy; decreased muscle coordination; decreased inhibitions
0.15%	Decreased sensory level; slurred speech; vertigo; ataxia; elevated pulse; diaphoresis
0.20%	Very decreased sensory level; marked decrease in reaction to stimuli; inability to walk; nausea, vomiting
0.40%	No response to stimuli; decreased deep tendon reflexes; decreased blood pressure; elevated pulse; cool, clammy, moist skin; seizures
0.50%	Death from primary respiratory arrest

Lactic acidosis
Decreased muscle coordination
Dehydration
■ **THERAPEUTIC INTERVENTIONS**
Airway management (**aspiration is a major cause of death in the acutely intoxicated)**
Oxygen
Cardiac monitor
ABCs, alcohol level, lytes, CBC, glucose
Drawing blood for medical/forensic purposes
Warming blanket
Chest x-ray film
Ipecac, if necessary, if alcohol was consumed within 1 to 2 hours, especially in children
Gastric lavage with charcoal if necessary
Control of seizures with diazepam (Valium)
IV D_5W or RL or D_5NS if hypovolemia or alcoholic ketoacidosis is suspected
Dextrose 50% and thiamin 100 mg (to prevent Wernicke-Korsakoff syndrome), naloxone, dextrose, and thiamine
Possible renal dialysis
Electrolyte replacement
Ruling out other causes of current status
Other appropriate therapeutic intervention, depending on findings (Figure 12-1)

Rum Fits/Alcohol Seizures

Rum fits are seizures that are concurrent with drinking alcohol, generally following 8 to 36 hours of abstinence. Typically 1 to 3 grand mal seizures occur over a 6-hour period. They may be caused by a severely decreased blood alcohol level, a decreased glucose level, or an electrolyte imbalance. The patient may progress to delirium tremens without intervention.

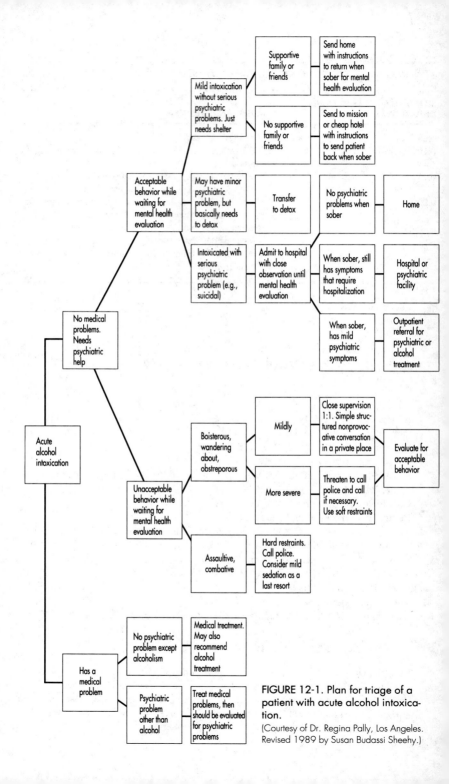

FIGURE 12-1. Plan for triage of a patient with acute alcohol intoxication.

(Courtesy of Dr. Regina Pally, Los Angeles. Revised 1989 by Susan Budassi Sheehy.)

■ **THERAPEUTIC INTERVENTIONS**
ABCs
Oxygen
Arterial blood gases
Diazepam
IV D_5W
Naloxone, dextrose, and thiamine
Use of anticonvulsants is controversial

Alcohol Withdrawal

Begins 6 to 48 hours after reduction or cessation of ethanol intake and lasts 2 to 7 days.

Minor

Less than 24 hours after cessation or reduction of alcohol consumption.

■ **SIGNS AND SYMPTOMS**
Hangover
Headache
Shaking
Nausea and vomiting
Insomnia
Irritability
Anxiety
Tachycardia
Mild ataxia
Hypertension

■ **THERAPEUTIC INTERVENTIONS**
Rest
Aspirin
Rehydration

Major

Severe alcohol withdrawal occurs in chronic alcoholics who have been without alcohol. It occurs from 24 hours to 5 days after cessation or reduction of alcohol consumption.

■ **SIGNS AND SYMPTOMS**
Seizures
Decreased level of consciousness
Nausea, vomiting, anorexia
Photophobia
Hallucinations (auditory and visual)
Slight lateral nystagmus
Diaphoresis
Ataxia
Fever

Disorientation
Anxiety
Irritability
Tremor
Tachycardia
Hyperreflexia
Hypertension
Delirium
■ **THERAPEUTIC INTERVENTIONS**
ABCs
Fluid and electrolyte replacement
Thiamine and dextrose IV
Multivitamins
Benzodiazepines
Dextrose 50%
Diazepam
Reassurance
Reorientation

Delirium Tremens

Delirium tremens (DTs) occurs after a severe drop in the amount of alcohol
consumed by an alcoholic usually after third day without alcohol. Delirium tremens is an acute medical emergency resulting in a 10% to 15% mortality rate.

■ **SIGNS AND SYMPTOMS**
Gross tremors
Increasing agitation
Hallucinations (auditory and visual)
Confusion
Fever
Incontinence
Mydriasis
Seizures
Decreased blood pressure
Elevated pulse
Dysrhythmias
■ **THERAPEUTIC INTERVENTIONS**
Haloperidol
Chlordiazepoxide
Careful airway management
Protection of head and limbs (padded bedsides)
IV with electrolyte additions

Disulfiram Reactions

Disulfiram is a drug given in some alcohol detoxification programs. Disulfiram may react with foods or medications containing alcohol, including cough syrups, fermented vinegar, and perhaps even the odor of rubbing alcohol or aftershave.

■ **SIGNS AND SYMPTOMS**

Severe nausea and vomiting (5 to 15 minutes following contact with alcohol) that may continue for 6 to 12 days

Flush of face, chest, and neck
Perspiration
Reddened conjunctiva
Headache
Increased pulse
Increased respirations
Decreased blood pressure
Decreased level of consciousness
Chest and abdominal pain
Vertigo

■ **THERAPEUTIC INTERVENTIONS**

ABCs
Oxygen
IV normal saline
Consider ascorbic acid
Chlorpheniramine
Diphenhydramine
Antiemetics

Metabolic emergencies require careful assessment, prompt diagnosis, and aggressive treatment of the acute problem. Follow-up management must include determination and treatment of the precipitating cause. Prevention of a future episode necessitates continued health care management and patient and family education. Emergency medical identification should be worn by individuals with chronic conditions that predispose them to acute metabolic crises.

REFERENCES

1. American Diabetes Association: Implications of the diabetes control and complications trial, *Clin Diabetes* 11(4):91, 1993.
2. Yealy DM, Wolfson AB: Hypoglycemia, *Emerg Med Clin North Am* 7(4):837, 1989.
3. Spittle L: Diagnoses in opposition: Thyroid storm and myxedema coma, *AACN Clin Issues Crit Care Nurs* 3(2):301, 1992.

Toxicologic Emergencies

Toxicology is the science of poisons. There are countless numbers of substances that can cause poisoning or overdose and only a few of these have specific antidotes. In general, therapeutic intervention is directed toward management of the airway, maintaining adequate ventilation and circulation, expediting the elimination of the toxic substance, and preventing further absorption of the substance.

General therapeutic intervention for poisonings and overdoses includes:
- ABCs (consider endotracheal intubation, if necessary)
- Oxygen
- Left lateral swimmer's position with head dependent
- IV Ringer's lactate or normal saline solution for possible fluid replacement
- Naloxone 0.4 mg up to 2 mg IV push or into the endotracheal tube
- Dextrose 50% 50 ml
- Thiamin 50 to 100 mg if the possibility of chronic alcohol ingestion exists
- Syrup of ipecac if not contraindicated and within 30 minutes of ingestion
- Gastric lavage
- Activated charcoal to adsorb the poison
- A cathartic to enhance excretion of the poison

Monitor:
ECG for dysrhythmias
Arterial blood gases
Urinary output
Vital signs

Try to ascertain the type of poison:
- What is the nature of the poison?
- How is it adsorbed?
- How is it catabolized?
- How is it excreted?
- How can it be detected?

POISON INFORMATION

Toxicology is a rapidly evolving science, and the standard of care changes as new interventions are found. Poison centers have assumed an increased role in the identification and management of poisonings and overdoses. Poison centers are located throughout every state and have access to information that is updated every three months on Poisindex and to other current toxicologic references. Poison centers should be contacted with each poisoned patient. The poison center will help the clinician assess the patient and implement the most current standard of care. Additionally, most poison centers collect and submit data to the American Association of Poison Control Centers. This data is used for support of product reformulations, repackaging, recalls, and bans as well as major prevention campaigns. Data also are used as postmarketing surveillance of newly released drugs and products.

THERAPEUTIC INTERVENTIONS FOR POISONINGS AND OVERDOSES

Induced Emesis

Although its role has significantly decreased, emesis remains a useful method of gastric emptying in certain patients.

Emesis is induced with syrup of ipecac, an emetic agent that causes irritation of the stomach lining and stimulates the emetic center in the medulla. It should only be given to patients with a gag reflex. It should not be given: (1) if there is altered mental status; (2) if there is predictable severe central nervous system depression within 30 minutes resulting in airway compromise; (3) if the substance can cause seizures to ensue at the same time ipecac begins to work; (4) in cases of acid ingestion; (5) in cases of alkali ingestion; (6) in cases of petroleum distillates ingestion; (7) in cases of aliphatic hydrocarbon ingestion; (8) when there are preexisting health problems—seizure disorder, cardiac history, or pregnancy; (9) when vagal reflexes from vomiting may worsen bradydysrhythmias in certain drugs, i.e., beta blockers, digoxin, calcium antagonist; and (10) to children younger than 9 months of age, who should be managed in a health care facility because of their immature gag reflex. It is imperative that liquids be given following ipecac administration and that the patient vomit until the stomach contents are clear.

SYRUP OF IPECAC DOSAGE

	Ipecac	Fluids
1 year old	10 ml	15 ml/kg
1 to 12 years old	15 ml	4 to 6 oz
>12 years old	30 ml	6 to 8 oz

Dose may be repeated once if emesis does not occur within 20 to 30 minutes.

Gastric Lavage

Perform gastric lavage when there is the possibility that a substance could be removed from the stomach.

Follow this procedure:

1. Protect the patient's airway.
   a. Consider endotracheal intubation if the patient has altered consciousness (CNS depression) or has no gag reflex.
   b. Place the patient in a left lateral decubitus (swimmer's) position and in Trendelenburg's position.
   c. Have suction readily available.
2. Select the proper size gastric tube.
   a. Preferably a 36-40 French gastric tube inserted via the oral route.
   b. Use a 24-32 French gastric tube for a child.
3. Lubricate the tube with a water-soluble lubricant.
4. If possible, have the patient cooperate by sitting up and taking sips of water while swallowing the tube.
5. Advance the tube.
6. Auscultate over the epigastric area while forcing some air into the tube to ensure proper placement.
7. Secure the tube with tape.
8. Place the patient in a left lateral position with the head dependent if this has not already been done.
9. Lavage with warmed normal saline solution (150 to 200 ml per rinse in an adult and 10 ml/kg in a child).
10. Allow for fluid return by gravity.
11. Repeat lavage until the fluid returned is clear.
12. Administer activated charcoal through the tube.
13. Administer a cathartic through the tube.
14. Remove the tube.
15. Provide oral hygiene.

Activated Charcoal

Activated charcoal is usually given by mouth or nasogastric tube following emesis or lavage. It adsorbs many substances and may even bind some agents in the proximal small bowel. There are some agents, however, that are not well adsorbed by activated charcoal. These are acids, alkalis, cyanide, ethanol, ferrous sulfate, methanol, and lithium. It may be given as a slurry, mixed with water, magnesium citrate, or sorbitol. It should be given slowly for best retention, and can be given via NG tube drip. The dosage is 1 to 2 g/kg body weight in children and 50 to 100 g in adults orally or through a gastric tube.

Multiple Dose Activated Charcoal

Multiple doses of activated charcoal have been shown effective in enhancing total body clearance and elimination in these drugs:

- Tricyclic antidepressants
- Phenobarbital
- Theophyllin
- Digoxin
- Phenytoin
- Carbamezapine
- Sustained release preparations

Repeat every 2 to 6 hours. Give 20 to 50 g in an adult and half that dose in a child. A cathartic should only be given with the first dose of activated charcoal. Do not repeat charcoal if an ileus is present.

Cathartics

Cathartics such as magnesium sulfate, magnesium citrate, sodium citrate, or sorbitol are used to enhance excretion of poisons. This should not be given to children less than 1 year old or if bowel sounds are absent.

Whole Bowel Irrigation

Whole bowel irrigation is the mechanical cleansing of the entire gastrointestinal tract by the instilling of large volumes of fluids. Commercially available solutions are Colyte or Golytely. Whole bowel irrigation produces a rapid catharsis, cleaning most matter from the GI tract in hours. Though it is not a substitute for activated charcoal, it seems to be most useful in agents not well adsorbed via charcoal (iron, lead, lithium, zinc), and in sustained-release products.

SOME COMMON POISONINGS AND OVERDOSES

Acetaminophen

Acetaminophen, a metabolite of phenacetin, is found in varying quantities in more than 200 miscellaneous remedies for pain, sleep, cough, and colds.

As few as 15 extra-strength acetaminophen tablets can produce hepatotoxicity in an adult. Greater than 7.5 g is potentially hepatotoxic in an adult, and greater than 140 mg/kg in a child (<100 pounds).

■ SIGNS AND SYMPTOMS

Initial stage (0 to 24 hours after ingestion)

Symptoms may be absent early even if severely toxic

GI irritation (nausea, vomiting, anorexia)

Lethargy

Diaphoresis

Coma and metabolic acidosis have developed in rare cases of poisoning when the $4°$ blood level is >800 mg/L

Middle stage (24 to 48 hours after ingestion)

This may be a symptom-free stage of toxicity.

Hepatic abnormalities of AST (SGOT), ALT (SGPT) bilirubin, and pro-thrombin time will develop.

Right upper quadrant pain.

Hepatic stage (3 to 4 days after ingestion)

Progressive hepatic encephalopathy develops characterized by:

Vomiting	Confusion
Jaundice	Lethargy
Right upper quadrant pain	Coma
Bleeding	

Hypoglycemia

Transient high levels of liver enzymes

Renal damage

If acetaminophen ingestion is suspected, draw blood for serum acetaminophen level, ideally done at 4 hours post ingestion, and plot it on the Rumack/Matthews Nomogram. Levels drawn prior to 4 hours have no clinical value. Also obtain baseline liver enzymes, prothrombin time, BUN, blood sugar.

Specific intervention

1. Gastric decontamination using ipecac or lavage should be done if ingested dose is >7.5 g in an adult or >140 mg/kg in a child. If there is a delay in GI decontamination (>30 minutes), lavage is preferred.
2. Activated charcoal should be given as soon as possible to prevent subsequent toxic acetaminophen level. Do not administer concomitantly with NAC.
3. Cathartic.
4. Antidote administration N-acetylcysteine (NAC).
   a. If plasma level is toxic—N-acetylcysteine is preferably initiated within 8 hours of ingestion, but has statistical efficacy when given up to 24 hours post ingestion.
   b. NAC dosage
       Loading dose: 140 mg/kg orally as a 5% solution in cola, Fresca, orange juice, or grapefruit juice.
       Maintenance dose: 70 mg/kg orally as 5% solution every 4 hours for a total of 17 doses.
   c. Note: If a plasma level is obtained (at least 4 hours post ingestion) and falls above the broken line on the nomogram, NAC should be completely administered until the entire 17 doses are completed. Do not discontinue NAC even if future levels fall below the broken line.
   d. If there are problems with retention of NAC:
       I. Make sure it is a 5% solution.
       II. Metoclopramide may be given.
       III. Insert a gastric tube and drip in slowly.
       IV. If any dose is vomited within 1 hour, the dose should be repeated.

Alcohols (Table 13-1)

Alcohol is the most common drug taken by patients today. Different forms of alcohol—ethanol, isopropanolol, methanol, and ethylene glycol—have varying degrees of toxicity. A table showing varying degrees of toxicity is provided.

TABLE 13-1   Alcohols

FORMULATIONS AND USES:

Use	Approx. Conc.
1. Methanol: Gas line antifreeze	95
Windshield washer fluid	35-95
Antifreeze	Varied
Industrial solvents (e.g., paint & varnish remover, shellac)	
Sterno	
Dry gas	
2. Ethanol/Isopropanol	
Ethanol: Beverages	(proof/2 = % ETOH)
A) Beer	4-6
B) Wine	10-20
C) Spirits	20-50
Rubbing alcohol	70
Aftershaves/colognes	40-60
Mouthwashes	Up to 75
Medicinal Preparations	Varied
Isopropanol: Rubbing alcohol	70
Pine disinfectants	5-30
Solvents	Varied
3. Ethylene glycol, car radiator antifreeze	95

Note: Longer chain glycols (i.e., propylene glycol, polyethylene glycol) are relatively nontoxic orally.

Continued

TABLE 13-1 Alcohols—cont'd.

	METHANOL	ETHANOL/ISOPROPANOL	ETHYLENE GLYCOL
Comparison of toxicity	"Highly toxic" By history death has been reported after 15 ml 40% methylhydroxide; blindness reported after 4 ml.	Isopropanol is approximately twice as intoxicating as ethanol at equivalent blood levels. (Severe toxicity with blood levels >150 mg%)	"Highly toxic" Ex 3.0 ml of 100% ethylene glycol in a 10 kg child produces a potential level of 50 mg%; one gulp (2-8 ml) can produce levels of 34-135 mg%
	Ex. 1.5 ml of 100% methanol in a 10 kg child produces a potential level of 20 mg%; one gulp (2-8 ml) can produce levels of 26-105 mg%	Ethanol (blood levels) 50-100 mg% = mild toxicity 100-300 mg% = moderate toxicity >300 mg% = severe toxicity, but 1 ml/kg of pure ethanol will result in a blood level of approximately 100 mg% at 2 hours postingestion.	
	Blood levels	**Blood levels**	
	All are potentially toxic depending on the time of ingestion and presence of signs and symptoms.	All are potentially toxic depending on the time of ingestion and presence of signs and symptoms.	
Presentation and onset of symptoms	Toxicity *delayed:* Usual latent period is 12-24 hrs (may be delayed during concurrent ethanol ingestion). Gastritis and "hang-over"-like effect followed by visual disturbances and an anion gap metabolic acidosis.	Rapid onset of intoxication (30-60 min) Gastritis possible from high concentrations.	**Phase I (½-12 hr)** CNS ethanol-like inebriation (no odor) Anion gap metabolic acidosis Calcium oxalluria
			Phase II (2-36 hr) Tachypnea, Tachycardia
	Anion gap = *Na minus (HCO3 + CL). Normal = 12 ± 4 Mnemonic for an anion gap metabolic acidosis.		**Phase III (2-3 days)** Renal failure

M-U-D-P-I-L-E-S

Methanol
Uremia
Diabetic ketoacidosis
Paraldehyde; phenformin
Iron, isoniazid
Lactic acidosis
Ethylene glycol, ethanol ketoacidosis
Salicylates, sympathomimetics

Toxicology	Metabolized by the liver via alcohol dehydrogenase, to formaldehyde, and then very quickly to formic acid. It is these two metabolites, rather than the methanol, that causes the visual and metabolic changes.	*Ethanol:* Direct-acting CNS (reticular activating system) depressant. *Isopropanol:* Direct-acting CNS depressant. Causes local gastritis. The metabolite acetone acts to prolong CNS effects. Produces a ketosis without an acidosis	Neurologic symptoms. Due to parent compound. Renal toxicity due to formation of oxalic acid metabolite.
Home management	Consider emesis while en route to hospital. All but minute amounts of dilute concentrations must be referred to hospital.	If ingestion accidental, home assessment for CNS changes.	Consider emesis while en route to hospital. All but minute amounts of dilute concentration: refer to hospital.
Referral to medical facility	All suicide gestures. All symptomatic patients. All but minute amounts of dilute concentrations.	All suicide gestures. Symptomatic patients with calculated ethanol level >100 mg%.	All suicide gestures. All symptomatic patients. All but minute amounts of dilute concentration.

*New York City Poison Center: *Syllabus,* 1993.

Continued

TABLE 13-1 Alcohols—cont'd.

	METHANOL	ETHANOL/ISOPROPANOL	ETHYLENE GLYCOL
Hospital Management	(1) ABCs	(1) ABCs	(1) ABCs
	(2) Gut decontamination (time dependent)	(2) Gut decontamination (time dependent)	(2) Gut decontamination (time dependent)
	(3) Labs, diagnostic	(3) Labs, diagnostic	(3) Labs
	Blood methanol	Ethanol/Isopropanol/Acetone Levels	Ethylene glycol (if possible)
	Lytes	Blood and urine ketones	Electrolytes—including calcium
	ABCs	Electrolytes	ABG
	Calculate anion gap	Glucose	Calculate anion gap
	Blood ethanol	Calculate anion gap	ECG
	Fundoscopic exam of the eye	(4) Supportive Care	Urine analysis for oxalate or hippurate crystals
	(4) Ethanol therapy:		Some brands of antifreeze may be fluorescent under Woods' lamp.
	Loading dose followed by maintenance dose.		Ethanol therapy—loading dose followed by maintenance. (Same indications and dosing as in methanol management.)
	(Ethanol has 20× the affinity for alcohol dehydrogenase compared to methanol.)		(5) Hemodialysis.
	Indications		(6) Possibly thiamine and pyridoxine.
	OR		
	(B) (+) Blood methanol level		
	OR		
	(C) Symptomatic patient and strong suspicion.		
	Load		
	7.6-10 ml/kg IV of 10% ethanol in D5W over 30 minutes to achieve blood ethanol level of 100-130 mg%.		
	Oral route acceptable.		

Maintenance

1.4 ml/kg/hr of 10% ethanol IV.
Requirements increase in chronic alcoholics and during hemodialysis.
Treat until level of methanol is zero.
(5) Hemodialysis
(6) Folinic or folic acid.

Physician consultant   All patients in hospital.   All patients with unstable vital signs (or acidosis-unrelated). Suspect MEOH or ethylene glycol.   All patients in hospital.

*New York City Poison Center: *Syllabus*, 1993.

Calcium Antagonists

This is rapidly becoming one of the most serious overdoses in toxicology today. Potentially any amount can be toxic in a patient with underlying cardiac disease. Dose relationships are not well established, and patients must be monitored for signs and symptoms. Hypotension and bradycardia generally occur within 1 to 5 hours postingestion. These effects may worsen over this time and persist more than 24 hours. Use caution with sustained-release products because although the onset may be rapid, peak effects may be delayed and prolonged. These drugs come as both prompt and sustained-release forms.

■ **SIGNS AND SYMPTOMS**
Hypotension
Cardiac disturbances (dysrhythmias and conduction abnormalities)
Confusion, drowsiness, mental status changes
Nausea and vomiting are common

■ **THERAPEUTIC INTERVENTIONS**
Lavage
Activated charcoal and cathartic
Multiple-dose activated charcoal for sustained release products
Consideration of whole bowel irrigation with sustained release products
Monitoring ECG and vital signs
If hypotensive and/or bradycardia, calcium chloride is antidotal by increasing the concentration gradient in the serum to lower intracellular calcium flow.

Carbon Monoxide

Carbon monoxide poisoning causes a multitude of effects due to tissue hypoxia and possible cellular poisoning. It has rapid onset of poisoning following acute exposure. Acute symptoms may be followed by delayed neuropsychiatric sequelae.*

■ **SIGNS AND SYMPTOMS**

MILD TO MODERATE	MODERATE TO SEVERE
Nausea	Agitation
Vomiting	Confusion
Mild throbbing headache	Severe headache
Malaise	Unconsciousness
Mimics flulike illness	Seizures
Should be suspect in outbreaks of "food poisoning"	Respiratory failure

■ **THERAPEUTIC INTERVENTIONS**
Give 100% oxygen by tight-fitting mask to reduce the half-life of carbon monoxide.
Monitor EKG.
Assess vital signs.
Draw carboxyhemoglobin level (before starting oxygen as long as this does not delay initiation of this treatment).

*Pregnant women are at high risk. The fetus has an affinity for carbon monoxide and the concentration of carboxyhemoglobin is 10% to 15% greater in the fetus than in the mother.

Concentrations frequently do not correlate well with the severity of the poisoning.

Consider hyperbaric oxygen therapy in severely poisoned patients who have altered mental status or coma, and in pregnant women.

Cyclic Antidepressants

Cyclic antidepressants are drugs that are used to treat depression. The major problems with these overdoses is seizure coma and fatal dysrhythmias. Ingesting 10 to 20 mg/kg of tricyclic antidepressant can result in moderate to serious exposure.

■ **SIGNS AND SYMPTOMS OF TOXICITY**

Confusion	Red, dry skin
Agitation	Urinary retention
Hallucinations	Decreased respirations
Seizures/coma	Mydriasis
Hypotension	Dysrhythmias (especially tachydysrhythmias and conduction
Fever	blocks)

■ **THERAPEUTIC INTERVENTIONS**

ABCs
Oxygen
IV Ringer's lactate
Do not give ipecac because of the risk of seizures
Gastric lavage
Multiple-dose activated charcoal
Cathartic

Sodium bicarbonate is the first-line drug for treatment of cardiac conduction defects and hypotension. If the patient is hypotensive keep his or her blood pH at 7.5. If the hypotension is unresponsive to $NaHCO_3$, norepinephrine is the drug of choice.

Give diazepam for seizures. Do not use phenytoin: it may worsen cardiac toxicity. If the QRS >0.10 seconds, there is an increased chance for seizures. If the QRS >0.16 seconds, there is an increased chance for dysrhythmias.

Digoxin

Digoxin can increase inotrophy (contractility), cause a prolonged AV node refractory period, and shorten the action potential of the Purkinje fibers. It enhances cardiac output and reduces cardiac rate. It is used most commonly to treat congestive heart failure, atrial fibrillation, atrial flutter, and, on occasion, paroxysmal atrial tachycardia. Toxicity should be suspected in the elderly when any of the following signs and symptoms appear.

■ **SIGNS AND SYMPTOMS**

MILD	**SEVERE**
Anorexia	Blurred vision
Premature ventricular contractions	Disorientation
Bradycardia	Diarrhea

MILD	**SEVERE**
Nausea and vomiting	SA or AV block
Headache	Ventricular tachycardia
Malaise	Ventricular fibrillation
Color disturbances (see yellow)	

The onset of peak manifestations of cardiac toxicity following acute digoxin poisoning may be as little as 30 minutes and as much as 3 to 12 hours, respectively.

■ **THERAPEUTIC INTERVENTIONS**

ABCs

Discontinuation of digoxin and diuretics

Lavage

Activated charcoal and cathartic

Multiple-dose activated charcoal

Correcting electrolyte imbalances (hypokalemia-enhanced digoxin toxicity)

Correcting dysrhythmias

Possible administration of digitalis-specific antidote (Digibind)

Monitoring serial serum digoxin and potassium levels

FOOD POISONING

Food poisoning occurs in two forms:

1. Food infection—Ingested food substances contain bacteria that produce illness following their multiplication in the intestinal tract.
2. Food intoxication—Ingested food substances contain toxins from previous multiplication of bacteria, resulting in poisoning from toxin released into the body system. The causative organism is usually *Staphylococcus aureus.*

For an overview of food toxins refer to Table 13-2.

■ **SIGNS AND SYMPTOMS**

Signs and symptoms usually occur 1 to 24 hours following ingestion of contaminated food. Onset is abrupt.

Nausea and vomiting

Diarrhea and abdominal cramping

■ **THERAPEUTIC INTERVENTIONS**

Obtain a history of the patient's food intake.

Ascertain if other individuals who ate the same foods have also been affected.

Monitor the patient's temperature (often subnormal).

Draw blood samples for electrolytes and osmolarity values.

Initiate IV fluids if dehydration is severe or if signs of shock are present.

Correct electrolyte imbalances.

Obtain stool culture.

TABLE 13-2 Differential Diagnosis of Bacterial Etiologies for Diarrhea and Food Poisoning

BACTERIAL DIARRHEA	PATHOGENESIS	SYMPTOMS					INCUBATION PERIOD	EFFECT OF HEAT	AGE GROUP	TRANSMISSION PATTERN	EXTRA INTESTINAL SYMPTOMS	CULTURE
		FEVER	DIARRHEA	DYSENTERY*	ABDOMINAL PAIN	VOMITING						
Clostridium perfringens	Enterotoxin	–	+	+†	++	±‡	8-24 hr	Thermostable organism Thermolabile toxin	Adults	Poultry, heat-processed meats (stews)	Volume depletion	Food, stool, vomitus
Escherichia coli	Enterotoxin	–	±	±	±	0§	24-72 hr	Thermostable toxin capsular-thermolabile toxin	All	Contact	Volume depletion	Stool
Salmonellae	Bacteria (Endotoxin)	+	+	±	±	±	8-48 hr	Thermolabile organism	All	Prepared foods, poultry, egg products, pet turtles and chicks	Headache, bacteremia	Food, stool, blood
Shigellae	Bacteria (Endotoxin)	±	+	+	+	±	24-72 hr	Thermolabile organism, thermolabile toxin	All	Institutions	Seizures, meningismus	Food, stool
Staphylococci	Enterotoxin	–	+	0	+	+	2-6 hr	Thermostable toxin	All	Prepared food, (salami, varied salads), fowl, pastry	Volume depletion	Food, stool

*Dysentery = diarrhea with blood and mucus.
† + = Occurs regularly. §0 = Does not occur.
‡ ± = May or may not occur. †† = Very consequential
(Modified after Grady GF, Keusch GT: Pathogenesis of bacterial diarrheas, *N Engl J Med* 285:831-841, 891-900, 1971.)

Continued.

TABLE 13-2 Differential Diagnosis of Bacterial Etiologies for Diarrhea and Food Poisoning—cont'd.

BACTERIAL DIARRHEA	PATHOGENESIS	SYMPTOMS FEVER	SYMPTOMS DIARRHEA	SYMPTOMS DYSENTERY*	SYMPTOMS ABDOMINAL PAIN	SYMPTOMS VOMITING	INCUBATION PERIOD	EFFECT OF HEAT	AGE GROUP	TRANSMISSION PATTERN	EXTRA INTESTINAL SYMPTOMS	CULTURE
Streptococci	Bacteria	+	±	–	–	–	24-72 hr	Thermolabile organism	All	Proteinaceous foods	Influenza-like pharyngitis	Food, stool, blood
Vibrio cholerae	Enterotoxin	±	+	0	±	±	24-72 hr	Thermolabile toxin	All	Water, food	Hypokalemic nephropathy	Stool
Clostridium botulinum	Neurotoxin	–	–	–	±	±	12-36 hr	Thermostable spor thermo-labile toxin	All	Diverse canned foods	Dysphagia, descending paralysis	Serum, stool, vomitus for toxin
Bacillus cereus												
Type I	Enterotoxin	–	+	–	+	++	1-6 hr	Thermolabile toxin	All	Fried rice	Limited	Food, stool
Type II	Enterotoxin	–	++	–	+	±	10-12 hr	Thermolabile toxin	All	Meats, vegetables	Volume depletion	Food, stool
Campylobacter jejuni	Enterotoxin	+	+	–	+	+	1-7 days	Thermolabile toxin	All	Poultry, meats, dairy produce	Limited	Food, stool, blood

*Dysentery = diarrhea with blood and mucus.
† + = Occurs regularly.
‡ ± = May or may not occur.
§0 = Does not occur.
†† = Very consequential
(Modified after Grady GF, Keusch GT: Pathogenesis of bacterial diarrhea, N Engl J Med 285:831-841, 891-900, 1971.)

Botulism

Suspect botulism in the presence of any neurologic signs and symptoms that mimic a stroke, Guillian-Barré syndrome, myasthenia gravis, or arsenic toxicity. Botulism is relatively rare, but occurs typically in a sporadic outbreak of a family or other group. The usual exotoxins causing poisoning are A, B, and E (E is commonly from fish); rare toxins C and F are also seen on occasion. Botulism is the most serious type of food poisoning. It can also occur following wound contamination with *Clostridium botulinum.*

The typical cause of botulism is poorly processed or spoiled home-canned vegetables, especially the nonacid types, such as green beans. Bulging can lids (resulting from expanding gases as the organisms grow) are often determined in the history-taking phase.

Signs and symptoms usually develop 8 to 36 hours following ingestion of contaminated food, but may be delayed for as long as 4 days.

■ **SIGNS AND SYMPTOMS**

Presenting signs and symptoms are often vague.

Lethargy/weakness
Constipation
Visual disturbances (double vision)
Impaired speech
Headache
Afebrile or subnormal temperature
Dry, sore throat with hoarseness; inability to swallow
Limited eye movement
Dilated pupils
Decreased tendon reflexes
Descending paralysis

■ **THERAPEUTIC INTERVENTIONS**

Ensure ABCs (the patient may require a tracheostomy and ventilatory assistance).

Induction of emesis may be of benefit in patients immediately following food *known* to contain botulism toxin.

Symptomatic patients should not be lavaged or made to vomit.

If the patient is asymptomatic or exposure is questionable: may follow closely as an outpatient.

Asymptomatic and probably exposed patients should be hospitalized under close observation and treated with antitoxin on appearance of symptoms.

Symptomatic patients should be admitted to ICU, the toxin type determined, and treated with the antitoxin.

If several hours have elapsed, administer sodium sulfate (250 mg/kg) orally or magnesium sulfate (250 mg/kg) orally as a cathartic because this toxin is slowly absorbed.

Salmonellosis

Salmonellosis is contracted through ingestion of contaminated foods. It may be found in raw meats, poultry, eggs, fish, and milk and products made with them.

■ **SIGNS AND SYMPTOMS**
Onset approximately 12 to 48 hours after eating
Diarrhea (severe)
Nausea and vomiting (severe)
Chills
Fever

■ **THERAPEUTIC INTERVENTIONS**
Treatment of symptoms
Fluid and electrolyte replacement
Antidiarrheal agents
Antiemetics
Antipyretics

Iron

The number one cause of death in pediatric poisonings in 1991 and 1992 was iron. A wide variety of drugs and chemical agents contain iron. Toxicity is based on mg/kg. Serious toxicity is also based on clinical findings in addition to the mg/kg calculation.

■ **SIGNS AND SYMPTOMS**

MINOR	MAJOR
Vomiting	Stupor
Diarrhea	Shock
Mild lethargy	Hematemesis
Hyperglycemia	Acidosis
	Bloody diarrhea
	Coma

■ **THERAPEUTIC INTERVENTIONS**
ABCs
Induced emesis (preferred especially in children)
Gastric lavage (most adult-strength pills will not fit through lavage tubes)
Cathartic
Abdominal and chest x-ray to view for tablets remaining in the gut and further lavage may be necessary (children's multiple vitamins are less likely to show up)
Whole bowel irrigation when there is radiographic evidence of iron tablets past the pylorus or if the tablets persist in the stomach after other attempts at decontamination
Serum iron drawn at 4 to 6 hours postingestion; if >350 mcg/dl in a symptomatic patient initiate deferoxamine. If SI cannot be obtained in a reasonable amount of time in a symptomatic patient, begin deferoxamine
IV D_5W
Treatment of acid/base abnormalities
Monitoring electrolytes
Administer deferoxamine (15 mg/kg/hr IV or IM [90 mg/kg every 8 hours]) until the vin rose color of the urine disappears. Be sure to get an initial urine

sample before deferoxamine therapy to compare because urine color change
may be very subtle.

Consider exchange transfusions in severely symptomatic patients.

Mushrooms

Mushroom species range from being nontoxic to lethal, depending on the type
of toxin present. It is important that the mushroom specimen be identified as
soon as possible by a competent mycologist if the patient has symptoms.

The clinical effects will vary with the type of mushroom toxin involved. A
good history may help to identify the mushrooms involved. Any poisoning
involving an unidentified mushroom in which the latent period between ingestion and onset of symptoms is 6 hours or more, should be presumed to be an
intoxication from mushrooms containing highly toxic amatoxins, and intensive
care should be initiated immediately.

■ **SIGNS AND SYMPTOMS**

Will vary with the different type or types of mushrooms ingested. Consult with
your local poison center.

■ **THERAPEUTIC INTERVENTIONS**

Emesis—if recent ingestion

Activated charcoal and cathartic

Save all emesis and stools in refrigerator (do not freeze) for possible microscopic study and analysis.

Observation for seizures, hypotension

Possible analgesics, sedatives, antispasmodics, and antiemetics

Supportive care

PESTICIDES

Organophosphates and carbamates are two very common pesticides available
that can cause serious toxicity. They have similar symptoms, but duration of
symptoms is usually less with carbamates.

These can be absorbed by all routes of administration—inhalation, dermal,
and oral.

■ **SIGNS AND SYMPTOMS**

Salivation

Lacrimation

Urination

Defecation

GI disturbances

Emesis

plus bradycardia and miosis

■ **THERAPEUTIC INTERVENTIONS**

Decontamination of eyes and skin (remove clothing and isolate; leather must be
discarded)

Lavage

Administering activated charcoal/cathartic

Protecting hospital personnel from exposure

IV access—(if sick) for fluids and electrolytes and antidotes

Administering antidotes: atropine—may need large doses, give until secretions are minimized and the airway is stable.

2 Pam is usually given only with organophosphate, but many exposures are mixed exposures. 2-Pam is synergistic with atropine, so use only with severe organophosphate poisoning and when exposure is unknown.

PETROLEUM DISTILLATES

Kerosene, charcoal lighter fluid, mineral oil, furniture polish, turpentine, gasoline, and many insecticides have petroleum-distillate bases. Complications usually occur as a result of aspiration or other pulmonary problems. Aspiration of hydrocarbons may also result in transient CNS depression or excitation.

■ **SIGNS AND SYMPTOMS**

Respiratory difficulty

Infiltrates on chest x-ray

Abnormal arterial blood gases

Dysrhythmias

■ **THERAPEUTIC INTERVENTIONS**

ABCs; intubate if necessary.

Give oxygen.

Wash surface areas that have been contaminated.

Gastric emptying is not indicated unless a history of large ingestion of hydrocarbons that may produce renal, liver or CNS toxicity (i.e., halogenated hydrocarbons or petroleum or petroleum distillates with additives).

Monitor ABGs in symptomatic patients (e.g., coughing, choking).

Obtain a chest x-ray film (should be diagnostic within 6 hours after ingestion).

SALICYLATES

With over 200 readily available over-the-counter preparations containing salicylates it is a common overdose seen in emergency departments. Diagnosis can be missed at admission, resulting in increased morbidity and mortality. Hallmark symptoms consist of metabolic acidosis with a concomitant respiratory alkalosis.

Toxicity

Greater than 150 to 300 mg/kg can cause moderate to serious exposure.

Greater than 300 to 500 mg/kg can cause severe toxicity.

■ **SIGNS AND SYMPTOMS**

Tachypnea

Tachycardia

Tinnitus

Volume depletion

GI (nausea, vomiting, hemorrhagic gastritis)

Altered mental status
Coagulation abnormalities
Fluid and electrolyte disturbances
■ **THERAPEUTIC INTERVENTIONS**
ABCs (consider endotracheal intubation, if necessary)
Oxygen
Inducing emesis if gag reflex present and recent ingestion
Lavage
Activated charcoal and cathartic
Multiple-dose activated charcoal
Obtain serum salicylate levels—stat level repeat serial levels every 2 to 4 hours
   in large overdose. Serum levels may rise for up to 24 hours when the patient
   will be absorbing the drug.
Lab studies—CBC, lytes, glucose, blood gases, PT, platelet count, BUN, creati-
   nine, LFTs and urinalysis
Supportive therapy consists of correcting acidosis, treating dehydration aggres-
   sively, replacing potassium, and alkalinizing the urine. Treat hemorrhage
   with vitamin K, and external cooling for fever.
Consider hemodialysis in severity toxic patients with progressive clinical deterioration despite conventional therapy. The inability to alkalinize the urine is a
   grave sign and hemodialysis should be considered.

THEOPHYLLIN

This drug is commonly used in treating both acute and chronic illness. Its repu-
tation for causing toxicity is great as it has a low therapeutic index. There are
many sustained-release preparations available that can cause prolonged CNS
and cardiovascular toxicity.
■ **SIGNS AND SYMPTOMS**
Protracted nausea and vomiting
Seizures
Cardiac arrhythmias
Hypotension
Metabolic acidosis
Hypokalemia
■ **THERAPEUTIC INTERVENTIONS**
Lavage (pill size may be too large to fit through orogastric tube)
Activated charcoal and cathartic
Multiple-dose activated charcoal—in serious overdoses repeat every 1 to 2
   hours.
Be aggressive with antiemetics—it is mandatory to keep the charcoal down.
Determine the theophyllin level and monitor serial levels frequently until the
   level is therapeutic.
Consider whole bowel irrigation.
Hemodialysis should be considered if there are seizures, cardiovascular instabil-
   ity, or rising theophyllin levels despite good attempts at GI decontamination.

DRUGS OF ABUSE

These are varied in different parts of the country. With the number of available illicit drugs increasing at a rapid rate, the poison center may be the only source of information for an overdose or poisoning with a brand new "designer" drug.

Cocaine

Cocaine is the recreational drug of choice in America today. Any dosage is potentially toxic. Clinical symptoms are a better indication of toxicity. Toxic reactions are hard to predict because of the variation in street impurities, adulterants, cocaine content, and individual tolerance. The greatest risk is for a myocardial infarction.

■ **SIGNS AND SYMPTOMS**
CNS—euphoria, hyperactivity, agitation, seizures, hyperthermia
Mydriasis
Cardiovascular—chest pain with or without tachycardia, hypertension, dysrhythmia, cardiac arrest

■ **THERAPEUTIC INTERVENTIONS**
If ingested, administer activated charcoal and cathartic.
Obtain an EKG on all patients (suspect myocardial insult; this finding may be delayed).
Administer glucose and thiamine for agitated patients.
Administer benzodiazepines for sedation and seizures.
Institute external cooling for hyperthermia.

Opioids/Opioid Antagonist

These drugs are used for analgesia, sedation, and mood altering. There is a great variation in toxicity, depending on a patient's tolerance. New designer opioids vary widely in toxicity. Infants and children are more susceptible than adults. Clinical symptoms are more useful to judge toxicity. Patients with significant opioid overdose merit close observation and supportive care for 24 to 48 hours.

■ **SIGNS AND SYMPTOMS**
Depression of all vital signs
Miosis
Hypotension
Mental status depression
Respiratory depression is most critical problem
Nausea/vomiting

■ **THERAPEUTIC INTERVENTIONS**
Gastric lavage
Activated charcoal and cathartic
Multiple-dose activated charcoal
Naloxone (Narcan)
IV fluids

CURRENTLY AVAILABLE ANTIDOTES

An antidote is a physiological antagonist that may reverse the signs and symptoms of poisoning and should be employed as soon as possible (Table 13-3).

This is only a very brief guide to some of the more common problems in toxicology. This field is emerging and changing rapidly. For the most current information and help in caring for your patient, contact your local Poison Information Center. They can give you more in-depth guidance for treatment of the poisoned patient.

REFERENCES

1. Ellenhorn MJ, Barceloux DG: *Medical toxicology—diagnosis and treatment of human poisoning.* New York, 1988, Elsevier.
2. Goldfrank L: *Goldfrank's toxicological emergencies.* East Norwalk, Conn, 1990, Appleton and Lange.
3. Haddad LM, Winchester JF: *Clinical management of poisoning and drug overdose,* ed 2. Philadelphia, 1990, Saunders.
4. New York City Poison Center. *Syllabus,* 1993.
5. Rumack BH, Spoerrke DG: *Poisindex information system.* Denver, Micromedex, Inc.

SUGGESTED READINGS

Markenson D, Greenberg D: Cyclic antidepressant overdose: mechanism to management, *Emergency Medicine* 25(11):49, 1993.

TABLE 13-3 Antidote Chart

POISON	ANTIDOTE	COMMENTS
Black widow	Antivenin	Latrodectus-mactans venom neutralizer; 1–2 vials IV over 1 hour
Rattlesnake		Crotalidae Polyvalent venom neutralizer; see P'dex for dosage.
Carbamates	Atropine	Antagonizes cholinergic stimuli at muscarinic receptors.
Organophosphate		
Physostigmine excess		
Synthetic choline esters and inocybe		
Mushrooms (clitocybe and inocybe)		
Neuroleptic drugs (Haloperidol, Phenothiazines, Thioxanthenes) and Metoclopramide	Benztropine	Reverses drug-induced dystonias through competitive inhibition of muscarinic receptors & blockade of dopamine reuptake.
Botulism	Botulism antitoxin	Contact CDC—404-329-3753; after hours—404-329-3644. Draw 10 ml of serum for determination of toxin before treatment is started.
Calcium channel blockers	Calcium chloride (drug of choice unless patient is acidotic) Calcium gluconate (use if patient is acidotic)	Large amounts may be required. Keep serum $Ca^{++} < 11$.
Hydrofluoric acid burns Black widow spider Hyperkalemia Hypermagnesemia	Calcium gluconate	2.5% gel for dermal exposure (calcium gluconate). 10% calcium gluconate local infiltration or arterial infusion for HF burns. IV calcium gluconate for hyperkalemia & hypermagnesemia
Lead	CaEDTA	
Cadmium Zinc Copper	Calcium disodium edetate	Precautions: adequate fluids, monitor urine output; avoid rapid IV. Not effective on mercury, gold or arsenic.

Poison/Toxin	Antidote	Comments
Cyanide Hydrogen sulfide (H₂SO)	Cyanide kit	Instructions are explicit in kit. Oxygen and methemoglobin levels need to be monitored closely. * Do not use methylene blue if excessive methemoglobinemia occurs. H₂SO. DO NOT use NaThiosulfate. Use nitrites only.
Iron	Deferoxamine	Deferoxamine mesylate forms excretable ferrioxamine complex. This red complex is water soluble and readily excreted by the kidneys. Passing of vin rosé urine indicates Fe present.
Cocaine LSD	Diazepam	
Digitalis Oleander Foxglove	Digoxin Immune Fab (Digibind®)	Antigen binding fragments bind with digoxin for digitalis overdose.
Arsenic Lead encephalopathy Gold Mercury	Dimercaprol (Bal)	Heavy metals inhibit sulfhydryl containing enzymes; the resulting chelated mercaptide product is less toxic and more easily excreted from the body than the heavy metals.
Phenothiazine Allergic reactions	Diphenhydramine	Will reverse drug-induced extrapyramidal effects.
Lead	DMSA (Dimercaptosuccinic acid)	Oral active chelating agent indicated for treatment of lead poisoning in children with lead levels >45 µg/dl.
Arsenic Lead Mercury Bismuth	D-Penicillamine	Contraindicated for penicillin allergic patients.
Methalon Ethylene glycol	Ethanol for IV administration	Reduces formation of toxic metabolites. Competitive inhibitors of alcohol dehydrogenase. Monitor blood glucose. Adjust dose if dialysis is performed.
Benzodiazepines	Flumazenil	Use caution if unknown drug ingestion. Seizures can occur with reversal of BZP effects, especially with TCA coingestion.
Methanol	Folic acid & Leucovorin	May be effective in adjunctive therapy stimulating the pathway for methanol metabolites. Allergic reaction may occur.
Beta-blocker	Glucagon	Bypasses beta adrenergic blockades by activating non-beta receptors; increasing contractility.

*Adapted from New Hampshire Poison Center's Protocols

Continued.

TABLE 13-3 Antidote Chart—cont'd

POISON	ANTIDOTE	COMMENTS
Aniline Nitrites Local anesthetics	Methylene blue	Reducing agent to convert methemoglobin to methemoglobin hemoglobin.
Acetaminophen	N-Acetylcysteine	Gluthathione substitute that prevents the formation of toxic intermediary metabolites. Best when given within 8 hours of ingestion; can be given within 24 hours of ingestion.
Opioids Ethanol-induced coma Clonidine Propoxyphene Diphenoxylate Pentazocine	Naloxone	Opioid antagonist that reverses the CNS and respiratory depressant effects.
Vacor Streptozocin	Nicotinamide	For best results should be given within 30 minutes of vacor ingestion.
Carbon monoxide	Oxygen	Administer 100% oxygen by tight-fitting mask to reduce half life of CO.
Anticholinergic (rarely) TCA (last resort)	Physostigmine	Inhibits the destructive action of acetylcholinesterase. Should not be used routinely for OD because of its potential adverse effects.
Warfarin Long-acting anticoagulants	Phytonadione (Vit K$_1$)	Reverses the inhibitory action of warfarin on blood clotting factors II, VII, IX & X in the liver.
Organophosphate	Pralidoxime	Cholinesterase reactivator for organophosphate OD. Should be given after adequate atropine therapy.
Heparin	Protamine	Protamine reacts with heparin to form a stable salt resulting in neutralization of heparin anticoagulant activity.
Isoniazid Monomethylhydrazine mushrooms	Pyridoxine	Pyridoxine is used to prevent & control isoniazid-induced seizures. Pyridoxine may reverse neurologic symptoms with this mushroom ingestion.
TCA	Sodium bicarbonate	Aside from gastric decontamination NaHCO$_3$ is the most useful single intervention for management of TCA.

*Adapted from New Hampshire Poison Center's Protocols

14

Environmental Emergencies

SNAKEBITES

There are over 3000 species of snakes; of these, 375 from five different families are venomous. These families are:

- Crotalidae—copperheads, rattlesnakes, cottonmouths
- Elapidae—coral snakes, cobras, mambas
- Viperidae (true vipers)—puff adders
- Hydrophidae—sea snakes
- Colubridae—boomslangs

Over 45,000 snakebites occur each year in the United States. Of these, 8000 are from poisonous snakes. There are, however, fewer than 15 deaths.

Many venoms contain toxins that are cardiotoxic, neurotoxic, or hemotoxic. Venom is injected by the fangs of the snake. The ducts of the fangs are filled with venom that is manufactured in the salivary glands.

The most common site for a snakebite is an extremity that is close to the snake (i.e., an arm or a leg).

■ **SIGNS AND SYMPTOMS**

Signs and symptoms of snakebite depend on several factors:

Size and species of the snake
Location of the bite
Depth of the bite
Number of bites inflicted
Amount of venom injected
Age of the patient
Size of the patient
Patient's sensitivity to venom
Number of microorganisms in the snake's mouth

Signs and symptoms can be divided into local and systemic reactions

Local reactions

Fang marks
Teeth marks
Edema (occurs within 5 minutes and may extend to 36 hours)
Pain at the site (usually correlated with the amount of edema)
Petechiae
Ecchymosis
Loss of function of the limb
Necrosis (16 to 36 hours after the bite)

Systemic reactions

Nausea and vomiting
Diaphoresis
Syncope
Metallic or rubber taste in mouth
Constricted pupil
Ptosis
Visual disturbances (mostly diplopia)
Muscle twitching
Paresthesias

Paralysis
Salivation
Difficulty speaking
Seizures
Epistaxis
Hematemesis
Hemoptysis
Hematuria
Melena

Severe systemic reactions

Pulmonary edema
Severe hemorrhage
Renal failure
Hypovolemic shock

■ THERAPEUTIC INTERVENTIONS

Ensure ABCs.
Keep the patient calm.
Remove potentially constricting jewelry.
DO NOT use ice. (Although cryotherapy has some strong proponents, most
   experts advise against the application of cold packs. In some cases, *cryother-*
   apy rather than the bite itself has necessitated amputation).
DO NOT give alcohol or substances containing caffeine to drink.
DO NOT allow patient to smoke.
Immobilize the limb.
Keep the limb at or below the level of the heart.
Place a *loose* constriction band 4 inches proximal to the bite if within 30 min-
   utes of the bite. (Once applied, do not remove in the field.)
Cleanse the wound.
Early incision and wound suction. (If done *immediately*, this can remove 25%
   to 50% of the venom. This is generally not effective after 10 to 15 minutes.)
   Suction wound with rubber suction cup or syringe. Avoid mouth suction to
   prevent absorption of venom via open areas in the mouth.
Give analgesia for pain management.
Initiate IVs (two) with Ringer's lactate or normal saline solution.
Place a central venous pressure line or an arterial pressure line.
Consider tetanus prophylaxis.

Consider surgical intervention.

Consider antivenin therapy.

Be sure to record the time of the bite and the times of any subsequent therapies. Identify or secure the snake if possible. (DO NOT HANDLE THE SNAKE!)

Antivenin. Antivenin administration should be reserved for life-threatening snakebites only because it carries a high incidence of sensitivity reactions and possible anaphylaxis. It should be administered in the hospital setting, where the patient can be closely monitored. (Antivenin administration is not a prehospital care procedure!) Follow these guidelines:

- Be sure equipment is readily available; be prepared for CPR situations.
- Obtain a careful allergy history.
- Do a conjunctival or skin test to test for sensitivity reaction: A positive reaction occurs within 5 to 30 minutes.
- If a reaction does occur (urticaria, wheezing, cyanosis, edema, anaphylaxis), administer 1:1000 epinephrine (0.2 to 0.5 ml) subcutaneously

Be sure to read the antivenin package insert thoroughly and follow the directions *precisely.*

SPIDER (ARACHNID) BITES

Most spider bites induce itching, swelling, and stinging pain as local complications. Spiders that induce systemic and local complications are the black widow and the brown recluse.

Black Widow Spiders (Latorodectus Mactans)

Black widow spiders are usually found in damp, cool places. They may be identified by their black bodies and the red hourglass-shaped figure on their abdomens. The venom of the black widow is *neurotoxic.*

■ **SIGNS AND SYMPTOMS**

Painful sting at the time of the bite followed by a dull, numb pain

Tiny red marks at the point of entry of the venom

Nausea and vomiting

Hypertension

Elevated temperature

Respiratory distress

Headache

Syncope

Weakness

Chest pain

Abdominal pain

Seizures

Shock

■ **THERAPEUTIC INTERVENTIONS**

If aggressive supportive therapy is given, signs and symptoms will usually be gone within 48 hours.

Treat the patient symptomatically.

Cool the area of the bite with ice packs to slow the action of the neurotoxin.

Give muscle relaxants—methocarbamol (Robaxin) or diazepam (Valium).

Administer calcium gluconate for muscle spasms (use 10 ml of 10% solution mixed in 100 ml of normal saline solution and run it in over 20 minutes).

Consider narcotic analgesics.

Consider antivenin; read antivenin literature carefully and thoroughly before administering.

Brown Recluse Spiders (Loxosceles Reclusa)

Brown recluse spiders are found in the southeastern, south-central, and southwestern states. They inhabit dark areas such as basements, garages, boxes, and closets. These spiders may be identified by their light brown color and the dark brown fiddle-shaped mark on their thoraxes.

■ **SIGNS AND SYMPTOMS**

Local reactions

Mild stinging at the time of the bite

Local edema

Bluish ring around the bite appears within 2 to 8 hours after the bite

Bleb formation

Erythema

Local ischemia

Tissue necrosis—appears on third or fourth day

Eschar/open sore—appears in 14 days

Wound healing—appears in 21 days

Systemic reactions

Fever	General malaise
Chills	Arthralgias/joint pain
Nausea and vomiting	Petechiae
Weakness	

Severe systemic reactions (seen in small adults and children)—very rare

Seizures

Disseminated intravascular coagulation (DIC)

Renal failure

Hemolysis

Cardiopulmonary arrest

■ **THERAPEUTIC INTERVENTIONS**

Consider antihistamines.

Consider antibiotics.

Consider systemic or local steroids.

Consider local debridement.

Consider skin grafting.

Rehydration (orally or intravenously).

Consider blood transfusions.

Perform dialysis.

Scorpion Stings

Scorpions are found in the warm southwestern states of California, Arizona, and Texas. Incidence of scorpion stings increases in the cool evening and night hours. Although there are several species of scorpions, *Centuroides sculpturatus* is the only species that injects a lethal venom. The tail of the scorpion contains the telson, in which venom is produced and stored, and the stinger, which injects the venom.

■ **SIGNS AND SYMPTOMS**

Local pain at the sting site	Wheezing stridor
Edema	Profuse salivation
Discoloration	Visual disturbances
Hyperesthesia	Ataxic gait
Numbness	Incontinence
Agitation or drowsiness	Jaw muscle spasms
Itching	Nausea and vomiting
Speech disturbances	Dysphagia
Tachycardia	Seizures
Hypertension	Anaphylaxis
Tachypnea	

■ **THERAPEUTIC INTERVENTIONS**

Support ABCs.

Treat the patient symptomatically.

Ensure tetanus prophylaxis.

Consider antivenin therapy.

(Avoid narcotic analgesics and barbiturates as these have been shown to increase the toxic effects of the venom.)

BEE, WASP, HORNET, AND FIRE ANT (HYMENOPTERA) STINGS

Hymenoptera stings can result in anything from a local reaction to anaphylactic shock. Reactions can occur from immediately to 48 hours after the sting. The greater the incidence of stings, the greater the possibility of a severe reaction.

■ **SIGNS AND SYMPTOMS**

Mild local reactions

Stinging and burning sensation at time of sting

Swelling

Itching

Severe local reaction

Total extremity edema

Systemic reactions

Urticaria

Pruritus

Edema (extremities and periorbital region)

Anaphylactic shock

Bronchospasm

Laryngeal edema

Hypotension

■ **THERAPEUTIC INTERVENTIONS**

For mild reactions

Scrape the stinger away with a dull object; do not grasp and pull it as this contracts the venom sac and releases more toxin.

Cleanse the sting site.

Apply antiseptic cream.

Consider oral antihistamines.

Consider steroids.

Apply ice.

Elevate the limb.

For severe reactions

Support ABCs.

Give epinephrine (1:10,000 IV for anaphylactic shock)

Initiate IVs.

Apply the PASG.

Consider vasopressors.

Antihistamines doses will vary.

Consider steroids.

Consider theophylline.

Fire ants have a painful sting that forms a wheal, which expands into a large vesicle. The area reddens and a pustule forms. As the pustule is reabsorbed, crusting and scar formation follow. This hymenopteran's sting may also cause anaphylaxis. Therapeutic intervention is the same as that for other hymenoptera stings.

■ **PREVENTIVE MEASURES AGAINST HYMENOPTERA STINGS**

Avoid areas where hymenoptera are usually present.

Avoid wearing bright colors.

Do not wear perfumes outdoors.

Wear shoes when walking outdoors.

People who have a sensitivity to hymenoptera venom should carry an anaphylaxis prevention kit that contains 1:1000 epinephrine and antihistamines. They should also be instructed to wear a Medic-Alert bracelet or some other type of medical identification tag stating their sensitivity. Desensitization is a possibility in some patients; it has been reported as 95% effective.

TICK BITES

Ticks may cause flaccid paralysis when they bite because of the neurotoxins they inject. Initially the patient will have paresthesias and pain in the lower extremities. Respiratory failure may result from bulbar paralysis.

■ **THERAPEUTIC INTERVENTIONS**

Support ABCs.

Remove the tick.

Observe for local reaction infection at the site.

Lyme Disease

Ticks are the vector for the spirochete that causes Lyme disease, so named for the geographic location of its original presentation. Due to the vague viral symptomatology, Lyme disease is often misdiagnosed.

- **SIGNS AND SYMPTOMS (generally occur 1 week after exposure)**
  Fatigue
  Lethargy
  Myalgias
  Headache
  Target rash (annular lesion with bright red borders and fading center, present in only 25% of cases)
  Second stage presentation (4 weeks after the bite)
  Bell's palsy (common)
  Meningitis
  Syncope/AV Block
  Third stage (6 months after the bite)
  Joint pain
  Arthritis, predominantly in large joints
- **THERAPEUTIC INTERVENTIONS**
  Symptomatic treatment (nonsteroidal antiinflammatory medicines)
  Doxycycline/tetracycline/Pen-VK/erythromycin for 30 days

INJURIES CAUSED BY COLD

Chilblains

Chilblains are localized areas of itching, painful redness, and recurrent edema, usually on the earlobes, fingers, and toes. Chilblains usually occur in climates that are cool and damp. It is a mild form of frostbite. Patients should be cautioned to avoid cold climates. There is no specific treatment as the symptoms are usually self-limiting.

Immersion Foot

Immersion foot occurs when there is constant contact of the foot with cold temperatures through moisture inside a boot. It is a common condition in foot soldiers and hunters who spend some time in the water and then later come to dry ground without changing their wet socks or boots. The foot begins to appear wrinkled and, if the condition is allowed to continue for a prolonged period, may develop tissue sloughing.

- **THERAPEUTIC INTERVENTIONS**
  Warm the affected foot in tepid water.
  Wear dry shoes and socks.

Frostbite

Frostbite is a traumatic condition induced when ice crystals form and expand in the extracellular spaces. The enlarging ice crystals compress the cells, resulting in cell membrane rupture and the interruption of enzymatic activity and metabolic processes. As histamine is released, capillary permeability is increased with red-cell aggregation and microvascular occlusion similar to that seen in burn patients. This is a condition that is not reversible once it has occurred. It is important, however, to protect the areas surrounding the frostbite to prevent further injury.

Frostbite is often accompanied by hypothermia. Depending on the degree of the hypothermia, it may take priority over frostbite for therapeutic intervention.

Superficial frostbite

Superficial frostbite usually involves the fingertips, ears, nose or cheeks, and toes.

■ **SIGNS AND SYMPTOMS**

Burning	Numbness
Tingling	Whitish color

■ **THERAPEUTIC INTERVENTIONS**
Apply warm (104° to 110° F [40° to 43.3° C]) soaks.
Do *not* apply friction (rubbing).

Deep frostbite

In deep frostbite the actual temperature of the injured part is lowered. This produces local vascular and tissue changes that can lead to the injury and death of the surrounding cells. Several factors can affect the possibility of sustaining frostbite:
Ambient temperature
Wind-chill factor (Figure 14-1)
Amount of time exposed
Whether or not the patient was wet or exposed to direct contact with metal objects
Type and number of layers of clothing worn
Other factors may contribute to the individual's predisposition to frostbite:
Darker-skinned people are more prone
Lack of acclimatization (moving abruptly from a warm area to a cold area)
Previous frostbite injury
Poor peripheral vascular status
Anxiety
Exhaustion
Frail body type

■ **SIGNS AND SYMPTOMS**
Whitish discoloration of the skin, followed by a waxy appearance
Slight burning pain, followed by a feeling of warmth, then numbness
Swelling and burning following numbness
Blisters (usually appear in 1 to 7 days)

Estimated wind speed (in mph)	Actual Thermometer Reading (°F)											
	50	40	30	20	10	0	−10	−20	−30	−40	−50	−60
	EQUIVALENT CHILL TEMPERATURE (°F)											
Calm	50	40	30	20	10	0	−10	−20	−30	−40	−50	−60
5	48	37	27	16	6	−5	−15	−26	−36	−47	−57	−68
10	40	28	16	4	−9	−24	−33	−46	−58	−70	−83	−95
15	36	22	9	−5	−18	−32	−45	−58	−72	−85	−99	−112
20	32	18	4	−10	−25	−39	−53	−67	−82	−96	−110	−124
25	30	16	0	−15	−29	−44	−59	−74	−88	−104	−118	−133
30	28	13	−2	−18	−33	−48	−63	−79	−94	−109	−125	−140
35	27	11	−4	−21	−35	−51	−67	−82	−98	−113	−129	−145
40	26	10	−6	−21	−37	−53	−69	−85	−100	−116	−132	−148
(Wind speeds greater than 40 mph have little additional effect)	LITTLE DANGER in <5 hr with dry skin Maximum danger of false sense of security				INCREASING DANGER Danger from freezing of exposed flesh within one minute				GREAT DANGER Flesh may freeze within 30 seconds			
	Trenchfoot and immersion foot may occur at any point on this chart.											

FIGURE 14-1. Cooling power of wind on exposed flesh expressed as an equivalent temperature.

Edema of entire extremity

Severe discoloration and gangrene appear later

■ **THERAPEUTIC INTERVENTIONS**

Prehospital (or in the wilderness)

Leave the affected part cold unless the temperature of thawing water can be ensured and maintained, and analgesics are available (thawing is extremely painful).

If the extremity is thawed, do not permit the patient to use it.

Do not use ice or snow and friction (this causes tissue damage).

Prevent any further heat loss:

Remove the patient's wet clothing.

Cover the patient with dry blanket or sheets.

Give warm non-caffeine liquids if the patient is conscious and has a gag reflex.

Protect the injured part from further damage.

Splinting and soft padding are advisable (avoid pressure).

Attempt to get to a place where there is a heat source and a supply of warm water.

If in the wilderness and walking to "civilization," the patient may walk on the frostbitten extremity unless it is thawed or begins to thaw; the patient must *not* walk on a thawed extremity.

In the emergency department

Immerse the frostbitten part in warm (104° to 110° F [40° to 43.3° C]) water.

Administer warm liquids by mouth if the patient is alert and has a gag reflex.

Cover the patient with warm blankets; be careful not to place any pressure on the frostbitten part.

Administer narcotic analgesics (rewarming is very painful).

After it has thawed, protect the part with bulky sterile dressings.

Ensure tetanus prophylaxis.

Consider antibiotics.

Consider escharotomy if vascular constriction is severe.

Amputation is not an emergency procedure; it may have to be performed several weeks after the injury.

■ **PREVENTIVE MEASURES AGAINST FROSTBITE**

Have proper dress for climate (layers of loose-fitting clothing).

Eat a diet high in carbohydrates and fats (a heat source).

Avoid smoking and drinking alcohol or beverages that contain caffeine.

Avoid bare skin contact with metal objects.

Keep dry.

Avoid exhaustion.

Protect previously frostbitten parts from exposure.

Hypothermia (Table 14-1)

Hypothermia is defined as a condition in which the core temperature of the body is less than 95° F (35° C). Severe hypothermia is defined as a core temperature of 90° F (32.2° C). It is at this temperature that severe physiologic detri-

TABLE 14-1   Signs and Symptoms of Hypothermia

TEMPERATURES	SIGNS AND SYMPTOMS
96°-99° F (35.6°-37.2° C)	Shivering, loss of manual coordination
91°-95° F (32.8°-35° C)	Violent shivering, slurred speech, amnesia
86°-90° F (30°-32.2° C)	Shivering decreases but is replaced by strong muscular rigidity and cyanosis
Below 86° F (30° C)	Possibility of developing rewarming shock, atrial fibrillation
81°-85° F (27.2°-29.4° C)	Irrational, stuporous; pulse and respirations decrease
78°-80° F (25.6°-26.7° C)	Coma, erratic heartbeat
Below 81° F (27.2° C)	Possibility of ventricular fibrillation
Below 78° F (25.6° C)	Cardiopulmonary arrest

ments occur. Death usually occurs when core temperature falls below 78° F (25.6° C). Early signs and symptoms of hypothermia are:

Fatigue
Slow gait
Muscle incoordination
Apathy

Pathophysiology of hypothermia

Many metabolic responses are temperature dependent. When hypothermia occurs, cellular activity drops. As the temperature drops by 18° F (10° C), the metabolic rate decreases by two to three times. Renal blood flow decreases, causing a decrease in glomerular filtration rate. As a result of this, water is not reabsorbed and dehydration occurs. In addition, respirations decrease, carbon dioxide is retained, and hypoxia and acidosis occur. Because of diminished glucose supply, the patient becomes hypoglycemic.

In addition to the cellular changes, the cells of the heart become more sensitive and prone to dysrhythmias as core temperature begins to fall. Osborne waves develop on the ECG. Be very careful not to cause any sudden movement of the hypothermia patient because movement may trigger fibrillation.

Mild hypothermia, in which the patient is shivering and still alert and oriented, should be treated by placing the patient in a warm (104° to 110° F [40° to 43.3° C]) bath and administering warm fluids that contain glucose or other sugar substances by mouth to provide heat through calories.

■ **THERAPEUTIC INTERVENTION FOR SEVERE HYPOTHERMIA**
Core rewarming is essential to prevent rewarming shock. Rewarming shock occurs when the peripheral areas are rewarmed faster than the core. This causes a large amount of lactic acid, which was located in the extremities, to be rapidly shunted back to the heart, where fibrillation may occur. It is also possible that peripheral vasodilation and hypotension will occur as a result of relative hypovolemia.

Protection of ABCs

Avoid endotracheal intubation if possible and manage the airway and

breathing with a bag-valve-mask device to avoid excess patient stimulation and the possibility of ventricular fibrillation.

Warm humidified oxygen

Core rewarming

by peritoneal lavage Two cannulas running warmed normal saline or Ringer's lactate solution into the peritoneal cavity and removing it by suction
can raise the core temperature 10.8° F (6° C)/hour.

by gastric lavage Not as effective as peritoneal lavage because of smaller
surface area of stomach; there is a risk of ventricular fibrillation when the
lavage tube is placed.

by warmed IV solutions This will not raise core temperature significantly,
but will prevent further heat loss.

by warm humidified oxygen with IPPB This will not raise the core temperature very much, but will prevent further heat loss.

by mediastinal lavage through two chest tubes or through direct contact of
warmed fluids on the mediastinum through a thoracotomy incision; this is
used only in the event of intractable ventricular fibrillation in which core
temperature elevation is the only hope of survival.

by renal dialysis or heart-lung bypass machine Although impractical in
most emergency settings, this may be done if the equipment is ready and
proper personnel are available to run the equipment.

Correct fluid and electrolyte status.

Administer IV fluids to compensate for hypovolemic state (avoid use of the
PASG).

Consider administration of steroids.

INJURIES CAUSED BY HEAT

Heat Cramps

Heat cramps occur when a person is doing hard work in hot weather causing
electrolyte loss from excessive perspiration.

■ **SIGNS AND SYMPTOMS**

Cramps (particularly in the shoulders, thighs, and abdominal wall muscles)

Weakness

Nausea

Tachycardia

Pallor

Profuse diaphoresis

Cool, moist skin

■ **THERAPEUTIC INTERVENTIONS**

Sodium chloride by mouth or intravenously (depending on degree of discomfort
and clinical status of patient), Gatorade or similar preparations

Cool environment

Rest

Heat Exhaustion

Heat exhaustion occurs when there is a prolonged period of fluid loss (e.g., from perspiration, diarrhea, or the use of diuretics) and exposure to warm ambient temperatures without adequate fluid *and* electrolyte replacement. It is particularly common in the very young and the very old.

■ **SIGNS AND SYMPTOMS**

Thirst	Anorexia
General malaise	Anxiety
Cramps in muscles	Syncope
Headache	Dehydration
Tachycardia	Muscle incoordination
Orthostatic hypotension	Possible elevated temperature
Nausea and vomiting	

■ **THERAPEUTIC INTERVENTIONS**
Rest
Cool environment
IV fluids to replenish fluids and electrolytes

Heat Stroke

Heat stroke can be exercise-induced, occurring when a person exercises strenuously in a very hot environment and is unable to dissipate the heat the body produces. It can also be nonexercise-induced, occurring in individuals who are vulnerable to high temperatures. Heat stroke can be precipitated by certain medications that affect heat production (thyroid extracts and amphetamines), decrease thirst (haloperidol), and decrease diaphoresis (antihistamines, anticholinergics, phenothiazines, and propranolol). As the body temperature rises to 105.8° F (41° C) there is depressed central nervous system, heart, and cellular function. Death will occur if the body temperature is not lowered.

For every 1.8° F (1° C) rise in temperature, the body's metabolism will increase by 13% (refer to the box on p. 346).

■ **SIGNS AND SYMPTOMS**

Tachycardia	Decreasing level of consciousness
Tachypnea	Decreased urinary output
Hyperpyrexia of 105.8° F (41° C) or more	Hot, dry skin
Hypotension	Seizures
Nausea and vomiting	Decerebrate posturing
Diarrhea	Dilated, nonresponsive pupils

■ **THERAPEUTIC INTERVENTIONS**
ABCs
Rapid cooling
IVs
Other supportive measures:
   Control shivering (will cause temperature to rise)
   Chlorpromazine
Hospital admission

If body temperature rises to 100.4° F (38° C), metabolism will be increased by 13%.

If body temperature rises to 102.2° F (39° C), metabolism will increase by 26%.

If body temperature rises to 104° F (40° C), metabolism will increase by 39%.

If body temperature rises to 105.8° F (41° C), metabolism will rise by 52%.

If body temperature rises to 107.6° F (42° C), there will not be enough oxygen available to meet the increased needs of the cells.

DIVING EMERGENCIES

In diving, a person is exposed to pressures greater than he or she is normally exposed to on land. These greater atmospheric pressures bring with them a whole array of medical problems unique to underwater diving and conditions that cause increased atmospheric pressures.

When a person is at sea level, the pressure exerted on the body is 1 atmosphere. At a water depth of 33 feet, the pressure exerted on the diver's body is 2 atmospheres. At a water depth of 66 feet, the pressure is 3 atmospheres.

WATER DEPTH (feet)	PRESSURE (atmosphere)
Sea level	1
33	2
66	3
100	4
133	5
166	6
200	7
300	10
400	13
500	16

Depth of Diver and Effect on Gas Volume

Boyle's law states: The volume of a gas varies inversely with the absolute pressure. In other words, as pressure increases, gas volume decreases. For example, if a normal pair of lungs contains 2000 cc of air at sea level, the volume of air decreases as the diver descends:

DEPTH	AIR IN BOTH LUNGS (cc)
Sea level	2000
33	1000
100	500
233	250

At a depth of 33 feet the total volume of air would be 1000 cc (half of normal), at 100 feet it would be 500 cc (one fourth of normal), and at 233 feet it would be 250 cc (one eighth of normal).

A scuba tank is added to the diver at sea level. If the diver forcefully inhales supplemental air from the tank, the lungs will still contain 2000 cc.

DEPTH (feet)	AIR IN BOTH LUNGS (cc)
Sea level	2000
33	2000
100	2000
233	2000

If the diver ascends but forgets to exhale on the way up, the atmospheric pressure will decrease as he ascends and the gas in his lungs will expand.

DEPTH (feet)	AIR IN BOTH LUNGS (cc)
233	2000
100	4000
33	8000
Sea level	16000

It is easy to see what will happen—as the gas expands, the lungs expand, to a limit. Then the lungs rupture, a spontaneous pneumothorax results, and air escapes into the circulation, producing an air embolism. The mechanism of injury is breath holding on ascent.

Air Embolism

■ **SIGNS AND SYMPTOMS**
Tightness of chest
Shortness of breath
Pink frothy sputum from nose and mouth
Vertigo (loss of visual point of reference)
Limb paresthesias or vertical (one-sided) paralysis
Seizures
Loss of consciousness
Other signs and symptoms of pneumothorax
This is an extremely serious condition. If the diver does not die before reaching the surface, he or she must receive extremely prompt therapy.

■ **THERAPEUTIC INTERVENTIONS**
Oxygen under positive pressure
If tension pneumothorax is present, needles inserted into anterior chest wall
Trendelenburg's position in left lateral decubitus position to avoid cerebral embolization
Prompt recompression in hyperbaric chamber

Nitrogen Narcosis

Nitrogen narcosis is a condition in which, in accordance with Henry's law,* nitrogen (which is 79% of air) is dissolved in solution because the person is breathing nitrogen under greater pressure than normal. Dissolved nitrogen pro-

---

*At a constant temperature, the solubility of any gas in a liquid is almost directly proportional to the pressure of the liquid.

duces effects similar to those of alcohol. The deeper one dives, the greater the narcosis. After 1 hour, the effects of nitrogen at various depths are as follows:

DEPTH	EFFECTS
125 to 150 ft	Narcosis begins
150 to 200 ft	Drowsiness, decreased mental functions
200 to 250 ft	Decreased strength, decreased coordination
300 ft	Diver becomes useless
350 to 400 ft	Unconsciousness, death

Therapeutic intervention consists of a gradual ascent to shallow water.

Decompression Sickness

If a diver is at a depth long enough for nitrogen to be dissolved and then ascends rapidly, there is not enough time for the nitrogen to reabsorb, and nitrogen bubbles form, producing decompression sickness (the bends, dysbarism, caisson disease, diver's paralysis). Exercise (such as swimming toward the surface) causes a rapid release of nitrogen bubbles, similar to the effect of shaking a bottle of a carbonated beverage, causing gas to be released from the solution.

■ **SIGNS AND SYMPTOMS**

Itch	Crepitus
Rash	Visual loss
Fatigue	Unconsciousness
Dizziness	Joint soreness
Paresthesias or paralysis	Shortness of breath
Seizures	

■ **FACTORS INCREASING SEVERITY OF SIGNS AND SYMPTOMS**

Extremes of water temperature	Poor physical condition
Increasing age	Alcohol consumption
Obesity	Peripheral vascular disease
Fatigue	Heavy work while diving

■ **THERAPEUTIC INTERVENTIONS**

Recompression

Oxygen at 10 L/min by mask

IV infusion

IV sodium bicarbonate

Transport in left lateral Trendelenburg's position to decrease the possibility of air embolization

■ **SPECIAL NOTES**

Any complaint of joint soreness 24 to 48 hours after a dive should be treated by decompression in a hyperbaric chamber.

Bends can occur at depths less than 33 feet (1 atmosphere).

OTHER MEDICAL PROBLEMS ENCOUNTERED IN DIVING

The "Squeeze"

The squeeze results from a compression of air trapped in hollow chambers, producing severe, sharp pain, when outside pressure is greater than inside pressure. It may occur in these areas:

Ears	Thoracic cavity
Sinuses	Teeth
Lungs and airways	Added air spaces (face mask or wet suit)
Gastrointestinal tract	

■ **SIGNS AND SYMPTOMS**

Pain	Rupture
Edema	Bleeding
Capillary dilation	

Hyperpnea Exhaustion Syndrome

Hyperpnea exhaustion syndrome usually results from diver fatigue.

■ **SIGNS AND SYMPTOMS**

Tachypnea
Anxiety
Feeling of impending doom
Difficulty floating
Exhaustion

■ **THERAPEUTIC INTERVENTIONS**

Ascent to the surface and rest aboard a flotation device or boat.

■ **THERAPEUTIC INTERVENTIONS (FOR GAS TOXICITIES)** (Table 14-2)

TABLE 14-2   Gas Toxicities in Diving

GAS	SIGNS AND SYMPTOMS	THERAPEUTIC INTERVENTIONS
Oxygen (from breathing 100% oxygen)	Twitching, nausea, dizziness, tunnel vision, restlessness, paresthesias, seizures, confusion, pulmonary edema, atelectasis, shock lung	ACBs, intubation, controlled ventilation to reduce FiO_2, decompression, PEEP
Carbon dioxide (from inhaling expired air; 8%-10% causes toxicity)	Dizziness, lethargy, heavy labored breathing, unconsciousness	Ascent to surface, ABCs, 100% oxygen
Carbon monoxide (from contaminated tank—filled too close to internal combustion engine)	Dizziness, pink or red lips and mouth, euphoria	Ascent to surface, ABCs (CPR if necessary), 100% oxygen in hyperbaric chamber at 3 atmospheres for 1 hour

The mechanism by which this occurs is breath held on descent or trapping of air in the hollow cavity.

Gradual ascent to shallower depths to decrease the pressure

Maintenance of airway, breathing, and circulation

Ear Squeeze or Sinus Squeeze

The cause of the ear squeeze is a blocked eustachian tube or paranasal sinus and an inability to equalize the pressures.

■ **THERAPEUTIC INTERVENTIONS**

Ascend to shallower water.

EMERGENCY INFORMATION

The following information should be kept readily available when treating an injured diver:

Hyperbaric chamber location and telephone number*

Name and telephone number (24-hour number) of a physician trained in underwater emergencies

Environmental emergencies can prove devastating to the patient and challenging to the emergency care provider. An in-depth understanding of the scope and unique presentation of all patient care situations represented in this chapter is essential to competently evaluate and intervene effectively.

SUGGESTED READINGS

Dickey LS: Baro-trauma. In Rosen P, Barkin RM, eds: *Emergency medicine concepts and clinical practice.* St Louis, 1992, Mosby, pp 875-93.

Herman JM, Sonntag VK: Diving accidents. Mechanism of injury and treatment of the patient, *Crit Care Nurs Clin North Am* 3(2):331, 1991.

Kol S, Weisz G, Melamed Y: Pulmonary barotrauma after a free dive—a possible mechanism, *Aviation, Space and Environmental Medicine* 3:236, 1993.

Martin D, Loth TS: Bite wounds to the upper extremity, *Orthopedics* 14(5):571, 1991.

Parell GJ, Becker GD: Inner ear barotrauma in scuba divers, *Arch Otolaryngol* 4:455, 1993.

Sheehy SB: *Emergency nursing, principles and practice,* ed 3. St Louis, 1992, Mosby.

Weaver DA et al: Timber rattlesnake bite to the hand with secondary coagulopathy and serum sickness, *JEN* 17(4):193, 1991.

*If this information is unavailable, call the U.S. Navy Experimental Diving Unit in Washington, DC (202-433-2790, 24 hours a day, 7 days a week). Ask for the duty officer, who will give you the name, location, and telephone number of the nearest decompression chamber. A useful reference book is the *Directory of Worldwide Decompression Chambers,* available from the Superintendent of Diving, U.S. Navy, Naval Ships Systems Command, National Center Building #3, Washington, DC 20360.

Genitourinary Emergencies

Traumatic Genitourinary Emergencies

This chapter outlines signs and symptoms, diagnostic aids, and therapeutic interventions for traumatic and nontraumatic genitourinary emergencies, non-emergency genitourinary conditions, and emergencies in dialysis patients such as clotted access, and cardiovascular and metabolic disorders.

Renal Trauma

Renal trauma (trauma to the kidneys) should be suspected in any injury that involves a blunt or penetrating blow to the anterior or posterior lower chest, a fracture of the 11th or 12th ribs or of the transverse process of L_1 to L_3 (Figure 15-1). It should also be suspected with fractures of the pelvis or in any patient who has sustained a multiple-systems injury. Of patients seen in the emergency department with abdominal trauma, it is estimated that 86% have injury to the kidney. Pedicle injuries are the most likely renal cause of poor outcome.[1]

■ **SIGNS AND SYMPTOMS**

History of trauma: *blunt*—motor vehicle crashes (MVC), falls, fights, contact sports; *penetrating*—associated with other intraabdominal and intrathoracic injuries (i.e., liver, small bowel, colon)

Abdominal, flank, suprapubic, and/or back pain

Ecchymosis or hematoma in flank area

Microscopic or gross hematuria

Prior history of renal abnormality

Possible

Abdominal rigidity

Swelling or mass in flank

Hypovolemic shock

Crepitus over lower rib cage or lumbar vertebrae

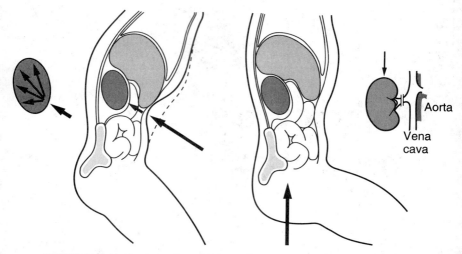

FIGURE 15-1. Mechanisms of renal injury. *Left,* Direct blow to abdomen. Smaller drawing shows force of blow radiating from the renal hilum. *Right,* Falling on buttocks from a height (contrecoup of kidney). Smaller drawing shows direction of force exerted upon the kidney from above. Tear of renal pedicle.

(From McAninch JW: *In* Smith DR, Ed: *General urology.* Los Altos, 1981, Lange Medical Publications, p 245. Used by permission.)

■ **DIAGNOSTIC AIDS**

Check urine for hematuria (use reagent papers specifically designed to check for blood). Degree of hematuria may bear no relationship to the severity of the injury. Hematuria is absent in 10% to 25% of all renal injuries.[2]

Urinalysis: if catheterization is required for male patient, this must be preceded by a rectal exam by the physician. A ''boggy'' or ''high riding'' prostate may indicate urethral damage.

Chest x-ray film

Abdominal x-ray film of kidneys, ureters, bladder (KUB)

Intravenous pyelogram (IVP). If an IVP and cystogram need to be obtained, the IVP is done first (to avoid dye extravasation and obscuring of lower ureteral injury). If immediate surgery is indicated, a KUB with contrast is obtained quickly to check for the presence of both kidneys.

Renal angiogram

CT scan

CBC, electrolytes, BUN, serum creatinine, possible type and crossmatch

■ **THERAPEUTIC INTERVENTIONS**

Close monitoring of vital signs, urine output

Penetrating injury: A culture of the site and tetanus and antibiotic prophylaxis are required in addition to previous interventions.

Renal Contusion

■ **SIGNS AND SYMPTOMS**
Flank ecchymosis
Subcapsular hematoma on x-ray film
Mild hematuria
Flank pain or pain upon palpation
Retroperitoneal hematoma (bruising at area of 11th and 12th ribs, Grey-Turner's
    sign (bruising around the umbilicus, and hematuria)
Perirenal hematoma (palpable flank mass)
■ **THERAPEUTIC INTERVENTIONS**
   Blunt
   Discharge to home
   Bed rest until the hematuria resolves
   Great volumes of fluids for a few days
   Penetrating
   There should be surgical exploration of all penetrating renal injuries because
of a high incidence of associated intraabdominal injuries.

Renal Laceration

A laceration is an actual disruption of renal tissue:
    Through the parenchyma
    Through the renal pelvis
    Through the capsule
■ **SIGNS AND SYMPTOMS**
Gross hematuria
Possible flank pain
Other signs of hypovolemia
Palpable flank mass
Possible shock
■ **THERAPEUTIC INTERVENTIONS**
Hospital admission
Observation
Bed rest
Possible surgical repair or partial/total nephrectomy

Renal Vascular Disruption

A renal vascular disruption involves the disruption of the renal arteries or veins.
Renal artery thrombosis is commonly associated with falls and motor vehicle
crashes and is usually unilateral.
■ **SIGNS AND SYMPTOMS**
Bruits auscultated at the first or second lumbar vertebra, near the midline
■ **DIAGNOSITC AID**
No kidney visualization on IVP and extravasation of contrast during procedure
■ **THERAPEUTIC INTERVENTIONS**
Surgical intervention for reanastomosis of the artery or vein

Renal Fracture

A renal fracture is considered the most critical injury involving fragmentation of the kidney or fracture extension into the renal pedicle. Often seen with penetrating trauma due to gunshot and stab wounds.

■ **SIGNS AND SYMPTOMS**
Severe blood loss
Shock
Expanding flank mass

■ **DIAGNOSTIC AID**
Angiography

■ **THERAPEUTIC INTERVENTIONS**
Surgical exploration. A complete rupture of the kidney requires nephrectomy.

Ureteral Injury

Ureteral injury is caused by blunt or penetrating trauma such as a gunshot wound or an iatrogenic injury such as occurs during abdominal surgery and urologic procedures.

■ **SIGNS AND SYMPTOMS**
Delayed presentation of flank pain
Abdominal pain or tenderness
Urinary sepsis
Ileus
Soft palpable mass
Fever
Leukocytosis

■ **DIAGNOSTIC AID**
IVP

■ **THERAPEUTIC INTERVENTIONS**
Therapeutic intervention is dependent upon the location of the injury. Surgical emergency treatment ranges from neoureteropyeloplasty, ureteroureterostomy with a stent or a neoureterocystostomy.

Bladder Trauma

Bladder trauma should be suspected with a fractured pelvis or direct suprapubic trauma. It also may be injured in penetrating trauma, where the bladder is in the path of the penetrating object.

■ **SIGNS AND SYMPTOMS**
Suprapubic pain
Urine extravasation
Possible hematuria
Possible shock
Possible anuria
Inability to void spontaneously

■ **DIAGNOSTIC AIDS**
Urinalysis

Retrograde cystogram
Abdominal x-ray film
■ **THERAPEUTIC INTERVENTIONS**
Surgical repair and drainage of the areas of extravasation
Urinary diversion from the injury

Penetrating Urethral Trauma

Penetrating urethral trauma is rare, but usually occurs as a result of a direct
penetrating injury or pelvic injury (most commonly a straddle injury). The
patient may have an iatrogenic injury or spontaneous rupture due to urethral
stricture.
■ **SIGNS AND SYMPTOMS**
Blood at meatus
Hematuria
Anuria
Flank pain
Urinary fistula
History of trauma
Prostate elevated above normal position
■ **DIAGNOSTIC AID**
Retrograde urethrogram
■ **THERAPEUTIC INTERVENTIONS**
Surgical repair to anastomose the urethra
Cystostomy with 3 to 6 month delayed closure

Obstructive Urethral Trauma

Obstructive urethral trauma may be caused either by a foreign body in the ure-
thral tract or by constricting objects around external urethral structures. These
types of injuries are commonly seen in young children, senile adults, victims of
sexual assault, and those who practice unusual methods of sexual stimulation.
■ **SIGNS AND SYMPTOMS**
Blood at urethral meatus
Swelling or discoloration of the genitalia (butterfly-shaped hematoma in the per-
    ineal area)
Inability to void (In males, ensure attempt to void while standing.)
Hematuria
Anuria
Edema
Urethral tears
Possible infection with purulent discharge
Report of specific foreign body implantation
Urinary tract infection
Necrosis
Distended bladder
Abdominal pain

■ **DIAGNOSTIC AID**
Retrograde cystourethrogram
■ **THERAPEUTIC INTERVENTIONS**
Analgesia or sedation
Local anesthesia
Removal of foreign body
Suprapubic urine aspiration if the bladder is severely distended
Possible administration of antibiotics
Possible surgical intervention

Fracture of the Penile Shaft

A fracture of the penile shaft is a traumatic rupture of the corpus cavernosum. It may occur when an erect penis is bent forcibly during intercourse. It occurs exclusively during erection as a result of direct blunt trauma.[3] Penile fracture should be suspected in any male with multiple trauma involving the pelvic region, especially when the mechanism of injury was a straddle incident, such as would occur in an accident on a motorcycle or a bicycle with a crossbar. It is considered a urologic emergency.

■ **SIGNS AND SYMPTOMS**
A penile shaft fracture may be discovered when meeting obstruction/resistance when attempting to insert a Foley catheter during resuscitation in a multiple trauma situation.
Hematoma
Hemorrhage
Swelling, distortion of penis
Discoloration
Patient reports cracking sound and severe pain
■ **DIAGNOSTIC AID**
Retrograde urethrogram if there is blood at the meatus, hematuria, or with difficulty voiding
■ **THERAPEUTIC INTERVENTIONS**
Splint
Ice packs
Urologic consultation—immediate surgical repair and placement of a catheter
Evacuation of hematoma
Placement of suprapubic catheter by urologist if studies are positive or inconclusive

Soft-Tissue Zipper Injury

Soft-tissue zipper injury occurs when the soft tissue of the penis gets caught in the teeth of a metal or plastic zipper.
■ **THERAPEUTIC INTERVENTIONS**
Remove the bottom tab from the zipper (this usually involves prying the four sharp metal teeth of the tab at the bottom of the zipper), or

Cut the distal end of the zipper with strong scissors; the zipper should then easily separate.

If the soft tissue is caught in the moving mechanism of the zipper, it may be necessary to apply regional anesthesia to the penis before removal.

Control any bleeding.

Apply ice packs.

NONTRAUMATIC GENITOURINARY EMERGENCIES

Pyelonephritis

Pyelonephritis is an inflammation of the kidneys that involves the tubules, glomeruli, and renal pelvis. It is usually caused by a bacterial infection.

■ **SIGNS AND SYMPTOMS**

Severe flank or back pain at CVA (costal-vertebral angle)
Fever
Nausea/vomiting
Chills
Urinary frequency
Urinary urgency

Nocturia
Dysuria
Tenderness over the affected flank area

Presence of pus in the urine
Presence of bacteria in the urine with a positive antibody on the surface of bacteria
Leukocytosis
Hematuria

■ **DIAGNOSTIC AIDS**

Urine and blood cultures
WBCs—Leukocytosis

■ **THERAPEUTIC INTERVENTIONS**

Forced fluids
Bed rest
Broad-spectrum antibiotics
Possible hospital admission (especially in cases of abscess, gram-negative septicemia, or severe signs and symptoms) with drainage of abscess

Perinephric Abscess

Patients with perinephric abscess usually offer a history of a recent skin infection, usually within 1 month of the abscess, or a urinary tract infection that has lasted for a prolonged time, or pyelonephritis.

■ **SIGNS AND SYMPTOMS**

High-grade or low-grade fever
Exquisite tenderness in the flank area
Palpation of a mass in the flank area
Spinal scoliosis (concave on the affected side) that has recently occurred

■ **DIAGNOSTIC AIDS**
Visualizing an elevated diaphragm on the affected side on x-ray film
Visualizing a decreased psoas shadow on x-ray film
Ultrasound
CT
■ **THERAPEUTIC INTERVENTIONS**
Incision and drainage
Antibiotics

Renal Carbuncle

A renal carbuncle is a cortical abscess in the periphery of the kidney usually caused by *Staphylococcus aureus*.

■ **SIGNS AND SYMPTOMS**
Severe flank tenderness or pain
Fever
Chills
If these signs and symptoms are present and urinalysis is normal, renal carbuncle is suspected.

■ **THERAPEUTIC INTERVENTIONS**
Incision and drainage
Antibiotics
NOTE: A relapse is common if the carbuncle is incompletely treated.

Renal Colic/Renal Calculi

Pain from renal colic or calculi radiates from the flank to the left or right lower quadrant and occasionally to the leg. This pain results from ureteral distension caused by the passage of a renal stone (calculus) or from blood clots. The size of the stone or clot does not relate to the severity of the pain.

■ **SIGNS AND SYMPTOMS**
Restlessness
Severe flank pain that radiates to the right or left lower quadrant (sudden onset)
Urinary urgency and frequency
Diaphoresis
Low-grade fever
Hematuria
Dysuria
Decreased blood pressure
History of renal calculi, presence of an ileal conduit, hypercalcemia

■ **DIAGNOSTIC AIDS**
Straining urine for calculi
Intravenous pyelogram
Urinalysis
X-ray films of KUB

■ **THERAPEUTIC INTERVENTIONS**
Forced fluids
Analgesics
Pharmacologic dissolution of stone
Urologic consultation
Antiemetic if patient experiences nausea and vomiting
IV fluids at rapid rate to flush stone and provide rehydration
Possible hospital admission
Possible extracorporeal shock wave lithotripsy (ESWL), laser lithotripsy, or surgical intervention

Urinary Retention

Urinary retention is the inability to void. It may be caused by urethral strictures, an enlarged prostate, blood clots, renal stones, a reflex neurogenic bladder (usually associated with a CVA), multiple sclerosis, congenital stenosis, foreign bodies, bladder stones, hysteria, or as a side effect of parasympatholytics and certain other drugs. Rapid drainage avoids stretch injury to bladder.

■ **SIGNS AND SYMPTOMS**
Lower abdominal discomfort
Mass palpated just above symphysis pubis
Bladder distension

■ **THERAPEUTIC INTERVENTIONS**
Insertion of an indwelling catheter
Possible urologic consultation

Hematuria

Blood can appear in urine from trauma, renal calculi, anticoagulants, blood dyscrasias, ruptured scrotal varices, ruptured cysts, renal or bladder tumors, or recent urologic surgery manipulation. If bleeding occurs at the beginning of urination, bleeding from the anterior urethral region is suggested. If bleeding occurs at the end of the urinary stream, bleeding from the posterior urethra or the point at which the bladder connects to the urethra is suggested. If bleeding occurs throughout urination, it is most likely from the upper urinary tract or from the bladder itself.

The caregiver should be cautious not to assume that all red-colored urine indicates hematuria. Red-colored urine may be caused by food colorings, medications, and the ingestion of beets. If bleeding occurs in a female, check to see if the bleeding is from the vagina.

■ **DIAGNOSTIC AIDS**
History
Urinalysis (if during menstruation, obtain the sample via catheter)
CBC

■ **THERAPEUTIC INTERVENTION**
Depends on the cause of the bleeding.

Oliguria/Anuria

Oliguria is defined as the excretion of less than 500 ml of urine per day. Anuria is the complete absence of urine. A patient with one of these conditions may complain of inability to void, yet little or no urine may be obtained on catheterization. Oliguria and anuria may be caused by fluid and electrolyte imbalances, urinary tract obstructions, acute tubular necrosis, tumors, trauma, or accidental laceration of a ureter during abdominal surgery.

■ **SIGNS AND SYMPTOMS**
Dehydration
Complaint of inability to void
Weakness
Uremic frost
Distended abdomen

■ **THERAPEUTIC INTERVENTIONS**
Urologic consultation
IVP or CT scan to rule out obstruction
Specific treatment for the cause

Acute Cystitis

Acute cystitis is an infection of the bladder that occurs as a result of the migration of bacteria from the urethra (also known as "honeymoon cystitis") or occurring secondary to acute prostatitis.

■ **SIGNS AND SYMPTOMS**
Urinary urgency/frequency
Nocturia
WBCs, RBCs, bacteria on urinalysis
Fever
Suprapubic pain
Tender prostate ⎫
Urinary retention ⎭ in males

■ **DIAGNOSTIC AIDS**
Urinalysis
Prostate examination in males

■ **THERAPEUTIC INTERVENTIONS**
Females
Nitrofurantoin or sulfonamides
Increased fluids
Warm baths
Males
Sulfa combination drugs (Septra) or tetracycline
Drainage of the abscess if one is present
Bed rest
Increased fluids

GENITOURINARY PROBLEMS UNIQUE TO MALES

Cryptorchidism

Cryptorchidism is an undescended testicle(s).
- **SIGNS AND SYMPTOMS**
  Mass in inguinal region
  Absence of a testicle in scrotum
- **THERAPEUTIC INTERVENTIONS**
  Gonadotropins
  Surgical intervention

Penile/Scrotal Edema

Penile/scrotal edema is often found in males with congestive heart failure or a recent abdominal surgery in which the pelvic lymph nodes were affected.
- **SIGNS AND SYMPTOMS**
  History of recent pelvic lymphadenectomy
  Diffuse edema in penile and scrotal skin
- **THERAPEUTIC INTERVENTIONS**
  Treatment of the congestive heart failure
  Elevation of the penis and scrotum on a towel
  Taping the penis to the abdomen

Acute Epididymitis

Acute epididymitis is an infection of the epididymis (a portion of the male reproductive system). It may occur as the result of a physical strain, after cystoscopic examination, after prostate surgery with a history of urethral discharge, or after urinary bladder catheterization. Commonly caused by *Neisseria gonorrhoeae* or *Chlamydia trachomatis.*
- **SIGNS AND SYMPTOMS**
  Swelling/enlargement of scrotum, epididymis
  Sudden tenderness in the scrotal area (unilateral), radiating up the spermatic cord
  Elevated temperature
  Sepsis
- **DIAGNOSTIC AID**
  Urethral smear for gram stain and culture
  Urine culture
- **THERAPEUTIC INTERVENTIONS**
  Antibiotics—ceftriaxone and doxycycline
  Bed rest
  Elevation of scrotum
  Forced fluids

Hematospermia

Hematospermia is a condition in which blood is present in semen. It may be caused by a rupture of varicosities.

■ **SIGNS AND SYMPTOMS**
Blood in the semen

■ **THERAPEUTIC INTERVENTIONS**
Reassurance
Urologic consultation if the condition recurs

Hydrocele

A hydrocele is a collection of fluid within the tunica vaginalis.

■ **SIGNS AND SYMPTOMS**
No pain or tenderness
Presence of a large scrotal mass

■ **DIAGNOSTIC AIDS**
Transillumination with a bright light
Scrotal ultrasound

■ **THERAPEUTIC INTERVENTIONS**
Drainage
Surgery, only if the mass is large and uncomfortable

Acute Orchitis

Acute orchitis is an inflammation of the testicle that may result from epidemic parotiditis (mumps) or other viral infection.

■ **SIGNS AND SYMPTOMS**
Unilateral testicular swelling
Unilateral tenderness
Elevated temperature

■ **THERAPEUTIC INTERVENTIONS**
Antibiotics
Bed rest
Scrotal support

Peyronie's Disease

Peyronie's disease is a syndrome in which a fibrous plaque forms on the corpora cavernosa of the penis. When the patient has an erection, he experiences considerable pain, and the penis curves.

■ **SIGNS AND SYMPTOMS**
Curved penis
Difficulty with intercourse

■ **THERAPEUTIC INTERVENTIONS**
There is no specific therapy for Peyronie's disease other than psychologic support and reassurance.

Priapism

Priapism is a prolonged erection that is not relieved by ejaculation. Physiological causes include spinal cord injury, sickle cell disease, tumors, or hematologic disorders. Pharmacologic treatment for impotence (papavarine/regitine, prostaglandin E_1 subcutaneously (SQ) given into corpus cavernosum) also may elicit priapism, which is considered an emergency state if erection lasts 4 hours.

■ **SIGNS AND SYMPTOMS**
Prolonged erection

■ **THERAPEUTIC INTERVENTIONS**
Analgesia/sedation
Possible surgical intervention if erection persists
Pharmacologic antidote: epinephrine 0.10 mg sq into corpus cavernosa if history of papavarine/regitine use.

Prostatitis

An inflamed prostate gland that is usually accompanied by cystitis.

■ **SIGNS AND SYMPTOMS**
Positive urine culture and analysis, positive urethral culture
Tenderness of the prostate
Pain in the lower abdomen and perineum
Elevated temperature
Possible urinary retention, irritative bladder symptoms
Hematospermia, hematuria

■ **DIAGNOSTIC AIDS**
Urine and urethral culture
Uroflowmetry
Prostate examination

■ **THERAPEUTIC INTERVENTIONS**
Antibiotics—if causative bacteria identified, trimethoprim, doxycycline, acyclovir for herpes proctitis[4]
Bed rest
Forced fluids
Possible incision and drainage if there is an abscess
Instruction to patient to increase ejaculation if possible

Testicular Torsion

Testicular torsion is the twisting of the testicle or the spermatic cord in the tunica vaginalis. It occurs most commonly in children and adolescents.

■ **SIGNS AND SYMPTOMS**
Severe scrotal pain and swelling (especially during physical activity) or testicular elevation
Swelling, especially during physical activity

Nausea and vomiting	Tense scrotal mass (epididymis cannot be palpated)
± High-riding testicle	Intense pain when the testicle is elevated

■ **DIAGNOSTIC AID**
Scrotal ultrasound
■ **THERAPEUTIC INTERVENTIONS**
Urologic consultation
Immediate surgical intervention is indicated for exploration

Testicular Tumor

Testicular tumor is most common in the 20- to 30-year age group. The chief complaint will be a scrotal mass with or without pain.

■ **SIGNS AND SYMPTOMS**
Swelling
A hard testicular mass with normal epididymis
Presence or absence of pain
■ **DIAGNOSTIC AID**
Scrotal ultrasound
■ **THERAPEUTIC INTERVENTIONS**
Surgical intervention

NON-EMERGENCY GENITOURINARY CONDITIONS

Nonspecific Urethritis/Nongonococcal Urethritis

Patients with nonspecific urethritis will frequently come to the emergency department with a chief complaint of urethral discharge.

■ **SIGNS AND SYMPTOMS**
Burning on urination and urinary frequency
Dysuria
Urethral discharge
■ **DIAGNOSTIC AID**
Gram stain shows no gram-negative intracellular diplococci in cases of nonspecific urethritis, abundant polymorphonuclear leukocytes. *C. trachomatis* implicated in about 50% of cases.[5]
■ **THERAPEUTIC INTERVENTIONS**
Doxycycline, Erythromycinbase
Treatment of sex partners

Varicocele

A dilation of the spermatic cord is known as a varicocele. It is caused by poor vascular drainage that results in dilation of the veins.

■ **SIGNS AND SYMPTOMS**
Scrotal mass above the testicle
Disappearance of the mass when the patient is supine
■ **THERAPEUTIC INTERVENTIONS**
Possible surgical intervention

VENEREAL DISEASES

Chancroid

A chancroid is a venereal disease that appears as an ulceration on the penis. Most patients with genital ulcers have genital herpes, syphilis, or chancroid. These patients may be at risk for HIV.

■ **SIGNS AND SYMPTOMS**

Genital lesions

Painful inguinal adenopathy 3 to 4 days after sexual intercourse

Positive culture of lesion

Positive skin test

■ **DIAGNOSTIC AID**

Exudate–dark field exam or direct immunofluorescence test for *Treponema pallidum:* serologic test for syphilis, culture for HSV, culture for *Haemophilis ducreyi*

Skin test

■ **THERAPEUTIC INTERVENTIONS**

Erythromycin base, Ceftriaxone, Trimethaprim/sulfamethoxazole, Amoxicillin

Treatment of sex partners

Follow-up with urologist

Gonorrhea

Gonorrhea is a venereal disease that appears like urethritis. Caused by *N. gonorrhoeae*. A coexisting chlamydial infection exists in 45% of gonorrhea cases *(C. trachomatis)*. Disseminated infection can lead to endocarditis or meningitis.[5]

■ **SIGNS AND SYMPTOMS**

Burning on urination

Positive gonococcus culture

White, creamy discharge 3 to 7 days after sexual intercourse

■ **DIAGNOSTIC AIDS**

Gram-negative diplococci on gram stain

Positive gonococcus culture, antibiotic sensitivity testing due to increased numbers of antibiotic resistant stains

■ **THERAPEUTIC INTERVENTIONS**

Antibiotics (penicillin or tetracycline), treatment for presumptive chlamydial infection

Follow-up care, counseling for HIV, HIV testing

Ceftriaxone plus doxycycline, spectinomycin, ciprofloxacin, tetracycline, erythromycin

Serologic testing for syphilis

Treatment of sex partners

Chlamydial Infections

Chlamydial infections are commonly found coexisting with gonorrheal infection; they may occur endocervically, rectally, or urethrally.

■ **SIGNS AND SYMPTOMS**
Same as gonorrhea
Positive *C. trachomatis* culture (available lab tests not sensitive enough)
■ **THERAPEUTIC INTERVENTIONS**
Doxycycline, tetracycline, erythromycin base
Treatment of sex partners

Genital Herpes Simplex Virus Infections

Genital herpes is a viral disease that may be chronic and recurrent.
■ **SIGNS AND SYMPTOMS**
Genital ulcers
■ **THERAPEUTIC INTERVENTIONS**
Acyclovir first clinical episode and for recurrent treatment and early suppressive
therapy
Counseling and treatment of sex partners

Syphilis

Syphilis is a type of venereal disease caused by the spirochete *T. pallidum*.
■ **SIGNS AND SYMPTOMS**
First stage early syphilis—primary and secondary
Painless ulcerations that appear several weeks after exposure through sexual
intercourse, or painless red pustules.
Positive serologic skin testing
Second stage (occurs in 2 months), early latent <1 year duration
General malaise
Anorexia
Nausea
Fever
Headache
Alopecia
Bone/joint pain
White sores in mouth
Third stage (may take 3 to 15 years to develop), latent >1 year
Soft rubbery tumors attacking all areas of the body, including the central
nervous system.
May also cause congenital syphilis.
■ **DIAGNOSTIC AIDS**
Serologic skin testing
HIV testing
Lumbar puncture and CSF examination dependent on stage
■ **THERAPEUTIC INTERVENTIONS**
Penicillin
Evaluation and treatment of sex partners
Counseling regarding risk of HIV
Follow-up

Granuloma Inguinale

Granuloma inguinale is a chronic venereal infection of the skin and subcutaneous tissue of the genitalia, the perineum, and the inguinal region.

■ **SIGNS AND SYMPTOMS**
Swelling
Ulceration
Pain

■ **THERAPEUTIC INTERVENTIONS**
Tetracycline

Lymphogranuloma Venereum

Lymphogranuloma venereum is a venereal disease caused by a virus *(C. trachomatis)*.

■ **SIGNS AND SYMPTOMS**
Transient genital lesion
Inguinal lymphadenopathy 1 to 3 weeks after exposure through sexual intercourse
Rectal stricture (in females)
Painful nodes

■ **THERAPEUTIC INTERVENTIONS**
Doxycycline or tetracycline, erythromycin or sulfisoxazole, or equivalent sulfonamide course

EMERGENCIES IN DIALYSIS PATIENTS

Dialysis patients often come to the emergency department with a variety of complaints. Some of the more common problem areas are discussed below.

CLOTTED ACCESS

There are two common types of access used for hemodialysis. A Cimino-Brescia fistula is a surgically created fistula made from a native artery and vein. Many patients have a temporary subclavian or femoral catheter placed for hemodialysis in an acute situation, or if they are awaiting surgery for a new fistula. They may have a peritoneal catheter.

Bleeding

■ **THERAPEUTIC INTERVENTIONS**
Uremic patients may have a platelet defect. Also, postdialysis it is important to know that the patient has been heparinized. Due to the short half-life of heparin, bleeding tends to occur soon after the dialysis run.

Fistula infection

■ **THERAPEUTIC INTERVENTIONS**
If a Cimino-Brescia fistula is infected, there are usually signs of systemic infection.

Administer antibiotics.

Evaluate blood cultures for definitive therapy.

With peritoneal dialysis the patient may be seen with symptoms of peritonitis, complain of blood in their exchanges, or have peritoneal bleeding.

Cardiovascular Problems/Metabolic Imbalance

Pulmonary embolus

Patients with temporary arterial-venous access may form thrombi that become emboli. A patient presenting with shortness of breath and a temporary or endogenous fistula should be evaluated for a pulmonary embolus.

Uremic pericarditis

Assessment of patients with renal disease should involve close attention to heart sounds, since uremic-induced pericarditis is a common finding. Tamponade and worsening effusion is another complication.

Dialysis patients may develop dysrhythmias, hypotension, hypertension, and cardiac arrest. Sequelae from hypervolemia (pulmonary edema, CHF) and hypovolemia may be seen before and after dialysis. For the most part, these emergencies are treated as they are in any other patient. Dysrhythmias usually occur as a result of hyperkalemia. In the typical scenario, the patient begins to develop dysrhythmias just *before* a dialysis treatment. This usually results from hyperkalemia. The patient may even develop cardiac arrest because of an intolerably high potassium level. If a dialysis arrest occurs, chances are that it is caused by either hypovolemia, for which fluid replacement is the therapeutic intervention of choice, or hyperkalemia, for which the administration of calcium chloride in large doses and other advanced life support measures are indicated.

REFERENCES

1. Landis JS: Emergency department evaluation of genitourinary trauma: an overview, *J Urol Nurs* (3):285, 1989.
2. Bland CA, Hood IG, Mascitti-Mazur J: Genitourinary trauma, *J Urol Nurs* 11, 1991.
3. Mansi KM: Experience with penile fractures in Egypt: long term results of immediate surgical repair, *J Trauma* 1:67, 1993.
4. DeLa Rosette JJMCH: Diagnosis and treatment of 409 patients with prostatitis syndromes, *Urology* 41(4):301, 1993.
5. U.S. Department of Health and Human Services: *Seminars in Urology,* vol IX, no 1, pp 40-70, 1993.

SUGGESTED READINGS

Innerarity SA: Electrolyte emergencies in the critically ill renal patient, *Crit Care Nurs Clin North Am* 2(1):89, 1990.

Reisman J, Naitoh J, Morgan AS: Genitourinary trauma, *Top Emerg Med* 15(2):22, 1993.

Infectious Diseases

Infection is the invasion and multiplication of an agent that causes a response in a host. Often therapeutic interventions must be initiated according to pertinent signs and symptoms without the benefit of confirming laboratory tests. Some of the more commonly seen infectious diseases are reviewed in this chapter.

UNIVERSAL PRECAUTIONS

The approach of treating all blood and body fluids as potentially infectious is termed *universal precautions.* The adoption of this practice is essential to the safe practice of all health care delivery. It is imperative that emergency nurses practice this when dealing with all patients (Table 16-1). Universal precautions includes the following:

- Use of gloves when contact with mucous membranes, nonintact skin, blood, or body fluids is anticipated. Gloves must be changed between patient contacts.
- Hand washing should occur after gloves are removed and if skin surfaces contacted blood or body fluids.
- Gowns should be worn during procedures that may generate splashes of blood or body fluids.
- Protective eyewear (goggles or glasses with solid side shields) and masks (or chin-length face shields) should be worn whenever there is risk of splashing or spraying of blood or body fluids to prevent exposure to mucous membranes. All health care workers should take precautions to prevent injuries from needlesticks or sharps (Figure 16-1).

AIDS

AIDS is caused by the human immunodeficiency virus (HIV). HIV infection causes an interference with the body's immune response, affecting both T-cell and B-cell immunity, thus allowing for opportunistic infections and diseases. HIV infection is chronic. The development of AIDS can range from 1 to 2 years after infection to more than a decade (Table 16-2). Transmission of HIV is known to occur through sexual intercourse, intravenous needle sharing, blood

TABLE 16-1 Emergency Department Isolation Techniques*

TYPE OF ISOLATION	COMMON DISEASES	GOWN	GLOVES	MASK	ISOLATION ROOM	LINEN PRECAUTIONS	EATING UTENSILS
Strict	Varicella Herpes zoster AIDS	A	A	A	A	A	A
Modified strict	Group A streptococci Staphylococci Streptococcal pneumonia	B	B	A	A	A	A
Respiratory	Tuberculosis Rubella Mumps Pertussis Meningococcemia Meningococcal meningitis	C	C	A	A	C	C
Protective	Leukemia Lymphoma Patient taking immunosuppressives	B	B	C	A	C	C
Enteric	Viral hepatitis Salmonella Shigella Gastroenteritis	B	B	B	C	A	A
Wound and skin†	Any draining wounds Skin infections Draining ulcers Abscesses	B	B	B	A	A	C

*A = always; B = only with direct contact with patient's secretions, excretions, urine, feces or blood; C = optional.
†Also, double-bag any waste materials or items that come into contact with drainage.

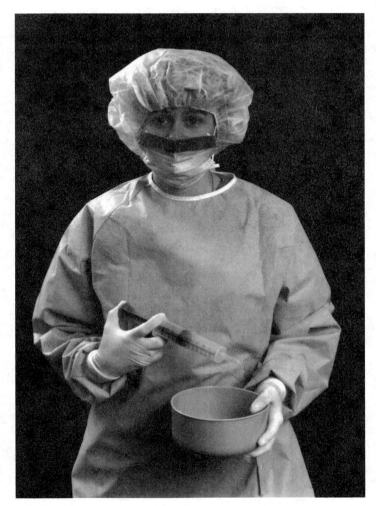

FIGURE 16-1. Universal precautions consist of eye protection, mask, gown, and gloves.

transfusions, exposures from an infected source, and in utero transmission of the virus from mother to infant. Historically, persons considered at high risk for contraction of AIDS are homosexual and bisexual men, hemophiliacs, intravenous drug abusers, prostitutes, and recipients of blood transfusions. There has also been an increase in HIV among heterosexuals. The mortality rate remains 100%.

■ **SIGNS AND SYMPTOMS**

Signs and symptoms of AIDS are highly variable and depend on the progression of the HIV infection and the amount of immunosuppression. Symptoms range from generalized and vague to diagnostic and fatal. The complex known as

TABLE 16-2   Incubation Periods*

DISEASE	DURATION OF INCUBATION
AIDS	Unknown
Bacillary dysentery (Shigellosis)	1 to 7 days; average of 4 days
Botulism (food poisoning)	Less than 24 hr.; several days after ingestion of food containing the toxin
Chickenpox (varicella)	14 to 16 days
Common cold	1 to 3 days
Diarrhea, viral	3 to 5 days
Diphtheria	2 to 6 days; may be longer
Encephalitis	5 to 15 days; range of 4 to 21 days; varies as to the type
Food infection with *Salmonella*	7 to 72 hours
Hepatitis	
Infectious (epidemic—virus A, catarrhal jaundice)	15 to 50 days
Serum (virus B)	2 to 6 months
Herpes simplex (cold sore, fever blister)	2 to 12 days; average of 4 days
Herpes zoster (shingles)	4 to 24 days; average of 4 days
Infectious mononucleosis (glandular fever)	Children, less than 14 days; adults, 33 to 49 days; average of 4 to 14 days
Influenza, epidemic	24 to 72 hours
Malaria	Varies with particular species; 12 to 14 days or as long as 30 days; some strains from 8 to 10 months
Measles (rubella, red measles)	9 to 14 days; about 10 days from exposure to onset of fever, and about 14 days to appearance of rash
Meningitis, bacterial	2 to 7 days
Mumps (epidemic parotiditis)	14 to 28 days
Pertussis (whooping cough)	5 to 21 days
Plague *(Pasturella pestis)*	
Bubonic	2 to 6 days
Pneumonic	2 to 4 days
Pneumococcal pneumonia (bacterial)	1 to 3 days
Poliomyelitis (infantile paralysis)	7 to 14 days
Rabies (hydrophobia)	Dogs, 3 to 8 weeks; man, 10 days to 2 years with an average of 2 to 6 weeks.
Rocky Mountain spotted fever (tick fever)	2 to 12 days; may be as long as 14 days; average of 7 days
Rubella (German measles)	14 to 21 days; usually 18 days after exposure
Scarlet fever (scarlatina) and septic sore throat	24 hours to 10 days, but first clinical signs generally appear between 2 to 5 days
Smallpox (variola)	7 to 16 days; average of 12 days
Tetanus	3 to 21 days; average of 10 days
Typhoid fever	10 to 14 days; may be as short as 7 days or as long as 21 days

*Modified from McInnes ME: *Essentials of communicable disease,* ed 2. St Louis, 1975, Mosby.

TABLE 16-2   Incubation Periods—cont'd

DISEASE	DURATION OF INCUBATION
Typhus fever	10 to 14 days; variation depending on the size of the dose of the infecting organism
Venereal diseases: syphilis, gonorrhea	10 to 90 days; average of 3 to 4 weeks, short as 2 to 10 days or as long as 21 days; average of 3 to 5 days
Viral pneumonia (atypical pneumonia)	Varies widely, depending on specific virus; may be from a few days to a week or longer

Classification of Commonly Used Antibiotics

Penicillin
Penicillin G
Penicillin G benzathine
Penicillin G procaine
Penicillin V potassium (Pen-Vee K)
Broad-spectrum antibiotics
Amoxicillin
Ampicillin
Azlocillin
Carbenicillin (Geopen)
Mezlocillin
Piperacillin
Ticarcillin
Synthetic antibiotics
Cloxacillin
Dicloxacillin
Methicillin
Nafcillin (Unipen)
Oxacillin (Prostaphlin)
Cephalosporins
Cefaclor (Ceclor)
Cefadroxil (Duricef)
Cefamandol (Mandol)
Cefazolin (Kefzol, Ancef)
Cefotaxime (Cloforan)
Cefotentan (Cefotan)
Cefoxitin (Mefoxin)
Ceftazidime

Ceftriaxone (Rocephin)
Cefuroxime axetel (Ceftin)
Cephalexin (Keflex)
Cephalothin (Keflin)
Cephradine (Velosef)
Moxalactam (Moxam)
Macrolides
Clindamycin (Cleocin)
Erythromycin (Ilosone, Erythrocin)
Aminoglycosides
Amikacin
Gentamicin (Garamycin)
Kanamycin (Kantrex)
Polymixin B (Aerosporin)
Polymixin E (Colistin)
Streptomycin
Tobramycin
Others
Chloramphenicol (Chloromycetin)
Ciprofloxacin
Horfloxacin
Methenamine (Mandelamine)
Metronidazole
Nalidixic acid (NegGram)
Nitrofurantoin (Macrodantin, Furadantin)
Sulfonamides
Tetracycline
Vancomycin

AIDS related complex (ARC) is generally recognized as a precurser to the life-threatening illness.

Fever	Headache
Extreme fatigue	Unexplained weight loss
General malaise	Lymphadenopathy
General weakness	Diarrhea
Myalgias	Arthralgias

Clinical disease manifestations include:

Persistent unexplained fever	Weight loss
Persistent unexplained diarrhea	Encephalopathies
Aseptic meningitis	Peripheral neuropathies

Complications such as secondary infections and secondary cancers include:
Pneumocystis pneumonia
Fungal infections
Toxoplasmosis
Disseminated herpes zoster
Salmonella bacteremia
Tuberculosis
Oral hairy leukoplakia
Disseminated cytomegalovirus (CMV)
Kaposi's sarcoma (a malignant endothelial tumor that can involve the visceral organs, skin, mucous membranes, lung, and GI tract) or non-Hodgkin's lymphomas as well as primary lymphomas of the brain.

■ **THERAPEUTIC INTERVENTIONS**
Therapeutic interventions for AIDS consist mainly of supportive care such as placement of indwelling venous catheter for frequent blood drawing and hyper-alimentation, along with much physical and psychological support. Prophylaxis and treatments for HIV infection with antiviral chemotherapy has recently become available due to intense research efforts internationally. These are not considered cures, although such agents help to prolong the person's life, decrease risk of opportunistic infections, and may prolong the HIV incubation period.

AIDS and Emergency Health Care Personnel

It remains essential that health care workers within the emergency department treat all patients as potentially infectious and thus follow universal precautions. Other specific isolation procedures are dependent upon other concurrent infections.

BACTEREMIA (GRAM-NEGATIVE)

The severity of bacteremia depends on the previous condition of the patient. The patient may have had an underlying disorder that precipitated the bacteremia, such as a gynecologic infection, a respiratory tract infection, a urinary

> **The CDC's recommendations for the prevention of occupational transmission of HIV include:**
>
> Use of latex gloves
> Gowns
> Protective eyewear and masks or face shields
> Safe, careful disposal of needles and other contaminated types of equipment and/or instruments

tract infection, or a burn injury, or the condition may have been compromised by agents such as immunosuppressants or antibiotics.

■ **SIGNS AND SYMPTOMS**

Fever	Extremes of underlying condition
Chills	Decreased blood pressure
Shortness of breath	Petechiae
Tachypnea	Cool, clammy, moist skin
Weakness	Cyanosis
Syncope	

■ **THERAPEUTIC INTERVENTIONS**

Prevention (aseptic technique and decreasing source of infection)
Antimicrobial agents
Oxygen
Volume replacement
Possible use of steroids
Possible use of naloxone
Possible use of dopamine
Incision and drainage if abscess is present

BACTERIAL VAGINOSIS (NONSPECIFIC-VAGINITIS)

The syndrome of bacterial vaginosis (BV) almost universally has the organism *Gardnerella vaginalis* present in the vagina of women, along with other infecting organisms. Recent studies suspect *G. vaginalis* to be the most common cause of vaginitis, more common among IUD users. Infection can lead to bacteremia and such conditions as postpartum endometritis and/or fever, chorioamnionitis, and postcesarean section infection.

■ **SIGNS AND SYMPTOMS**

Increased vaginal discharge
Pruritis

■ **THERAPEUTIC INTERVENTIONS**

Metronidazole
Antibiotics (for suspected *G. vaginalis* alone)

CELLULITIS

Cellulitis is an acute spreading disease of the skin that extends to the subcutaneous tissues, and in severe cases to the lymphatics and blood stream. Inciting causes include lacerations, crush injuries, and puncture wounds. Incubation period is within several days, generally 3 to 4. Common etiologic agents include Group A streptococcus and *S. aureus*.

■ **SIGNS AND SYMPTOMS**
Local tenderness/pain
Local erythema
Local edema
Foul-smelling exudate
Dirty wound
Patient may appear otherwise healthy
Malaise, fever, chills may develop

■ **THERAPEUTIC INTERVENTIONS**
Antibiotics
Needle aspiration (for diagnostic purpose)
Immobilization
Elevation
Cool compresses/moist heat
Incision and drainage

CONDYLOMA ACUMINATA (GENITAL WARTS)

Condyloma acuminatum is a papilloma caused by the human papillomavirus (HPV). Condyloma acuminata is usually sexually transmitted and is seen in sexually active young adults. Genital warts have occasionally become malignant and have been associated with higher rates of HIV infection.

Condyloma acuminata are papillary or sessile, cauliflower-like, pink growths. They develop around the anus, anal canal, glans penis, urethra, vulva, vagina, or cervix.

■ **THERAPEUTIC INTERVENTIONS**
Tincture of benzoin mixed with 10% to 25% podophyllin *(do not use on pregnant women)*
Cryotherapy
Curettage
Intralesional recombinant interferon alpha-2b (Interon A, Shering) C-section should be considered for cases of extensive papillomatosis in the genital tract.

DIPHTHERIA

Diphtheria is caused by the endotoxin *Corynebacterium diphtheria*. The usual sites of entry are the oropharynx, the nasopharynx, or skin lesions.

■ **SIGNS AND SYMPTOMS**
If immunized:

Low-grade fever and mild sore throat
If not immunized:
  Fever
  Severe sore throat
  Cervical lymph node edema
  Nonproductive cough
  Respiratory stridor
  Respiratory embarrassment from edema
  Gray-black diphtheritic membrane
■ **THERAPEUTIC INTERVENTIONS**
ABCs
Antitoxin
Consider tracheostomy
Antibiotics

EPIGLOTTITIS

Epiglottitis is a rapidly progressive cellulitis caused by a bacterial infection, usually *Haemophilus influenzae* type b. The epiglottis enlarges and causes airway obstruction. It may be a life-threatening condition. Epiglottitis most commonly appears in children aged 2 to 7 years, but may occur in adults.

■ **SIGNS AND SYMPTOMS**

Sore throat	Muffled voice
Drooling	Stridor
Progressive dysphagia	Difficulty breathing
Low-grade temperature	Cyanosis
Upright sitting position, leaning forward	

■ **THERAPEUTIC INTERVENTIONS**
Oxygen
Endotracheal intubation or cricothyrotomy
IV therapy
Antibiotics
Possible use of racemic epinephrine

GAS GANGRENE (CLOSTRIDIAL MYONECROSIS)

Gas gangrene is a soft-tissue infection caused by the organism *Clostridium perfringens*. It may occur after trauma, infection, or ischemia where an anaerobic environment exists. It is characterized by muscle necrosis and systemic toxicity. Clostridium infections are often accompanied by infections with other bacteria, such as *Streptococci* or *Staphylococci*. Many of these organisms produce gases that are secreted into soft tissues. Gas gangrene may develop within hours of bacterial invasion, although usually within 1 to 4 days.

■ **SIGNS AND SYMPTOMS**
Swelling
Local pain and pain when touched

Oozing serosanguinous material (initially brown or red and sweet smelling, then green or black)

Diaphoresis

Pallor

Low-grade fever

Delirium

Blebs

Inability of muscle to contract

■ **THERAPEUTIC INTERVENTIONS**

Antibiotics

Fasciotomy

Surgical intervention (debridement of necrotic tissue or amputation)

Possible use of hyperbaric oxygen therapy

Possible polyvalent antitoxin

GONORRHEA ("CLAP," "DRIP")

Gonorrhea is the most common of the reportable infectious diseases. It is caused by the organism *Neisseria gonorrhoeae*. Gonorrhea can infect any area of the genitourinary or reproductive system and may also infect the eyes or limb joints. The highest incidence is in persons 15 to 24 years old. Complications include meningitis, septicemia, epididymitis, pharyngitis, pelvic inflammatory disease, newborn conjunctivitis, sterility, polyarthralgias, skin lesions, and endocarditis.

■ **SIGNS AND SYMPTOMS**

Dysuria

Urethritis

Urinary frequency

Purulent discharge from the urethra (especially in females)

Vaginal discharge

Cystitis

Pruritis, tenesmus, and discharge in rectal infection

Some patients are asymptomatic

■ **THERAPEUTIC INTERVENTIONS**

Antibiotics

Probenecid

Treatment of sexual contact also

GRANULOMA INGUINALE

Granuloma inguinale is caused by the gram-negative coccobacillus *Donovania granulomatis*. It is rarely seen in the United States. Complications include urethral strictures, engorged pelvic glands, and (rarely) elephantiasis.

■ **SIGNS AND SYMPTOMS**

Very red lesions that are granulating and painless

■ **THERAPEUTIC INTERVENTIONS**

Antibiotics

HEPATITIS A (INFECTIOUS HEPATITIS, HA)

Hepatitis A is an infectious disease of the liver that may be mild or disabling in severity, often seen as an acute self-limiting disease caused by the hepatitis A virus. It is frequently found among children and young adults, transmitted generally by the fecal-oral route (commonly via contaminated food/water). Direct transmission is seen among homosexuals. It often requires prolonged convalescence, although a complete recovery without sequelae is normal.

■ **SIGNS AND SYMPTOMS**
Abrupt onset
Fever
Malaise
Abdominal pain
Nausea
Anorexia
Jaundice

■ **THERAPEUTIC INTERVENTIONS**
Treat symptomatically.
Take enteric precautions for 2 weeks from start of signs and symptoms (no longer than 1 week after development of jaundice).

VIRAL HEPATITIS B (SERUM HEPATITIS, HEPATITIS B, HB)

Hepatitis B is an inflammatory liver condition caused by the Hepatitis B virus. Infection can be transmitted via blood (and serum-derived fluids), semen, vaginal fluids, and saliva. Complications include cirrhosis and death. Vaccination is recommended for health care providers who are at high risk of contracting hepatitis B.

■ **SIGNS AND SYMPTOMS**

Abdominal pain	Jaundice
Nausea and vomiting	Erythema
Headache	Urticaria
Fever	Arthralgias
Anorexia	Hepatomegaly
Myalgias	Hepatic tenderness

■ **THERAPEUTIC INTERVENTIONS**
Treat symptomatically.

VIRAL HEPATITIS C (PARENTERALLY TRANSMITTED NON-A NON-B HEPATITIS, HC)

Hepatitis C is an inflammatory liver condition. As yet the causative agent is unidentified, and the diagnosis is based on the exclusion of other causes. This form of serum hepatitis is the most common post-transfusion hepatitis and is frequently seen among IV drug users, dialysis patients, hemophiliacs, and health care workers. Transmission is also thought to occur through sexual, intimate, or intrafamilial exposure. This disease is frequently insidious and chronic in nature with death as a rare complication.

■ **SIGNS AND SYMPTOMS**
Anorexia
Vague abdominal discomfort
Nausea and vomiting
Jaundice (less frequently than with hepatitis B)
Cirrhosis (possibly)

■ **THERAPEUTIC INTERVENTIONS**
Treat symptomatically.

DELTA HEPATITIS (VIRAL HEPATITIS D)

Delta hepatitis is an inflammation of the liver caused by the delta hepatitis virus, which is present always in a coexistent state with hepatitis B. The disease may be self-limiting or chronic. Transmission is through blood, serous body fluids, or sexual contact.

■ **SIGNS AND SYMPTOMS**
Similar to HBV, abrupt onset

■ **THERAPEUTIC INTERVENTIONS**
Treat symptomatically.

VIRAL HEPATITIS E (ENTERICALLY TRANSMITTED NON-A NON-B HEPATITIS)

Viral hepatitis E is an inflammatory liver disease similar to hepatitis A, frequently found linked to feces-contaminated water, considered to be caused by a hepatitis E virus. Outbreaks are generally self-limiting though they are associated with high mortality rates in pregnant women. Thought to be the most common cause of jaundice and acute hepatitis in third world countries.

■ **SIGNS AND SYMPTOMS**
Fever
Malaise
Abdominal discomfort
Jaundice

■ **THERAPEUTIC INTERVENTIONS**
Treat symptomatically.
Take enteric precautions for 2 weeks from start of signs and symptoms (but no longer than 1 week after the onset of jaundice).

HERPES SIMPLEX TYPE 1 (ORAL HERPES, HERPES LABIALIS)

Oral herpes simplex is caused by herpes virus type 1. In severe cases, usually in immunocompromised patients, it may present as CNS involvement. It is a common cause of meningoencephalitis.

- **SIGNS AND SYMPTOMS**
  Small fluid-filled blisters on facial area
  Burning
  Itching
  Low-grade fever
  Cervical lymphadenopathy
  Headache
  Leukocytosis
  Meningeal irritation
  Drowsiness
  Stupor
  Coma
- **THERAPEUTIC INTERVENTIONS**
  Washing hands with soap and water to avoid spreading
  Contact isolation for disseminated or neonatal infections
  Drainage/secretion precautions for recurrent lesions
  Possible use of antiviral agents (such as Acyclovir)

HERPES SIMPLEX TYPE 2 (GENITAL HERPES)

Genital herpes is caused by herpes virus type 2. Complications include infection of the neonate (if herpes virus is present in the birth canal at the time of vaginal delivery), kernicterus, encephalitis, aseptic meningitis, and radiculitis.

- **SIGNS AND SYMPTOMS**
  Tender vesicles on penile shaft
  Vesicles on prepuce or glans penis
  Vesicles on scrotum or perineum
  Grayish-colored lesions
  Vulvular, perineal, vaginal, or cervical lesions
  Dyspareunia (painful intercourse)
  Erythema
  Pain
  Lymphadenopathy
  Fever
  Lethargy
  Dysuria
  Headache
  Recurrent infection
  Anorexia
- **THERAPEUTIC INTERVENTIONS**
  At this time there is no known absolute therapeutic intervention. Consider Acyclovir (currently considered antiviral drug of choice).

HERPES ZOSTER (SHINGLES)

Herpes zoster is caused by the organism varicella-zoster virus. Once lesions are crusted, virus is no longer present.

■ **SIGNS AND SYMPTOMS**
Skin eruptions that follow a cranial or spinal nerve tract
Severe pain along the nerve tract
Paresthesias
Fever
Headache
General malaise

■ **THERAPEUTIC INTERVENTIONS**
Topical antipruritics
Analgesics
Bed rest
Acyclovir currently considered the antiviral drug of choice

HISTOPLASMOSIS

Histoplasmosis is caused by the fungal organism *Histoplasma capsulatum,* which is found in the excrement of birds and bats. This disease has an appearance much like that of pulmonary tuberculosis.

■ **SIGNS AND SYMPTOMS**
Fever
Nocturnal diaphoresis
Ulcerations on mucosal surfaces
Anorexia
Weight loss
Lymphadenopathy
Hepatomegaly

■ **THERAPEUTIC INTERVENTIONS**
Amphotericin B for disseminated cases
Oral Ketoconazole

LYMPHOGRANULOMA VENEREUM

Lymphogranuloma venereum is caused by the parasite *Chlamydia trachomatis.* It most often occurs in warm tropical regions and is rarely seen in the United States.

■ **SIGNS AND SYMPTOMS**
Genital ulcer that is painless and not indurated
Regional lymphadenopathy
Fever
Chills
Headache
Joint pains
Anorexia
Arthritis
Meningitis (rare)

■ **THERAPEUTIC INTERVENTIONS**
Antibiotics
Possible aspiration of affected glands

MALARIA

Malaria is a parasitic infection caused by the one of four different species of *Plasmodium.* Transmission to humans is caused by the bite of an infected mosquito or occasionally by blood transfusion or in utero transmission from mother to fetus.

■ **SIGNS AND SYMPTOMS**
Fever
Flulike symptoms
Chills
Headache
Myalgias
Malaise
Anemia
Jaundice
Renal failure, coma, death with *P. falciparum* infection

■ **THERAPEUTIC INTERVENTIONS**
Supportive
Chloroquine/quinine/primaquine depending upon specific form of malaria

MENINGITIS (BACTERIAL)

The causative bacterial organism of meningitis are *Neisseria meningitiditis, Haemophilus influenzae,* and *Streptococcus pneumoniae.* Children under the age of 5 are extremely susceptible. It is often preceded by a bout of influenza or a urinary tract infection.

■ **SIGNS AND SYMPTOMS**

Fever	Respiratory distress
Lethargy	Nuchal rigidity
Headache	Positive Kernig's sign
Projectile vomiting	Positive Brudzinski's sign
Anorexia	Papilledema
Febrile seizures	Petechiae over anterior trunk
Restlessness	

■ **THERAPEUTIC INTERVENTIONS**

ABCs	Antipyretics
Antibiotics	Diagnostic lumbar puncture
Anticonvulsants	

INFECTIOUS MONONUCLEOSIS

Infectious mononucleosis ("mono") is a mildly contagious disease caused by the Epstein-Barr herpetovirus. It is transmitted by droplet cross-infection. It most often affects young people, but when it affects older people the symptoms are more severe. Once infected, a person is immune to further infection.

■ **SIGNS AND SYMPTOMS**
Fever
Sore throat
Lymphadenopathy (especially cervical)
Splenomegaly
Hepatomegaly
■ **THERAPEUTIC INTERVENTIONS**
Symptomatic
Rest
Fluids
Analgesics
Warm saline solution gargles

MYCOPLASMA INFECTION

Mycoplasma are very small bacteria that can cause pneumonia, tracheobronchitis, pharyngitis, or myringitis. Mycoplasma pneumonia usually occurs in children and young adults. Complications include sinusitis, myocarditis, polyneuritis, and Stevens-Johnson syndrome.

■ **SIGNS AND SYMPTOMS**
Upper respiratory tract infection
Dry cough
Weakness
Fever
Decreased breath sounds
Inspiratory rales
Pulmonary infiltrates
■ **THERAPEUTIC INTERVENTIONS**
Antibiotics
Rest
Fluids
High-protein diet

NECROTIZING FASCIITIS

Necrotizing fasciitis is a severe infection of subcutaneous tissue and fasciae. This condition may be life-threatening. The most common sites of infection are the anterior abdominal wall and the perineal area. *Streptococci* and *Staphylococci* are the most common causative organisms.

■ **SIGNS AND SYMPTOMS**
Fever

Hyperesthesia
Decreased blood pressure
Edema
Crepitus
Blebs

■ **THERAPEUTIC INTERVENTIONS**
Surgical intervention
Antibiotics

PAROTIDITIS (MUMPS)

Parotiditis is edema of the parotid glands caused by the *Paramyxovirus* contracted from the saliva of an infected person. It usually affects children between 4 and 16 years old. When it occurs in adults, it may be critical. It is a seasonal disease, with its highest incidence in late winter and early spring. Complications include orchiditis (usually unilateral with testicular atrophy), arthritis, oophoritis, myocarditis, pancreatitis, nephritis, thyroiditis, sterility, and mumps meningitis. Incubation period is from 12 to 25 days and is contagious from 7 days before to 9 days after the parotid swelling is evident.

■ **SIGNS AND SYMPTOMS**

Headache	Painful chewing
Earache	Sore throat
Anorexia	General malaise
Swelling of parotid glands	Fever

■ **THERAPEUTIC INTERVENTIONS**

Airway management	Fluids
Analgesics	Consider IV fluid replacement
Antipyretics	Cool sponging

PEDICULOSIS PUBIS ("CRABS")

Pediculosis pubis is the infestation of the *pthirus pubis* louse, an insect that is initially gray in color and later turns red or brown when it has filled with blood. Complications are rare but include eczema, impetigo, or furunculosis. Pediculosis pubis can occur in any age group. It is contracted by direct contact with clothing, bedding, or a person who is infested with the louse.

■ **SIGNS AND SYMPTOMS**
Visualization of lice in pubic, anal, or abdominal hair
Itching
Erythema

■ **THERAPEUTIC INTERVENTIONS**
1% lindane and 25% benzyl benzoate lotion or shampoo (Kwell)

PERTUSSIS (WHOOPING COUGH)

Pertussis is caused by the gram-negative coccobacillus *Bordetella pertussis*. Infants and children up to 4 years old who have not been immunized are most commonly affected. Complications include atelectasis, bronchiectasis, otitis media, seizures, intracranial hemorrhage, epistaxis, dehydration, asphyxia, hernia, pneumonia, and death.

■ **SIGNS AND SYMPTOMS**
Paroxysmal cough with loud end-cough whooping noise
Sneezing
Possible fever
Irritability
Weakness
Vomiting
Anorexia
Large amounts of viscous sputum
Vomiting

■ **THERAPEUTIC INTERVENTIONS**
Oxygen
Suction
Rest
IVs
Adequate diet
Antibiotics
Possible endotracheal intubation

PLAGUE

Plague is transmitted to humans by a bite from a flea that has been contaminated by a rat infested with the bacillus *Yersinia pestis*.

Bubonic Plague

Bubonic plague is also known as "black death."

■ **SIGNS AND SYMPTOMS**
Lymphadenopathy
Fever greater than 106° F (41.1° C)
Tachycardia
Hypotension
Hemorrhage into skin
Delirium
Buboes

■ **THERAPEUTIC INTERVENTIONS**
Antibiotics
Supportive care
Prevention by vaccination

Pneumonic Plague

Pneumonic plague has a high mortality rate. Primary pneumonic plague is defined as bubonic plague with lung involvement. Secondary pneumonic plague is contracted through inhalation of droplets from an infected person.

Septicemic Plague

Septicemic plague is the development of septicemia with meningitis from bubonic plague. It occurs before bubo formation.

POLIOMYELITIS

Poliomyelitis is caused by the virus *Poliovirus hominis*. The most severe complications are respiratory and muscular paralysis. Prevention is by immunization.

■ **SIGNS AND SYMPTOMS**
Nonparalytic
Fever
Malaise
Headache
Nausea and vomiting
Abdominal pain
Neck pain
Paralytic
Fever
Malaise
Headache
Generalized pain, weakness, and muscle spasm
Paralysis of limbs
Paralysis of muscles
■ **THERAPEUTIC INTERVENTIONS**
ABCs
Respiratory support
Rest
Range of motion exercises

RABIES

Rabies is an acute viral encephalitis caused by a rhabdovirus that can infect animals as well as humans. Transmission occurs through nonintact skin or mucous membranes. If the disease develops, it is usually fatal.

■ **SIGNS AND SYMPTOMS**
Sense of apprehension
Headache
Fever
Malaise
Paresis
Paralysis
Hydrophobia (caused by spasm of muscles of deglutition on trying to swallow)
Delirium
Convulsions
■ **THERAPEUTIC INTERVENTIONS**
Clean and flush wound immediately.
Seek prompt medical attention.

Consult public health official if animal escaped.

If bitten by known rabid domestic animal or by wild carnivore (skunk, fox, bat, coyote, bobcat, or raccoon), then proceed with:

Passively immunize with rabies immune globulin as soon as possible after exposure.

Actively immunize with human diploid cells rabies vaccine (HDCV).

Consider tetanus prophylaxis.

Consider antibiotics.

RHEUMATIC FEVER

Rheumatic fever is infestation of the upper respiratory tract with the organism b-*Hemolytic streptococcus.* It most commonly occurs in young children. It affects the skin, joints, heart, and brain.

■ **SIGNS AND SYMPTOMS**

History of sore throat or scarlet fever within 5 weeks
Fever
Abdominal pain
Epistaxis
Nausea and vomiting
Polyarthritis
Carditis (chest pain, palpitations, heart failure)
Syndenham's chorea (awkwardness)
Erythema marginatum
Anemia
Leukocytosis

■ **THERAPEUTIC INTERVENTIONS**

Rest
Antibiotics
Analgesics
Fluids

ROCKY MOUNTAIN SPOTTED FEVER

Rocky Mountain spotted fever is a tick-borne disease for which the causative agent is *Rickettsia rickettsii.* Complications include renal failure and shock.

■ **SIGNS AND SYMPTOMS**

Chills
Fever
Severe headache
Myalgias
Hemorrhagic lesions, petechiae
Constipation
Abdominal distension
Decreased level of consciousness
Maculopapular rash (initially on wrists and ankles, then on extremities, trunk, face, palms, and soles of feet)

■ **THERAPEUTIC INTERVENTIONS**
Removing tick
Antibiotics

RUBELLA (MEASLES, GERMAN MEASLES)

Rubella is a viral illness that is contracted by droplet infection. There is a 10- to 12-day incubation period. It is contagious from the fifth day of incubation through the first few days of the rash. Once a patient has contracted rubella, he or she is immunized for life. Rubella is dangerous in the first trimester of pregnancy, because it may cause fetal injuries that lead to deafness, mental retardation, cataracts, and heart defects.

■ **SIGNS AND SYMPTOMS**
Fever
Possible cough and conjunctivitis
Upper respiratory infection
Red maculopapular rash (lasting 1 week to 10 days)
Lymphadenopathy
Arthralgias

■ **THERAPEUTIC INTERVENTIONS**
Antipyretics
Fluids
Cool compresses

SALPINGITIS AND OOPHORITIS

Salpingitis and oophoritis are bacterial infections of the fallopian tubes and ovaries, respectively. Usually these infections are recurrent, and they eventually cause scarring and contractures of the tubes. As the scarring becomes severe and adhesions form, the tubes become filled with exudate and eventually abscesses form. If rupture occurs, peritonitis will result.

■ **SIGNS AND SYMPTOMS**
Fever
Tachycardia
General malaise
Lower-quadrant abdominal pain (bilateral)
Palpated abdominal adnexal masses

■ **THERAPEUTIC INTERVENTIONS**
Cultures
Antibiotics
Possible surgical intervention

SCABIES

Scabies is caused by the mite *Scarcoptes scabiei* when it burrows into the skin in the area of the ankles, elbows, wrists, fingers, and penis. The mite is transmitted via close body contact, particularly sexual intercourse, and via infested clothing and bedding. Complications include impetigo and pustular eczema.

■ **SIGNS AND SYMPTOMS**
Burrows 1 to 10 ml in length
Small red papule at end of burrow
Itching

■ **THERAPEUTIC INTERVENTIONS**
25% benzyl benzoate emulsion and lindane with crotamiton (Kwell lotion/shampoo)

SCARLET FEVER (SCARLETINA)

Scarlet fever is caused by group A hemolytic streptococcus.

■ **SIGNS AND SYMPTOMS**

Sore throat	Bright red, diffuse rash
Fever	Prostration
Cervical lymphadenopathy	

■ **THERAPEUTIC INTERVENTIONS**

Antipyretics	Fluids
Rest	Antibiotics

SYPHILIS

See Chapter 15 on genitourinary emergencies.

TETANUS

Tetanus is caused by the exotoxin *Clostridium tetani,* an anaerobic bacillus that is found in abundance in soil, human and animal excrement, and household dust. It forms hardy spores that can resist extremes of temperature and strong antiseptic solutions. Under proper conditions, the spores will germinate and infect the injured soft-tissue areas. The bacillus excretes a neurotoxin that is absorbed into the circulation and affects the central nervous system. The incubation period may vary from 3 days to several months, with 3 to 10 days after the invasion of the organism being most common. Cases of tetanus are rare in the United States because of the high immunization rate, but mortality is high, particularly in the elderly and infants.

■ **SIGNS AND SYMPTOMS**
History of penetrating injury or burn
General malaise
Muscle rigidity
Low-grade fever
Headache
Trismus (lockjaw)
Inability to swallow

Distortion of facial muscles
Sardonic grin *(risus sardonicus)*
Opisthotonos
Seizures
Respiratory arrest
Clostridium tetani cultured from wound
■ **THERAPEUTIC INTERVENTIONS**
ABCs
Much supportive care
Dark room with low stimulation
Possible tracheostomy
Diazepam (Valium)
Possible use of neuromuscular blocking agents
Careful fluid and electrolyte balance
Antibiotics
Tetanus immune globulin (preferably human) *or*
Possible intrathecal administration of TIG (Tetanus immune globulin)
Wound excision and debridement
Active immunization concurrent with therapy
Horse serum antitoxin
Possible use of sodium nitroprusside for severe hypertension
Possible use of propranolol for tachydysrhythmias

TRICHOMONIASIS

Trichomoniasis is caused by the protozoan organism *Trichomonas vaginalis.*
■ **SIGNS AND SYMPTOMS**
May be asymptomatic
Erythema of external genitalia
Edema of external genitalia
Vaginal discharge (greenish gray and frothy), foul smelling
Possible urethritis in males
■ **THERAPEUTIC INTERVENTIONS**
Metronidazole (contraindicated in first-trimester pregnancy)
No alcohol consumption while taking medication
Treatment of sex partners

TUBERCULOSIS

Tuberculosis is caused by the bacteria *Mycobacterium tuberculosis,* and *Mycobacterium africanum* from humans, and *Mycobacterium bovis* from cattle. The bacteria typically locates itself in the lungs and spreads systemically. It is contracted by inhalation of tuberculosis-infested droplets. The infection has the appearance of a form of bacterial pneumonia. The organism may pass into the lymphatic vascular systems and then infect the entire body. Common sites for tuberculosis infection besides the lungs are the spine and other bony areas, the meninges, the kidneys, the liver, and the spleen. Susceptibility to disease is increased in those with HIV infection or other causes of immunocompromise.

■ **SIGNS AND SYMPTOMS**

Fever of undetermined origin
Pleuritic chest pain
Tachypnea
Productive cough
Abdominal pain
Nuchal rigidity
Delirium
Positive chest x-ray examination
Positive sputum test
Positive biopsy
Positive tuberculin skin test
Meningeal signs
Other signs and symptoms specific to areas of involvement

■ **THERAPEUTIC INTERVENTIONS**

Antituberculin medications (isoniazid, rifampin; consider addition of pyrazinamide)
Antibiotics
Oxygen
Possible BCG administration of tuberculin-negative household contacts

TYPHOID

Typhoid is an infection caused by the bacterium *Salmonella typhi,* which can be found in contaminated food, water, or milk. Typhoid has a high mortality. Complications include thrombophlebitis and intestinal hemorrhage.

■ **SIGNS AND SYMPTOMS**

Headache	Maculopapular rash on abdomen
Cough	Diarrhea
High fever	Splenomegaly

■ **THERAPEUTIC INTERVENTIONS**

Antibiotics	Cool sponging
Antipyretics	Prevention by vaccination
Possible use of steroids	

NONSPECIFIC URETHRITIS

Nonspecific urethritis may be caused by the organisms *C. trachomatis, Ureaplasma urealyticum, T. vaginalis,* or herpes virus. The most common age group affected is from 15 to 24 years. Complications include cervicitis, salpingitis, prostatitis, epididymitis, proctitis, Reiter's syndrome, and ophthalmia neonatorum.

■ **SIGNS AND SYMPTOMS**

Urethral discharge

Dysuria
Some males may be asymptomatic
■ **THERAPEUTIC INTERVENTIONS**
Antibiotics

VAGINITIS (FROM HAEMOPHILUS VAGINALIS)

Vaginitis is usually caused by the gram-negative organism *Haemophilus vaginalis*. This particular organism is found in up to 96% of women with vaginitis. There are no known complications.

■ **SIGNS AND SYMPTOMS**
May be asymptomatic
Frothy, thin, grayish white vaginal discharge
Vulvar irritation
■ **THERAPEUTIC INTERVENTIONS**
Antibiotics

VARICELLA (CHICKENPOX)

Varicella is caused by the virus *Varicella zoster*. The incidence is higher in young children. It has a 14- to 16-day incubation period. It is contagious from 1 day before the appearance of the rash to 5 to 6 days after. Children with varicella appear mildly sick.

■ **SIGNS AND SYMPTOMS**
Purulent vesicular skin eruptions, initially on back and chest, then on head and
    limbs
Urticaria
Fever
Lymphadenopathy
Headache
Anorexia
General malaise
■ **THERAPEUTIC INTERVENTIONS**
Rest
Fluids
Topical antipruritics
Antihistamines
Topical antibiotic ointment to vesicles
Immunization: Zoster immune globulin (ZIG)
Cutting child's fingernails short to avoid bacterial infection when child scratches
    lesions
Possibly using Acyclovir as the antiviral drug of choice in treating varicella zoster infections.

VULVOVAGINITIS CANDIDIASIS

Vulvovaginitis candidiasis is caused by the gram-positive fungus *Candida albi-*

cans. This organism can be found in approximately 20% of nonpregnant women. There are no known complications from candidiasis infections.

■ **SIGNS AND SYMPTOMS**

May be asymptomatic

Erythema of vulva

Edema of vulva

Vaginal discharge (normally whitish and thick, with the appearance of cottage cheese, but may be thin and watery)

Groin lesions

Balanitis found in male sexual partners

Lesions on penis

■ **THERAPEUTIC INTERVENTIONS**

Nystatin vaginal suppositories or niconazole vaginal cream

LUMBAR PUNCTURE (SPINAL TAP)

A lumbar puncture is performed to measure cerebrospinal fluid pressure, remove cerebrospinal fluid, to decrease pressure, for laboratory analysis in order to detect meningitis versus bleeding. A lumbar puncture should *NOT* be done if there is potential for intracranial bleeding, which may lead to brainstem herniation.

■ **PROCEDURE**

1. Explain the procedure to the patient if possible.
2. Have the patient breathe deeply and straighten legs and neck.
3. Open the stopcock and record an opening pressure measurement (lowest level during fluctuations).
4. Collect cerebrospinal fluid samples in serially numbered tubes.
5. Remove the needle and place a sterile dressing over puncture site.
6. Keep the patient on bed rest for at least 1 hour after the procedure.
7. Obtain a consent for the procedure.
8. Obtain baseline vital signs.
9. Empty the patient's bladder.
10. Position the patient on his or her side with neck flexed and knees drawn up to abdomen (Figure 16-2).
11. Prepare the tap site with antiseptic solution.
12. Drape the site with sterile towels.
13. Introduce 1% lidocaine into the space between L4 and L5.

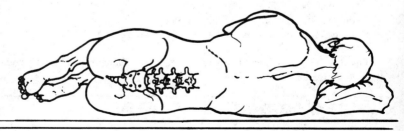

FIGURE 16-2. Position of patient for lumbar puncture.

14. Introduce a 20- or 22-gauge spinal needle with a stylet into the subarachnoid space (Figure 16-3).
15. Remove the stylet after piercing the dura mater; spinal fluid will drip out at this point (Figure 16-4).

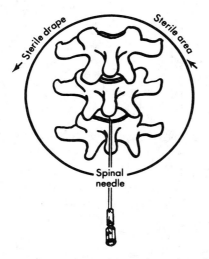

FIGURE 16-3. Introduction of spinal needle.

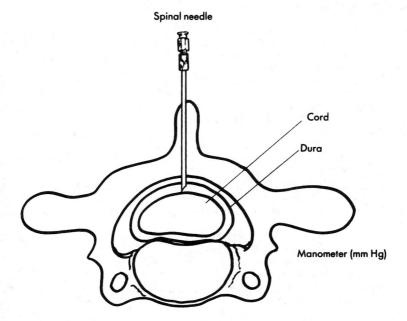

FIGURE 16-4. Spinal needle in subdural space.

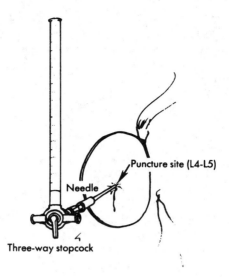

FIGURE 16-5. Spinal needle and manometer.

16. Rotate the needle to direct the bevel rostrally (to prevent obstruction).
17. Attach a three-way stopcock with manometer (Figure 16-5).

SUGGESTED READINGS

Baraff LJ, Talan DA: Compliance with universal precautions in a university hospital emergency department, *Ann Emerg Med* 18(6):654, 1989.

Benenson AS, ed: *Control of communicable diseases in man,* Washington, DC, 1990, American Public Health Association.

CDC health information for international travel 1992. Washington, DC, 1992. U.S. Department of Health and Human Services Public Health Services.

Emergency Nurses Association position statement: infectious diseases and the emergency care setting, *J Emerg Nurs* 17(3):31A, 1991.

Fassbinder B: Profiles HIV positive: the story of one "ordinary" emergency nurse, *J Emerg Nurs* 18(1):84, 1992.

Jordan KS: Assessment of the person with AIDS in the emergency department, *Int Nurs Rev* 36(2):57, 1989.

Schwartzm GR, Cayten CG, Mayer TA et al, eds: *Principles and practice of emergency medicine,* vol II, ed 3. Philadelphia, 1992, Lea and Febiger.

Somerson SW: Triage decisions: a 57 year-old-man with muscle spasms, *J Emerg Nurs* 17(5):351, 1991.

Stoner Halpern J: Clinical notebook: respiratory cyncytial virus (RSV): a common health problem, *J Emerg Nurs* 18(1):61, 1992.

Talan DA, Kennedy CA: The management of HIV-related illnesses in the emergency department, *Ann Emerg Med* 20(12):1355, 1991.

Wilson ME: *A world guide to infections, diseases, distribution, diagnosis.* Oxford, 1991, Oxford University Press.

Trauma Emergencies

CHAPTER

Wound Management

GENERAL

There are two basic principles in the management of wounds:
- To decrease the likelihood of infection
- To promote optimal wound healing

Several other important factors to consider in wound management are:
- What caused the injury?
- How did the injury happen?
- What were the circumstances surrounding the injury?
- When did the injury occur?
- On what part of the body is the wound?
- In what condition is the tissue surrounding the wound?
- Can the edges of the wound be approximated?
- What is the patient's age?
- What is the patient's occupation?
- What is the patient's physical condition?
- Is the patient taking any medications?
- Does the patient have any other pertinent medical history?
- What is the condition of the patient's skin?
- Was there any care given to the wound before arrival in the emergency department?
- Is there movement and sensation distal to the wound?
- Is vascular status intact distal to the wound?

THE PROCESS OF WOUND HEALING

When an injury occurs, there is immediate vasoconstriction. This causes sludging of blood and then vasodilation, resulting in redness and swelling in the subepithelial layer of the skin. Epithelial cells begin to migrate 24 hours after the injury, and fibrin begins to form. This period of wound healing is known as the proliferative phase. During the subsequent days and over the next year, collagen is continually laid down at the areas around the wound that sustain the greatest amount of stress. The tensile strength of a wound is weakest 3 days after the initial injury.

Factors that Affect Wound Healing

Preexisting illness
Infection
Vascular supply
Obesity
Altered electrolytes
Oxygen levels
Poor nutritional state
Age
Stress
Certain medications

General Principles of Wound Management

Ensure airway, breathing, and circulation.
Control bleeding.
Treat shock.
Check the wound itself.
Check the area distal to the wound to assess neurovascular status (color, temperature, pulse, sensation, movement).
Splint any possible fractures or dislocations.
Determine the mechanism of injury.
Notify the police if foul play is suspected.
Prepare wound culture if wound is from a contaminated object.
Apply local anesthetic prior to procedures.
Avoid soaking, except for puncture wounds; soak puncture wounds for 10 to 15 minutes.
Cleanse wound and surrounding tissue with an antiseptic solution (Table 17-1). DO NOT USE toxic solutions in the wound itself.
Irrigate the wound with isotonic solution (normal saline).
Remove all foreign material.
If there is much hair around the wound, such as on the scalp, consider clipping the hair surrounding the wound.
Never shave eyebrows (they may not grow back).
Debride devitalized tissue.
Close the wound; use suture, skin staples, or skin tapes.
Dress the wound with antibiotic ointment.
Cover the wound with nonadherent dressing.

CATEGORIES OF WOUNDS

There are six basic types of wounds:
Abrasion

TABLE 17-1 Antiseptic Solutions

AGENTS	ANTIMICROBIAL ACTIVITY	MECHANICS OF ACTION	TISSUE TOXICITY	INDICATIONS AND CONTRAINDICATIONS
Povidone-iodine solution (iodine complexes) (Betadine)	Available as a 10% solution with polyvinyl-pyrolidine (povidone) containing 1% free iodine with broad rapid-onset antimicrobial activity	Potent germicide in low concentrations	Will decrease PMN migration and life span at concentration >1%	Probably a safe and effective wound cleanser at a 1% concentration
			May cause systemic toxicity at higher concentrations; questionable toxicity at 1% concentration	10% solution is effective to prepare the skin about the wound
Povidone-iodine surgical scrub	Same as the solution	Same	Toxic to open wounds	Best as a hand cleanser; never use in open wounds
Nonionic detergents Pluronic F-68 Shur Clens	Ethyleneoxide is 80% of its molecular weight It has no antimicrobial activity	Wound cleanser	No toxicity to open wounds, eyes or intravenous solutions	It appears to be an effective, safe wound cleanser
Hydrogren peroxide	3% solution in water has brief germicidal activity	Oxidizing agent that denatures protein	Toxic to open wound	Should not be used on wounds after initial cleaning, may be used to clean intact skin
Hexachlorophene (pHiso Hex) (polychlorinated bis-phenol)	Bacteriostatic (2% to 5%) Greater activity against gram-positive organisms	Interruption of bacterial electron transport and disruption of membrane-bound enzymes	Little skin toxicity; the scrub form is damaging to open wound	Never use scrub solution in open wounds Very good preoperative hand preparation
Alcohols	Low-potency antimicrobial most effective as a 70% ethyl and 70% isopropyl alcohol solution	Denatures protein	Will kill irreversibly and function as a fixative	No role in routine care
Phenols	Bacteriostatic >.2% Bactericidal >1% Fungicidal 1.3%	Denatures protein	Extensive tissue necrosis and systemic toxicity	Never use >2% aqueous phenol or >4% phenol plus glycerol

From Rosen P et al: *Emergency medicine*, ed 2. St Louis, 1992, Mosby.

Abscess
Avulsion
Contusion
Laceration
Puncture

Abrasion ("brush burn")

An abrasion is a wound caused by the rubbing of skin against a hard surface. The friction removes at least the epithelial layer of the skin, exposing the dermal or epidermal layer. Abrasion is physiologically the same as a second-degree burn. Be concerned about large body surface area abrasions that may result in fluid loss.

■ **THERAPEUTIC INTERVENTIONS**

Consider local infiltration or topical application of an anesthetic agent. If area of abrasion is extremely large, consider IV administration of medications for sedation and pain control.

Cleanse the wound by scrubbing and irrigating.

Remove any foreign bodies.

Apply topical antibiotic ointment.

Apply a nonadherent dressing or leave open.

Change the dressing once each day until formation of an eschar.

Instruct the patient to avoid direct sunlight to the area for at least 6 months.

Abscess

An abscess is localized collection of pus.

■ **THERAPEUTIC INTERVENTIONS**

Prepare the area.

Anesthetize the area.

Drain the abscess using a needle and syringe.

Remove an elliptical area of tissue.

Cleanse the wound.

Pack the wound loosely to allow for drainage.

Cover the wound with a loose dressing.

Have the patient return for follow-up care every 2 days until wound is almost completely healed.

If the patient is febrile, consider antibiotics.

Avulsion

An avulsion is a full-thickness skin loss where it may not be possible to approximate wound edges. A degloving injury is a severe type of avulsion wound.

■ **THERAPEUTIC INTERVENTIONS**

Consider local infiltration or topical application of an anesthetic agent. If the avulsion is extensive, consider IV administration of medication for sedation and pain control.

Cleanse the wound by scrubbing.

Irrigate the wound.

Debride devitalized tissue.

Repair injured muscles or tendons.

Apply a split-thickness graft or flap if necessary, depending on extent of avulsion.

Apply a bulky dressing.

Contusion

A contusion is an extravasation of blood into the tissues without disruption of the skin that usually results from a blunt injury.

■ **THERAPEUTIC INTERVENTIONS**

Assess neurovascular status.

Apply cold packs.

Administer analgesia if necessary.

No dressing is usually necessary.

If hematoma is extensive, observe closely for the development of compartment syndrome.

Laceration

A laceration is an open wound that extends at least into the deep epithelium and will vary considerably in length and depth. A *superficial* laceration refers to a laceration that involves only the dermis and epidermis. A *deep* laceration is a laceration that extends through tissues deeper than the epidermis.

■ **THERAPEUTIC INTERVENTIONS**

Control bleeding with direct pressure.

Evaluate neurovascular status distal to the wound.

Anesthetize the wound.

Cleanse the wound by scrubbing and irrigation.

Remove any foreign bodies.

Excise any necrotic tissue.

Approximate the wound edges.

Close the wound using sutures or skin tapes.

Apply antibiotic ointment.

Apply a nonadherent dressing.

If a laceration is deep and there is question of damage to underlying structures, explore the wound in either the emergency department or the operating suite.

PUNCTURE AND PENETRATING TRAUMA

A puncture wound results from penetration of tissue by an object such as a knife blade, bullet, or piece of glass, or injection of material from a high-pressure paint gun or similar device. Damage to underlying structures may be great even though the wound appears benign. Gross contamination is also possible.

■ **THERAPEUTIC INTERVENTIONS**

Therapeutic intervention of puncture wounds depends on the depth of penetration, the amount of underlying damage, and the level of contamination. General guidelines to follow are:

Soak the wound twice a day for 2 to 4 days.

If the wound is known to be contaminated, soak the wound, anesthetize it, and inspect it.

If the foreign body is still in place and is small enough that removal will not cause further damage, remove it.

If there is necrotic tissue, debride it, place a drain, and dress the area.

If the foreign body is deep enough that removal may cause further damage, decide whether the object should be removed in surgery or left in place.

In cases of penetrating trauma in which the penetrating object is still in place, *do not remove the object.* The only exception to this rule is if the patient is in shock and the object must be removed to enable PASG placement. If the penetrating object is cumbersome, it may be shortened if possible to allow for transport of the victim. Be sure that the penetrating object is secured to the victim so there is no chance of dislodging it.

General Principles Concerning Gunshot Wounds

The amount of trauma in a gunshot wound depends on the mass, size, and velocity and angle of yaw of the bullet.

The position of the victim at the time of injury may help determine the track of the bullet.

Muscle has a high density; damage is usually severe.

Bone may change the direction of the missile.

A small entrance wound with a large, explosive exit wound usually indicates a high-velocity missile fired at close range. The energy dissipated by a high-velocity missile is equal to the difference between the energy present when the missile enters the body and that left when it exits. Usually there is a violent expansion of the missile track, which ruptures arteries, veins, and nerves, and fractures bones.

A small entrance wound with no exit wound indicates a low-velocity missile that is retained within the tissue.

Forensic Considerations in Management of Gunshot Wounds

Report all gunshot wounds to the police, regardless of the circumstances surrounding the incident.

Document the exact condition of the patient *and the wound* on arrival at the emergency department.

Prehospital personnel should note the environment of the patient, including the patient's position in relation to objects, doorways, and so on.

Disturb the scene as little as possible, but do not permit this consideration for preserving evidence to interfere with emergency care.

Life-saving procedures take precedence over forensic considerations. Do not touch or move weapons, furniture, or other environmental clues to the incident unless it is absolutely imperative for patient care.

Place the patient on a catch-all sheet, since bullets and other items may dislodge during changes in the patient's body position.

Cut or tear clothing, preferably along a seam, avoiding any tears a penetrating object could have made.

Do not drop the clothing onto the floor, but hang it up, taking care to handle it as little as possible. Later, place all clothing in a brown paper bag (not plastic) and seal the bag with all patient identification attached. Allow any blood to dry before bagging.

Do not shake clothing.

Keep all clothing as evidence, and do not give it to the family. (All clothing is examined for powder residue, metallic traces, and other foreign material.)

Avoid scrubbing powder away from the skin; the area of powder dispersal is a clue to the distance between the patient and the weapon fired. If the skin must be scrubbed before forensic pathologists examine it, carefully document the appearance of the wound and the surrounding skin, and include a photograph whenever possible.

Save any tissue debrided from the wound for forensic pathology.

To remove a bullet use gloved fingers or padded forceps. Ordinary surgical clamps or similar devices can alter a bullet's markings and render it useless for evidence.

When it is removed, mark the bullet on the nose or base with identifying letters or numbers for later identification. This identification can facilitate testimony that a particular bullet was indeed removed from the patient's body as described.

Place the bullet in a small padded container (e.g., a urine specimen cup) to prevent marring. Do not place bullets in bottles or basins, because their rolling causes dulling of the barrel markings.

When more than one bullet is removed, place them in separate containers that are sealed and labeled with the physician's name, time, date, exact site of removal, and pertinent patient identification.

Turn over all bullets to the police pathology department at once. If this is not feasible, place the bullet in a locked box.

Always obtain a police receipt when surrendering any item of evidence.

Shotgun wounds may exhibit wadding, pellets, and the inner lining of the cartridge. These may assist in matching the wound to the weapon fired. Place such evidence in a properly marked sealed envelope and retain it for police study.

If the patient dies, *do not* clean the body.

Leave all invasive tubing and apparatus in the body cavities (e.g., endotracheal tubes, catheters, IV lines).

Mark any sites where IVs or other invasive procedures were attempted, where there is no longer a cannula.

Place brown paper bags over the patient's hands to protect potential sources of evidence, such as fingernail scrapings, foreign hair, blood, and gunpowder. (Do not use plastic bags, because condensation destroys evidence.)

Do not probe the wound further after the death in an attempt to locate the bullet. Unnecessary probing could create false or misleading forensic reports.

High-Pressure Paint Gun Injuries

High-pressure paint gun injuries deserve special mention because a seemingly benign injury may turn out to be devastating. This injury occurs when the patient attempts to clean the tip of the paint gun. If the gun releases, a large amount of paint may be injected into the fingertip and perhaps up into the hand and arm. The results will be much tissue swelling, decreased circulation, ischemia, and necrosis.

■ **SIGNS AND SYMPTOMS**

Small puncture wound on the tip of the finger
Swelling of the extremity
Extremity appears mottled
Focal tenderness
Extremity cool to the touch

■ **THERAPEUTIC INTERVENTIONS**

DO NOT soak the wound in warm water. These measures may increase swelling and ischemia and induce vasospasm.
DO NOT inject local anesthesia.
Obtain an x-ray film to observe the paint, which is radiopaque.
Provide tetanus toxoid immunization.
Consider tetanus immune globulin.
Give antibiotics.
Consider surgical debridement (in the operating suite) with possible fasciotomy preceding in the emergency department.

TYPES OF ANESTHESIA FOR WOUND MANAGEMENT

Lidocaine is the most commonly used anesthetic for both local and regional anesthesia in wound management. It may be used with or without epinephrine. Lidocaine is used with epinephrine when the area to be repaired is highly vascular and bleeding must be controlled. Ounce for ounce, lidocaine is more potent than any other anesthetic agent. It is also, however, more toxic than the others. It is not a very irritating agent, and it appears to have a longer effect than other anesthetic agents.

Other agents used for anesthesia include procaine, mepivacaine (Carbocaine), bupivacaine (Marcaine), and tetracaine (Pontocaine).

The caregiver may elect to administer regional anesthesia. To do this, inject an anesthetic agent intravenously distal to the injury. Apply a tourniquet and inflate it proximal to the body on the affected extremity.

Another option is to apply a local nerve block. To do this, inject the anesthetic agent along the course of the nerve, abolishing conduction of afferent and efferent impulses for a limited time.

Topical anesthesia (TAC = 0.25% tetracaine, 0.025% epinephrine, 5.9% cocaine) can be effective for lacerations. The solution is administered by placing several drops of solution into the wound. A small piece of sterile cotton or gauze is placed in the wound with 25% to 50% of the material overlapping the wound edges. Then slowly drip the TAC solution onto the material to saturate it. Using gloves, hold material onto the wound. After 10 to 15 minutes the wound may be checked for adequate anesthesia. The maximum total dose of TAC should be 3 cc. DO NOT ALLOW TAC TO CONTACT MUCOUS MEMBRANES. The solution should not be used for lacerations involving the mucous membranes, tip of the nose, external ear, penis, or digits.

Consider the use of nitrous oxide gas for procedures that are short but may be painful, such as scrubbing cinders from a wound. Also consider IV sedative or narcotic administration if wounds are extensive.

SUTURING

Suturing is the art of proximating and fixing wound edges to promote a decreased incidence of infection, good healing, and minimal scar formation. The type of suture material and suture technique used depends on the extent of the wound injury. If suturing is required, consider the possibility of using skin staples instead of suture material, depending on the location and extent of the wound (Table 17-2).

The location of the wound and the state of wound healing determine when sutures are removed. See Figure 17-1.

Lacerations involving extensor surfaces of joints should be kept in longer.

TETANUS

Tetanus is caused by the organism *Clostridium tetani,* a gram-positive, spore-forming, anaerobic bacillus. It is highly resistant to any measure taken against it, including sterilization, because of its tendency to form spores when conditions for its survival are not favorable. The incubation period is from 2 days to 2 weeks or more. The organism is present in soil and garden moss, on farms, and anywhere else animal and human excreta can be found. It enters the human circulation through an open wound and attaches itself to cells within the central nervous system. Tetanus causes depression of the respiratory center in the medulla.

■ **SIGNS AND SYMPTOMS**

Mild tetanus

Local joint stiffness

Mild trismus (inability to open jaw)

Moderate tetanus

Generalized body stiffness	Difficulty swallowing
Moderate trismus	Decreased vital capacity

TABLE 17-2 Suture Materials for Wound Closure

TYPE	DESCRIPTION	SECURITY	STRENGTH	REACTION	WORKABILITY	INFECTION	COMMENT
Nonabsorbables							
Silk		++++	+	++++	++++	++	Nice around mouth, nose, or nipples, but too reactive and weak to be used universally
Mersilene	Braided synthetic	++++	++	+++	++++		Good tensile strength; some prefer for fascia repairs
Nylon	Monofilament	++	+++	++	++	+++	Good strength, decreased infection rate; but knots tend to slip, especially the first throw
Prolene Polypropylene	Monofilament	+	++++	+	+	++++	Good resistance to infection; often difficult to work with; requires an extra throw
Ethibond	Braided coated polyester	+++	++++	++½	++	+++	Costly
Stainless steel wire	Monofilament	++++	++++	+	+	+	Hard to use; painful to patient; some prefer for tendons

Absorbables

Gut (plain)	From sheep intima	+	+++	+			Loses strength rapidly and is quickly absorbed; rarely used today
Chromic (gut)	Plain gut treated with chromic salts	++	++	+++	+		Similar to plain gut; often used to close intraoral lacerations
Dexon	Braided co-polymer of glycolic acid	++++	++++	+	++++		Braiding may cause it to "hang up" when tying knots
Vicryl	Braided polymer of lactide and glycolide	+++	++++	+	+++		Low reactivity with good strength; therefore, nice for subcutaneous healing; good in mucous membranes
Polydioxanone	Monofilament	++++	++++	+	Excellent	Unavailable	First available monofilament synthetic absorbable sutures; appears to be excellent

From Swanson NA, Tromovitch TA: *Int J Dermatol* 21:373, 1982.
From Rosen P et al: *Emergency medicine*, ed 2. St Louis, 1987, Mosby.

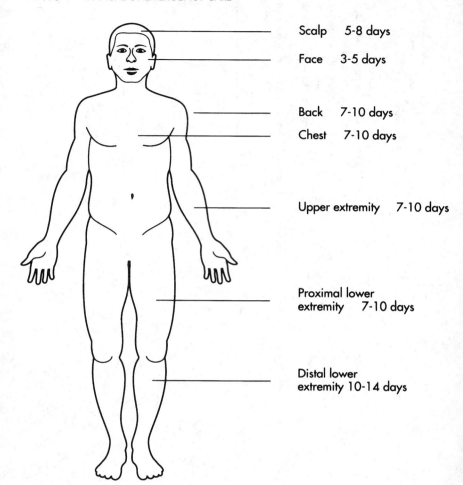

FIGURE 17-1. Guide for suture removal.

Scalp   5-8 days

Face   3-5 days

Back   7-10 days

Chest   7-10 days

Upper extremity   7-10 days

Proximal lower extremity   7-10 days

Distal lower extremity 10-14 days

Severe tetanus

Severe trismus	Hypertension
Pain in back	Dysrhythmias
Pain in penis	Hyperpyrexia
Seizures	Usually mental alertness until
Opisthotonos	cardiopulmonary arrest occurs
Tachycardia	

■ **THERAPEUTIC INTERVENTIONS**
ABCs
Oxygen at high flow rate

Hyperalimentation
Antibiotics
Ventilatory support

Tetanus Prophylaxis*

Initial immunization series

In an infant and young child give diphtheria/tetanus/pertussis (DPT) injections:
  0.5 ml at 2 months
  0.5 ml at 4 months
  0.5 ml at 6 months
  0.5 ml at 18 months
  0.5 ml at 4 to 6 years
For persons aged 6 years and older, give tetanus/diphtheria toxoid (TD)
absorbed injections:
  0.5 ml initially
  0.5 ml 4 to 6 weeks later
  0.5 ml 6 months to 1 year later
  0.5 ml booster every 10 years
Fully immunized (last dose within 10 years)
  Non–tetanus-prone wound—No prophylaxis required
  Tetanus-prone wound—If last dose was given more than 5 years ago, administer 0.5 ml absorbed toxoid. (May be omitted if patient has had many absorbed toxoid injections.)
Partially immunized (two or more previous injections, with last dose given more than 10 years ago)
  Non–tetanus-prone wound—0.5 ml absorbed toxoid
  Tetanus-prone wound—0.5 ml absorbed toxoid (passive immunization considered unnecessary)
Not adequately immunized (one or no previous injections or if infection history is unknown)
  Non–tetanus-prone wound—0.5 ml absorbed toxoid
  Tetanus-prone wound—0.5 ml absorbed toxoid plus 250 units (or more) TAT† (tetanus antitoxin), and consider antibiotics.

Tetanus-Prone Wounds

Wounds that are tetanus-prone are those that:
  Are greater than 6 hours old
  Are stellate or avulsed
  Have been caused by a missile
  Have been caused by a crushing mechanism

---

*Recommendations of the American College of Surgeons Committee on Trauma.
†*Equine* tetanus antitoxin should only be given if *human* tetanus antitoxin is not available, and only if the possibility of tetanus outweighs the danger of a reaction to the equine tetanus antitoxin.

Have been caused by heat or cold
Have signs of infection
Have signs of devitalized tissue
Contain contaminants

HUMAN AND ANIMAL BITES

All bite wounds, whether inflicted by a human, a domestic animal, or a wild animal, are considered contaminated. Most bites will result in puncture wounds, possible crush injuries, and possible lacerations.

Factors to Consider

Origin of the bite
Age of the patient
General physical condition of the patient
Site of the wound
Severity of the wound
  Location
  Size
  Depth
  Amount of contamination
Time between the bite incident and when the patient first sought medical assistance
First aid given at the scene of the incident
The potential for wound infection

Complications

Infection
Abscess
Cellulitis
Septicemia
Osteomyelitis
Tenosynovitis
Pyarthrosis
Rabies
Loss of injured part

Aftercare Instructions for All Bite Patients

Keep the injured part elevated above the heart if possible.
Take medications as ordered.
Return to your private physician, the clinic, or the emergency department if:
  A fever develops.
  Redness appears.
  Swelling occurs.

Streaks appear.
The site becomes very hot.
There is increasing pain at the site.
A foul odor develops.
Drainage occurs.

Human Bites

A human bite may be self-inflicted or inflicted by another person. The many organisms normally present in the human mouth may cause a severe infection and other complications.

The most common location of human bites is on hand and fingers. The mouth contains greater than 10 bacteria per ml of saliva.[1] Gram-positive organisms are commonly *Staphylococcus aureus* and *Streptococcus*. Gram-negative organisms may be *Proteus, Escherichia coli, Pseudomonas, Neisseria,* or *Klebsiella.* More than 3% of these organisms are coagulase-positive, penicillin-resistant *Staphylococcus aureus.*

■ **SIGNS AND SYMPTOMS**

History (the patient may be hesitant to admit a human bite)
Teeth marks
Laceration across the knuckles (caused by impact with the tooth)

■ **THERAPEUTIC INTERVENTIONS**

Evaluate neurovascular status.
Administer local anesthesia.
Obtain a culture and gram stain.
Irrigate and scrub the wound thoroughly.
Debride devitalized tissue.
Do *not* suture the wound (facial wounds are the exception).
Administer broad-spectrum antibiotics.
Ensure tetanus prophylaxis.
Start strict follow-up care.

■ **ANTIBIOTIC REGIMEN**

Human bites should be treated with prophylactic antibiotics. Treatment should be for 3 to 5 days with penicillin 250 mg four times a day. Patients with a PCN allergy can be treated with erythromycin 250 mg four times a day.

Complications of human bites include:
Abscess
Cellulitis
Osteomyelitis
Pyarthrosis

Dog and Cat Bites

Approximately 1/2 to 1 million persons in the United States are bitten by dogs or cats each year.[2] The organism that is usually present is *Pasteurella multocida.*[3] A dog's jaws and teeth can exert a pressure of up to 400 pounds per square inch.[4] Factors that will place a patient at greater risk for infection are:[5]

Age less than 4 years
Age greater than 50 years
Increased time before medical assistance is sought
Anatomic location of the wound in a poorly vascularized area (e.g., the earlobe)
Puncture wounds

■ **SIGNS AND SYMPTOMS**
History of bite
Visible puncture wound(s)
Infection
Pain
Swelling
Inflammation
Regional lymphadenopathy
Low-grade fever

■ **THERAPEUTIC INTERVENTIONS**
Culture and gram stain.
Consider topical or local anesthesia.
Irrigate and scrub wound thoroughly.
Debride devitalized tissue.
Suture if necessary (many practitioners prefer to leave the wound open).
Administer antibiotics (especially penicillins).
Ensure tetanus prophylaxis.
Dress wound (optional).
Consider rabies prophylaxis.

RABIES AND RABIES PROPHYLAXIS

Rabies is caused by a virus that can be found in the saliva of many mammals. The rabies virus is highly neurotoxic. The incubation period for rabies is from 10 days to several months.

■ **SIGNS AND SYMPTOMS**
History of bite (type, animal, geographic region, whether or not animal was provoked)
Malaise for 2 to 4 days
Fever
Headache
Granulomatous lymphadenitis
Photophobia
Muscle spasm
Coma

■ **THERAPEUTIC INTERVENTIONS**
Ensure ABCs.
Culture the wound.
Consider topical or local anesthesia.
Irrigate and scrub the wound.
Debride and devitalize tissue.

Consider suturing the wound (very controversial).
Administer antibiotics.
Ensure tetanus prophylaxis.
Follow rabies prophylaxis procedures.
NOTE: Bite incidents must be reported to local health authorities.

RABIES PROPHYLAXIS GUIDELINES[6]

Domestic dogs and cats
- If animal is healthy and can be observed for 10 days without signs of rabies, no prophylaxis is required.
- If the animal shows signs of rabies, the animal must be destroyed and laboratory analysis of the animal accomplished. If the animal is unavailable, the patient must also be treated.
- Administer the Human Rabies Immunoglobulin (RIG) and Rabies Human Diploid Cell Vaccine (HDCV).

Wild animals
- Animals included in this category are wolves, fox, coyotes, bobcats, skunks, raccoons, bats, and other carnivorous animals. They should be considered rabid unless proven otherwise by laboratory analysis.
- Patient should be treated with RIG and HDCV.

Domestic animals, rodents, and rabbits
Animals such as cattle, rodents, rabbits, squirrels, gerbels, hamsters, and guinea pigs usually are considered nonrabid. One should consult with local health authorities for recommendations.

Usually no intervention is required.

SUMMARY

With any type of wound, patients must be given careful after-care instructions in an attempt to prevent complications or detect early signs of complications. Instructions should include:

Elevation of injured part, if possible
Cleansing or dressing change instructions
Immobilization instructions
Signs of infection

Redness   Pain
Swelling red streaks   Temperature

Wound follow-up instructions, including date, time, and place of follow-up.

REFERENCES

1. Doan-Wiggins L: Animal bites and rabies. In Rosen P, Barkin R, eds: *Emergency medicine: concepts in clinical practice,* ed 3. St Louis, 1992, Mosby.
2. Simon B: *Principles of wound management.* In Rosen P, Barkin R, eds: *Emergency medicine: concepts in clinical practice,* ed 3. St Louis, 1992, Mosby.
3. Zukin D, Simon R: *Emergency wound care: principles and practice.* Rockville, Md: Aspen Publications, 1987.

SUGGESTED READINGS

Aghababian RV, Conte JF: Mammalism bite wounds, *Ann Emerg Med* 9:79, 1980.

Baron MC: The skin and wound healing, *Topics Clin Nurs* 5:11, 1983.

Beran GW, Crowley AJ: Towards worldwide rabies control, *WHO Chron* 37:192, 1983.

Bruno P: The nature of wound healing: implications for nursing practice, *Nurs Clin North Am* 14:667, 1979.

Bruno P, Craven RF: Age challenges to wound healing, *J Geront Nurs* 8:686, 1982.

Bucknall TE: The effect of local infection upon wound healing and experimental study, *Br J Surg* 67:851, 1980.

Callaham ML: Treatment of common dog bites: infection risk factors, *JACEP* 7:11, 1978.

Carrico TJ, Mehrohf AI, Cohen IK: Biology of wound healing, *Surg Clin North Amer* 64: 721, 1984.

Delancy V, North C: Skin assessment, *Topics Clin Nurs* 5:5, 1983.

Flynn ME, Rovel DT: Promoting wound healing, *Am J Nurs* 82:1544, 1982.

Goldstein EJ, Citron DM, Finegold SM: Dogbite wounds and infection, *Ann Emerg Med* 9:508, 1980.

Haas J: Emergency management of soft tissue injuries, *J Emerg Nurs* 6:20, 1980.

Haury B et al: Debridement: an essential component of traumatic wound care, *Am J Surg* 135:238, 1978.

Henrich JJ et al: Human bites, *JEN* 2:21, 1976.

Immunization practices advisory committee, *MMWR* July 20, 1984, 33:399.

Jaffe AC: Animal bites, *Pediatr Clin North Am* 30:405, 1983.

Neuberger GB, Reckling JB: A new look at wound care, *Nursing '85*, 15(2):34, 1985.

Parks B, Hawkins L, Horner P: Bites of the hand, *Rocky Mount Med J* 71:85, 1974.

Peacock EE: *Wound repair.* Philadelphia, 1984, Saunders.

Peeples E, Boswick JA Jr, Scott FA: Wounds of the hand contaminated by human or animal saliva, *J Trauma* 20:383, 1980.

Pryor GJ, Kilpatrick WR, Opp DR: Local anesthesia in minor lacerations: topical TAC vs lidocaine infiltration, *Ann Emerg Med* 9:568, 1980.

Robinson DA: Dogbites and rabies: an assessment of risk, *Br Med J* 1:1066, 1976.

Scarcella J: Management of bites: early definitive care of bite wounds, *Ohio State Med J* 65:25, 1969.

Silver IA: The physiology of wound healing. In Hunt TK, ed: *Wound healing and wound infection.* New York, 1980, Appleton-Century-Crofts.

Statt NA: The most effective method of wound irrigation, *Focus Crit Care* 10:45, 1983.

Stillman RM: Wound closure: choosing optimal materials and methods, *Emerg Room Rep* 2:41, 1981.

Thompson HG, Sviter V: Small animal bites: the role of primary closure, *J Trauma* 13:20, 1973.

Wiggins LD: Animal bites and rabies. In Rosen P et al, eds: *Emergency medicine: concepts and clinical practices.* St Louis, 1988, Mosby.

Head Trauma

In 1988, motor vehicle crashes on public roads in the United States injured an estimated 4.88 million people.[1] Of the injured, 47,000 died (National Highway Traffic Safety Administration, NHTSA 1989).[1]

Over one half of all trauma deaths in the United States each year are caused by head trauma. More than 4000 victims of head trauma are children.[2] More than 80,000 people sustain head or spinal cord injuries that result in disabilities. Of these people, 2000 remain in a vegetative state.[3] In the United States, up to 75% of serious injuries are attributed to high-speed motor vehicle crashes.[4] The most severe head injuries occur to those people who are riding in the front passenger's seat.[5] Of children with multiple trauma, 75% have a head injury.[5] The etiology of head injury is as follows[5]:

1. Motor vehicle crashes
2. Falls
3. Recreation injuries
4. Gunshot wounds
5. Stab wounds

ANATOMY (Figure 18-1)

The brain is protected by hair, the scalp, the skull, the meningeal layers, and cerebrospinal fluid. The scalp has five layers: **S**kin, **C**onnective tissue, **A**poneurotica, **L**igaments, and **P**eriosteum. Because the scalp is very vascular, disruption causes profuse bleeding.

The skull is the bony structure that protects the brain. It is composed of the frontal, parietal, occipital, and temporal regions. It is divided into two major parts—the calvarium (the cranial vault) and the base.

The three meningeal layers provide protection for the brain and spinal cord. The layers are the pia mater, the arachnoid, and the dura mater (forming the mnemonic PAD, because they "pad" the brain). The pia mater is very thin and adheres to the cortex of the brain. The arachnoid layer is also very thin. Major arteries are located in the subarachnoid space. The dura mater adheres to the internal skull surface. The meningeal arteries are between the internal surface of the skull and the dura in the area known as the epidural space.

417

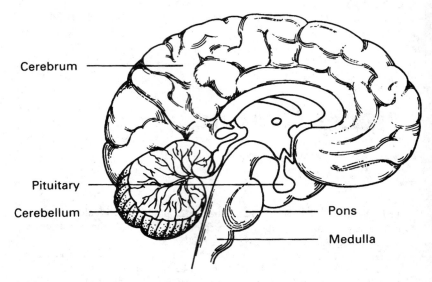

FIGURE 18-1. Some key anatomic landmarks of the brain.

Cerebrospinal fluid (CSF) is produced in the ventricles of the brain and acts as a cushion for the brain and spinal cord. CSF is located in the subarachnoid space. The brain comprises 80% to 85% of the intracranial mass. It is composed of a collection of very delicate tissues and water. The main part of the brain, the cerebrum, is divided into two hemispheres and each hemisphere is subdivided into four lobes—frontal, parietal, temporal, and occipital.

The frontal lobe's function is primarily to conceptualize, abstract, and form judgments. Injury to this area may result in impaired judgment and reasoning, and the patient may frequently use foul language.

The parietal lobe is the area of highest integration and coordination of perception and interpretation of sensory phenomena. If a patient's parietal lobe suffers an injury, the patient will have difficulty with receptive communication.

The occipital lobe is the area responsible for vision. If there is injury to this area, the patient may develop blurred vision, diplopia, or even blindness.

The temporal lobe (the lobe that looks like the thumb of a boxing glove) is thought to be responsible for memory. Injury to this area may affect recent memory.

The brainstem, which contains the reticular activating system, is responsible for consciousness. The lower part of the brainstem, the medulla, contains the cardiorespiratory center.

The cerebellum, located under the cerebrum and next to the brainstem, is responsible for movement and coordination. The tentorial notch, often the site of herniation, is located where the cerebrum and the midbrain meet.

THE CRANIAL NERVES

There are twelve pairs of cranial nerves. A description of each pair follows.

Olfactory (I)

This nerve is responsible for smell. It is tested by checking the patient's ability to smell. Injury to the olfactory nerve, common in head injury, will result in the ability to discern sweet and bitter taste only, due to the loss of sense of smell.

Optic (II)

The optic nerve controls sight. If the optic nerve is intact, the patient will be able to count fingers, perceive light, or blink when the eyes are threatened.

Oculomotor (III), Trochlear (IV), Abducens (VI)

Check the patient's pupil size, shape and reactivity, and extraocular movement to assess the function of these nerves. The third cranial nerve passes through the tentorium. Brain herniation through the tentorium will produce pressure on the third nerve, causing the pupil to dilate and fix on the ipsilateral (same) side as the herniation. One millimeter difference in pupil size may be significant; however, 10% of the population normally have unequal pupils (anisocoria).

Trigeminal (V)

The trigeminal nerve controls facial sensation and jaw movement. Check for facial sensation, strength of mastication muscles, and jaw movement.

Facial (VII)

The facial nerve controls facial expression and taste in the anterior two thirds of the tongue. Have the patient raise his eyebrows, close his eyelids tightly to resistance, show his teeth, smile, frown, and puff his cheeks. If there is a peripheral ipsilateral injury, both the upper and lower face will be involved. If there is a central injury, the brow of the controlateral (opposite) side will be spared.

Acoustic and Auditory (VII)

The eighth nerve is responsible for hearing and balance. It has two branches—the acoustic branch, which controls balance, and the auditory branch, which controls hearing. Assess the auditory branch by having the patient respond to a loud voice or clap. The eighth nerve can also be tested by using ice water calorics.

Glossopharyngeal (IX), Vagus (X)

These nerves are evaluated together because they are closely related anatomically and functionally. The glossopharyngeal nerve controls taste in the posterior two thirds of the tongue and sensation in the pharynx and nostrils. The vagus nerve controls the soft palate, pharynx and larynx, the heart, the lungs, and the stomach. Both nerves are tested by checking the gag and swallow reflexes and by assessing the patient's ability to discriminate between a salty taste and a sweet taste.

Spinal Accessory (XI)

The spinal accessory nerve controls movement of the sternocleidomastoid and trapezius muscles. To test this nerve, have the patient turn his head against resistance or shrug his shoulders. Do not test this nerve until the likelihood of cervical spine injury has been ruled out.

Hypoglossal (XII)

The hypoglossal nerve controls tongue movement. It can be tested by having the patient stick out his tongue. If, when the patient sticks out his tongue, his tongue is in midline, the nerve is considered intact.

THE BRIEF NEUROLOGICAL EXAMINATION

It is essential to obtain an initial neurological evaluation as soon as possible in the care and evaluation of the head-injured patient. The evaluation should then be repeated frequently. Using the DERM neurologic evaluation and the Glasgow Coma Scale, the caregiver can perform a brief neurologic examination in a consistent, precise manner, observing both clinical changes and measuring calculated improvements or deteriorations.

DERM

D = Depth of Coma
Use a stimulus/describe the response:

STIMULUS	RESPONSE (describe)
Voice	Appropriate (Inappropriate)
Touch	Appropriate (Inappropriate)
Pain	Appropriate (Inappropriate)

E = Eyes
Note pupillary response to light and accommodation. If the corpus callosum is intact, there will be simultaneous consensual reaction of the unstimulated pupil with light stimulation. (Note that 10% of the population have unequal pupils (anisocoria) with no disease.)

R = Respirations
Note regular or irregular rate, rhythm, and depth.

M = Motor/Movement
Does the patient move extremities? All?

Glasgow Coma Scale*

The Glasgow Coma Scale has been designed to quantitatively relate consciousness to motor response, verbal response, and eye opening. Coma is defined as no response and no eye opening. Scores of 7 or less on the Glasgow Scale qualify as "coma"; all scores of 9 or more do not qualify as "coma." The examiner determines the best response the patient can make to a set of standardized stimuli. Higher points are assigned to responses that indicate increasing degrees of arousal.

1. **Best motor response.** (Examiner determines the best response with either arm.)
   a. *6 points.* Obeys simple commands. Raises arms on request or holds up specified number of fingers. Releasing a grip (not grasping, which can be reflexive) is also an appropriate test.
   b. *5 points.* Localizes noxious stimuli, fails to obey commands, but can move either arm toward a noxious cutaneous stimulus and eventually contacts it with the hand. The stimulus should be maximal and applied in various locations, for example, sternal pressure or trapezius pinch.
   c. *4 points.* Flexion withdrawal. Responds to noxious stimulus with arm flexion, but does not localize it with the hand.
   d. *3 points.* Abnormal flexion. Adducts shoulder, flexes and pronates arm, flexes wrist and makes a fist in response to a noxious stimulus. Previously known as decorticate posturing.
   e. *2 points.* Abnormal extension. Adducts and internally rotates shoulders, extends forearm, flexes wrist and makes a fist in response to a noxious stimulus. Previously known as decerebrate posturing.
   f. *1 point.* No motor response.

A problem with the Glasgow Coma Scale is that it scores "best motor response." How should we interpret the findings if we see flexion in one arm and extension in the other?

2. **Best verbal response.** (Examiner determines the best response after arousal. Noxious stimuli are employed if necessary.) Omit this test if the patient is dysphasic, has oral injuries, or is intubated. Place a check mark after the other two test category scores after totaling to indicate omission of the verbal response section.
   a. *5 points.* Oriented patient. Can converse and relate who he is, where he is, the year, and the month.
   b. *4 points.* Confused patient. Is not fully oriented or demonstrates confusion.
   c. *3 points.* Verbalizes. Does not engage in sustained conversation, but

---

*Adapted from Teasdale G, Jennett B: *Lancet* 2:81, 1974.

uses intelligible words in an exclamation (curse) or in a disorganized manner that is nonsensical.

d. *2 points.* Vocalizes. Makes moaning or groaning sounds that are not recognizable words.

e. *1 point.* No vocalization. Does not make any sound, even in response to noxious stimulus.

3. **Eye opening.** (Examiner determines the minimum stimulus that evokes opening one or both eyes.) If the patient cannot realistically open the eyes because of bandages or lid edema, write "E" after the total test score to indicate omission of this component.

a. *4 points.* Eyes open spontaneously.

b. *3 points.* Eyes open to speech. Patient opens eyes in response to command or on being called by name.

c. *2 points.* Eyes open to noxious stimuli.

d. *1 point.* No eye opening in response to noxious stimuli.

The examiner should remember that the Glasgow Coma Score may not be valid in patients who have used alcohol or other mind-altering drugs, are hypoglycemic, in shock (with systemic blood pressure less than 80 mm Hg), or who are hypothermic (below 34° C).[5]

DIAGNOSTIC EXAMINATION TECHNIQUES/ DEVICES USED IN HEAD INJURY

Cross-Table Lateral Cervical Spine X-ray

Of all patients with significant head trauma, 10% have concurrent spinal cord trauma.[6] The caregiver must ensure that the C-spine is immobilized and protected while radiographic studies are obtained to rule out fracture. If a cross-table lateral film cannot adequately visualize the entire C-spine, to include T1, a "swimmer's view" should be obtained. (Figure 18-2).

Skull X-rays

Skull x-rays offer the least amount of clinically useful information in terms of treatment intervention. The patient should be treated systematically and not on the basis of the x-ray film. If, however, CT is not available, a skull x-ray may confirm the diagnosis of skull fracture.

Computerized Axial Tomography (CT Scan, CAT Scan, EMI Scan)

CT scans detect 90% of head trauma accurately. It should be done quickly if the patient has an altered level of consciousness, hemiparesis, or any kind of aphasia.

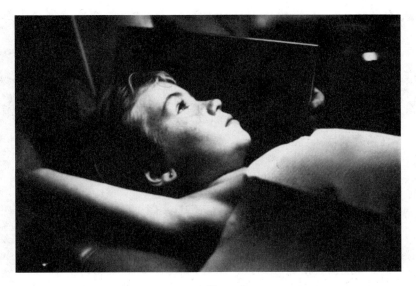

FIGURE 18-2. X-ray film; swimmer's view.

Magnetic Resonance Imaging (MRI, NMR)

The atoms of the body broadcast signals from which images may be created. These broadcasts can be tracked through nuclear magnetic resonance, using ionizing radiation or sound waves as a noninvasive method to obtain a visual image. By using NMR, the caregiver can also chemically analyze cellular content by measuring phosphorous emissions. It is a procedure not generally used in trauma, because it cannot be used if the patient is unstable, uncooperative, and unable to remain still.

Pupillary Responses

Normal reactions
Pupils constrict when exposed directly to light.
Light shined into one pupil causes the other pupil to constrict as well.
Abnormal reactions
Fixed pinpoint pupils indicate pons involvement or use of opiates.
Ptosis may indicate third cranial nerve involvement.
Dilated fixed pupil (unilateral) indicates third cranial nerve involvement (early).
Dilated fixed pupils (bilatera) indicate third cranial nerve involvement (late).

Reflexes

Corneal

Touch the cornea with a wisp of cotton from a swab.
Normal reaction—blinks eye
Abnormal reaction—no response

Gag

(Cranial nerves IX and X)
Normal reaction—intact
Abnormal reaction—loss of gag reflex

Deep tendon

Scored from 0 to 4.
0 = Absent
1 = Decreased
2 = Normal
3 = Increased
4 = Hyperactive
Normal reaction—normal reflexes
Abnormal reaction—hypoactivity or absence of reaction indicates cerebellar
    lesions or intricate peripheral nerve or anterior horn cell disease; hyperactiv-
    ity indicates pyramidal tract lesions and sometimes psychogenic disorders.

Babinski

Checked by applying cutaneous stimulation to the plantar surface of the foot.
Normal reaction—Great toe and other toes flex.
Abnormal (positive) reaction—Great toe extends upward and other toes fan out
    toward the head (''it points to where the problem is''). This is a normal
    reaction in children under age 2. No response at all is also considered an
    abnormal reaction.

Posturing

Elicited by verbal or painful stimulation.
Abnormal flexion (Figure 18-3)—arms flex, wrists flex, legs and feet extend.
    Indicates a lesion *above* midbrain. This is also known as decorticate postur-
    ing.
Abnormal extension (Figure 18-4)—arms extend, wrists flex, legs and feet
    extend. Indicates brainstem herniation. This is also known as decerebrate
    posturing.

SPECIFIC HEAD INJURY CONDITIONS

Scalp Lacerations

A scalp laceration is one of the most frequently seen types of head injuries. If
the scalp is lacerated, it may bleed profusely because of its ample vascular supply. A scalp laceration may be caused by any blunt or penetrating trauma to the

FIGURE 18-3. Abnormal flexion.

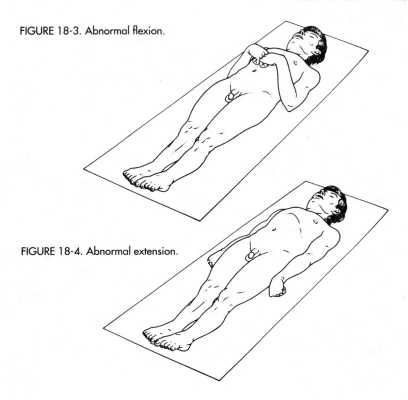

FIGURE 18-4. Abnormal extension.

head. When the head hits the car windshield, the scalp will absorb the first 33% of the force.[5]

■ **SIGNS AND SYMPTOMS**

Direct observation of the laceration

Bleeding

■ **DIAGNOSIS**

Clinical observation of the laceration

■ **THERAPEUTIC INTERVENTIONS**

Apply direct or peripheral pressure to control bleeding.

Palpate underlying skull for fractures.

Protect cervical spine. (It is imperative to rule out cervical spine injury with any head injury.)

Cleanse laceration area with surgical prep solution.

Debride devitalized tissue.

Suture the wound if indicated.

closure of galea with 2-0 or 3-0 absorbable suture

nylon or prolene suture for skin

Apply small sterile dressing or open to air and Bacitracin ointment.

Ensure tetanus prophylaxis.

Give aftercare instructions for both wound management and head trauma.

Skull fracture

Examine the patient's skull for bumps, defects, bruises, or lacerations. The presence of a skull fracture does not necessarily indicate that a cerebral injury has occurred. There are three types of skull fractures:

Simple
Depressed
Basilar

Simple skull fractures (linear/nondisplaced)

A simple skull fracture is a linear crack in the surface of the skull. The bone is not displaced, and therapeutic intervention involves observation of the patient for other associated injuries. If there are no other obvious findings and the patient has a good support system (family or friends), he may be discharged to home with careful head trauma aftercare instructions.

Depressed skull fracture

A depressed skull fracture is a depression of a segment of the bony skull. If the fragment is depressed beneath the table of the adjacent bone by more than 5 mm, surgery must be performed to elevate the depression and decrease the possibility of intracranial infection. If the depression overlies the sinuses (sagittal or lateral), there may be profuse bleeding, underlying brain contusion, or tears of the cerebral tissue.

■ **SIGNS AND SYMPTOMS**
Observation/palpation of the deformity
Bleeding
Altered level of consciousness

■ **DIAGNOSIS**
Observation/palpation of the deformity
X-ray
CT scan

■ **THERAPEUTIC INTERVENTIONS**
Ensure airway management, cervical spine protection.
Control external bleeding.
Place sterile dressing over wound.
Surgical intervention to:
Elevate the depressed segment.
Remove fragments.
Debride necrotic brain tissue.
Remove hematomas.
Repair lacerations.
Consider antibiotics.
Ensure tetanus prophylaxis.

Basilar skull fracture

A basilar skull fracture is a fracture at the base of the skull. On impact, all forces go to two bones: the sphenoid (causing periorbital ecchymosis), or the petrus temple (causing Battle's sign). The danger of a basilar skull fracture is that it may cross the course of the middle meningeal artery, disrupting it and causing:

A hematoma of the scalp

An epidural hematoma (cause of 90% of epidurals)

A subarachnoid hemorrhage

An intracerebral bleed

In addition, a cerebrospinal fistula may occur. The mechanism of injury is usually a significant blow to the head.

■ **SIGNS AND SYMPTOMS**

Headache

Nausea and/or vomiting

Scalp laceration

Periorbital ecchymosis ("raccoon eyes") (Figure 18-5)

Unilateral or bilateral periorbital ecchymosis that occurs as a result of

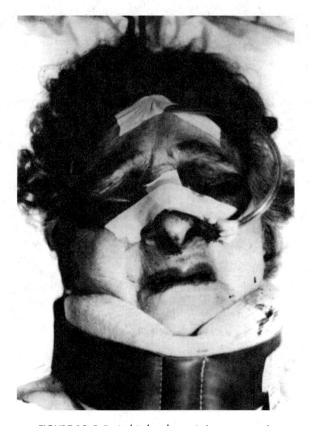

FIGURE 18-5. Periorbital ecchymosis (raccoon eyes).

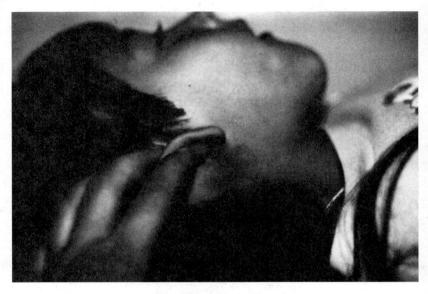

FIGURE 18-6. Battle's sign.

intraorbital bleeding from an intraorbital root fracture or a cribiform plate fracture.

Battle's sign (Figure 18-6)

Formation of an ecchymosis behind the ear in the mastoid region. It usually occurs 12 to 24 hours after injury.

Hematotympanum

Blood behind the eardrum caused by temporal bone fracture near the tympanic membrane.

Cerebrospinal fluid leak (CSF rhinorrhea, CSF otorrhea)

Caused by a fracture of part of the cranial vault that creates an opening between the cranium and the outside of the cranium. CSF otorrhea is caused by a crack in the petrus temple bone. If the tympanic membrane is intact, CSF may exit via the eustachian tube. The patient may complain of a salty taste in his mouth. CSF contains 15.9 mEq of sodium chloride. A scar formation from an old basilar skull fracture may dislodge, forming an open fistula into the cranium and a CSF leak. Blood and CSF separate to form two distinct rings, known as a "target sign," "ring sign," or "halo sign" on filter paper or bed clothing.

■ **THERAPEUTIC INTERVENTIONS**

Protect cervical spine.

Do *not* attempt to stop CSF leak.

Do *not* put nasogastric tube or endotracheal tube through the nose—use the oral route.

Do a baseline neurologic exam.

Obtain an x-ray film (basilar skull fractures are not seen on 25% of routine skull films).

Consider antibiotics.

Ensure tetanus prophylaxis.

Admit patient to hospital for observation.

Concussion

A concussion usually occurs as a result of a direct blow to the head or from an acceleration/deceleration injury where brain tissue impacts with the inside of the bony skull. A brief interruption of the reticular activating system occurs, causing a short period of amnesia. This is a transient, limited process that usually requires no therapeutic intervention, but the patient may take up to 3 months to fully recover. Concussion is often accompanied by a coup/contrecoup injury (Figure 18-7 *A, B*).

■ **SIGNS AND SYMPTOMS**

Nausea and vomiting

Possible brief loss of sight or ''seeing stars'' (precipitated by occipital lobe involvement)

Uncontrolled use of foul language (caused by frontal lobe involvement)

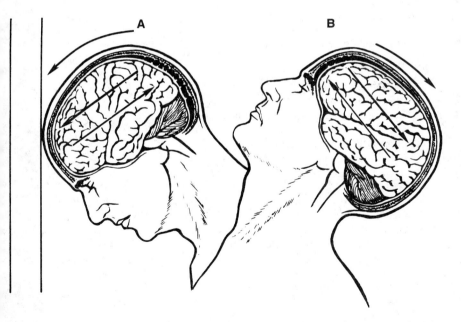

FIGURE 18-7. **A**, Coup: the brain impacts with the skull at the point of impact of the skull with another force. **B**, Contrecoup: the brain accelerates forward after the initial impact and causes an additional injury as the interior brain impacts with the skull.

Headache
Loss of consciousness
Flaccid paralysis
Hypertension or hypotension
Apnea

■ **THERAPEUTIC INTERVENTIONS**

Protect cervical spine.

If nausea and vomiting are severe and dehydration results, admit to hospital for rehydration.

If loss of consciousness is more than 2 to 3 minutes, admit to hospital for observation.

If the skull is fractured, admit to hospital for observation.

Administer *non*narcotic analgesics for headache to observe level of consciousness.

If family member and/or friend is reliable, patient may be discharged to home with careful verbal and written aftercare instructions.

Postconcussion syndrome

Late sequelae of concussion may include:

Headache	Syncopal episodes
Nausea	Loss of coordination
Memory loss	Numbness
Decreased concentration	Tinnitus ("ringing" in ears)
Decreased organizational skills	Diplopia (double vision)
Difficulty handling more than one task at once	Loss of menstrual periods
	Breast secretions

■ **DIAGNOSIS**

Reevaluation
CT scan (may be normal, but will be evident on MRI)
MRI

■ **THERAPEUTIC INTERVENTIONS**

Treat in accordance with findings.

Contusion

A contusion is an actual bruise on the surface of the brain causing a structural alteration of the brain.

■ **SIGNS AND SYMPTOMS**

Altered level of consciousness for more than 6 hours
Nausea and vomiting
Vision disturbances
Neurologic dysfunction
    Weakness
    Ataxia

Hemiparesis
Confusion
Speech problems
Seizures (5% of patients)
■ **DIAGNOSIS**
Clinical signs and symptoms
CT scan
MRI
■ **THERAPEUTIC INTERVENTIONS**
Protect cervical spine.
Admit to hospital for observation.
Give antiemetics.

Intracranial Bleeding

The three meningeal layers of the brain are the pia, the arachnoid, and the dura. Lesions or bleeding sites in the head are named according to their location in respect to these meningeal layers (Figure 18-8).

One compensatory mechanism for increasing edema or blood in the cranial vault is for fluid to be squeezed out of the cerebral sinuses and the cerebral sinuses to compress. This mechanism can accommodate approximately 75 ml of edema or fluid before more serious consequences occur.

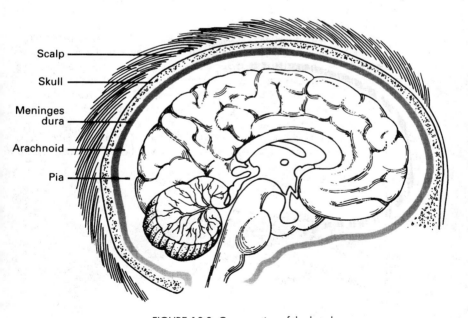

FIGURE 18-8. Cross-section of the head.

Epidural (extradural) hematoma

An epidural hematoma is a collection of blood between the skull and the dura mater (Figure 18-9) in the epidural space. This bleeding may be venous, but is usually arterial. Venous bleeding is rare and may be manageable medically. Epidural bleeds occur in 1% to 2% of all head injuries.[4] The usual etiology is a middle meningeal artery rupture or a tear of a dural sinus. Death is often rapid because the bleed is usually arterial, causing much pressure and uncal herniation. It is most commonly seen with a temporal or parietal skull fracture near the middle meningeal artery. Of patients with epidural bleeds, however, 50% will show no evidence of skull fracture. Mortality rate is between 25% and 50%, and morbidity rate is equally high.[4]

■ **SIGNS AND SYMPTOMS**

Short period of loss of consciousness, caused by a concussion, followed by a lucid period, followed by a loss of consciousness, caused by the bleed. There may be loss of consciousness without a lucid period.

Prior to unconsciousness, complaint of severe headache

Hemiparesis

Ipsilateral (same side) dilated pupil

Bradycardia

Increased blood pressure

■ **DIAGNOSIS**

CT scan

■ **THERAPEUTIC INTERVENTIONS**

Airway management.

Protecting cervical spine

Ventilation with 100% oxygen

Positive pressure to maintain Pco_2 at 26 to 28 torr. (deliberate hypocapnia). When Pco_2 rises, vasodilation occurs and blood volume in the brain is increased. When this occurs, intracranial pressure increases and heightens the possibility of brainstem herniation. If Pco_2 level is reduced, intracranial pressure will be decreased. Hyperventilation is usually only effective to decrease intracranial pressure the first 48 hours following injury.

Oral intubation

Administer 25 mg lidocaine before endotracheal intubation. Lidocaine causes a very transient (2 to 3 minutes) decrease in intracranial pressure that may

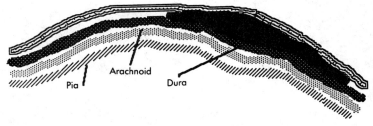

FIGURE 18-9. An acute epidural hematoma.

Pia

Arachnoid

Dura

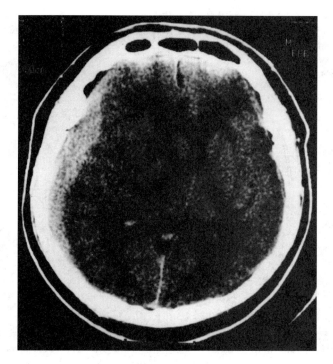

FIGURE 18-10. Subdural hematoma.

prevent the possibility of increased intracranial pressure as a result of the process of endotracheal intubation.[5]

Diuretic agent

Furosemide, a loop diuretic, and/or mannitol, an osmotic diuretic

Head of bed elevated to 30 degrees

IVs at a maintenance rate (125 to 150 ml/hr)

Possible surgical intervention

Subdural hematoma

A subdural hemorrhage is bleeding between the dura mater and the arachnoid membrane in the subdural space (Figure 18-10). It is usually caused by severe blunt trauma, such as an acceleration/deceleration incident, where a venous bridge (where it crosses the subdural space) or cortical artery is torn. It is the most frequently seen type of intracranial bleed and carries a 73% mortality rate and a 90% morbidity rate.[5]

It may occur rapidly (acute) or develop over a period of days, weeks, or months (chronic). If a subdural hemorrhage is seen in a child less than 1 year of age, the etiology should be considered child abuse until proven otherwise.

If a subdural hemorrhage is not rapidly surgically controlled, transtentorial herniation and death may ensue (Figure 18-11). If there is an operative delay of 4 or more hours on operable subdural hemorrhages, mortality rate increases to

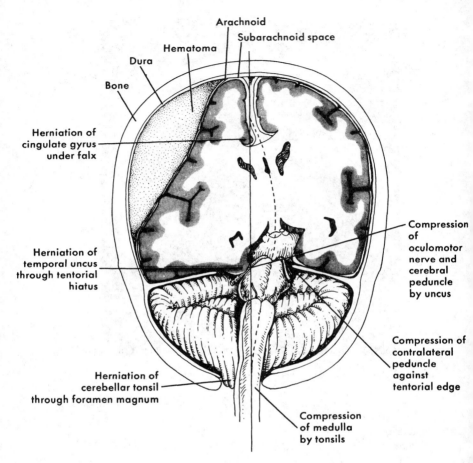

FIGURE 18-11. Mechanism of injury in subdural hematoma.

94%.[5] If the bleeding is bilateral, the diagnostic ''ventricular shift'' may not be seen on computerized tomography. Chronic subdural hemorrhage may occur nontraumatically in the elderly and in chronic alcoholics.

■ **SIGNS AND SYMPTOMS**

Loss of consciousness
Positive Babinski reflex
Fixed dilated pupil(s)
Hemiparesis
Hyperreflexia to abnormal flexion to abnormal extension to flaccidity
Abnormal respirations (type depends on level of herniation)
Elevated temperature

Chronic subdural hematoma

■ **SIGNS AND SYMPTOMS**
Headache
Ataxia
Incontinence
Increasing dementia
Decreasing level of consciousness

■ **DIAGNOSIS**
Clinical findings
CT scan
MRI

■ **THERAPEUTIC INTERVENTIONS**
Airway management
Protecting cervical spine
  Oral intubation
Ventilation with 100% oxygen
Diuretic agents
  Furosemide (Lasix) and/or mannitol
IVs at maintenance rate (125 to 180 ml/hr)
Nonaspirin antipyretics
Surgical intervention
  If the patient is an infant with retinal hemorrhage and abnormal flexion, consider the option of subdural tap in the emergency department.

Subarachnoid hemorrhage

A subarachnoid hemorrhage occurs between the arachnoid membrane and the pia mater (Figure 18-12). It may result from severe head trauma, severe hypertension, aneurysm, or an arteriovenous malformation rupture. The most common cause is trauma.

■ **SIGNS AND SYMPTOMS**
Severe, "piercing" headache
Meningismus
Nausea and vomiting
Delirium, abtundation, syncope, coma
Photophobia
Respiratory abnormalities
  Type depends on level of herniation
Fixed dilated pupils
Papilledema, retinal hemorrhage
Focal motor signs
Seizures

■ **DIAGNOSIS**
Clinical signs and symptoms
CT scan
MRI

■ **THERAPEUTIC INTERVENTIONS**
Airway management.
Protecting cervical spine if suspected trauma

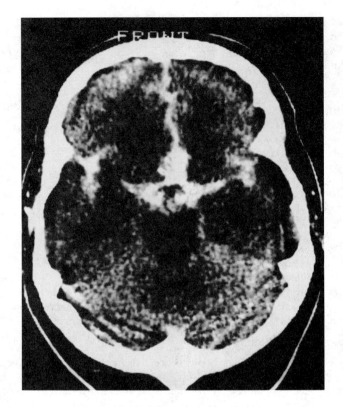

FIGURE 18-12. Subarachnoid hemorrhage.

Ventilation with 100% oxygen
Diuretics
Furosemide (Lasix) and/or mannitol
Surgical intervention
IVs at a maintenance (125 to 150 ml/hr)

Intracerebral (brain) hemorrhage

An intracerebral hemorrhage (Figure 18-13) is a hemorrhage into the brain tissue or the cerebral/ventricular sinuses. It may result from a penetrating injury, a diffuse injury, or a laceration, particularly in the basilar area of the skull where there are bony prominences. In addition to the hemorrhage, there is usually an additional area of edema. Overall prognosis is poor.

■ **SIGNS AND SYMPTOMS**
Loss of consciousness
Fixed dilated pupils
Abnormal respirations
　　Type in accordance with level of herniation

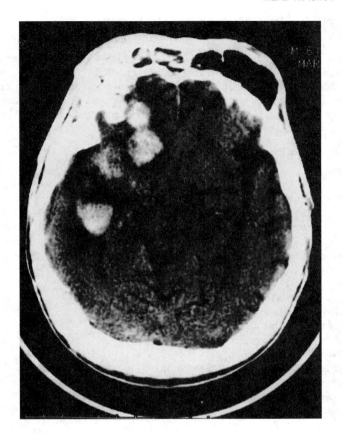

FIGURE 18-13. Intracerebral (brain) hemorrhage.

Abnormal motor function
   Type in accordance with level of herniation
■ **DIAGNOSIS**
Clinical observation
CT scan
MRI
■ **THERAPEUTIC INTERVENTION**
Airway management
Ventilation with 100% oxygen
Diuretics
   Furosemide (Lasix) and/or mannitol
Surgical intervention
IVs at a maintenance rate (125 to 150 ml/hr)

Brainstem Herniation

Brainstem herniation occurs when the brainstem herniates through the tentorial notch or the foramen magnum or the cerebellar tonsils jam into the foramen magnum causing severe permanent neurologic deficits. It occurs as a result of an expanding hematoma in a meningeal space or in cerebral tissue or cerebral/ vascular sinuses, cerebral edema or a mass that propels brain and brainstem tissue toward the path of least resistance, which is usually the tentorial notch or the foramen magnum (Figure 18-14).

Transtentorial (uncal) herniation

A transtentorial herniation occurs when lesions or bleeds at the lateral middle fossa or the temporal lobe cause the inner edge (basal edge) of the uncus and the hippocampal gyrus to be pushed toward the midline and into the lateral edge of the tentorial notch. Pressure builds at the tentorial notch, causing the midbrain to be pushed into the opposite side of the tentorial notch. At this point, the third cranial nerve (oculomotor) and posterior cerebral artery may become caught between the part of the uncus that has herniated and the edge of the tentorial notch.

■ **EARLY SIGNS OF TRANSTENTORIAL HERNIATION**
Decreased level of consciousness
Ipsilateral or bilateral dilated pupils
Cheyne-Stokes breathing
Contralateral hemiparesis
Positive Babinski sign

■ **LATE SIGNS OF TRANSTENTORIAL HERNIATION**
Unconsciousness
Bilateral fixed dilated pupils
Central neurogenic breathing
Abnormal extension

Central herniation (rostral-caudal deterioration)

When intracranial pressure increases and is uniformly distributed throughout the brain, the cerebral tissue is forced downward, causing the cerebellar tonsils to herniate through the foramen magnum, compressing the medulla.

The brain, cerebrospinal fluid, and blood are contained in the skull, which allows very little space for expansion of these substances. When one of these substances increases in volume, the others compensate by decreasing their volume, thereby maintaining a constant intracranial pressure. This compensation can only occur when there is a slight increase in volume. If volume increase is excessive, intracranial pressure will rise.

When intracranial pressure increases beyond mean arterial pressure, the brain cells become anoxic because of inadequate perfusion of brain tissue and eventually suffer irreparable damage. The brain tissue itself begins to shift, compressing the ventricles and forcing brain tissue into the tentorial notch. This compresses the brainstem and the third cranial nerve.

It is therefore necessary to avoid, or at least moderate, those activities that cause an increase in intracranial pressure in those patients who are already at risk of increased pressure.

Signs and symptoms of supratentorial herniation are: coma from impairment of the reticular activating system; changes in pupil size and reaction to light, including the dilated, fixed pupil; decreased motor response, decerebrate posturing if the herniation is at the midbrain level or decorticate posturing if the herniation is at the thalamic level, and flaccidity if the herniation has reached the level of the lower pons; and Cheyne-Stokes, central neurogenic, or ataxic respirations.

Intracranial pressure monitoring may be indicated when there is suspicion of increased intracranial pressure, such as may be found when there has been head trauma resulting in cerebral edema, increased intracranial pressure caused by a tumor or other expanding lesion, and increased intracranial pressure may have occurred as a result of an obstruction in the path of the cerebrospinal fluid.

A A subarachnoid screw is shown on the left with a catheter in the lateral ventricle.

The most common devices used to monitor intracranial pressure are the subarachnoid screw and a ventricular cannula. The subarachnoid screw is passed through a small threaded drill hole in the skull into the subarachnoid space. The screw is connected to a saline-filled transducer via a stopcock and pressure tubing, which converts mechanical impulses from the subarachnoid space into electrical impulses that are displayed on a digital readout or as a visible wave form on an oscilloscope. If a catheter is used, it is passed through a burr hole into the lateral ventricle and connected to a saline-filled transducer via a stopcock and pressure tubing. It transmits impulses in the same manner as the subarachnoid screw.

An alternate method, using a sensor implanted in the epidural or subdural space (through a burr hole) provides a constant monitor pattern. This approach to intracranial pressure monitoring is safer in terms of electrical hazards and potential infection, and there is no risk of uncontrolled loss of CSF from ventricles.

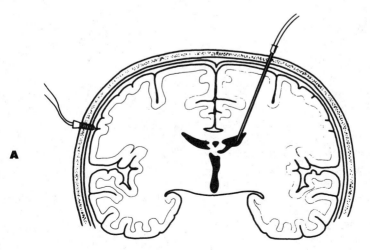

FIGURE 18-14. Intracranial pressure monitoring.

Continued.

B Sensor implantation.

Normal intracranial pressure is 5.8 to 13 mm Hg (70 to 190 mm H_2O). It is quite normal to have brief intracranial pressure elevations of greater than 13 mm Hg with such activities as suctioning, turning, or sneezing. A prolonged intracranial pressure reading of greater than 13 mm Hg, however, is abnormal. If intracranial pressure increases to 50 mm Hg or greater for over 20 minutes, the patient has a very poor prognosis.

C A strain relief loop prevents damage if the patient rolls his head.

Cerebral perfusion pressure can be calculated by subtracting intracranial pressure from mean arterial pressure. A result of less than 60 mm H_2O will indicate cerebral ischemia and a cerebral perfusion pressure of less than 30 mm H_2O will result in death.

Administration of osmotic diuretics, such as mannitol or urea, or the use of steroids may increase cerebral perfusion pressure. Fluids can also be decreased by limiting those taken by mouth or by the parenteral route. Cerebrospinal fluid can be removed via ventriculostomy or lumbar puncture. Pressure can be reduced by temporal decompression or by pharmacological measures to increase the mean arterial pressure, and the patient can be hyperventilated to blow off CO_2.

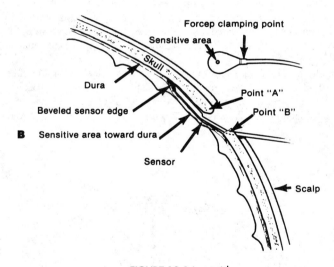

FIGURE 18-14, cont'd

■ **EARLY SIGNS OF CENTRAL HERNIATION**
Restlessness to lethargy
Pupils constricted, but equal and reactive
Cheyne-Stokes breathing with yawns and sighs that deteriorate to central neurogenic breathing

■ **LATE SIGNS OF CENTRAL HERNIATION**
Unconsciousness
Midpoint to dilated fixed pupils

Central neurogenic to ataxic breathing
Abnormal flexion to abnormal extension to flaccidity
    NOTE: Oval-shaped pupils indicate increased intracranial pressure and incipient herniation.

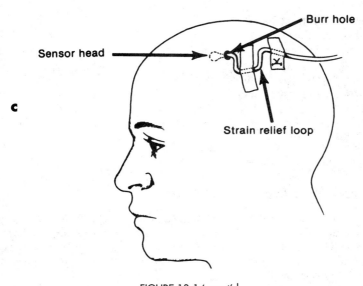

FIGURE 18-14, cont'd
From: Budassi SA: *JEN,* May, 1979.

■ **DIAGNOSIS**
Clinical observation
CT scan
Increased intracranial pressure
■ **THERAPEUTIC INTERVENTIONS**
Airway management. Protect cervical spine
    Oral tracheal intubation
    Consider lidocaine IV just before intubation
Hyperventilation using 100% oxygen with positive pressure
Diuretics
    Furosemide
    Mannitol
Surgical intervention

SPECIAL CONSIDERATIONS

Impaled Objects

An object that is impaled into the skull and cranial vault may or may not produce a severe injury. The extent of trauma depends on the location of the wound and the caliber and velocity of the impaled object.

■ **DIAGNOSIS**
Observation
X-ray
CT scan

■ **THERAPEUTIC INTERVENTIONS**
Airway management.
Protect cervical spine.
Provide oxygen.
Do not remove impaled object!
Secure impaled object.
Control bleeding.
Apply sterile dressing around impaled object.
Give psychological support.
Treat for other associated findings.
Ensure tetanus prophylaxis.

Seizures Following Head Trauma

Patients often develop seizures after a head trauma incident. The seizures may result from a direct injury to the brain or increased intracranial pressure. Seizure activity will cause PCO_2 to rise and PO_2 to fall, resulting in cerebral edema and cerebral hypoxia.

■ **SIGNS AND SYMPTOMS**
Seizure activity
Other neurologic findings

■ **DIAGNOSIS**
Clinical observation
Clinical history

■ **THERAPEUTIC INTERVENTIONS**
Airway management
Oxygen
Diazepam (Valium) IV as prescribed to control seizure activity (usually 2.5 to 5 mg IV, titrated to effect)
   If the seizure continues, administer 1g phenytoin IV.
   Consider phenobarbital and/or general anesthesia (a neuromuscular blocking agent) if seizures remain uncontrolled.

SUMMARY OF THERAPEUTIC INTERVENTIONS FOR ALL PATIENTS WITH SEVERE HEAD INJURIES

Maintain airway.
Protect cervical spine.
Give 100% oxygen with positive pressure.
   Maintain PCO_2 at 26 to 28 torr (first 48 hours after injury).
Provide diuretics
   Furosemide and/or Mannitol

Obtain cervical spine x-ray film.

Restrict fluids unless hypovolemic shock is evidenced.

Monitor and record baseline and serial neurologic exams.

Maintain head in midline position.

Keep head elevated at 30 degrees unless contraindicated by spinal injury.

Foley and hourly urine output

Monitor temperature.

> Keep patient normothermic (use cooling blanket or alpha blockade [2.5 to 3 mg thorazine] if necessary).

Consider neurosurgery consult.

Assess for other injuries.

Consider transfer to appropriate facility.

Minimize external stimulation.

Consider dextrose 50% and naloxone 0.8 mg IV if unsure if unconscious state is caused by trauma.

Draw toxicology or alcohol screen if indicated.

Victims of head trauma often have serious to life-threatening injuries. The patient's prognosis and outcome will depend upon how quickly the patient is diagnosed and treated. It is imperative, therefore, for emergency nurses to be familiar and comfortable with identification and treatment of head trauma.

REFERENCES

1. Miller TR et al: Costs and functional consequences of U.S. roadway crashes, *Accident Analysis and Prevention* 25:593, 1993.
2. Kraus JF et al: The incidence of acute brain injury and serious impairment in a defined population, *Am J Epidemiol* 119:186, 1984.
3. Kraus JF: Epidemiology of brain injury. In Cooper PR, ed: *Head injury,* ed 2. Baltimore, 1986, Williams and Wilkins.
4. Rosen P et al: *Emergency medicine,* ed 2. St. Louis, 1988, Mosby.
5. Sheehy SB: *Emergency nursing,* ed 4, St Louis, 1994, Mosby.

SUGGESTED READINGS

Adler JS et al: Inadvertent intracranial placement of a nasogastric tube in a patient with severe head trauma, *Canadian Med Assoc J* 147(S):668, 1992.

Henderson A et al: A survey of interhospital transfer of head injured patients with inadequately treated life-threatening extracranial injuries, *Austral N Ze J Surg* 62(10):759, 1992.

Pons P: Concussion and skull fracture in blunt head trauma. In Calliham ML: *Current concepts in emergency medicine.* Toronto, 1987, Decker.

Pons P: Head trauma. In Rosen P et al, eds: *Emergency medicine,* ed 2. St Louis, 1987, Mosby.

Sefrin P: Current level of prehospital care in severe head injury—potential for improvement, *Acta Neurochirurgica* 57:141, 1993.

Wesson DE et al: The physical, psychological and socioeconomic costs of pediatric trauma, *J Trauma* 33(2):252, 1992.

Spinal Cord and Neck Trauma

The annual incidence of spinal cord injury in the United States is 50 persons per 1 million population.[1]

The higher-risk population for spinal cord injury is primarily young adult males between the ages of 15 and 30, those who are impulsive or risk takers in daily living.[2]

Motor vehicle crashes account for most spinal cord injuries, followed by falls, sporting injuries, diving, penetrating wounds, and assaults.

There appears to be a high relationship between spinal cord injuries and alcohol and drug abuse. The spinal cord and vertebrae may be injured as a result of fractures, dislocations, or subluxations that produce abnormal anatomic movements:

Hypertension	The head is forced back and the neck is placed in an overextended position.
Hyperflexion	The head is forced forward and the neck is placed in an overflexed position.
Axial loading	A severe blow to the top of the head that results in a blunt force into the spinal column.
Compression	A force from above and a concurrent force from below.
Lateral bend	The head and neck are bent to one side, beyond normal limits.
Overrotation	The head and neck turn beyond normal limits.
Distraction	The vertebrae are pulled out of alignment.

THE SPINAL CORD

A weight as little as 400 mg (approximately the weight of a Kennedy half-dollar) dropped onto the spinal cord from a 7 inch height can cause permanent injury.[3] In 93% of cord injuries the cord is not severed. The problem results from intramedullary bleeding and edema.[3]

The spinal cord is an integral part of the central nervous system. It controls consciousness, regulates body movement and function, and transmits nerve impulses. It has both voluntary and involuntary functions. It is enclosed in a canal that extends the length of the vertebral column. Spinal nerves extend through openings in the vertebrae. The anterior part of the spinal cord contains motor tracts. The posterior part of the spinal cord contains sensory tracts. It is possible to have an incomplete lesion, where motor function below the level of the lesion is gone but sensation remains intact.

The spinal cord transmits nerve impulses to and from the brain and the body to regulate function and movement. It is, like the brain, protected by the three layers of meninges, the pia, the arachnoid and the dura, the vertebrae, and the paravertebral muscles. The openings in the vertebrae form the canal through which the spinal cord passes. The spinal cord itself may be concussed, contused, or transected. A concussed cord produces transient changes that will resolve from a few minutes to hours. A contused spinal cord may result in a structural defect and permanent disability. Spinal cord transection causes permanent disability or death. The disability causes loss of motor and sensory functions below the level of the injury. An acute transection may also cause spinal shock (see Chapter 6).

The immediate problems with cervical spine injury are to ensure airway maintenance and adequate breathing. Cervical vertebrae 3, 4, and 5 contain the phrenic nerve. Injury at or above this area causes loss of control of the diaphragm (the main muscle of respiration). Survival from such an injury is rare—lesions above C3 or C4 usually result in death.

Innervations at the level of the vertebrae include the following:

C2 to C4	—diaphragm, neck muscles
C5, C6	—biceps brachii, deltoid, triceps brachii, wrist extensors
C6 to T1	—latissimus dorsi, hand muscles
T2 to T7	—intercostal muscles
T6 to L1	—abdominal muscles
T12 to L2	—quadratus lumborum
L1 to L5	—leg muscles
L2 to L3	—psoas muscles
L2 to L4	—quadriceps
L4 to L5	—tibialis anterior
S1	—bowel and bladder

LESIONS OF	**PRODUCE**
C3, C4, or above	Respiratory arrest; flaccid paralysis; quadriplegia
C5, C6	Reduced respiratory effort; almost total dependence; flaccid paralysis; quadriplegia
C7	Reduced respiratory effort; almost total dependence; splints necessary for forearms to function; quadriplegia
T1	Reduced respiratory effort; partial dependence; paraplegia
T1, T2	Reduced respiratory effort; complete independence; paraplegia
T7	Complete independence; walk with long leg braces; paraplegia
L4	Complete independence; walk with foot braces; paraplegia

INCOMPLETE CORD LESIONS

Central Cord Syndrome

The most common cause of central cord syndrome (Figure 19-1) is hyperextension. It is commonly seen in the elderly following a fall. This type of injury produces loss of function (lower motor neuron disease) in the upper extremities; bowel and bladder function are maintained.

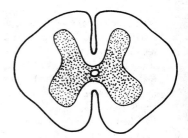

FIGURE 19-1. Central cord syndrome.

Anterior Cord Syndrome

Anterior cord syndrome (Figure 19-2) is usually seen in flexion injuries. This results from an occlusion of the anterior spinal artery, a herniated nucleus pulposus (ruptured disc), or a transection of the anterior portion of the cord. The patient experiences hyperesthesia, hypoalgesia, and either incomplete or complete paralysis. The patient is able to feel vibrations and proprioception because of a preserved posterior column function.

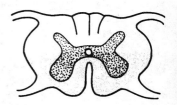

FIGURE 19-2. Anterior cord syndrome.

Brown-Sequard Syndrome

Involvement of the hemisection of the cord in the anterior-posterior plane is known as Brown-Sequard syndrome (Figure 19-3). It is most often caused by penetrating objects, such as those that occur with gunshot wounds or stab wounds. Hallmarks are ipsilateral (same side) paresis or hemiplegia and contralateral (opposite side) reduced sensation to pain and temperature. A person with

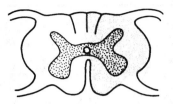

FIGURE 19-3. Brown-Sequard syndrome.

Brown-Sequard syndrome can feel on one side but not the other, and can move on the opposite side but not the side with sensation loss.

Root Injuries

Injuries to the nerve roots (Figure 19-4) often occur with spinal cord trauma. Most common findings are hypoalgesia, pain, or referred pain.

Posterior Cord Syndrome

The less common finding is usually related to extension injury. Below the level of injury there will be decreased sensations of proprioception, vibration, and light touch.

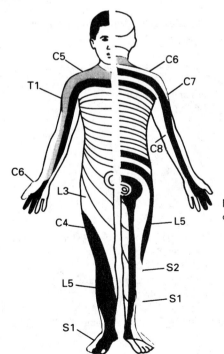

FIGURE 19-4. Nerve roots and the muscles they innervate.

THE VERTEBRAE

The human body has seven cervical, twelve thoracic, and five lumbar vertebrae; the sacrum, five fused sacral vertebrae, and one or two coccygeal segments (Figure 19-5). Vertebrae may become subluxed, fractured, compressed, or dislocated.

A Jefferson fracture is a fracture of the first cervical (atlas) vertebral arch. Initially, there may be no neurologic deficit. This patient will require traction and surgical fixation. A Hangman's fracture is a bilateral arch fracture of the second cervical vertebrae (axis).

There are three major types of spinal injury: injury to the cord itself, fracture of the vertebrae, and injury to the spinal nerves. Be sure to document all findings and changes that would indicate a specific type of injury.

Assessment

Before assessment immobilize the patient's spine completely and ensure that there will be minimal movement.

Assess for patent airway.

Check respiratory rate, rhythm, and depth. Pay particular attention to the use of accessory muscles of respiration, especially the diaphragm.

Evaluate blood pressure, pulse, and skin vitals (color, temperature, and moisture).

Observe patient's level of consciousness; check for neurologic deficits.

Check for a cerebrospinal fluid leak from the nose or the ears.

Palpate the spine.

Assess for the presence of pain, tenderness, step-off deformity, and/or edema.

Assess motor strength or weakness and document.

Assess sensory levels (Figure 19-6) and document

to touch, pain

for paresthesias and paralysis

Check for ecchymosis.

Check for tracheal deviation.

Check for a hematoma in the posterior pharyngeal area.

Check sphincter tone.

Check for priapism.

Check for diaphoresis.

Injuries above T4 usually cause sympathetic nervous system disruption. When this occurs, vasodilation occurs below the level of the injury because of inability to vasoconstrict. If the patient is diaphoretic, this is evidenced above the level of the injury and not below.

Check for other associated injuries, especially:

Head injuries

27% of patients with spinal cord injuries have concurrent head injuries[3]

Skull and facial bones

Chest

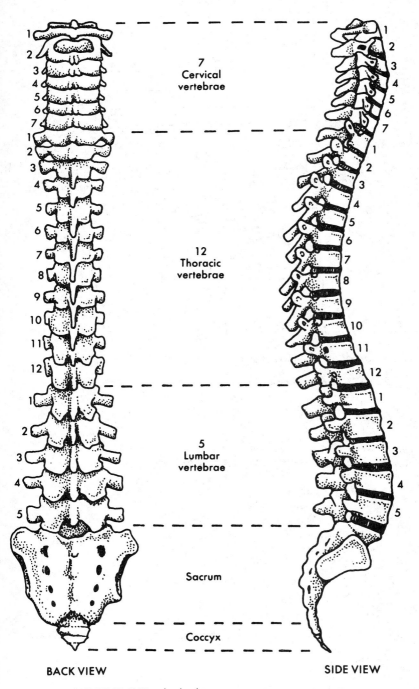

FIGURE 19-5. Vertebral column.
(From Rosen P et al: *Emergency medicine,* ed 2. St Louis, 1988, Mosby.)

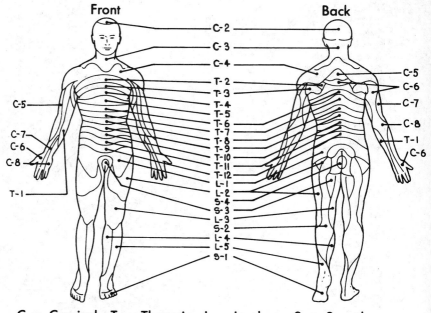

Front   **Back**

C-2
C-3
C-4
T-2
T-3
T-4
T-5
T-6
T-7
T-8
T-9
T-10
T-11
T-12
L-1
L-2
S-4
S-3
L-3
S-2
L-4
L-5
S-1

C-5
C-6
C-7
C-8
T-1
C-6

C-5
C-7
C-6
C-8
T-1

C = Cervical T = Thoracic L = Lumbar S = Sacral

FIGURE 19-6. Dermatome chart demonstrating sensory and motor levels.

Abdomen
Pelvis

■ **SIGNS AND SYMPTOMS OF SPINAL CORD INJURY**
Neck tenderness and pain
Weakness of extremities
Numbness and tingling or paralysis
Decreased motor activity distal to the injury
Unexplained hypotension
Altered level of consciousness
Pain upon palpation
Local edema
Deformity
Priapism
Cough tenderness (coughing produces neck pain)
Feeling of ''electric shock'' or ''hot water'' running down the patient's back
Ptosis
Patient holding head
Mouth breathing (Gautman's position)
 The patient laps air due to loss of diaphragm control

Cock Robin appearance
    May indicate C1-C2 injury
Arms folded across chest
    May indicate C5-C6 injury

■ **DIAGNOSIS**

Diagnosis is made by clinical findings, x-rays, CT scan, and other findings.

    X-rays (Figure 19-7). Obtain a cervical spine series that includes a cross-table lateral cervical spine film. One must be able to visualize all seven cervical

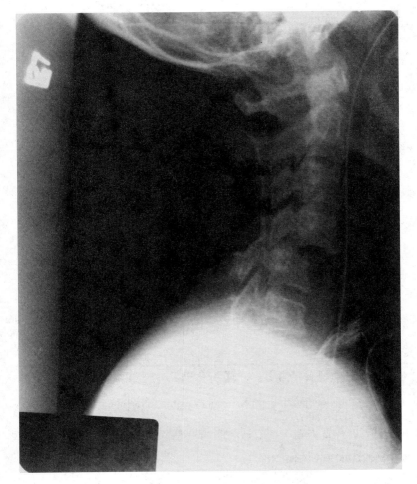

FIGURE 19-7. Visualizing only six cervical vertebrae is inadequate. One must be able to visualize all seven cervical vertebrae on a cross-table cervical spine film.

vertebrae and the top of T-1. X-rays may demonstrate subluxations, fractures, dislocations, and narrowing of paravertebral spaces.

In order to truly clear the cervical spine, four x-ray views are necessary: cross-table lateral, anterior-posterior, oblique, and open-mouth odontoid. If T1 cannot be visualized on the cross-table lateral view, obtain a swimmer's view, with the x-ray being shot through the axilla. If there is a high probability of injury, one should also include flexion-extension views (if the patient is conscious and can tell you if she or he is having pain—when the procedure is stopped) to check for soft-tissue injury that would compromise ability to maintain vertebral column alignment.

The patient's arms may need to be pulled downward to cause the shoulders to drop to ensure adequate visualization of the C-spine. Ensure adequate C-spine immobilization during this procedure. Assess the films for:

Anterior-posterior column alignment
Anterior/posterior diameter of the spinal canal
Presence of bone fragments or bone displacement
Presence of linear fractures or comminuted fractures
Soft-tissue edema at or below C-3
Presence of a retropharyngeal hematoma
Vertebral inclination

An angle that is greater than 11 degrees or one that exceeds one fourth of the vertebral body is considered "unstable."

NOTE: If a patient has an associated head injury, alcohol or drug ingestion, even if cervical spine radiographs are read as negative for fracture, it is very important for the patient to remain in a collar until flexion/extension views are completed to rule out ligamentous injury.

Bulbocavernosus reflex. Place a finger in the patient's rectum and compress the glans or the clitoris or tug on the Foley catheter. With a normal finding the anal sphincter contracts. If this reflex is absent initially and then returns within 24 hours, it is indicative of a total lesion.

Anal "wink" or contraction. The anal sphincter should contract when a pin prick is applied in close proximity. When there is spinal cord injury, there is no response.

MEASURES TO PREVENT FURTHER INJURIES

Have a sufficient number of personnel available so that the patient can be moved carefully.

Immobilize the cervical, thoracic, and lumbar spine in accordance with local protocol.

■ **THERAPEUTIC INTERVENTIONS**

Ensure airway, breathing, and circulation.

The airway is always at risk secondary to edema.

Of persons with neck fractures 96% can be safely orally intubated.[4]

Consider cricothyrotomy or tracheostomy.

Problems with circulation may be directly related to the presence of spinal shock.

Immobilize the cervical, thoracic, and lumbar spine.

Consider placement of tongs (Figure 19-8, *A, B*) and cervical traction.

Closed reduction for injuries (below C_3) begin with No. 15 then increase by No. 5 until reduction is accomplished.

Initiate at least two large-bore IV lines with Ringer's lactate solution, and run at a keep-open rate unless hemodynamic signs indicate otherwise.

Place a urinary catheter to straight drainage and monitor urinary output hourly. Prevent urinary retention.

Consider steroids to reduce edema; prevent posttraumatic ischemia by increasing blood flow. Give methylprednisolone, initially 30 mg/kg bolus with 5.4 mg/kg/hr for 24 hours within 12 hours of acute spinal cord injury.[5]

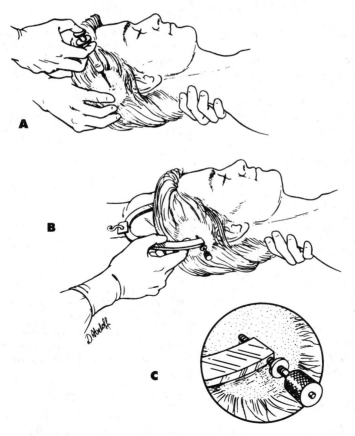

FIGURE 19-8. **A,** Anesthetizing pin sites. **B,** Placing the tongs. **C,** Tightening the pins.

Place a nasogastric tube; consider oral gastric when there is a head or facial injury present.

If patient presents hypothermic, use caution not to overcorrect as spinal-cord-injured patient's normal temperature regulating mechanisms may not be functioning.[6]

Pad pressure points.

One hour on an unpadded board provides an 80% chance of significant skin problems later.[7]

Administer tetanus prophylaxis and antibiotics if appropriate.

Facilitate early neurosurgical consultation.

Consider transfer to facility with neurosurgical and/or rehabilitation capabilities.

If transferring a patient in tongs and traction, do *not* tape the hanging weights to anything.

Give hopeful, but not false, psychological support.

CERVICAL SPINE IMMOBILIZATION

Cervical spine immobilization should be considered simultaneously with airway management as one of the first priorities of care of a patient with multiple injuries, a patient with known or suspected trauma to the cervical spine, or a patient whose mechanism of injury suggests the possibility of cervical spine injury. This needs to be done regardless of subjective cervical spine pain. The responsibility of "doing no further harm" cannot be overemphasized. Extreme caution and a high index of suspicion are recommended when handling trauma patients before a cervical spine injury has been ruled out.

Equipment List

Semi-rigid cervical collar
Kedrick extrication device
Short spine board with straps
Long spine board with straps
Sandbags
Blankets, towels for padding
2- or 3-inch adhesive tape
Cervical extrication device

Equipment used to immobilize the neck may be as varied as the situation in which it is being utilized (Figure 19-9). If it is being applied in the hospital or in the field by prehospital rescue personnel, there are many commercial devices available. However, if cervical spine immobilization is indicated in the absence of this equipment, everyday materials on hand are adequate for achieving the necessary stabilization.

Procedure

1. Assess airway; ensure patency by using jaw thrust or chin lift (Figure 19-10); do not hyperextend neck; if endotracheal intubation is necessary and not pos-

sible without hyperextension, consider nasotracheal or digital intubation or cricothyrotomy to ensure the airway.

2. Evaluate cervical spine by observation; palpate each spinous process; note deformity, crepitus, pain, and instability. (Talk to the patient; also remember to inform the patient of each step of the procedure to alleviate anxiety and movement and to elicit the patient's cooperation.)

3. Gently apply inline manual stabilization by placing the hands on either side of the head and stabilizing the head and neck in a neutral, vertical position; in children this is defined as the "sniffing" position. (Once this stabilization is applied it must be maintained until a comparable alternative has been implemented or until cervical spine injury has been ruled out by x-ray.)

4. Have other members of the team assist by gently placing a spine board under the patient while one caregiver continues to maintain stabilization. (Synchronized logroll with absolute cervical spine protection by manual stabilization may be the best way, but adequate personnel manpower is essential to avoid further harm.)

5. Secure the patient to the board by:

Using chest, hip, and leg straps across the patient, snugly attached to handles or cutouts in board (remember to undress patient completely if possible, or at least remove any sharp or bulky items that may cause soft-tissue pressure areas; pad bony prominences liberally).

Securing straps diagonally from legs to chest.

Padding behind the head and neck to support the cervical spine (always

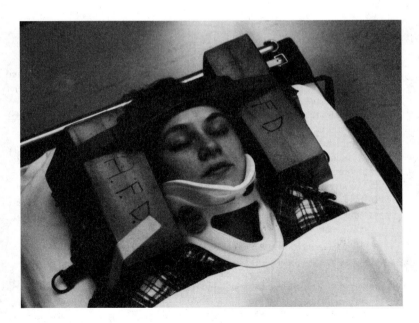

FIGURE 19-9. Full cervical spine immobilization, utilizing long board, C-blocks, straps, and stiffneck collar.

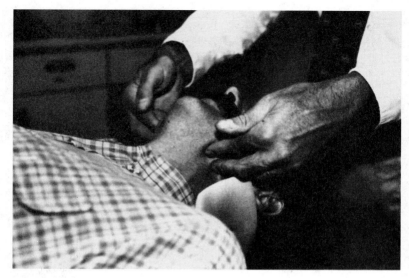

FIGURE 19-10. Maintenance of airway may involve jaw thrust technique allowing the examiner to monitor the airway closely and ensure protection of the cervical spine.

maintaining the neutral, vertical position of the manual stabilization). Securing the patient's head to the spine board using 2- or 3-inch tape applied across the eyebrows and across the chin; this tape must be secured snugly to both sides of the spine board. Exercise caution to prevent any of the securing devices from interfering with respirations or emesis.

6. When you are satisfied with the absolute immobility of the patient's cervical spine, you may release manual stabilization.

7. Be prepared to logroll the patient using the backboard if vomiting occurs; have suction on hand.

8. If a short spine board or other short device is used, also use a long board or scoop stretcher for extrication and further movement.

9. If the patient has a helmet on (e.g., motorcycle, football), leave it in place, provided airway is not compromised, until the condition of the cervical spine is confirmed and measures can be taken to remove the helmet safely.

Helmet Removal

There are a variety of helmets available for those sports that recommend head protection—motorcycling, bicycling, kayaking, ice hockey, football, and auto racing are just a few. The careful removal of this gear is imperative for protection of the cervical spine.

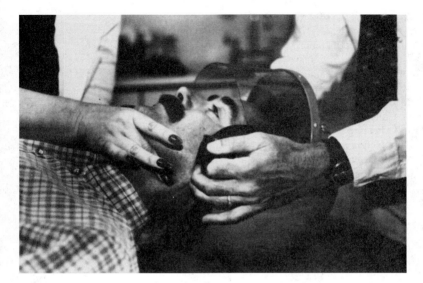

FIGURE 19-11. Helmet removal should be done with manual control of the cervical spine by one individual while the other person spreads the helmet laterally and removes it.

Procedure

1. *Never attempt to remove a helmet alone:* airway protection can be achieved with most helmets in place and the potential for complicating an injury with a difficult removal is great.
2. One person should apply inline traction by placing hands on each side of the helmet with fingers on the patient's mandible, exerting careful pulling; remember to loosen or cut the chin strap (Figure 19-11).
3. A second person should then receive the weight of the patient's head by placing one hand behind the head, resting on the occiput, and placing the front hand on the angles of the mandible, thumb on one side, fingers on the other *(the second person is now in control of the head and neck)*.
4. The first person should then remove the helmet by pulling laterally on the sides and sliding it off. If the helmet has full face protection, special consideration must be given to the eye covering, which must be removed first; if it cannot be removed, tilt the helmet (not the head) back to pass the face protector over the patient's nose.

SOFT-TISSUE INJURIES OF THE NECK

Fractured Larynx

The most common cause of a fractured larynx is blunt trauma, such as occurs in a sudden impact with the steering wheel, a deceleration caused by a rope or wire, a hanging, or a karate chop.

■ **SIGNS AND SYMPTOMS**
Hoarse voice
Cough with hemoptysis
Progressive respiratory stridor
Difficulty breathing/respiratory distress
Subcutaneous emphysema
■ **DIAGNOSIS**
Clinical observation
   Feeling subcutaneous emphysema
   Noting progressive stridor
Displacement of landmarks
■ **THERAPEUTIC INTERVENTIONS**
Emergency cricothyrotomy (in emergency department) or tracheostomy (in surgery). (See Chapter 4.)
High-flow oxygen before and after procedure
Broad-spectrum antibiotics

Penetrating Neck Wounds

Penetrating objects, such as bullets and knife blades, can cause trauma to the tissues of the neck. The extent of injury depends on the type of penetrating object, the force of the object, and the location and angle of the penetration.
■ **SIGNS AND SYMPTOMS**
Obvious penetrating wound
Airway obstruction or stridor
Signs of hypovolemia, hemothorax, or shock
Presence of a large or expanding hematoma
■ **DIAGNOSIS**
Clinical observation
Arteriography
Exploratory surgery
■ **THERAPEUTIC INTERVENTIONS**
Airway management
   Consider surgical procedure
Breathing
   Ensure adequate oxygenation
Circulation
   Control bleeding
   Replace volume (2 large-bore, 16-gauge or larger IVs with Ringer's Lactate)
Consider surgery

REFERENCES

1. Domzalski F: Spinal cord injury and cord syndromes. In Hamilton G, ed: *Presenting signs and symptoms in the emergency department: evaluation and treatment.* Baltimore, 1993, Williams and Wilkins.
2. Walleck CA: Peripheral nerve and spinal cord problems. In Lewis S, Collier I, eds: *Medical-surgical nursing: assessment and management of clinical problems.* St Louis, 1992, Mosby.
3. Shea J: Lecture presentation, Emergency Nurses Association Annual Meeting, Orlando, Fla, 1992.
4. Bauer D, Errico T: Cervical spine injuries. In Errico T, Bauer D, Waugh T: *Spinal trauma.* Philadelphia, 1991, Lippincott.
5. Bauer D, Errico T: Pharmacologic therapy of acute spinal cord injury. In Errico T, Bauer D, Waugh T: *Spinal trauma.* Philadelphia, 1991, Lippincott.
6. Mangiardi JR et al: Spinal injuries. In Schwartz G, Cayten CG, Mangelsen MA et al: *Principles and practice of emergency medicine.* Philadelphia, 1992, Lea and Febiger.
7. American College of Surgeons, Committee on Trauma: *ATLS Manual,* Chicago, 1992, ACS.

SUGGESTED READINGS

Athey AM: A 3-year-old with spinal cord injury without radiographic abnormality (Sciwora), *JEN* 17:380, 1991.

Brown VL, Espinosa J: Near hanging injury: two case studies and an overview, *JEN* 17: 386, 1991.

Browner C, Prendergast V: Spinal cord damage with diving injuries: consideration for nursing care, *Crit Care Nurs Clin North Am* 3:339, 1991.

Burchiel KJ: Emergency management of stable and unstable injuries. In Tollison CD, Satterthwaite JR, eds: *Painful cervical trauma: diagnosis and rehabilitative treatment of neuromusculoskeletal injuries.* Baltimore, 1992, Williams & Wilkins.

Herman J, Sonnatas VKH: Diving accidents: mechanism of injury and treatment of the patient, *Crit Care Nurs Clin North Am* 3:331, 1991.

Lewis AM: A 17-year-old male with traumatic laryngeal fracture, *JEN* 16:135, 1990.

Orenstein JB et al: Delayed diagnosis of pediatric cervical spine injury, *Pediatrics* 89: 1185, 1992.

Roberge RJ: Facilitating cervical spine radiography in blunt trauma, *Emerg Med Clin North Am* 9:733, 1991.

Selivanov V, Martinez R: Clinical clearance of the cervical spine, *JEN* 18:79, 1992.

Shagoury C, Fazio J: A 23 year-old with an unusual impalement injury, *JEN* 16:379, 1990.

Sweeney TA, Marz JA: Blunt neck injury, *Emerg Med Clin North Am* 11:71, 1993.

Wright S et al: Cervical spine injuries in blunt trauma in patients requiring emergent endotracheal intubation, *Am J Emerg Med* 10:104, 1992.

Facial Trauma

Facial trauma may cause severe complications, such as airway obstruction and respiratory distress, and may mask other problems, such as spinal cord injury or intracranial bleed. Most cases of facial trauma result from motor vehicle accidents, but they may also be the result of domestic violence or physical assault, contact sports, or a blow by any mechanism that can cause blunt or penetrating trauma to the face.

ASSESSMENT

Always begin assessment and therapeutic intervention of facial trauma with the following:

Airway

Ensure that there is an open airway. Avoid tilting the head; assume that there is a concurrent cervical spine injury until proven otherwise. If one must manually control the airway, first use the jaw thrust maneuver and consider using airway adjuncts (see Chapters 3 and 4).

Breathing

Always remember that noisy breathing means obstructed breathing. Administer supplemental oxygen.

Circulation

Control any obvious bleeding. The patient may lose enough blood to develop hypovolemic shock. Consider initiating an IV line.

Cervical Spine

Assume that a cervical spine injury exists until it can be proven otherwise. IMMOBILIZE THE NECK. Check for a laryngeal fracture.

Level of Consciousness

Evaluate level of consciousness, pupillary reaction, and movement.

Eyes

Check each eye individually. Note loss of vision, diplopia (double vision) in each of four quadrants, and check for intraocular hemorrhage and penetration by a foreign body.

Malocclusion of Teeth

Assess that teeth meet properly as the patient closes mouth and "bites down" on back molars. (Generally malocclusion indicates mandible fracture.)

Point Tenderness

Assess for specific area of palpable tenderness.

Asymmetry

Infraorbital rim
Zygomatic arch
Anterior wall of antrum
Angles of the jaw
Lower borders of the mandible

Cerebrospinal fluid leak

From the nose (CSF rhinorrhea)
From the ear (CSF otorrhea)
Complaint of a salty taste

It is important to remember that facial injuries are diagnosed through astute clinical assessment and confirmed via appropriate radiographs.

FACIAL LACERATIONS

Facial lacerations can bleed profusely and may cause severe disfigurement. They may be caused by penetrating objects such as glass, metal, or knives.

■ **THERAPEUTIC INTERVENTIONS**

Local anesthesia (with epinephrine to control bleeding) or regional anesthesia.
Cleanse the laceration.
   Use normal saline or antibacterial solution.
   Remember to rinse the laceration thoroughly after cleansing.
   Debride the wound, if necessary.
   Remove foreign bodies.
Suture the wound.
   Wounds may be sutured up to 24 hours postinjury.
   Suturing is usually performed by a physician.

A plastic surgery consultation may be appropriate due to extent or type of injury, or when requested by patient/family.

■ **SPECIAL NOTES**

When there is a lip laceration, the vermilion border must be carefully approximated.

Eyebrows should be carefully approximated. (Never shave eyebrows!)

If there is a laceration of the cheek, check carefully for a parotid duct laceration and arrange for repair if lacerated.

ABRASIONS AND CONTUSIONS

(See Chapter 17, Wound Management.)

■ **THERAPEUTIC INTERVENTIONS**

Anesthetize.

Cleanse and debride devitalized or grossly contaminated tissue conservatively. Carefully remove foreign bodies to avoid "tattooing."

Suture.

Dress with a topical antibiotic.

FACIAL FRACTURES

When a patient suffers multiple trauma injuries, facial fractures do not usually receive a high priority until other more life-threatening injuries can be treated. Unlike treatment of a laceration, treatment of a facial fracture can often be delayed for up to 10 days without serious consequences.

Nasal Fractures

The mechanism of injury for a nasal fracture is usually blunt trauma to the front or side of the nose. Diagnosis may be made clinically by obtaining a good history and observing for swelling, deformity, crepitus, and pain on palpation. Nasal fractures usually cause bleeding both externally and internally. If the patient is not treated immediately following the incident, reduction usually must be delayed until swelling has subsided. Treat any fracture of the nose as an open fracture; administer antibiotics and ensure tetanus prophylaxis. Also check and treat for a septal hematoma, since a septal hematoma that is not excised and packed may become infected or necrotic.

■ **THERAPEUTIC INTERVENTIONS**

Apply cold pack.

Splint.

Control bleeding.

Administer anesthetic.

Infraorbital area, anterior nasal spine, and dorsum of nose—use 1% lidocaine with epinephrine.

Mucosa—pack with cotton pledgets soaked in 5% lidocaine.

Manipulate the impacted bone and cartilage to "free" them, using fingers and forceps.

Mold the fractured parts with fingers.

Pack the inside to decrease bleeding; if the septum is fractured, pack both sides.

Splint for 2 weeks.

Zygomatic Fracture (Tripod Fracture)

The zygomatic arch often will be fractured in three places: at the arch itself, at the zygomatic suture line, and at the posterior half of the infraorbital rim (Figure 20-1). This injury is caused by a blunt force to the front and side of the face.

■ **SIGNS AND SYMPTOMS**

Palpable infraorbital rim fracture (step defect)

Facial edema

Change in consensual gaze

Trismus

Infraorbital hyperesthesia

Diplopia—use mnemonic "TIDES"

Epistaxis

Absence of symmetry

Possible CSF rhinorrhea

Periorbital edema and ecchymosis

Subconjunctival hemorrhage

■ **DIAGNOSIS**

Palpable infraorbital rim fracture

Clinical observation

X-ray (Water's, Caldwell, and submental vertex views)

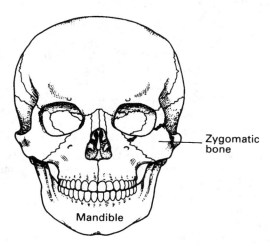

FIGURE 20-1. Zygomatic (tripod) fracture.

■ **THERAPEUTIC INTERVENTIONS**
Airway management
Cervical spine precautions
Cold pack
Surgery for fixation (usually delayed 3 to 4 days, until edema is reduced)
Ophthalmic consult

Orbital Blow-out Fractures

A fracture of the orbital floor occurs when the globe of the eye is struck by a blunt force, forcing the globe inward and causing a fracture of the very thin orbital floor bone. There is *not* usually a concurrent fracture of the orbital rim.

■ **SIGNS AND SYMPTOMS**
Diplopia
Enophthalmos
Epistaxis
Infraorbital paresthesia
Periorbital ecchymosis
Subconjunctival hemorrhage

■ **DIAGNOSIS**
Good history of mechanism of injury
Clinical observation
X-ray (Water's view)
CT scan

■ **THERAPEUTIC INTERVENTIONS**
Ophthalmologic consultation
Surgery for reduction

Maxillary Mid-Face Fracture

French pathologist René LeFort identified in 1901 that facial bones often fracture in specific patterns when blunt trauma occurs. The most common cause is severe blunt trauma to the face, with the most common etiology being motor vehicle accidents involving unrestrained occupants.

These fractures are categorized into three levels, LeFort I, LeFort II, and LeFort III, depending on the pattern of fracture. Patients may also have combinations of these fractures.

LeFort I fracture

A LeFort I fracture (Figure 20-2) is a fracture of the transverse alveolar process at the nasal floor. It extends from the upper teeth into the nose.

■ **SIGNS AND SYMPTOMS**
Malocclusion of teeth, anterior open bite
Moveable maxilla
Epistaxis

■ **DIAGNOSIS**
History of mechanism of injury

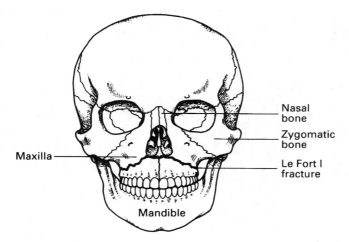

FIGURE 20-2. LeFort I facial fracture.

Clinical observation
X-ray
■ **THERAPEUTIC INTERVENTIONS**
Airway management
Cold pack
Surgery for fixation
Check for other associated injuries

LeFort II fracture

A LeFort II fracture (Figure 20-3) is a pyramidal fracture that extends through the central part of the maxilla up through the superior nasal area. It also usually involves the orbits.
■ **SIGNS AND SYMPTOMS**
Nose and dental arch move together when manipulated
Epistaxis
Periorbital edema and ecchymosis
Subconjunctival hemorrhage
Infraorbital paresthesia
■ **DIAGNOSIS**
History of mechanism of injury
Nose and dental arch move together when manipulated
Clinical observation
Extraocular muscle entrapment
X-ray (Water's view)
■ **THERAPEUTIC INTERVENTIONS**
Airway management; consider endotracheal intubation
Cold pack

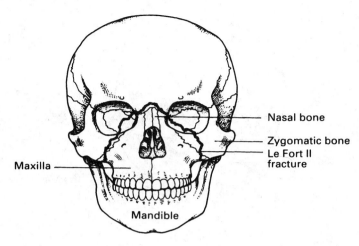

FIGURE 20-3. LeFort II facial fracture.

Surgery for open reduction and internal fixation
IV antibiotics
Check for other associated injuries

LeFort III fracture

A LeFort III fracture (Figure 20-4, *A, B*) is a major fracture that is usually caused by a major blunt trauma to the face. When fracture occurs, a total craniofacial separation results. It usually involves the maxilla, zygoma, nasal bones, ethmoids, vomer, and all lesser bones of the base of the cranium.

■ **SIGNS AND SYMPTOMS**
Massive bleeding
Loss of consciousness (usually)
Facial bones move without frontal bone movement when manipulated
CSF rhinorrhea
Epistaxis
Periorbital edema and ecchymosis
Subconjunctival hemorrhage
Infraorbital paresthesia

■ **DIAGNOSIS**
History of mechanism of injury
Facial bones move without frontal bone movement when manipulated
Extraocular muscle entrapment
Clinical observation
X-ray (Water's view)
CT scan

■ **THERAPEUTIC INTERVENTIONS**
Airway management; consider endotracheal intubation
Cervical spine protection

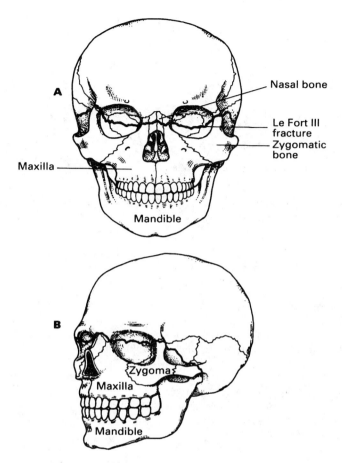

FIGURE 20-4. LeFort III facial fracture. **A,** Frontal view. **B,** Lateral view.

Cold pack
Surgery for open reduction and fixation
IV antibiotics
Check for other associated injuries

Mandibular fracture

The most common causes of mandible fractures (Figure 20-5) are domestic violence altercations and contact sports. Because the mandible is arch-shaped, in most cases, when it is fractured, it will fracture in two places. Often these are open fractures as evidenced by obvious intraoral bony fragments or simply bleeding around the teeth.

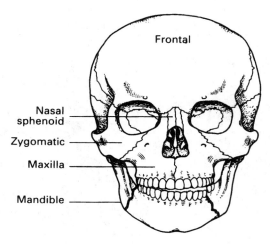

FIGURE 20-5. Mandibular fracture.

■ **SIGNS AND SYMPTOMS**
Palpation of the fracture(s)
Clinical observation of malocclusion of the teeth
Complaint of facial pain, especially in mandible area
Trismus
■ **DIAGNOSIS**
Palpation of the fracture(s)
Clinical observation of malocclusion of the teeth
X-ray (also observe condyles, because they are often fractured as well)
■ **THERAPEUTIC INTERVENTIONS**
Airway management
Cold pack
Immobilize jaw (use a Barton dressing—a large bulky kerlex dressing that surrounds the head)
Surgery for open reduction and internal fixation

Facial trauma is frequently associated with complications that may prove life threatening. Airway occlusion, respiratory distress, as well as associated C-spine injuries can prove devastating. Astute, systematic, thorough patient assessment and rapid, effective intervention are critical to positive patient outcome.

SUGGESTED READINGS

Dolin J et al: The management of GSW to the face, *J Trauma* 33(4):508, 1992.
Guyette RF: Facial injuries in basketball players, *Clin Sports Med* 12(2):247, 1993.
Huelke DF, Moore JL, Ostrom M: Airbag injuries and occupant protection, *Trauma* 33(6):894, 1992.

McDermott FT, Lance JC et al: The effectiveness of bicyclist helmets: a study of 1710 casualties, *J Trauma* 34(6):834, 1993.

McGregor RS et al: Rooster attacks in childhood, *Pediatr Emerg Care* 8(4):216, 1992.

Ochs MW, Tucker MR: Current concepts in management of facial trauma, *J Oral Maxillofac Surg* 51:42, 1993.

Sheehy SB: *Emergency nursing principles and practice,* ed 3. St Louis, 1992, Mosby.

Steinman R: A 40-year old woman with an airbag-mediated injury, *JEN* 18(4):308, 1992.

Steuer K: Facial fractures: diagnosis to discharge, *AORN* 54(4):774, 1991.

Tanz RR, Christoffel KK: Tykes on bikes: injuries associated with bicycle mounted child-seats, *Pediatr Emerg Care* 7(5):297, 1991.

CHAPTER | 21

Eye, Ear, Nose, Throat, and Dental Emergencies

Eye Emergencies

There are many occasions when rapid, careful assessment and intervention can prevent permanent or temporary loss of vision.

BASIC ANATOMY AND PHYSIOLOGY OF THE EYE (Figure 21-1)

body rim The bony process that protects the eyeball.

eyelid The covering that closes to protect the eyeball, distribute tears, and regulates light.

eyelashes Hairs that minimize the number of dirt particles that enter the eye area.

sclera The tough protective coating of the eyeball.

cornea The cornex, transparent anterior portion of the eye.

retina The inner lining of the posterior eyeball that collects and focuses light rays.

choroid The middle layer of the eyeball that supplies the retina with blood, oxygen, and other nutrients.

macula The area of the retina most sensitive to light and color.

lens The normally transparent disc through which light is refracted. Light passes through the cornea, the anterior chamber, the lens, and the vitreous humor to the retina.

iris Colored diaphragm that controls the amount of light entering the posterior chamber by means of expanding and contracting its opening (the pupil).

oculomotor muscles The six muscles that control eyeball movement.

lacrimal glands Glands that secrete fluid (tears) to soothe the eyeball and reduce friction.

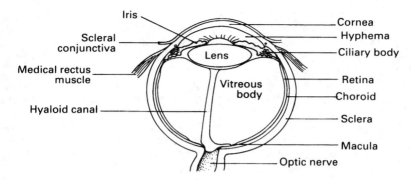

FIGURE 21-1. Horizontal section of left eye seen from above.

tears   Fluid that coats the eyeball; tears are distributed by blinking of the eyelids. Tears are secreted by the lacrimal glands and through the lacrimal puncta into the lacrimal and nasolacrimal ducts

meibomian glands   Glands that secrete the oil that lines the eyelid margins and prevents tears from running out of the conjunctival sac.

visual acuity   Central vision; stimuli on macula; a measure of the resolving power of the eye.

peripheral vision   Vision in which stimuli are on an area of the retina other than the macula.

There are certain conditions that should be given priority treatment in the emergency department. They are the following:
- Loss of vision without pain (may be caused by central artery occlusion or central vein occlusion, intraocular hemorrhage, or retinal detachment)
- Chemical burns
- Foreign bodies
- Painful eyes (may be caused by conjunctivitis, iritis, or keratitis)
- Laceration of the globe
- Hyphema

EXAMINATION OF THE EYE

Make sure that lighting is good.

If there is much pain, a topical anesthetic agent, such as proparacaine (Ophthaine) or tetracaine, may assist in examination of the eye.

Be gentle and explain the procedure to the patient.

VISUAL ACUITY EXAMINATION

Whenever possible, perform a visual acuity examination before examination of the eye, since manipulation may increase blurring and decrease acuity.

If the patient wears glasses, test vision first with glasses, then without.

If the patient's glasses are not available, have him or her read the chart through a pinhole poked in a piece of cardboard.

Check each eye separately, then both eyes together.

Follow specific instructions on how to conduct the examination according to the chart to be used:

The Snellen chart is read at 20 feet.

The Rosenbaum Pocket Vision Screener is read 14 inches from the tip of the nose.

If a Snellen or other vision chart is not available, have the patient read newsprint, and record the distance from the eye the paper must be held for the patient to read it.

If the patient cannot see newsprint, hold up a specific number of fingers and record the distance at which the patient can see the fingers (and be able to tell how many are being held up).

If the patient cannot see fingers, record the distance at which he can perceive hand motion.

If the patient cannot see hand motion, record the distance at which he or she can perceive light.

If the patient cannot perceive light, record this on the chart.

Examples of Visual Acuity Examination Scores

20/20   When standing 20 feet from the Snellen chart, the patient can read what the normal eye can read at 20 feet.

20/40−2   When standing 20 feet from the Snellen chart, the patient can read what the normal eye can read at 40 feet (and, in this example, has also missed two letters).

20/200   When standing 20 feet from the Snellen chart, the patient can read what the normal eye can read at 200 feet.

10/200   If the patient cannot read any of the letters on the Snellen chart, have him stand half the distance (10 feet) and read what he can; record this as the distance he actually is standing from the chart over the smallest line he can read.

CF/3 feet   The patient can count fingers at a maximum distance of 3 feet.

HM/4 feet   The patient can see hand motion at a maximum distance of 4 feet.

LP/position   The patient can perceive light and determine from which direction it came.

LP/no position   The patient can perceive light, but cannot determine from which direction it came.

NLP   The patient cannot perceive light.

When recording information about the eyes, use the following abbreviations:

ABBREVIATION	LATIN WORD	ENGLISH TRANSLATION
OD	oculus dexter	right eye
OS	oculus sinister	left eye
OU	oculus uterque	each eyes
gt	guttae	drops

Otherwise simply write ® or Ⓛ or both eyes.

EYE TRAUMA

In addition to obvious eye trauma, search for associated eye trauma when there is head or facial trauma. If there is great pain, sometimes it will help to patch both eyes. This minimizes movement and may decrease pain.

If the patient is unconscious, be sure to check for contact lenses and be sure to protect the cornea from drying by instilling an ophthalmic ointment and taping the eyelids shut or frequently instilling artificial tears.

When dealing with a patient with eye trauma, it is important to obtain a good history:

- What happened?
- How did it happen?
- Is there something in the eye? What?
- Were chemicals involved? What chemicals?
- Where did it happen?
- Did anyone see it happen? Who?
- Was care given at the scene? By whom?
- Was patient wearing safety glasses?
- Is patient on any medication (hormones, in particular)?
- Does the patient wear corrective lenses?
- Was the patient wearing contact lenses at the time of the injury? Are they in now?
- Does the patient have a history of glaucoma, diabetes, hypertension, or previous eye problems?

Lacerated Eyelid

The care provider will be able to diagnose a lacerated eyelid simply by observing it.

■ **THERAPEUTIC INTERVENTIONS**

Irrigation

Wound approximation and suturing

If a section of tissue is missing, consulting a plastic surgeon to reconstruct the section so the cornea will be protected

Checking for laceration of the lacrimal duct

Orbital Rim Trauma

This type of injury may occur as a result of blunt or penetrating injury to the face. The main sign of orbital rim trauma is periorbital ecchymosis.

■ **THERAPEUTIC INTERVENTIONS**

Ice pack

Examination for fracture and eyeball trauma

Visual acuity examination

If there is a fracture of the prominent supraorbital rim and frontal sinus, checking for cerebrospinal fluid leak in the form of CSF rhinorrhea.

If there is a visual disturbance, checking for a fracture of the orbital roof resulting in entrapment of the optic nerve

Hyphema

Blunt trauma to the eye may cause aqueous humor to depress the diaphragm of the iris or the ciliary bodies, causing a tear in the iris vasculature. When this occurs, hyphema results (a hemorrhage into the anterior chamber of the eye). This condition requires immediate ophthalmologic consultation.

■ **SIGNS AND SYMPTOMS**
Visible blood in the anterior chamber
Decrease in vision
Pain

■ **THERAPEUTIC INTERVENTIONS**
Strict bed rest: head of bed up at least 60 degrees
Heavy sedation
Diuretic to reduce ocular pressure
Acetazolamide or other carbonic anhydrate inhibitor if increased intraocular pressure

Massive hemorrhage can occur at any time up to 2 weeks after blunt trauma. It can cause corneal blood staining, secondary glaucoma, loss of vision, and maybe even loss of the eye.

An 8-ball hemorrhage is a condition in which old, clotted blood is found in the anterior chamber. Therapeutic intervention for this condition is to remove the clot surgically. Retrobulbar hemorrhage may occur as a result of ruptured intraorbital vessels. It can be diagnosed by the presence of a protruding eyeball (exophthalmos) and diplopia (double vision).

Subconjunctival Hemorrhage

A subconjunctival hemorrhage is common after trauma to the eye. It is usually left untreated and will resolve in about 2 weeks.

Blow-out Fracture

Blow-out fracture results from direct blunt trauma to the eyeball, which causes an increased intraocular pressure that fractures the orbit floor.

■ **SIGNS AND SYMPTOMS**
Periorbital hematoma
Subconjunctival hemorrhage
Periorbital edema
Enophthalmos/exophthalmos
Upward gaze
Diplopia
Anesthesia of infraorbital nerve

Crepitus (from orbital and lid subcutaneous emphysema
Possible epistaxis
■ **THERAPEUTIC INTERVENTIONS**
Ice packs
Reduction of fracture (if there is bony displacement)
Packing of maxillary sinus
Possible surgery
Analgesia
Antibiotic ointment
Patch

Foreign Bodies

Foreign bodies in the conjunctiva

The foreign body most commonly found in the conjunctiva is an eyelash.
■ **THERAPEUTIC INTERVENTIONS**
Give topical anesthesia, visual acuity examination.
Evert the eyelid (Figure 21-2, *A,B,C,D*).
Irrigate with normal saline.
Gently remove the foreign body with a moist cotton swab.
Administer local antibiotics 4 times a day for 5 days.
An eye patch may be applied, depending on the nature of the injury and the
    amount of damage.
The patient should return for follow-up care in 1 day if no improvement.

Foreign bodies in the cornea

The presence of a foreign body in the cornea is very painful. As the eyelid
moves up and down over the foreign body, pain increases.
■ **THERAPEUTIC INTERVENTIONS**
Topical anesthesia, visual acuity exam
Irrigation of eye with normal saline
Removal of foreign body with moistened swab
Checking for more than one foreign body
Slit lamp examination to look for corneal abrasion
If the foreign body is metal, it will form a rust ring that must be removed, usu-
    ally by an ophthalmologist.

Intraocular foreign bodies

Intraocular foreign bodies are usually caused by a small object moving at a high
speed that penetrates the eyeball and comes to rest somewhere within the posterior chamber. Pain may be minimal. The entrance wound may be very small and
difficult to locate. Finding the wound requires a high index of suspicion. This
condition constitutes an extreme emergency.
■ **THERAPEUTIC INTERVENTIONS**
Surgical intervention to prevent further injury.
All foreign bodies should be considered contaminated, and antibiotics should be
    considered.

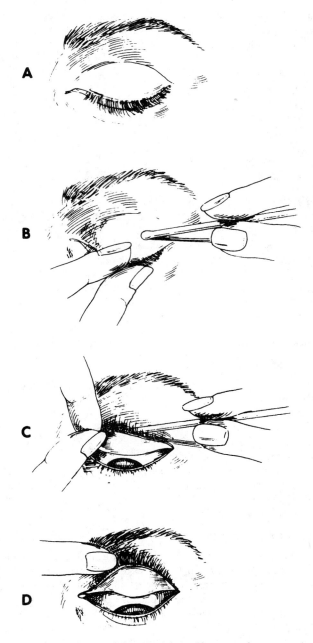

FIGURE 21-2. Steps in everting eyelid. **A**, Eyelid. **B**, Placement of cotton swab, pulling eyelashes down and over swab. **C**, Eyelid everted over swab. **D**, Examination of inside of eyelid and eye.

Ensure current tetanus immunization status.
Obtain x-ray film of the eye to inspect for the foreign body.
Cover both eyes to decrease movement.

Perforating and Penetrating Injuries to the Eyeball

Therapeutic intervention is essential in the early stages of the injury, and will decrease the likelihood of further injury. This condition constitutes an ophthalmologic emergency.

■ **THERAPEUTIC INTERVENTIONS**
Consider parenteral analgesia.
Secure the impaling object.
Cover both eyes to decrease eye movement.
Reserve detailed examination for an ophthalmologist.
Usually requires surgical intervention.
Start antibiotics—parenterally (do not manipulate eye to put in medications).
Start tetanus prophylaxis.

Corneal Lacerations

If a corneal laceration is small, it is usually not sutured. Therapeutic intervention for small corneal lacerations is antibiotic ointment and eye patch. If the laceration is large, it is usually sutured by an ophthalmologist with 8-0 silk or 7-0 chromic suture on a very fine needle prior to a dressing application.

Corneal Abrasions

Corneal abrasion occurs when the epithelium is denuded by a foreign object, such as a contact lens. It is important to obtain a history from the patient as to what caused the injury.

■ **SIGNS AND SYMPTOMS**
Tearing
Eyelid spasm
Pain on the surface of the eye (sensation of a foreign body)
Photophobia
Corneal abrasions can be diagnosed by staining the surface of the eye with fluorescein dye and observing the cornea with a cobalt lamp and magnification.

How to use fluorescein strips to stain the cornea (Figure 21-3)
1. Explain the procedure to the patient.
2. Use local anesthesia before exam.
3. Use individually wrapped sterile fluorescein strips (fluorescein is easily contaminated by *Pseudomonas*).
4. Moisten the end of the sterile strip with normal saline.
5. Pull down on the lower eyelid.
6. Touch the strip to the inner edge of the lower eyelid.
7. Ask the patient to blink to distribute the dye.

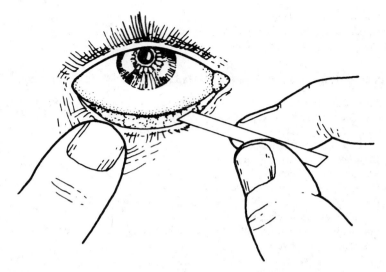

FIGURE 21-3. Placement of fluorescein strip to stain cornea.

    8. Examine the cornea using a cobalt lamp (an abrasion will be highlighted by the fluorescein).

■ **THERAPEUTIC INTERVENTIONS**

Local anesthesia during examination
Visual acuity examination
Local antibiotics
Patching of injured eye(s) for 24 hours
Follow-up visit in 1 day if no improvement
Instructing the patient not to use local anesthetic agents at home because they will delay healing

Conjunctival Lacerations

The main symptom of conjunctival laceration is swelling and bleeding from the conjunctiva.

■ **THERAPEUTIC INTERVENTIONS**

Local antibiotics
Application of an eye patch
Close observation
If the laceration is longer than 5 cm, an ophthalmologic consultation is needed for suturing.

Corneal Ulcer

Corneal ulcer is commonly found in the unconscious patient or the patient who has left contact lenses in place for an inordinately long period.

■ **SIGNS AND SYMPTOMS**
Whitish spot on the cornea
Pain
Photophobia
Profuse tearing
Vascular congestion
Blue-green cast on fluorescein staining
NOTE: If *Pseudomonas* is present, the patient may lose the eye within 48 hours.
■ **THERAPEUTIC INTERVENTIONS**
Antibiotics
Warm compresses
Eye patch

Optic Nerve Avulsion

Optic nerve avulsion usually results from severe trauma to the eye. The nerve avulses at the level where the optic nerve enters the eyeball. A partial tear will result in partial blindness; a total tear will result in total blindness. An immediate ophthalmologic consultation is indicated.

Iris Injury

Traumatic iridocyclitis is an inflammation of the iris and ciliary body following contusion of the eye. The main sign is the presence of uveal pigment and lens tissue in the anterior chamber.
■ **THERAPEUTIC INTERVENTIONS**
Treatment with topical cycloplegics
Topical systemic steroids
Ophthalmology consultation

Lens Injury

Injuries that can occur to the lens include partial dislocations (subluxations), total dislocations (luxations), and opacifications (cataracts). Surgical intervention is indicated for all of these conditions.

Retina and Choroid Injury

Trauma to the retina and choroid may produce a white ellipse where the sclera is visible through the rupture. If the macula is injured, a decrease in visual acuity will result. Surgical intervention is indicated for these injuries.

Problems with Contact Lenses

The most common problem experienced by the wearer of contact lenses is the presence of dirt particles or chemical irritants under the lenses, causing irritation of the cornea. The second most common problem results when the lenses are

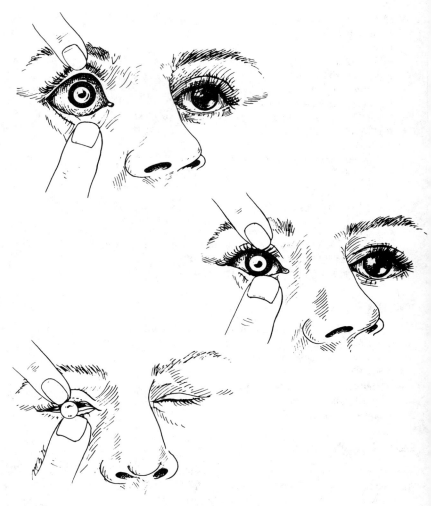

FIGURE 21-4. Techniques for removing hard corneal contact lenses from an individual's eye.

worn too long. This causes redness, swelling, pain, and corneal abrasions (Figure 21-4). Therapeutic intervention is removal of the lens and cleansing of lens and the eye.

■ **THERAPEUTIC INTERVENTION FOR PROLONGED CONTACT LENS USE**
Instruct the patient to refrain from wearing the lenses for 24 to 48 hours. Check for and treat corneal abrasions.

If a contact lens is lost in the eye, it is usually in the cul-de-sac of the upper
eyelid. Evert the eyelid, and remove the lens.

Look at the eye tangentially with a flashlight.

Check for a Medic-Alert bracelet.

Check for an identification card.

To remove a contact lens

Corneal hard lens. Use removal technique as demonstrated in Figure 21-4
or use a suction tip designed especially for removing contact lenses.

Soft lens. Locate the lens, slide the lens laterally onto the sclera, grasp it
between the thumb and forefinger, and lift it off the cornea. If the lens does not
remove easily, place a few drops of irrigating solution onto the eye to moisten
it. Place soft lenses in an isotonic solution without preservatives.

Burns of the Eye
Chemical burns
■ **THERAPEUTIC INTERVENTIONS**
Immediate therapeutic intervention for any type of chemical burn to the eye is
irrigation with copious amounts of saline solution or water, followed by careful
examination.

Acid burns
Tissue denatures from acid and denatured tissue neutralizes acid.
■ **THERAPEUTIC INTERVENTIONS**
Topical anesthetic
Irrigation with copious amounts of normal saline solution or water
Topical antibiotics and cycloplegics
Analgesics may be indicated

Alkali burns
An alkali burn is a **serious emergency** situation, because alkalis cause great tis-
sue destruction. Initially the burn may appear as white spots in the eye, and
severe damage may not be evident until 3 to 4 days after the initial injury.
■ **THERAPEUTIC INTERVENTIONS**
Irrigate with copious amounts of normal saline solution or water for 30 minutes,
then check pH; continue irrigation until pH is 7.0.
Antibiotics
Cycloplegics
Analgesics may be indicated
Ophthalmology consultation
■ **COMPLICATIONS OF ACID AND ALKALI BURNS**
Adhesion of globe to eyelid
Corneal ulceration
Entropion (eyelashes that turn in toward the eyeball)
Iridocyclitis
Glaucoma

Thermal burns

When facial burns are present, it is rather common to find associated burns of the eyelids. It is not common, however, to see burns of the eyeballs unless the burning agent was steam, metal, or gasoline.

■ **THERAPEUTIC INTERVENTIONS**

Topical anesthetic before exam
Analgesia
Sedation
Eye irrigation
Antibiotics
Cycloplegics
Bilateral eye patches
Ophthalmology consultation

Radiation burns

There are two types of radiation burns—ultraviolet and infrared.

Ultraviolet burn

Ultraviolet burns are seen with welder's flash and in snow skiers, ice climbers, people who read on the beach, and people who use sunlamps. The burn is caused when ultraviolet radiation is absorbed by the cornea. Keratitis or conjunctivitis or both result. Symptoms develop 3 to 6 hours after exposure.

■ **SIGNS AND SYMPTOMS**

Feeling of a foreign body
Tearing
Excessive blinking
Possible associated facial and eyelid burns

■ **THERAPEUTIC INTERVENTIONS**

Topical antibiotics
Analgesics
Cycloplegics
Bilateral eye patches
Signs and symptoms should be relieved within 24 hours after these measures are taken.

Infrared burn

An infrared burn is a severe type of burn. It may cause permanent loss of vision, because infrared rays are absorbed by the iris. This results in an increase of the temperature of the lens, which produces cataracts. When the lens is damaged, the repair process is very slow, and the lens remains much more vulnerable to injury during the healing process.

Common types of infrared burns

Glassblower's cataracts. Result from prolonged exposure to intense heat.

Focal retinitis. Caused by eclipse blindness or exposure to nuclear energy; the lens condenses heat, causing retinal scarring and blindness.

X-ray burns. Proportional to the amount of exposure and penetration of the x-rays; grenz rays are soft rays that produce superficial keratoconjunctivitis and dermatitis; gamma rays are hard rays that produce retinal damage and cataracts.

Irrigating the Eye

Instill topical anesthetic.

Cleanse the external area around the eye and eyelid.

Have the patient lie down or adjust the treatment chair so that the patient is in a supine position.

Have the patient turn his head with the affected side down.

Pull down on the lower eyelid of the affected side.

Run irrigation fluid directly over the globe of the eye and into the cul-de-sac of the lower eyelid from the inner to the outer canthus.

Have the patient blink occasionally to distribute the irrigation solution over the globe.

Irrigate for about 30 minutes (more if pH indicates).

Irrigation Using the Morgan Therapeutic Lens

The Morgan Therapeutic Lens (Figure 21-5, *A, B*) is a specially designed lens that is placed on the eye and is used to provide continuous ocular lavage or medication. It is a scleral lens made of hard plastic (polymethyl methacrylate). The tubing is made of soft silicone plastic and has a female adapter at the distal end.

1. Explain the procedure to the patient.
2. Instill anesthetic ocular medication.
3. Ask the patient to look down.

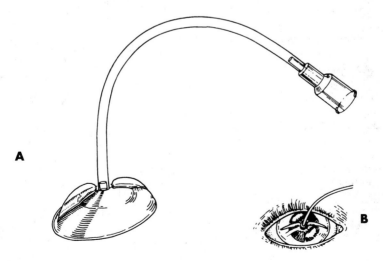

A

B

FIGURE 21-5. **A**, Morgan therapeutic lens. **B**, Lens in place for continuous irrigation.

4. Retract the upper eyelid.
5. Grasp the lens by the tubing and the small finlike projections.
6. Slip the superior border of the lens up under the upper eyelid.
7. Have the patient look up.
8. Retract the lower eyelid and place the lower border of the lens beneath it.
9. Have the patient turn the head toward the affected side, and place a folded towel under the head to collect irrigation solution.
10. Attach the female adapter at the end of the lens tubing to:
    a. A syringe filled with the solution of choice, and instill the solution at the desired rate, or
    b. Intravenous tubing that is connected to the solution of choice in an IV bottle or bag instilled at the selected drip rate.
11. To remove the lens, follow steps 3 through 8 in reverse order.
12. Dry the patient's face and eye area with a dry towel.
13. Dispose of the lens.

NOTE: The Morgan lens should be used for chemical burns of the eye. It should not be used for foreign bodies since the foreign body may become entrapped under the Morgan lens.

MEDICAL PROBLEMS INVOLVING THE EYE

Blepharitis

Blepharitis is an inflammation of the lid margin, usually caused by *Staphylococcus aureus*.

■ **THERAPEUTIC INTERVENTIONS**
Cool, moist compresses
Antibiotic ophthalmic ointment

Hordeolum

A hordeolum or "sty" is an infection of the upper or lower eyelid at the accessory gland. It is caused by *Staphylococcus aureus*.

■ **SIGNS AND SYMPTOMS**
Small external abscess
Pain
Redness
Swelling

■ **THERAPEUTIC INTERVENTIONS**
Warm compresses four times a day until the abscess points
Antibiotic ophthalmic ointment
Abscess may be incised by a physician when it points

Chalazion

A chalazion is a cyst that forms on the inside surface of the eyelid. It results from congestion of the meibomian gland.

■ **SIGNS AND SYMPTOMS**

Small mass beneath the conjunctiva of the lid

Redness

Swelling

Extreme pain

■ **THERAPEUTIC INTERVENTIONS**

Antibiotic ophthalmic ointment

Incision and drainage by a physician

Keratitis

Keratitis is an inflammation of the cornea.

■ **SIGNS AND SYMPTOMS**

Light sensitivity

Redness of the cornea

Pain

Profuse tearing

■ **THERAPEUTIC INTERVENTIONS**

Culture and sensitivity

Warm compresses

Antibiotic ophthalmic ointment

Uveitis

Uveitis is a uveal tract inflammation that usually includes the iris, ciliary body, and choroid.

■ **SIGNS AND SYMPTOMS**

Signs and symptoms of uveitis appear unilaterally.

Photophobia

Tearing

Pain

Blurred vision

Headache

■ **THERAPEUTIC INTERVENTIONS**

Warm compresses

Systemic analgesics

Antibiotic ophthalmic ointment

Topical steroids

Mydriatics to dilate the pupil

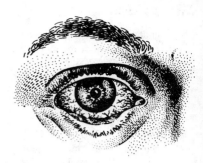

FIGURE 21-6. Conjunctivitis.

Acute Conjunctivitis (Pinkeye)

Acute conjunctivitis (Figure 21-6) is most commonly a bacterial infection of the conjunctiva. It may be caused by *Staphylococcus, Gonococcus, Pneumococcus, Haemophilus,* or *Pseudomonas.* Other causes may include: chlamydia, urreal chemical irritation, allergies, and systemic disease (Kawasaki disease, Stevens-Johnson syndrome).

■ **SIGNS AND SYMPTOMS**

Eyelids ''stick together'' on waking

Scratchy sensation, purulent discharge, infected conjunctiva

■ **THERAPEUTIC INTERVENTIONS**

Application of antibiotic ophthalmic ointment after a culture is obtained.

If chlamydia is suspected, tetracycline or erythromycin should be given topically and systemically.

Acute conjunctivitis is a *contagious* condition. Careful aftercare instructions should be given to the patient about how to avoid spreading the infection.

Acute Iritis

Acute iritis is an inflammatory condition of the iris. It is not an infectious process.

■ **SIGNS AND SYMPTOMS**

Acute pain

Constricted pupil

Photophobia

Tenderness of the globe

■ **THERAPEUTIC INTERVENTIONS**

Cold compresses

Mydriatics, cycloplegics

Analgesics

Dark glasses

Central Retinal Artery Occlusion

Central retinal artery occlusion produces painless sudden blindness. It is usually

embolic in origin. Prognosis for regaining sight is very poor
lasted longer than 1 hour.

■ **THERAPEUTIC INTERVENTIONS**
Anticoagulants may be indicated.
tPA may be given IV within 60 minutes of onset.
Gentle ocular massage.
Rebreathing CO_2 from a paper bag may decrease the blood pH and dilate the
artery.
Surgical intervention by ophthalmologist.

Cavernous Sinus Thrombosis (Orbital Cellulitis)

Cavernous sinus thrombosis is a pneumococcal, staphylococcal, or streptococcal
infection that spreads from an infected sinus or throat to the orbital area. It usually begins unilaterally and can spread to the other cavernous sinus.

■ **SIGNS AND SYMPTOMS**
Facial and globe edema
Vascular congestion in eyelids
Aching pain
Pain in globe
Exophthalmos
Conjunctival chemosis
Fever
Decreased visual acuity
Decreased pupil reflexes
Papilledema
Paralysis of extraocular muscles

■ **THERAPEUTIC INTERVENTIONS**
Antibiotic ophthalmic ointment
Parenteral antibiotics
Bed rest, hospitalization
Warm compresses
Ophthalmology consultation

Retinal Detachment

When the retina is torn, vitreous humor seeps between it and the choroid, resulting in the separation of the retina from the choroid, which decreases blood and
oxygen supply to the retina. This decreased blood and oxygen supply renders
the retina unable to perceive light.

■ **SIGNS AND SYMPTOMS**
Flashes of light
A "veil" or "curtain" effect in the visual field
A dark spot or particles in the visual field

■ **THERAPEUTIC INTERVENTIONS**
Strict bed rest
Bilateral eye patches

Tranquilizers
Possible surgical intervention

Glaucoma (Figure 21-7 A, B)

Glaucoma occurs when aqueous humor cannot escape from the anterior chamber, causing a rise in anterior chamber pressure. This increase in pressure causes a decrease in circulation to the retina and an increase in pressure on the optic nerve. Blindness may eventually result.

Acute glaucoma

Acute (closed-angle) glaucoma results when there is blockage in the anterior chamber angle near the root of the iris. ACUTE GLAUCOMA IS AN EMERGENCY SITUATION! It may cause blindness in just a few hours.

■ **SIGNS AND SYMPTOMS**
Acute eye pain

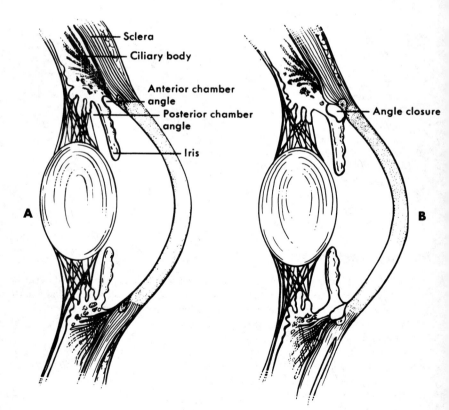

FIGURE 21-7. **A,** Normal eye. **B,** Closed-angle glaucoma.

Fixed and slightly dilated pupil
Hard globe
Foggy-appearing cornea
Severe headache
Halos around lights
Decreased peripheral vision
Nausea and vomiting

■ **THERAPEUTIC INTERVENTIONS**

Therapeutic intervention for acute glaucoma is aimed at decreasing pupil size to allow for aqueous humor drainage.

Frequent (every 15 minutes) instillation of miotic eyedrops (usually 1% or 4% pilocarpine)—the strength of the solution is not as important as frequent instillation
Systemic analgesia (usually morphine sulfate)
Sedation
Drugs such as acetazolamide (Diamox, mannitol, or glycerin) in an attempt to decrease intraocular pressure
Possible surgery

Chronic glaucoma

Chronic (open-angle or wide-angle) glaucoma occurs gradually and is caused by an obstruction of Schlemm's canal. Because it comes on very slowly, the patient may be unaware of its development.

■ **THERAPEUTIC INTERVENTIONS**

Instillation of miotic eyedrops
Possible surgery

Secondary glaucoma

Secondary glaucoma is an increase in intraocular pressure resulting from surgery, trauma, hemorrhage, inflammation, tumor, or various other conditions that may interfere with aqueous humor drainage. Therapeutic intervention will vary with the cause.

■ **HOW TO MEASURE INTRAOCULAR PRESSURE WITH A TONOMETER**

Tonometric examination is used to measure intraocular pressure. The Schiotz tonometer is the most commonly used type in the emergency department. It has a plunger that, when placed on the eye, measures the amount of indentation pressure on the cornea.

To properly use the tonometer, anesthetize the globe with an ophthalmic anesthetic agent.
Explain the procedure to the patient.
Have the patient lie down.
Have the patient stare upward at a spot on the ceiling.
Place a sterile (previously calibrated) tonometer on the globe.
Measure intraocular pressure.

How to read a Schiotz indentation tonometer

If intraocular pressure is high, tonometer scale will read low because the plunger cannot indent the globe very much.

If intraocular pressure is low, tonometer scale will read high because the plunger will indent the globe more than normal.

A normal indentation tonometer reading is 11 to 22 mm Hg. A lower reading indicates increased intraocular pressure and a higher reading indicates decreased intraocular pressure.

Eyedrops and Ophthalmic Ointments

Eyedrops are used to decrease pain, provide antibiotic therapy, increase or decrease the size of the pupil, decrease allergic reactions of the eye, or cleanse the eye.

Procedure for instilling eyedrops

1. Explain the procedure to the patient.
2. Pull the lower eyelid downward.
3. Have patient look upward.
4. Instill one or two drops of solution into the cul-de-sac (the center of the lower lid).
5. Have the patient blink to distribute the solution.
6. Instruct the patient not to squeeze his eyelids shut tightly, because this will cause the solution to leak out.

Procedure for instilling ophthalmic ointment

1. Explain the procedure to the patient.
2. Pull the lower eyelid downward.
3. Have the patient look upward.
4. Apply ointment in a thin line into the inner aspect of the lid from the inner to the outer canthus.
5. Have the patient blink to distribute the ointment.
6. Instruct the patient not to squeeze his eyelids shut tightly, as this will expel the ointment.

Ear Emergencies

There are three requirements for proper ear care:
- Good illumination
- Magnification
- Adequate physical control of the patient, including proper positioning and sedation, if necessary

Simple Lacerations

Simple lacerations of the outer ear are commonly seen in the emergency department.

■ **THERAPEUTIC INTERVENTIONS**
Cleanse the wound (scrub and irrigate).

Debride the wound.
Rejoin cartilage edges.
Cover the cartilage with skin.

Auriculectomy

An auriculectomy (Figure 21-8) is an amputation of the outer structures of the ear. Good results can be obtained if strict attention is paid to detail when reanastomosing the ear.

■ **THERAPEUTIC INTERVENTIONS (USUALLY PERFORMED BY A PLASTIC SURGEON)**
Reanastomose cartilage and skin.
Give IV antibiotics.

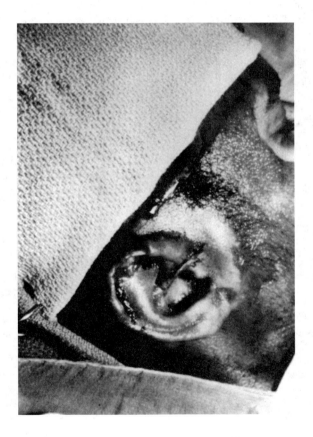

FIGURE 21-8. Repair of partial traumatic amputation of the pinna.
(Courtesy Dr. Daniel Cheney.)

Hematoma of Pinna

Hematoma of the pinna usually results from blunt trauma.

■ **THERAPEUTIC INTERVENTIONS**

Anesthetize the area.

Aspirate the hematoma with an 18-gauge or larger needle.

Place a drain if necessary.

Apply a pressure dressing (cotton soaked in mineral oil or petrolatum gauze).

Bleeding from External Ear

Bleeding from the external ear is usually a result of a ruptured eardrum, a foreign body, or a canal laceration. Other sources of bleeding are basilar skull fracture or temporal bone fracture. Canal lacerations result from the ear being probed by sharp items. If the temporal bone is fractured, there may be cerebrospinal fluid otorrhea, a ruptured tympanic membrane, or a lacerated facial nerve.

■ **THERAPEUTIC INTERVENTIONS (FOR LACERATIONS ONLY)**

Cleanse the wound.

Apply antibiotic ointment.

Otolaryngologic consultation may be indicated.

If there is any question of CSF leakage, a neurosurgeon should be consulted and nothing should be placed in or over the ear.

Ruptured Tympanic Membrane

Ruptured tympanic membrane (eardrum) occurs as a result of positive pressure over the tympanic membrane or a penetrating foreign body. It may be caused by a slap over the ears (pressure from the outside), a diving injury (vacuum from the inside), or an aircraft or altitude injury (expanding air inside).

■ **SIGNS AND SYMPTOMS**

Sharp pain

Vertigo

Bleeding

Tinnitus

Slight hearing impairment

May be asymptomatic

■ **THERAPEUTIC INTERVENTIONS**

Leave the area alone (do not probe it). Instruct the patient to do so as well.

Most small perforations will heal spontaneously; large perforations should be repaired by reapproximating the fragments with a suction apparatus; anesthesia is needed.

Antibiotics should be given if there is history of seawater or other contaminated water in the ear.

Note that diving injuries may cause a permanent loss of hearing and associated infection.

If associated with severe tinnitus or complete hearing loss, hospitalize the patient and obtain an otolaryngologic consultation.

Foreign Body

Cerumen is a natural foreign body of the ear. Other common foreign bodies include beans, beads, and bugs. Children are especially prone to putting foreign bodies in their ears. Bleeding may occur when the patient attempts to remove the foreign body.

■ **THERAPEUTIC INTERVENTIONS**

If there is no perforation, remove the foreign body (visualize it first).

It may be necessary to administer general anesthetic to a child.

Remove round objects with an ear hook or rubber-tipped suction.

Do not push the object deeper in the ear canal.

If the foreign body is an insect, shine a flashlight into the ear. The insect will usually go toward the light. (Do not try to remove it while it is alive; the insect may struggle and cause more damage.) Live insects may be immobilized by instilling a few drops of lidocaine, mineral oil, or ether.

If there is a perforation, make sure that the object is clearly visualized, and remove the object with suction.

Do not instill anything into the ear if it is draining any type of fluid.

Acute External Otitis

Acute external otitis, or ''swimmer's ear,'' is an infection of the external ear caused by bacteria or fungus. It is a common finding in children.

■ **SIGNS AND SYMPTOMS**

Severe pain

Ear tender to touch

Swelling to the canal

Cellulitis of the pinna and other structures

Occasionally, purulent discharge

■ **THERAPEUTIC INTERVENTIONS**

Culture.

Give analgesics.

Drain the abscess, if present.

Insert a wick soaked in antibiotic solution or ointment.

Apply hot compresses.

Acute Otitis Media

Otitis media is an inflammation of the middle ear lining. As fluid builds up in the middle ear, pain becomes severe.

■ **SIGNS AND SYMPTOMS**

Sharp pain

Sensation of fullness in the ear

Difficulty hearing

Bulging of tympanic membrane

Elevated temperature

Nausea and vomiting

History of upper respiratory infection

■ **THERAPEUTIC INTERVENTIONS**
Decongestants
Antibiotics
Analgesics
Myringotomy
■ **COMPLICATIONS**
Tympanic membrane rupture
Acute mastoiditis

Acute Mastoiditis

Acute mastoiditis is the most common middle ear infection.
■ **SIGNS AND SYMPTOMS**
Pain in the mastoid area
Elevated temperature
Tenderness in the mastoid area
Difficulty hearing
Local swelling
Vertigo
Possible history of acute external or internal otitis
■ **THERAPEUTIC INTERVENTIONS**
Heat packs
Analgesia
Antibiotics
Otolaryngologic consultation (in case surgical drainage is required)

Nose Emergencies

Foreign Bodies

Foreign bodies in the nose are common in children and often are discovered
only after a purulent discharge is seen draining from one of the nostrils.
■ **THERAPEUTIC INTERVENTIONS**
Decongestant nose drops
Topical anesthetic
Place the patient in Trendelenburg's position
Remove the object with a ring curette or alligator forceps

Epistaxis (Nosebleed)

Epistaxis can be a relatively minor problem, or it can turn into a life-threatening
emergency. It commonly occurs in the following groups:
Children
Adults 50 to 70 years old
Patients with blood dyscrasias, hypertension, or arteriosclerotic heart disease

Patients on anticoagulant therapy
Alcoholics
Patients with allergies
Patients with hereditary hemorrhagic telangiectasia (Rendu-Osler-Weber disease)

Anterior epistaxis

Anterior epistaxis is common at Kiesselbach's area or in the anterior and inferior turbinates.

■ **THERAPEUTIC INTERVENTIONS**

Give much reassurance.
Place the neck in slight hyperextension.
Suction clots.
Check for bleeding site.
Soak cotton pledgets in a vasoconstrictor agent (usually 10% cocaine solution).
Insert pledgets into the nostril.
Apply pressure for 5 to 10 minutes.
Cauterize bleeding sites with silver nitrate.
NOTE: In patients with blood dyscrasias or immunosuppression, use a wedge of salt pork in place of the cotton pledgets; this is much more comfortable and appears much more effective.

Posterior epistaxis

Posterior epistaxis is a more serious problem. It usually results from hypertension, arteriosclerotic heart disease, a blood dyscrasia, or a tumor.

■ **THERAPEUTIC INTERVENTIONS**

Check blood pressure.
Give volume replacement if necessary.
Ask about the medical history.
Check coagulation studies.
Anesthetize the nose (10% cocaine).
Check the bleeding site, if possible.
Pack as described below.
If bleeding continues, ligation of the internal maxillary or anterior ethmoid
    artery may be necessary (usually done by otolaryngologist).

■ **PACKING FOR POSTERIOR NOSEBLEED**

Analgesia and/or sedation is usually required during packing for posterior nosebleed. The patient should be given antibiotics and admitted to the hospital for 3 to 5 days following packing.

Equipment

No. 18 or 20 Foley catheter with balloon or specially designed nasal balloon
    catheter or tampon (tonsil or vaginal) with three ties or rolled 4 × 4-inch
    sponge with three ties
Antibiotic ointment
Rubber catheter
Half-inch selvage-edge petrolatum gauze

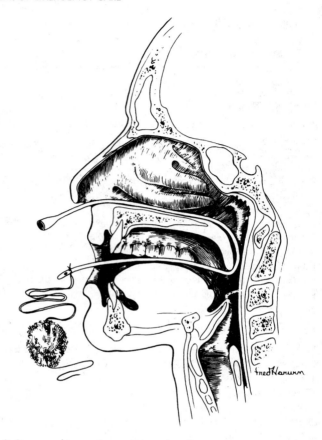

FIGURE 21-9. Steps used in passing a postnasal pack.
(From DeWeese DD, Saunders WH: *Textbook of otolaryngology*, ed 6. St Louis, 1982, Mosby)

Bayonet forceps
Gauze pad
Eye pad
Procedure with tampon
1. Pass the rubber catheter through the nostril to the back of the palate and forward out of the mouth.
2. Tie two of the ties of the tampon to the catheter (Figure 21-9).
3. Pull the catheter out of the nose; the tampon will seat near the choana.
4. With the fingers, push the tampon into place (Figure 21-10).
5. Bring the other tie, which is dangling in the back of the mouth, forward and secure it to the outside of the face with tape.
6. Pack the nasal cavity bilaterally from the anterior openings through a

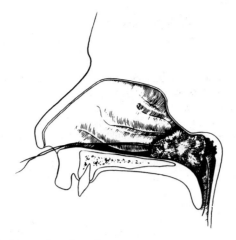

FIGURE 21-10. Postnasal pack in place.

(From DeWeese DD, Saunders WH: *Textbook of otolaryngology,* ed 6. St Louis, 1982, Mosby)

nasal speculum with bayonet forceps with 1/2-inch selvage-edged petrolatum gauze, layering front to back. (Be sure to count and record the number of packs used.)

7. Tie the ties from the tampon around a gauze pad outside of the nostril.
   (Make sure both strings are coming out of the same nostril; never have
   one string coming out of each nostril, because this will cause necrosis.)

Procedure with catheter

1. Pass the Foley catheter into the nostril and to the palate area.
2. Inflate the Foley balloon (with 10 ml saline).
3. Pull the catheter forward until the balloon seats near the choana.
4. Hold the catheter firmly and pack the anterior chambers with 1/2-inch selvage-edged petrolatum gauze, layering front to back. (Be sure to count
   and record the number of packs used.)
5. Place an eye pad or 4 × 4-inch sponge around the Foley catheter.
6. Clamp the Foley catheter distal to the eye pad with an umbilical clamp.

Epistaxis nasal balloon. This is a short (5-inch) catheter designed for control
of epistaxis, and employs two separately inflatable balloons.

1. Insert the catheter into the nose until the posterior balloon in located in
   the nasopharynx.
2. Fill the posterior balloon with 10 cc sterile saline or water.
3. Pull the catheter gently forward until the balloon is set.
4. Inflate the anterior balloon with 30 cc sterile saline or sterile water.
5. To remove, deflate both balloons and withdraw the catheter gently.

Throat Emergencies

Foreign Bodies

Foreign bodies in the throat may be penetrating, obstructing, or aspirated.

■ **THERAPEUTIC INTERVENTIONS**

Visualize the foreign body.

Remove it with the appropriate instrument.

If the foreign body is totally obstructing the airway:

Give four abdominal thrusts (Heimlich maneuver)

Attempt to breathe for the victim

If this is unsuccessful, do an emergency cricothyreotomy.

Fractured Larynx

A fractured larynx is usually caused by a direct blow to the neck. Often the patient comes to the emergency department with multiple injuries, making this injury easy to overlook. A fracture of the larynx produces edema and consequently blocks the upper airway. Fracture of the larynx is a surgical emergency.

■ **SIGNS AND SYMPTOMS**

Shortness of breath	Respiratory stridor
Vocal changes	History of throat trauma
Subcutaneous emphysema	Respiratory arrest

■ **THERAPEUTIC INTERVENTION**

Perform cricothyrotomy or tracheostomy (see Chapter 4).

Upper Respiratory Tract Infection or Pharyngitis ("The Common Cold")

■ **SIGNS AND SYMPTOMS**

Sore throat	Malaise
Difficulty swallowing	Foul breath odor
Pain referred to the ears	Enlarged tonsils
Elevated temperature	Enlarged cervical nodes
Feeling of fullness in the head	

■ **THERAPEUTIC INTERVENTIONS**

Throat culture

Warm saline gargles

Aspirin or acetaminophen

Antibiotics

Peritonsillar Abscess

A peritonsillar abscess is a collection of pus in the peritonsillar fascial planes and most commonly follows an episode of pharyngitis or tonsillitis.

■ **SIGNS AND SYMPTOMS**
Initially, pharyngitis
Difficulty speaking
Trismus
Difficulty swallowing
Drooling
Possible airway difficulties
Soft palate swollen on affected side
Deviation of uvula toward unaffected side
■ **THERAPEUTIC INTERVENTIONS**
Parenteral antibiotics
Otolaryngology consult
Possible irrigation and debridement

Dental Emergencies

Dental Pain

The most common cause of dental pain is tooth decay or pulpal disease. Pulpal disease has three phases:

Hyperemic—the vascular system responds to an external stimulus, such as dental caries (cavity) or dental trauma; this is a reversible condition.

Pulpitis—the pulp becomes infected.

Pulpal necrosis—the pulp dies; fluid and pressure build, causing pain.

Therapeutic intervention for these conditions consists of analgesia, antibiotics, and referral to a dentist.

Other causes of dental pain

Exposed root surfaces as a result of receding gums
Fractured teeth
Periodontal disease (in the supporting tissues)
Foreign bodies (such as a toothbrush bristle embedded in tissues)
Dry socket
Pressure from a prosthetic device
Mandibular fractures
Vincent's angina, or "trench mouth" or necrotizing ulcerative gingivitis (ulcers of the gingiva)
Pericoronitis (pain of wisdom teeth erupting)
Sinusitis
Trigeminal neuralgia
Glossodynia (a burning pain in the tongue)
Fractured styloid process
Hematomas (usually resulting from trauma, which may include injections of anesthetic)
Coronary artery disease (referred pain to jaw)
Carcinoma (hemostomatitis and radiation therapy)

Teeth in process of eruption
TMJ dysfunction

Toothaches

The most common cause of toothaches is pulpal disease or dental caries. This type of pain is paroxysmal and usually begins with a heat or cold stimulus. The pain usually occurs spontaneously and continues to worsen, especially at night when intracranial pressure increases.

■ **THERAPEUTIC INTERVENTIONS**
Topical oil of clove or other analgesia
Referral to a dentist

Dental Abscess

Abscesses in the periapical areas usually result from pulpal necrosis secondary to caries or trauma. Periodontal abscesses usually result from bony destruction at the periodontal membrane, which can form a pocket resulting in abscess formation.

■ **THERAPEUTIC INTERVENTIONS**
Drainage of the abscess
Antibiotics
Analgesics
Hot packs on the area
Warm saline rinses every 2 hours
Aspirin or other antipyretic for fever above 101° F (38.3° C)
Referral to a dentist

Periodontal Emergencies Requiring Dental Referral

gingivitis   Inflammation of the gums characterized by redness, swelling, pain, and bleeding.
periodontal disease   Loss of periodontal bone; symptoms more severe than gingivitis; definitive diagnosis is made on x-ray films.
necrotizing ulcerative gingivitis (Vincent's angina or "trenchmouth")   Painful bleeding, foul-smelling breath, lymphadenopathy, chills, fever, and malaise.
pericoronitis   Painful eruption of wisdom teeth accompanied by swelling, lymphadenopathy, and trismus; therapeutic intervention is by removal of tissue over the tooth, warm saline rinses, antibiotics, and dental referral for possible tooth extraction.

Postoperative Bleeding

Often a patient comes to the emergency department bleeding from the mouth, with a history of recent tooth extraction or other oral surgery. Usually all that is needed is to apply a pressure pack over the area of hemorrhage. If the bleeding persists, a hemostatic dressing such as absorbable gelatin sponge (Gelfoam), oxidized cellulose (Surgicel), or thrombin should be packed into the socket. A home remedy that may also be effective is to place a wet teabag over the socket. (The tannic acid may help produce hemostasis.) If the packing is unsuccessful, sutures may be placed or the bleeding vessels may be cauterized. Caution the patient to avoid mouth rinses until the bleeding has completely stopped, to eat a soft diet, to use intermittent ice packs, to avoid hot liquids, and not to drink through a straw.

Dry Socket (Postextraction Alveolitis)

Dry socket usually occurs 3 to 5 days after surgery, when a blood clot is lost and bone is exposed.

■ **THERAPEUTIC INTERVENTIONS**

A pledget soaked in oil of clove packed into the socket
Analgesia
Dental referral

Chipped (Broken) Teeth

Chipped or broken teeth are the most frequently seen dental emergencies in the emergency department. The four center upper teeth are the teeth most frequently injured.

Check for bleeding from gums and from pulp. Bleeding from pulp requires emergency dental consultation. Because these injuries are frequently associated with head injuries, be sure to check the mouth and pharynx area for pieces of teeth and debris that may obstruct the airway.

Avulsed Teeth

Avulsed teeth are teeth that have been totally dislodged from the socket by trauma. If found, these teeth may be reimplanted.

■ **THERAPEUTIC INTERVENTIONS**

Place the tooth in saline solution, milk, or water. If the patient is conscious, the tooth may be placed between the gum and up in the patient's mouth.
Refer patient to a dentist or oral surgeon.
Irrigate the wound.
Anesthetize the wound area.
Reimplant the tooth as soon as possible.
NOTE: Blood supply to the tooth comes via the pulp, so the viability of the tooth depends on the patency of the pulp.
Teeth that have been driven into the gums, especially in children, should be left alone. Patient should be referred to dentist.

NOTE: Remember to look for teeth and foreign bodies such as prostheses and bridges in the mouths of trauma patients and to remove these objects to avoid airway obstruction.

SUGGESTED READINGS

Eye

Karesh J, Keyes B: Ocular trauma. In Cardona V, Hurn P, Mason P et al, eds: *Trauma nursing: from resuscitation through rehabilitation.* Philadelphia, 1988, Saunders.

Ortiz J, Antoszyk J, Daniels M: Orbital and ocular injuries, *Top Emerg Med* 13(4):67, 1991.

Rogers J, Osborn H, Pousada L: Ophthalmologic emergencies. In Rogers J et al, eds: *Emergency nursing: a practice guide.* Baltimore, 1989, Williams & Wilkins.

Tabbara K: Eye emergencies. In Saunders C, Ho M, eds: *Current emergency diagnosis and treatment.* E. Norwalk, Conn, 1992, Appleton and Lange.

Ear, Nose, Throat, and Dental

Domzalski F: Otalagia. In Hamilton G, ed: *Presenting signs and symptoms in the emergency department: evaluation and treatment.* Baltimore, 1993, Williams & Wilkins.

Finkelstein J, Schaffer S, Dresner D: Otologic injuries, *Top Emerg Med* 13(4):60, 1991.

Hunt R: Epistaxis. In Hamilton G, ed: *Presenting signs and symptoms in the emergency department: evaluation and treatment.* Baltimore, 1993, Williams & Wilkins.

Lanzi G: Mandibular and dental injuries, *Top Emerg Med* 13(4):27, 1991.

Renicks M: Sore throat. In Hamilton G, ed: *Presenting signs and symptoms in the emergency department: evaluation and treatment.* Baltimore, 1993, Williams & Wilkins.

Rogers J, Osborn H, Pousada L: Ear, nose and throat disorders. In Rogers J et al, eds: *Emergency nursing: a practice guide.* Baltimore, 1989, Williams & Wilkins.

Schlesinger J: Dental disorders. In Hamilton G, ed: *Presenting signs and symptoms in the emergency department: evaluation and treatment.* Baltimore, 1993, Williams & Wilkins.

Serio J: Ear, nose and throat emergencies. In Cosgriff J, Anderson D, eds: *The practice of emergency care,* ed 2. Philadelphia, 1984, Lippincott.

Sheehy S: Ear, nose, throat, facial, and dental emergencies. In Sheehy S, ed: *Emergency nursing: principles and practice,* ed 3. St Louis, 1992, Mosby.

Tami T, Crumley R, Mills J: Disorders of the ears, nose, sinuses, oropharynx and teeth. In Saunders C, Ho M, eds: *Current emergency diagnosis and treatment,* ed 4. E. Norwalk, Conn, 1992, Appleton and Lange.

Ziter W: Dental emergencies. In Cosgriff J, Anderson D, eds: *The practice of emergency care,* ed 2. Philadelphia, 1984, Lippincott.

Chest Trauma

Many patients who suffer blunt or penetrating trauma to the chest will have severe and perhaps life-threatening injuries. Of all trauma deaths in the United States, 25% result from injuries to the chest.[1] It is essential that the patient's condition be assessed rapidly and life-saving therapeutic interventions applied concurrent with findings in order to reduce morbidity and mortality. Many life-threatening conditions can be reversed if they are identified early and interventions are rapid.

THORACIC CAVITY ANATOMY

The thoracic cavity (Figure 22-1) extends from the first rib under the clavicle, to the diaphragm. The diaphragm can elevate as high as the fourth intercostal space anteriorly upon exhalation and as low as the tenth intercostal space upon inhalation (Figure 22-2). Injuries between the fourth and tenth intercostal spaces should be considered both chest and abdominal until one or both are ruled out, because the diaphragm is so mobile and separates the thoracic cavity from the abdominal cavity. A gunshot or stab wound just below the right nipple may involve the skin, connective tissue, muscle, ribs, pleura, lungs, *and* liver.

The thoracic cavity contains the lower airway: the mainstem and right and left bronchi, the lungs, and the heart, the great vessels, and the esophagus. It is surrounded by twelve pairs of ribs that provide protection and structure. At the inferior border of each rib run the intercostal vein, artery, and nerve. It is important to note that chest procedures should be performed at the superior border of the ribs or at the sternum or subxyphoid, as intercostal arteries bleed a lot when disrupted.

The Angle of Louis is the most constant landmark on the anterior chest wall. The second intercostal space is at the Angle of Louis in the midclavicular line just below the clavicle (Figure 22-3).

The lungs are elastic in nature and have a natural tendency to collapse. Normally, with the presence of negative pressure (a ''vacuum'') in the intrathoracic

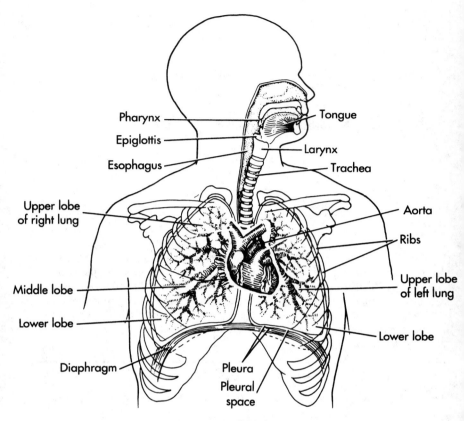

FIGURE 22-1. Anatomy of the thoracic cavity.

space, the lungs do not collapse. When there is an inspiratory effort, the intercostal muscles pull the ribs upward, the diaphragm drops downward, and negative pressure increases. The lungs respond to this negative pressure by filling with air. If negative pressure (the vacuum) is lost, the lungs collapse because of their elasticity. The normal tidal volume of the lungs is 5 to 7 ml per pound of body weight.

The intrathoracic space expands when the intercostal muscles lift the ribs and the diaphragm drops down. This process is assisted by the accessory muscles of respiration: the abdominal wall muscles, the pectoralis muscles, and the sternocleidomastoid muscles.

The phrenic nerve runs through the diaphragm. Irritation of the phrenic nerve by blood or other sources may cause hiccoughs or referred pain to the shoulder.

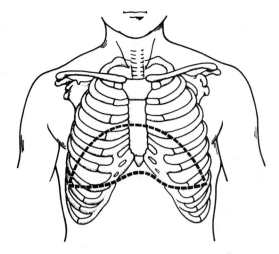

FIGURE 22-2. Level of diaphragm on inspiration and expiration.

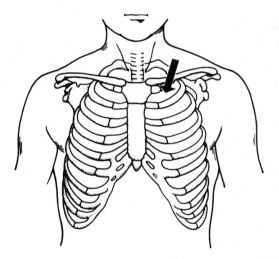

FIGURE 22-3. The Angle of Louis and the second intercostal space.

When assessing and treating a patient with chest trauma, *always* assume that the injury is serious until it is proven otherwise. Of people with chest trauma, 85% require nonsurgical intervention to improve their condition. There is usually a problem with hypoxia, circulation, or obstruction.[2] Hypoxia is a major cause of death in chest trauma. It may be caused by one of four states: perfusion (blood circulating) of an unventilated lung; ventilation of an unperfused lung; an abnormal airway/lung relationship, which may be due to a mechanical or physiological obstruction; or hypovolemia (and therefore decreased oxygenation).

PRIORITIES IN THE TREATMENT OF PATIENTS WITH CHEST INJURIES

- To maintain an adequate airway
  Assure that there are no obstructions.
- To ensure good ventilation
  Administer supplemental O_2 via non-rebreather mask or endotracheal tube. You must see the chest rise.
  Listen for bilateral breath sounds. When air enters the lungs, it enters the bases first. So, listen at the fifth or sixth intercostal space at the midaxillary line. Breath sounds only on the right side may indicate the presence of an endotracheal tube in the right mainstem bronchus or a pneumothorax. Check SaO_2.
  Check tidal volume. Place your hands on the patient's chest with fingers spread and thumb tips touching on exhalation. If the thumbs spread apart on inspiration, the patient is breathing a tidal volume of at least 78% of normal. With loss of intercostal muscles 50% of tidal volume is lost.[3]
  If the ribs do not move on inspiration, there may be a spinal injury with diaphragmatic breathing.
- To ensure adequate circulation
  Check skin vitals (color, temperature, moisture).
  Check capillary refill (greater than 2 seconds—the time it takes to say "capillary refill"—is abnormal).
  Check vital signs.
  Start one or two large-bore IV lines—16 gauge or larger; run warmed lactated Ringer's solution.
- To protect the cervical and thoracic spines
  Assume spinal injury until proven otherwise.
  Immobilize from the top of the head to the hips.
- To perform a rapid assessment for life-threatening injuries of the chest
  These include flail chest, tension pneumothorax, pericardial tamponade, massive hemothorax, open pneumothorax, and a dissecting or ruptured aorta.
  Potentially life-threatening conditions include pulmonary contusion, tracheobronchial rupture, esophageal rupture, diaphragmatic rupture, myocardial contusion, and a dissecting aorta.

In addition:

Get a good history, especially of the mechanism of injury and prehospital events.

Obtain an upright chest x-ray film (if possible). NOTE: If the chest x-ray film is done in a supine position, the mediastinum will appear widened.

Check for entrance and exit wounds.

Consider chest tube(s) placement.

Consider autotransfusion.

Obtain arterial blood gases.

Place the patient on a cardiac monitor and obtain a 12-lead ECG.

Consider emergency thoracotomy.

Consider any therapeutic intervention specific to the injury.

Measure urinary output.

TYPES OF CHEST INJURIES

Rib Fractures

Rib fractures are the most common type of chest injuries. A rib consists of the head, where it attaches to the vertebrae, the tubercle, the angles, and the body. Ribs fracture most commonly at the angles. The fifth through ninth ribs on the left and the fifth through tenth ribs on the right are the ribs most commonly fractured. If there is a first rib fracture, a flail chest, or multiple rib fractures, one must suspect that there has been a severe injury. Rib fractures may cause decreased ventilation, increased secretions, atelectasis, and pneumonia.

A first rib fracture is often associated with a clavicle fracture and sometimes a scapular fracture. First, second, and third rib fractures should be considered serious. Fractures of these ribs carry a 15% to 30% mortality rate caused by the proximity of those ribs to the subclavian artery, subclavian vein, aorta, and the tracheobronchial tree.[4]

When there are lower rib fractures, consider the possibility of damage to underlying structures. Fractures of ribs 5 through 9 on the right are dangerous because they overlie the liver. Ribs 9 through 11 on the left overlie the spleen and may cause it to rupture when the ribs are fractured.

■ **SIGNS AND SYMPTOMS**

Mechanism of injury that could cause chest trauma

Pain that increases with inspiration

(Bone spicules irritate the parietal pleura)

Splinting of the chest

Crepitus or subcutaneous emphysema at the fracture site

Possible palpation of the fracture

■ **DIAGNOSIS**

Chest x-ray film

■ **THERAPEUTIC INTERVENTIONS**

For simple fractures

Rest

Intermittent ice for first 24 hours, then heat

Simple analgesia or regional anesthesia

For displaced rib fractures or any rib fractures in the elderly

Hospital admission

Regional anesthesia for severe pain

    Local infiltration

    Intercostal nerve block

Flail Chest (Figure 22-4)

When two or more adjacent ribs are fractured in two or more places or the sternum is detached, the segment becomes flail. This segment loses continuity with the rest of the chest wall and responds directly to intrathoracic pressure changes; paradoxical chest wall motion results. When negative pressure increases (on inhalation), the flail segment is drawn inward (Figure 22-5, *A*). When negative pressure decreases (on exhalation), the segment is pushed outward (Figure 22-5, *B*). The flail segment moves in the opposite direction from the rest of the chest wall (paradoxical motion). This injury is usually caused by a massive blunt force to the chest. A major danger of a flail chest is that complications will arise, particularly hypoxia, from the underlying pulmonary contusion that is caused by the great force that caused the ribs to fracture.

■ **SIGNS AND SYMPTOMS**

Observed paradoxical motion of the chest wall

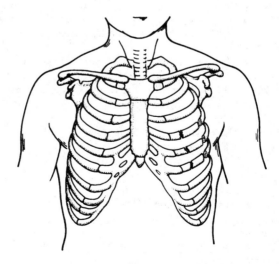

FIGURE 22-4. Flail chest. Two or more ribs fractured in consecutive places.

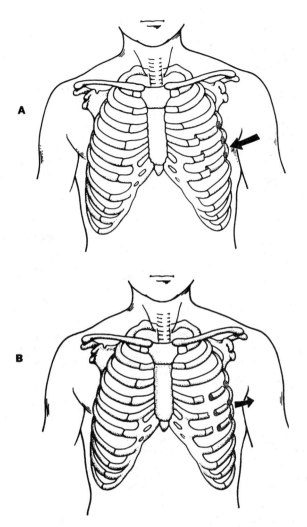

FIGURE 22-5. **A,** Flail chest; when diaphragm is drawn down and respiratory effort is made, flail segment pulls in. **B,** Flail chest; when diaphragm rises and exhalation occurs, flail segment moves outward.

Respiratory distress
Palpation of subcutaneous emphysema

■ **DIAGNOSIS**
Clinical observation
Chest x-ray
Arterial blood gases/SaO$_2$

■ **THERAPEUTIC INTERVENTIONS**
The goal of therapeutic intervention is to provide good ventilation; treat the pulmonary contusion.
Selective endotracheal intubation
Oxygen with positive pressure
    Consider positive end expiratory pressure (PEEP)
Consider stabilizing the flail segment
IVs
    Carefully administering crystalloids
    Consider using arterial pressure or pulmonary wedge pressure valves to guide
        fluid replacement
Pain control
Admission to ICU for close observation and pulmonary stabilization

Sternal Fracture

It takes a great force to fracture the sternum—most commonly an impact with a steering wheel or following CPR. A totally detached sternum is considered a flail segment and is treated accordingly. With sternal fractures, the most common underlying injury is a myocardial contusion.

■ **SIGNS AND SYMPTOMS**
Chest pain
Dysrhythmias/ECG changes
    Especially premature ventricular contractions, arterial fibrillation, right bundle
        branch block, and ST segment elevation
Pain on inspiration

■ **DIAGNOSIS**
Palpation of the fracture
Chest x-ray film

■ **THERAPEUTIC INTERVENTIONS**
Close observation
Pain control
Treat dysrhythmias
Consider surgery for fixation

Fractured Clavicle

A fractured clavicle is usually not a serious injury. However, a jagged fracture may lacerate the subclavian artery or vein. This injury is usually caused by a blunt force and is commonly seen as an athletic injury, where the blunt force is received laterally.

■ **SIGNS AND SYMPTOMS**
Pain (especially on palpation)
■ **DIAGNOSIS**
Clinical observation of the deformity
Chest x-ray film
Consider arteriogram to rule out vascular damage
■ **THERAPEUTIC INTERVENTIONS**
Figure-of-eight
Pain control

PNEUMOTHORAX

Simple Pneumothorax

A simple pneumothorax (Figure 22-6) is a condition that causes a ventilation defect when air enters the chest cavity, causing a loss of negative pressure (the vacuum) and a partial or total collapse of the lung. It may be caused by a hole in the chest wall or a hole in the lung tissue, the bronchus, or the trachea. A spontaneous pneumothorax is the occurrence of a pneumothorax without evidence of trauma. It is thought to be caused by a ruptured bleb or a ruptured cyst.

■ **SIGNS AND SYMPTOMS**
History of blunt or penetrating trauma to the chest
Sudden onset of sharp pleuritic chest pain
Decreased breath sounds on the affected side

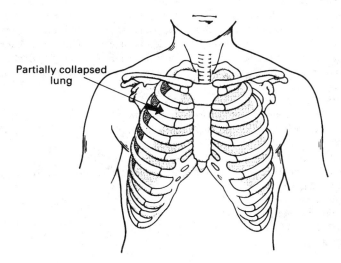

Partially collapsed lung

FIGURE 22-6. Simple pneumothorax; partial collapse of a lung.

Shortness of breath

Tachypnea

Syncope

Hamman's sign (a crunching sound with each heartbeat, caused by mediastinal air accumulation)

Hyperresonance on percussion

■ **DIAGNOSIS**

Clinical observation

Chest x-ray film

■ **THERAPEUTIC INTERVENTIONS**

Close observation

Oxygen by nonrebreather mask

Semi-Fowler's position

Consider placement of a large-bore needle through the anterior chest wall in the second intercostal space

Consider placement of a chest tube

Tension Pneumothorax

A tension pneumothorax (Figure 22-7) is a life-threatening condition. Usually there is good perfusion, but inadequate ventilation that eventually leads to poor perfusion. When air enters the pleural space during inspiration and is trapped during exhalation, pressure in the intrathoracic space begins to build, forming what is known as a *tension pneumothorax.* This usually occurs as the result of a penetrating injury, but may also be caused by blunt trauma, use of mechanical ventilation with positive end expiratory pressure (PEEP), a nonsealing puncture, or a ruptured bleb.

Pressure forces the heart and great vessels to be pushed toward the opposite side (Figure 22-8). This event is known as mediastinal shift. This shift causes the great vessels to kink, which results in a backup of blood into the venous system. This is demonstrated by distension of the neck veins and a decreased blood return to the heart, causing a decreased cardiac output. The trachea will also be pushed toward the uninjured side, causing an event that is known as tracheal deviation.

■ **SIGNS AND SYMPTOMS**

Difficulty breathing; severe shortness of breath

Deviated trachea (toward the unaffected side)

Mediastinal shift

Jugular vein distension

Decreased blood pressure and other hemodynamic deterioration signs

Increased pulse

Restlessness

Paradoxical movement of the chest

Cyanosis

Distant heart sounds

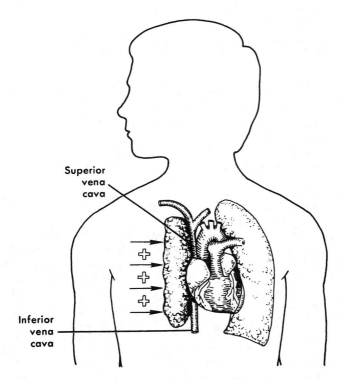

FIGURE 22-7. Tension pneumothorax.

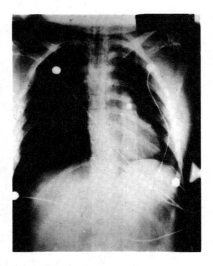

FIGURE 22-8. Right tension pneumothorax as seen on x-ray.

Hyperresonance on percussion

Chest on the side of the pneumothorax always bigger

■ **DIAGNOSIS**

Clinical observation

Chest x-ray film

■ **THERAPEUTIC INTERVENTIONS**

NOTE: If the patient is severely symptomatic, do not wait for chest x-ray film results before providing therapeutic intervention.

Airway

Oxygen at high-flow rate (be careful not to administer oxygen under positive pressure until the chest tube is placed because this may increase the tension)

Needle thoracotomy

Chest tube placement

IV Ringer's lactate or normal saline

Needle thoracotomy. The definitive therapy for tension pneumothorax is the placement of a chest tube. If a patient is in the field or it will be a while before a chest tube can be placed, consider placing a needle into the anterior chest wall of the affected side to partially relieve the tension until a chest tube is placed. This procedure may "buy some time," but must be followed by chest tube insertion.

The procedure.

1. Rapidly prepare the area in which the needle will be placed with alcohol or Betadine; use the second intercostal space at the midclavicular line.
2. Insert a needle (at least a 16-gauge, preferably metal) over the superior portion of the rib (the vein, artery, and nerve, and located behind the inferior border) and through the tissue covering the pleural cavity.
3. When the needle has entered the pleural cavity, there will be a hissing sound.
4. If desired, the needle may be attached to a flutter valve or a syringe filled with saline.
5. Leave the needle in place until the chest tube is placed.
6. Continue to ventilate the patient or provide supplemental oxygen.

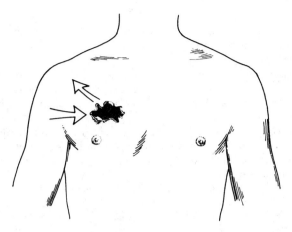

FIGURE 22-9. Sucking chest wound—open pneumothorax.

Sucking Chest Wound (Open Pneumothorax)

A sucking chest wound (Figure 22-9) is a chest wall defect that results in an open pneumothorax. It is usually caused by a penetrating force, such as a high-velocity missile. If there is a two-way flap, air will pass into the pleural space and back out again with inspiration and expiration. If the diameter of the hole in the chest wall is greater than two thirds the diameter of the trachea, there will be preferential flow of air through the chest wall defect (the path of least resistance).[5] This causes a simple pneumothorax as negative pressure is lost, which may be overcome with positive pressure ventilation. If there is a one-way flap, air can enter the pleural space but cannot escape. Pressure will build with each inspiratory effort until a tension pneumothorax has formed.

■ **SIGNS AND SYMPTOMS**

Dyspnea
Chest pain
Visualization of the defect
Sucking sound
Possible signs of tension pneumothorax

■ **DIAGNOSIS**

Clinical findings

■ **THERAPEUTIC INTERVENTIONS**

Ensure ABCs.

Oxygen under positive pressure

It is not necessary to cover the wound if the defect is less than two thirds the diameter of the trachea and the patient is intubated and being ventilated with positive pressures.

Consider covering wound with an occlusive dressing if that is local policy, sealed on three sides. Leave one side open for flutter valve effect.

Observe for the development of a tension pneumothorax. If a tension pneumothorax develops:

Remove the occlusive dressing. This should convert the tension pneumothorax to a simple pneumothorax.

If this does not relieve the tension pneumothorax, follow the steps for therapeutic intervention for tension pneumothorax.

Consider chest tube placement.

Consider autotransfusion.

Chest tube placement. Chest tubes are placed so that air and blood can be removed from the intrathoracic cavity. The procedure involves placing the chest tube in the appropriate space so that air is removed and the tension pneumothorax is relieved, or to drain blood and/or fluids by gravity drainage or with the assistance of suction.

■ **INDICATIONS**

Hemothorax

Pneumothorax

Empyema

■ **EQUIPMENT NEEDED** (Figure 22-10)

Betadine or other prep solution

Prep sponges

2 large curved Kelly clamps

6×10 ml syringes with 18- and 25-gauge needles

Scalpel and blade

1% lidocaine

Suture to secure chest tube

Suture for wound approximation

Needle holder

Appropriate size chest tube

Chest drainage collection device

Sterile surgical gloves

Occlusive dressing material

Sterile drape

Wide adhesive tape

Benzoin

■ **PROCEDURE**

1. Monitor the patient throughout procedure.
2. Determine chest tube placement site—usually the second intercostal space,

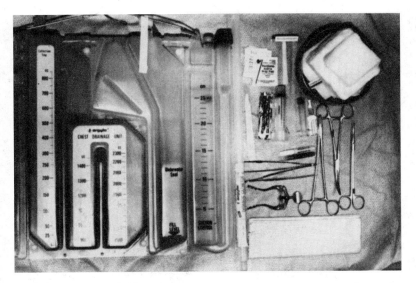

FIGURE 22-10. Equipment for chest tube thoracostomy and drainage collection.

midclavicular line for a pneumothorax, or fifth intercostal space, slightly anterior to the midaxillary line for a hemothorax.

3. Prep and drape the site.
4. Infiltrate the skin and rib periosteum with lidocaine.
5. Using a scalpel and blade, make a 2 to 3 cm transverse incision through the skin.
6. Using a Kelly clamp, bluntly dissect and spread through the subcutaneous tissue over the superior edge of the rib.
7. Puncture the tip of Kelly clamp (carefully) through the pleura (if there is a pneumothorax, air will rush out of the puncture hole).
8. Explore the intrathoracic area to free adhesions or clots with the sterile gloved index finger of the dominant hand.
9. Place half of the tip of a Kelly clamp through a perforation on the distal end of the chest tube, so that the tip of the tube is firm.
10. Advance the distal tip of the tube into the intrathoracic cavity, ensuring that it is situated well past the most proximal fenestration.
11. Once the tube is determined to be in the proper place, secure it using silk suture attached to the tube and to the skin.
12. Close the skin edges with nonabsorbable suture.
13. Apply Benzoin to the skin surrounding the chest tube.
14. Apply an occlusive dressing around the tube.
15. Secure the dressing and the chest tube with adhesive tape.
16. Attach the tube to a closed chest drainage system (Figure 22-11).

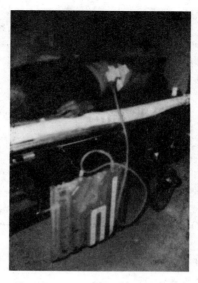

FIGURE 22-11. Chest tube in place, attached to a water seal chest drainage unit.

17. Note the amount of the initial drainage and any subsequent drainage directly on the collection chamber and on nurses' notes/flow chart.
18. Obtain a chest x-ray film to ensure proper placement of the tube.

Hemothorax

A hemothorax is a collection of blood in the intrathoracic space. It generally occurs when a lung or vessel is lacerated as the result of a blunt or penetrating trauma. Because hemothorax will cause a hypovolemic state, observe the patient carefully for signs and symptoms of shock. Hemothorax is often seen in conjunction with a simple or tension pneumothorax. Greater than 1500 ml of blood in the intrathoracic cavity is considered a *massive hemothorax*.

■ **SIGNS AND SYMPTOMS**
Similar to those of simple or tension pneumothorax
Signs of shock (including cool clammy skin, decreased capillary refill, decreased blood pressure, tachycardia, tachypnea, restlessness, anxiety, agitation, confusion, or unconsciousness)

■ **DIAGNOSIS**
Clinical observation
Chest x-ray film

■ **THERAPEUTIC INTERVENTIONS**
Treat shock condition
Oxygen
IVs

Chest tube placement
Consider autotransfusion
Consider emergency thoracotomy or surgery

> If initial drainage is 1000 ml or greater, followed by at least 200 ml of blood for each of four consecutive hours, or if there is an initial drainage of 1500 ml of blood or greater, this may indicate the need for emergency thoracotomy.[6]

Autotransfusion. Autotransfusion is a technique that is used to collect blood from an exsanguinating chest wound through a chest tube. The blood is filtered, anticoagulated, and reinfused into the patient. There are several types of autotransfuser set-ups. Caregivers should be familiar with the particular type of autotransfusion equipment used at their own facility.

In the emergency setting only blood from the chest can be used because it is considered relatively uncontaminated. This procedure has the advantage of having immediately available blood that is warm, perfectly cross-matched, and free from infectious diseases other than those the patient may already be carrying.

Autotransfusion may be indicated with the following conditions:
Massive hemothorax
Myocardial rupture
Great vessel rupture
Other chest trauma when there is:
    Nonavailability of banked blood
    A history of transfusion reactions
    Refusal of blood for religious reasons
Autotransfusion is contraindicated:
When wounds are more than 4 hours old
When the patient has inadequate kidney or liver function
When there is contamination of blood by:
    Outside sources
    Abdominal/intestinal contents
    Cancer cells

LUNG INJURIES

Pulmonary Contusion

Pulmonary contusion is the most common potentially life-threatening problem that occurs with chest trauma.[7] It is also one of the most common injuries in major trauma. It is often seen with flail chest and usually results from severe blunt trauma to the chest.

In pulmonary contusion, blood extravasates into the parenchyma of the lung because of an injury to the lung tissue. That causes the lung tissue to become anoxic and more permeable. Occasionally pulmonary contusion can cause tracheal obstruction.

■ **SIGNS AND SYMPTOMS**

The diagnosis of pulmonary contusion is usually made by suspecting it based on the mechanism of injury and looking for specific signs and symptoms to confirm one's suspicions.

Increasing hyperpnea

Dyspnea

Ineffective cough

Restlessness and agitation

Presence of other severe chest injuries

NOTE: Pulmonary contusion may be slow to develop (1 to 4 hours).[8]

■ **DIAGNOSIS**

High index of suspicion

Clinical observation

Chest x-ray film

Arterial blood gases

O_2 saturations

■ **THERAPEUTIC INTERVENTIONS**

Airway management; selective endotracheal intubation

Oxygen at high flow (humidified)

Consider ventilator

Limit fluids during resuscitation, unless there is associated injury causing hypovolemic shock.

Use whole blood products to replace lost blood, maintain oncotic pressure, and decrease pulmonary edema.

Consider diuretics.

Consider steroids.

Pain control

Morphine sulfate may be given in 1- to 2-mg increments IV.

Pay close attention to a decreased respiratory rate and to increased hypoxia.

Laceration of Lung Parenchyma

Lacerations of the parenchyma are usually caused by penetrating trauma or jagged rib fractures. They are usually self-limiting and rarely require surgical intervention.

■ **SIGNS AND SYMPTOMS**

Small hemothorax or pneumothorax

Hemoptysis

Subcutaneous emphysema

■ **DIAGNOSIS**

Clinical observation

Chest x-ray (showing hemothorax, pneumothorax, or subcutaneous emphysema)

Arterial blood gases

■ **THERAPEUTIC INTERVENTIONS**

Usually none necessary

Consider surgery if signs and symptoms are severe

Injury to Tracheobronchial Tree

Injury to the tracheobronchial tree usually involves the trachea or mainstem bronchus, most commonly near the bifurcation of the mainstem bronchus, 1 inch from the carina. This injury is usually caused by blunt or penetrating trauma. Signs and symptoms may not appear for up to 5 days following injury, and they may be subtle. There is a 50% mortality rate in the first hour.[9]

■ **SIGNS AND SYMPTOMS**
Airway obstruction
Atelectasis
Hemoptysis (massive)
Mediasternal and subcutaneous emphysema (progressive)
Air leak "somewhere in the chest"
Possible signs and symptoms of tension pneumothorax

■ **DIAGNOSIS**
Clinical findings
If the disruption is below the carina, chest x-ray film will demonstrate mediastinal air
Bronchoscopy

■ **THERAPEUTIC INTERVENTIONS**
Maintaining airway
Oxygen at high flow
Chest tube
Semi-Fowler's position
Surgical repair

Diaphragmatic Rupture

Diaphragmatic rupture may be a life-threatening injury. Disruption of the diaphragm, the main muscle of respiration, causes major interference with ventilation.[10] Consider the possibility of diaphragmatic injury when there is an injury below the level of the nipples caused by a forceful blow to the left side of the abdomen or by increased intraabdominal pressure (e.g., a motor vehicle crash where the victim was using a lap seat belt only). Blunt trauma usually causes large tears. A ruptured diaphragm is usually associated with other major injuries.

■ **SIGNS AND SYMPTOMS**
Chest pain referred to the shoulder
Severe shortness of breath
Difficulty breathing
Decreased breath sounds
Undigested food or fecal material in chest tube
Bowel sounds in the thoracic cavity

■ **DIAGNOSIS**
Chest x-ray film (supine—demonstrating bowel that herniated into the thoracic cavity and an elevated left hemi-diaphragm) (Figure 22-12), or the presence of the nasogastric tube in the thoracic cavity, or loss of the costophrenic angle on the side opposite the injury.[11]

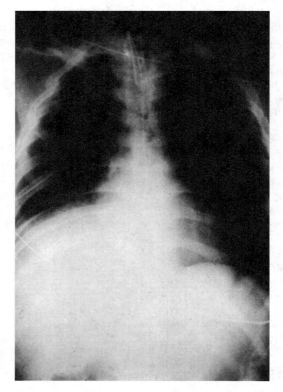

FIGURE 22-12. Bowel herniating through ruptured diaphragm.

GI series demonstrating stomach and/or intestines in the thoracic cavity

■ **THERAPEUTIC INTERVENTIONS**

Placement of a gastric tube

Surgery

CARDIAC INJURIES

Myocardial Contusion

Myocardial contusion probably occurs more frequently than it is diagnosed. It may be overlooked because of other, more obvious, severe injuries. Always suspect myocardial contusion in any patient who gives a history of blunt trauma to the chest or a severe acceleration/deceleration force, in any motor vehicle crash where a bent steering wheel has occurred, and in any patient who has recently had cardiopulmonary resuscitation/chest compressions.

■ **SIGNS AND SYMPTOMS**
Suspicion of myocardial contusion leading to its diagnosis
Severe chest pain
Chest wall contusion and ecchymosis (Figure 22-13)
Dysrhythmias/ECG changes
    Usually within the first hour, but up to 24 hours
    Usually premature ventricular contractions, atrial fibrillation, right bundle
       branch block, or elevated ST segment
Tachycardia
Hypotension
Dyspnea
Other associated signs of shock

■ **DIAGNOSIS**
High index of suspicion
Signs of injury on ECG
Elevated ST segment in V1, V2, V3 if injury is on the left
Elevated cardiac isoenzymes
Echocardiography

■ **THERAPEUTIC INTERVENTIONS**
Therapeutic interventions for myocardial contusion are similar to those for an
acute myocardial infarction. The patient should be treated symptomatically.
    Oxygen
    Semi-Fowler's position

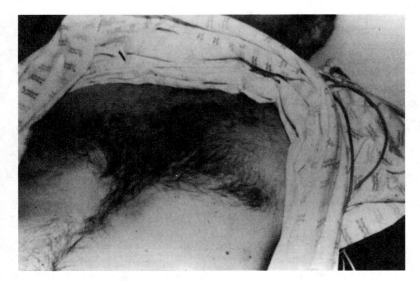

FIGURE 22-13. Mechanism of injury and chest abrasion suggest potential myocardial contusion.

Pain control
Treatment of dysrhythmias
Admission to monitored intensive care unit bed for at least 48 hours

Penetrating Cardiac Injuries

Penetrating injuries to the heart carry a high mortality rate. If the patient survives the prehospital phase of care and arrives at the emergency department, immediate thoracotomy and surgical repair are indicated.[12]

■ **SIGNS AND SYMPTOMS OF MYOCARDIAL DISRUPTION**
Severe hypotension
Elevated central venous pressure
Distended jugular veins
Decreased ECG voltage
Decreased heart sounds

■ **SIGNS AND SYMPTOMS OF AORTIC OR MITRAL VALVE DISRUPTION**
Sudden onset of severe chest pain
Severe dyspnea
Hemoptysis
Loud "roaring" murmur
Other associated signs of severe congestive heart failure and/or pulmonary
    edema

■ **DIAGNOSIS**
High index of suspicion
Chest x-ray film
Direct visualization

■ **THERAPEUTIC INTERVENTIONS**
Oxygen
Immediate surgery
    To repair rupture
    To replace valve

Pericardial Tamponade

Pericardial tamponade occurs when a wound of the heart, such as a pericardial laceration or a ruptured coronary artery, bleeds into the pericardial sac. Blood accumulates in the sac, causing pressure within the sac to rise. This interferes with ventricular filling and consequently with cardiac output. The heart attempts to compensate by activating the sympathetic nervous system, which causes the heart rate to increase. Because this compensation cannot continue for very long, the efficiency of the heart begins to deteriorate. As the heart rate increases, venous pressure increases, blood pressure falls, and heart sounds diminish.

A pericardial tamponade is usually caused by severe blunt trauma to the chest. It is often confused with tension pneumothorax. Consider the possibility of pericardial tamponade when there is unexplained pump failure that is not responsive to volume replacement.

■ **SIGNS AND SYMPTOMS**
Decreased blood pressure ⎫
Distended jugular veins ⎬ Beck's triad—the hallmark of pericardial tamponade
Muffled heart sounds ⎭
Increased heart rate
Dyspnea
Paradoxical pulse
Cyanosis
Other associated signs of shock
■ **DIAGNOSIS**
High index of suspicion
Clinical observation
Chest x-ray film (demonstrating a widened mediastinum)
Pericardiocentesis
Echocardiography
■ **THERAPEUTIC INTERVENTIONS**
Oxygen at high flow
IVs
High Fowler's position
Periocardiocentesis and/or pericardial window

AORTIC DISRUPTION

Tears of the aorta are usually the result of a blunt force such as occurs in motor vehicle accidents or falls from great heights. The aorta usually tears at the points of attachment, particularly at the ligamentum arteriosum and the aortic root. Patients who sustain aortic tears are usually in quite critical condition and rarely survive. There is a 90% at-the-scene mortality rate.[13] Of the remaining 10% of survivors, there is a 50% mortality rate with each day of treatment delayed.[14] The cause of death from aortic disruption is usually the result of a pericardial tamponade or massive exsanguination.

■ **SIGNS AND SYMPTOMS**
Signs of hypovolemic shock
Signs of pericardial tamponade
Chest wall bruise
First or second rib fracture
Sternal fracture
Scapula or multiple rib fractures
Large murmur heard best at the left parascapular region
Upper extremity blood pressure higher than lower extremities
Tracheal deviation to the right
Paraplegia
Trauma arrest
■ **DIAGNOSIS**
High index of suspicion
Chest x-ray film

Widened mediastinum
Obliteration of aortic knob
Presence of a pleural cap
Hemothorax
Esophageal deviation (by N/G tube on x-ray film)
Elevated right mainstem bronchus/lower left mainstem bronchus
Thoracic aortogram
CT scan
Transesophageal echo cardiogram (TEE)
■ THERAPEUTIC INTERVENTIONS
CPR
Oxygen at high flow
IVs (with whole blood as soon as possible)
Thoracotomy and surgical repair

Ruptured Esophagus

A ruptured esophagus is a rare event, but when it does occur, the mortality rate is high if the diagnosis is missed.[15] It usually occurs as a result of penetrating trauma or a severe blunt epigastric blow. When the cause is blunt trauma, the rupture often occurs just above the diaphragm. Consider esophageal rupture whenever there is evidence of a first or second rib fracture. It may be seen in conjunction with a pneumothorax or a hemothorax without evidence of fracture. It also may occur iatrogenically, during esophagoscopy.

■ SIGNS AND SYMPTOMS
Sudden onset of severe chest pain or upper abdominal pain following trauma
Signs and symptoms of pneumothorax
Pain on swallowing
Mediastinitis
Subcutaneous emphysema
Mediastinal ''crunch'' sound (Hamman's sign)
Increased respiratory effort
Pleural effusion
Gastric contents or bile in chest tube
Shock without associated pain
Elevated temperature
■ DIAGNOSIS
Clinical observation
Upper GI series
Endoscopy
■ THERAPEUTIC INTERVENTIONS
Oxygen at high flow
IVs
Immediate surgical intervention

SUMMARY

Chest trauma is potentially life-threatening; the primary focus of therapeutic intervention should be on maintenance of an airway, adequate breathing/ventilation, and adequate circulation. All injuries to the chest should be considered severe until proven otherwise.

REFERENCES

1. American College of Surgeons/Committee on Trauma: *Advanced trauma life support manual.* Chicago, 1992, American College of Surgeons.
2. Lawrence P: *Essentials of general surgery,* Baltimore, 1988, Williams and Wilkins.
3. Shea J: Lecture presented at The Emergency Nurses Association Annual Meeting, Orlando, Florida, Sept 1992.
4. Rosen P et al, eds: *Emergency medicine,* ed 3. St Louis, 1992, Mosby.
5. American College of Surgeons/Committee on Trauma: *Advanced Trauma Life Support Manual.* Chicago 1992, American College of Surgeons.
6. Sheehy SB, Jimmerson CL: *Manual of clinical trauma care: the first hour,* ed 2. St Louis, 1993, Mosby.
7. Jachimczyk K: Blunt chest trauma, *Emerg Med Clin North Am*11(1):81, 1993.
8. Lawrence P: *Essentials of general surgery,* Baltimore, 1988, Williams and Wilkins.
9. American College of Surgeons/Committee on Trauma: *Advanced trauma life support manual.* Chicago, 1992, American College of Surgeons.
10. Lawrence P: *Essentials of general surgery.* Baltimore, 1988, Williams and Wilkins.
11. American College of Surgeons/Committee on Trauma: *Advanced trauma life support instructor manual,* Chicago, 1992, American College of Surgeons.
12. Galliard M, Herve C, Mandin L, Raymond P: Mortality prognostic factors in chest injury. *J Trauma* 30(1):93, 1990.
13. Piano G, Turney SZ: Traumatic rupture of the thoracic aorta: surgical management, *Trauma Q* 4:2, 1988.
14. Lawrence P: *Essentials of general surgery,* Baltimore, 1988, Williams and Wilkins.

SUGGESTED READINGS

Brooks SW, Young JC, Cmolik B et al: The use of transesophageal echo in the evaluation of chest trauma, *J Trauma* 32(6):761, 1992.

Calhoun JH, Grover FL, Trinkle JK: Chest trauma: approach and management, *Clin Chest Med* 13(1):55, 1992.

Dee PM: The radiology of chest trauma, *Radiol Clin North Am* 38(2):291, 1992.

Gelman R, Mirvis SE, Glens D: Diaphragmatic rupture due to blunt trauma: sensitivity of plain chest radiographs, *J Roentgen* 156(1):51, 1991.

Hammond SG: Chest injuries in the trauma patient, *Nurs Clin North Am* 25(1):35, 1990.

Hefti D: Chest trauma, *RN,* 54(5):28, 1991.

Jorden RC: Penetrating chest trauma, *Emerg Med Clin North Am* 11(1):97, 1993.

Liev J, Kerstein MD: Role of three hour roentgenogram of the chest in penetrating injuries of the chest, *Surg Gynecol Obstet* 175(3):249, 1992.

Mansour MA, Moore EE, Moore FA, Read RR: Exigent postinjury thoracotomy analysis of blunt vs. penetrating trauma, *Surg Gynecol Obstet* 175(2):97, 1992.

Ruth-Sahd L: Pulmonary contusion: the hidden danger in blunt chest trauma, *Criti Care Nurse* 11(6):46, 1991.

Wolfman NT, Gelpin JW, Bechtold RE et al: Occult pneumothorax in patients with abdominal trauma: CT studies, *J Comput Assist Tomogr* 17(1):56, 1993.

Abdominal Trauma

There are two mechanisms of injury for abdominal trauma: *blunt* and *penetrating*. Blunt trauma results from a force to the abdominal wall that causes energy to diffuse into the abdominal cavity without causing an open injury. The abdominal organs are injured either by compression (squeezing the organ between the vertebral column and the impacting object), or deceleration (abdominal organs move forward with gravitational force until impacting an object, rupturing, or tearing away from supporting structures). The organs most commonly injured are the liver, spleen, and kidneys as they are solid organs and more likely to rupture when struck by a force. "Seatbelt syndrome," due to use of a lap belt only, may cause rupture of viscera or compression injuries.

Penetrating trauma results when an object such as a bullet, knife blade, or metal fragment pierces the abdominal wall and enters the abdominal cavity. Stab wounds often do not penetrate the peritoneal cavity and have a surprisingly low mortality rate (1% to 2%). Gunshot wounds, however, usually cause significant injury to abdominal organs and require surgical intervention.

Knowledge of the mechanism of injury, diligent physical exam, and maintaining a high degree of suspicion of injury are essential to reduce the morbidity and mortality related to abdominal trauma.

BLUNT TRAUMA

Blunt trauma most frequently occurs as a result of a motor vehicle crash, contact sports, falls, and child maltreatment. In the emergency care setting it is most important to determine whether the patient requires surgery and/or hospital admission for observation; it is not as important to determine which structures have been injured. Keeping this concept in mind, care is directed at frequent assessment and diagnostic tests in addition to keeping the patient stabilized through the use of emergency care adjuncts such as airway management and fluid replacement.

Give special consideration to those patients who are not reliable for diagnostic information, such as patients with spinal cord injuries, those who are unconscious or who have used mind-altering drugs or alcohol, and small children. The absence of signs and symptoms does not rule out abdominal injury. Further diagnostic studies are essential to reduce morbidity and mortality.

■ **SIGNS AND SYMPTOMS**

Bruises or abrasions
Distension (not a reliable sign)
Pain
Involuntary guarding
Rigidity
Crepitus
Masses
Signs of shock
    Decreased level of consciousness
    Cool, clammy skin
    Poor capillary refill
    Tachycardia
    Tachypnea
    Hypotension
Other associated severe injuries

■ **DIAGNOSIS**

Diagnosis may be difficult in the patient with blunt abdominal trauma. The importance of obtaining a good history of the mechanism of injury cannot be stressed enough.

The diagnostic examination should include:
Clinical observation with special attention to pain, rigidity, guarding, bruising
Peritoneal lavage to rule out intraabdominal injury; or
Abdominal CT to rule out intraabdominal or peritoneal bleeding
Arteriogram to rule out vascular injury
Cystogram to rule out bladder injury
Intravenous pyelogram (IVP) to rule out kidney and ureter injury
Retrograde urethrogram to rule out penile shaft injury
Rectal exam to rule out rectal injury
Nasogastric tube to rule out gastric injury and to decompress the stomach
Urinalysis to rule out renal and urinary tract injury
Laboratory studies (CBC, serum amylase, liver enzymes, renal function studies)
Surgery (indicated when involuntary guarding, abdominal expansion, hemodynamic instability, or gastrointestinal blood is present)

■ **THERAPEUTIC INTERVENTIONS**

Provide airway management and 100% supplemental oxygen.
Start IVs (two large-bore with crystalloids).
Stabilize cervical, thoracic, and lumbar spine.
Consider PASG (very controversial at the time of this printing).
Place nasogastric or orogastric tube.
Place Foley catheter.
Prepare patient for surgery.

Diagnostic Peritoneal Lavage

Indications for diagnostic peritoneal lavage (DPL) include:

- Evidence of blunt trauma to the abdomen in which shock ensues *but immediate CT scan is not possible.* It may also be done in the operating room if there is an urgency to take the patient to surgery for a severe head or chest injury and abdominal trauma has not yet been ruled out.
- Cases in which the patient is not conscious and cannot tell of abdominal tenderness, and signs of abdominal guarding and so on cannot be elicited.
- Patients who are inebriated or have spinal cord injury, from who it would be almost impossible to elicit signs and symptoms of blunt abdominal trauma.
- Diagnostic peritoneal lavage is not recommended for children.

The only absolute contraindication to the procedure is a distended bladder (Figure 23-1). The bladder must be emptied and the stomach decompressed prior to diagnostic peritoneal lavage.

■ RELATIVE CONTRAINDICATIONS

A gravid uterus

An abdominal wall hematoma

Abdominal scars from previous surgery

In all of these instances, the location of the incision should be changed, but the procedure may still be performed. If there is evidence of penetrating injury, diagnostic peritoneal lavage should not be performed, as the wound should be explored surgically.

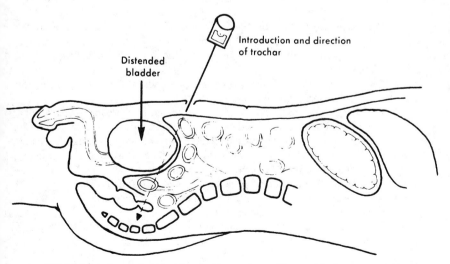

FIGURE 23-1. Distended bladder may be perforated by trochar for peritoneal lavage.

■ **EQUIPMENT**

Surgical antiseptic solution
Sterile drapes
Sterile gloves
1% lidocaine with epinephrine
No. 11 scalpel
No. 15 peritoneal dialysis catheter (with or without trocar)
Syringe with small-gauge needle
Ringer's lactate (1000 ml, warmed) and IV tubing
Nasogastric tube
Foley catheter
Skin retractors
4-0 nylon suture and needle
Antibiotic ointment
Small dressing for covering stab wounds

■ **PREPARATION OF PATIENT**

Explain the procedure to the conscious patient and give instruction about how to cooperate with the procedure.
Empty the bladder with a Foley catheter (Figure 23-1).
Empty the stomach with a nasogastric or orogastric tube.

■ **PROCEDURE**

1. Prepare the anterior abdominal wall by cleansing with a surgical solution such as 1% povidone-iodine (Betadine) and draping with sterile towels.
2. Inject 5 ml of 1% lidocaine with epinephrine in a subcutaneous wheal to 2 to 3 cm below the umbilicus.
3. Make a 2 cm or larger incision through the skin and subcutaneous adipose tissue to the linea retractor. Provide *absolute* hemostasis. If blood from the incision is allowed to escape, it can give a false indication to the lavage.
4. Engage the trochar into the linea alba at a 30° to 45° angle. (Instruct the patient to tense the abdomen if possible.) Apply rotary motion and pressure until the peritoneum is perforated or place the trochar through a surgical incision.
5. Direct the trochar tip toward the caudad pelvis and slide off the catheter 15 to 20 cm into the peritoneal cavity.
6. Attach a 20 ml syringe and aspirate the catheter. If aspiration yields 20 ml of blood, the tap is considered positive, and the procedure is terminated. If little or no blood is obtained, attach the IV line of 1000 ml Ringer's lactate and infuse over 15 minutes. Manually manipulate the abdomen to permit the solution to mix with abdominal cavity fluids.
7. Place the IV solution flask on the floor to siphon off the infused fluid.
8. When the majority of the fluid is returned, remove the catheter.
9. Close the skin with a 4-0 nylon suture.
10. Dress stab wounds with antibiotic ointment and a small sterile dressing.

Analysis of Findings

- **LABORATORY METHOD**
  The laboratory method requires three samples for analysis.

Hematocrit and red blood cell (RBC) count.	The level of hematocrit and RBCs that is considered significant for surgery will depend upon institutional policy.
White blood cell count	500/cu mm or more
Amylase	200 Somogyi units or more
Bile	Any free bile
Culture and Gram's stain	Any significant quantity of bacteria indicates perforation of the intestine.

Indications for Exploratory Laparotomy

Unexplained hemorrhagic shock
Peritoneal perforation
Increasing abdominal tenderness or rigidity
Evidence of peritonitis
Visualized free air in the abdomen
Definitive diagnostic peritoneal lavage or CT scan
Enlarging abdominal mass in the absence of pelvic or vertebral fractures
Progressive drop in hemoglobin and hematocrit in the absence of hypotension, especially in the second 24 hours after injury

Blunt abdominal trauma is rarely a singular event. Head and chest trauma or other life-threatening injuries may complicate assessment. Abdominal injuries account for 10% of all trauma-related deaths in the U.S.; hemorrhage is the most common cause of death.

PENETRATING TRAUMA

Civilian violence, particularly in urban settings, accounts for most penetrating abdominal trauma, with gunshot wounds being the most lethal. A thorough inspection of the patient's front and back should allow for examination and documentation of all entrance and exit wounds. Surgical exploration is recommended, as 96% to 98% of penetrating abdominal gunshot wounds produce significant intraabdominal injury. Stab wounds cause less significant injury, most often to the intestine, and require surgical intervention less frequently.

As with all major trauma patients, treat the patient with the standards of:
Airway management
Supplemental oxygen
Control of bleeding
Initiation of two large bore IVs
Protection of the cervical, thoracic, and lumbar spine
Saline-to-dry dressings on eviscerated tissue
Consideration of PASG (in accordance with institutional protocol)
Preparation for surgery

In the prehospital setting, most of these therapeutic interventions should be accomplished en route to the hospital. While therapeutic interventions are ongoing, someone should be trying to ascertain the type and size of weapon used, the amount of elapsed time since the injury, and the amount of estimated external blood loss.

THE ORGANS IN ABDOMINAL TRAUMA

The Stomach

Because the stomach is a hollow organ and can readily be displaced, it is rarely injured in blunt trauma to the abdomen. It is, however, often injured when trauma to the abdomen is penetrating. To check for stomach damage, insert a nasogastric tube and examine the aspirate. An abdominal x-ray might also prove useful if free air is seen, which is indicative of stomach or intestinal injury.

The Liver

The liver is the largest solid organ in the body. It is often injured in both blunt and abdominal trauma because it is located anteriorly, is large, very dense, and part of it is relatively unprotected. Be particularly suspicious of a liver injury when the eighth through twelfth ribs on the right are damaged and when trauma has involved the upper central abdomen.

Liver injury is diagnosed definitively on CT scan and at surgery. Large stellate lacerations must be surgically repaired, but small lacerations may be self-healing.

The Spleen

The spleen is the intraabdominal organ most frequently injured by blunt force. It is a very dense, encapsulated organ located behind the eighth through tenth ribs in the left upper abdominal quadrant, and injury should be suspected following any blow to the left upper quadrant. Pain and tenderness in the left upper quadrant that radiates to the left shoulder (Kehr's sign), along with peritoneal irritation and hypotension, aid in the diagnosis. Definitive diagnosis is made by CT scan or surgery. On occasion it may be advised to observe a patient with a splenic injury, provided that the patient is hemodynamically stable. Close observation and repeated CT scans are in order. Splenic preservation may prevent future immune response problems in the future.

The Pancreas

The pancreas is rarely injured in blunt abdominal trauma, but may be injured in penetrating trauma. The pancreas is a solid organ that is well protected by the stomach and the liver. It is located retroperitoneally, so that damage will not be evidenced on peritoneal lavage. Pancreatitis, a main concern of pancreatic injury, exhibits the delayed symptoms of pain, nausea/vomiting, abdominal distension, and altered vital signs. Serum amylase will elevate over 24 to 48 hours.

The Kidneys

The kidneys are located retroperitoneally in the flank area. They may be contused, which is usually self-limiting, or lacerated (fractured), which may require surgery. Contusion is usually treated with forced fluids and bed rest. A lacerated kidney may cause hemorrhage or may cause urine to extravasate, depending on the location and extent of the laceration. Diagnosis of the laceration is made by IVP or CT scan and urinalysis. Surgery may range from repair to nephrectomy.

The Ureters

Because the ureters are hollow and quite flexible, they are not usually injured in blunt trauma to the abdomen. They may, however, be disrupted in penetrating trauma. Diagnosis is made by IVP. If disruption occurs, surgery for reanastomosis is indicated.

The Bladder

The bladder, although a hollow organ, often contains urine, which essentially converts it to a solid organ, making it more vulnerable to injury in blunt trauma to the abdomen. It is also at great risk for injury when pelvic fractures occur. Bladder rupture is diagnosed by cystogram. If there is a laceration or rupture, surgical repair is indicated.

The Urethra

Urethral disruptions are more common in males than in females because of the external location of the urethra in males. It usually results from a straddle injury, such as occurs with impact of the crossbar on a bicycle or a motorcycle. Diagnosis is made by retrograde urethrogram. If disruption is present, urology consult is indicated.

The Intestines

The large and small intestines are hollow organs, but they are frequently injured in both blunt and penetrating trauma because of their size, anterior and relatively unprotected position, points of fixation, and vascularity. Intestinal disruptions must be repaired to control hemorrhage and to cleanse the abdominal cavity of abdominal contents that may later cause peritonitis and severe infections. Although abdominal x-rays, peritoneal lavage, and abdominal CT scan are used in diagnosis, definitive diagnosis is made by exploratory laparotomy.

The Diaphragm

Diaphragmatic ruptures may cause severe complications and even death because abdominal contents may herniate into the chest cavity, causing severe respiratory difficulty. In addition, the diaphragm is the main muscle of respiration and is required in order for respiration to occur. Diagnosis is made by observing bowel in the chest cavity or the distal end of the nasogastric or orogastric tube in the chest on chest x-ray.

The Abdominal Aorta, Inferior Vena Cava, and Hepatic Veins

These are the major blood vessels of the abdomen. If disrupted, hemorrhage will occur; and death will ensue if the injury is not corrected. They can be diagnosed by diagnostic peritoneal lavage, CT scan, and aortography. If disruption is present, immediate surgery is indicated.

SOME CONSIDERATION FOR THE PREGNANT PATIENT WITH ABDOMINAL TRAUMA

• A fetus may cause compression of abdominal vasculature and result in obstructive hypovolemia. Whenever possible, elevate the woman's right hip or manually displace the uterus to allow for venous return to the right side of the heart.
• If the woman is hypovolemic and requires volume replacement, administer blood products as soon as possible. Both the woman and the fetus require the oxygen-carrying capacity of the blood.
• Remember to shield the uterus with a lead shield as much as possible during x-ray procedures.
• Continue to monitor the fetus throughout the resuscitation and treatment period.
• Consider inflating only the leg chambers of the PASG, if PASG is local protocol for abdominal trauma.

Abdominal trauma is a frequent finding, especially following motor vehicle crashes. Careful attention to physical examination and diagnostic findings is essential.

SUGGESTED READINGS

Hanna, S: Diagnosis of abdominal trauma. In McMurtry R, McLellan B, eds: *Management of blunt trauma.* Baltimore, 1990, Williams and Wilkins.

Morgan A, Pepe J, eds: Diagnostic techniques in blunt and penetrating abdominal trauma, *Topics Emerg Med* 15(1):8-21, 1993.

Sklarov D, Kidd P: Elimination, metabolism and sexuality: gastrointestinal and genitourinary. In Neff J, Kidd P, eds. *Trauma nursing: the art and science.* St Louis, 1993, Mosby.

Trunkey D, Hill A, Schecter W: Abdominal trauma and indicators for celiotomy. In Moore E, Matton K, Feliciano D: *Trauma.* E. Norwalk, Conn, 1991, Appleton and Lange.

Extremity Trauma

Limb trauma can occur in any age group and at almost any time. It is probably the greatest source of disability in the United States. Prompt, accurate management may not only save life and limb, but may also prevent later severe disability.

DEFINITIONS

Skeleton

The skeleton forms the framework of the body; it provides both support and protection.

Bone

There are two types of bone: (1) cancellous (spongy) bone, which can be found in the skull, vertebrae, pelvis, and long-bone ends; and (2) cortical (dense) bone, which is found in the long bones. Bone has its own blood and nerve supply and is usually capable of healing itself. Bones serve to protect vital organs and serve as levers for movement.

Ligament

Ligament is fibrous connective tissue that connects bone to bone.

Tendon

Tendon is fibrous connective tissue that connects muscle to bone.

Cartilage

Cartilage is dense connective tissue found between the ribs; in the nasal septum, ear, larynx, trachea, and bronchi; between vertebrae; and on the articulating surfaces of bones. Cartilage has no neurovascular supply.

Joints

A joint is the connection of two bones for mobility and stability; it may provide flexion and extension, medial and lateral rotation, and abduction and adduction. A joint consists of articulating bone surfaces that are covered with cartilage, a two-layered sac containing synovial membranes (to lubricate), and a capsule that thickens and becomes a ligament. Muscles that overlie joints attach the bone surfaces to one another and provide movement.

EMERGENCY MANAGEMENT

In the prehospital treatment of a patient with limb trauma, it is important to obtain a brief history and discover the mechanism of injury. Early treatment includes:

ABCs

Quick assessment for other major trauma (head, cervical spine, chest, and abdomen)

Protection of the head and cervical spine

Immobilization of the traumatized limb above and below the trauma site

Evaluation of the vascular status of the limb, before and after immobilization:

Pulses distal to the trauma

Color

Temperature

Capillary refill

Evaluation of the neurologic status of the limb before and after immobilization

Elevation of the limb if possible

Cold pack application to the area

Transportation to the hospital

Immobilization is accomplished before movement or transport to prevent further damage and to reduce the amount of pain.

Note must be made of any swelling, discoloration, contusions, abrasion, or obvious deformities. If the trauma is obviously an open fracture:

Culture the wound site.

Irrigate the wound site with normal saline.

Apply a dry, sterile dressing over the wound.

Apply a slight compression dressing.

Splint the limb.

Do not attempt to reduce the fracture in the field.

If a puncture wound is present but no bone is protruding, assume that the wound was made by a jagged bone end or missile, and treat it as an open fracture. To control bleeding:

Apply pressure over the bleeding site or on the edges of the wound.

Elevate the extremity if possible.

Use tourniquet only as a life-saving measure.

Retrieve any bone fragments at the scene and transport to hospital. Place all fragments in clean plastic bag with ice.

SOFT-TISSUE INJURIES

Soft-tissue injuries include injuries to the skin and underlying tissues, muscles, tendons, cartilage, ligaments, veins, arteries, or nerves.

Immediate General Treatment of Soft-Tissue Injuries

Ensure ABCs.
Control bleeding.
Secure any impaling object.
Apply a dry, sterile dressing.
Elevate the injured part if possible.
Apply a cold pack.
Check the patient's tetanus prophylaxis status.

Abrasion

An abrasion is caused by rubbing of skin against a hard surface, scraping the epithelial layer away and exposing the epidermal or dermal layer; it is similar to a second-degree burn.

■ **THERAPEUTIC INTERVENTIONS**
Wound cleansing (scrub and irrigate)
Removal of foreign bodies
Topical antibiotic ointments
Nonadherent dressing
Dressing change once a day until eschar forms
Avoiding sunlight to damaged area for 6 months because of hypopigmentation

Avulsion

Avulsion is full-thickness skin loss; a cutting or gouging injury resulting from penetration of a sharp object or "pulling away" of a section of skin.

■ **THERAPEUTIC INTERVENTIONS**
Wound cleansing (scrub and irrigate)
Debridement
Restoration of divided deep structures (muscles and tendons)
Split-thickness skin graft of flap
Bulky dressing

Contusion

A contusion is extravasation of blood into tissues where vessels are damaged, but skin is not disrupted.

■ **THERAPEUTIC INTERVENTIONS**
Cold pack
Analgesia
No dressing

Laceration

Laceration is an open wound or a cut through the dermal layer.
■ **THERAPEUTIC INTERVENTIONS**
Control of bleeding (pressure and elevation)
Evaluation of neurovascular status
Anesthesia
Inspection
Cleansing (scrub and irrigate)
Removal of foreign bodies
Excision of necrotic margins
Approximation
Closing (steri-strip or suture)
Dressing

Puncture

Puncture is the penetration of the skin by a pointed or sharp object. It may appear innocent but may have damaged underlying structures, or may be grossly contaminated. A puncture wound rarely bleeds.
■ **THERAPEUTIC INTERVENTIONS**
Depends on depth of penetration and amount of contamination
Generally:
    Soaking in surgical soap solution twice a day for 2 to 4 days
    Removal of foreign bodies (taped to chart)
If contaminated:
    Soaking
    Anesthesia
    Cleansing (scrub and irrigate)
    Inspection
    Removal of foreign bodies
    Excision of necrotic tissue
    Drain placement
    Packing
If the object is impaled, leave it in place until it can be thoroughly evaluated.

Abscess

An abscess is localized collection of pus.
■ **THERAPEUTIC INTERVENTIONS**
Anesthesia
Drain in dependent position
Removal of elliptical area
Loose packing to allow for drainage
Loose dressing
Antibiotics if patient is febrile

SPECIAL NOTES: Do not wait until an abscess ''points''; if abscess is suspected, drain with a needle if assessment reveals fluctuant mass.

Hematoma

Hematoma is the escape of blood into subcutaneous space.
- **THERAPEUTIC INTERVENTIONS**
Varies, depending on location

COMMON TYPES OF SOFT TISSUE INJURIES

Wringer Injury

- **MECHANISM OF INJURY**
Machine wringer causes a crush injury.
- **THERAPEUTIC INTERVENTIONS**
Check of distal pulse
Check of neurologic status
Wound cleansing
Sterile bulky dressing
Elevation of injured part
Tetanus prophylaxis
Careful observation and follow-up due to possibility of neurovascular impairment (compartment syndrome)

Missile Injury, Gunshot Wound

- **MECHANISM OF INJURY**
These injuries or wounds are usually caused by bullet or explosion fragments or wadded pieces of clothing.
- **THERAPEUTIC INTERVENTIONS**
Check of distal pulse
Check of neurologic status
Assessment of limb if possible
Wound cleansing
Dry, dressing
Tetanus prophylaxis
Further surgical assessment

Impaling Injury

- **MECHANISM OF INJURY**
This type of injury is caused by a fall onto a sharp, immobile object.
- **THERAPEUTIC INTERVENTIONS**
Immobilization of extremity
Securing of impaling object (not to be removed if possible)
Check of neurovascular status of limbs distal to injury
Tetanus prophylaxis
Consider surgical intervention

Crush Injury

■ **MECHANISM OF INJURY**
This injury is caused by a heavy object falling on a body part.

■ **THERAPEUTIC INTERVENTIONS**
Check of distal pulses
Check of neurologic function
Control of bleeding
Dry, sterile bulky dressing
Elevation of limb if possible
Cold pack
Tetanus prophylaxis

Knee Injury (Figures 24-1 and 24-2)

■ **MECHANISM OF INJURY**
Knee injuries are caused by rotational or hyperflexion trauma.

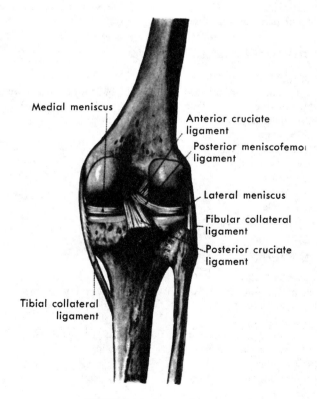

Medial meniscus

Anterior cruciate
ligament

Posterior meniscofemoi
ligament

Lateral meniscus

Fibular collateral
ligament

Posterior cruciate
ligament

Tibial collateral
ligament

FIGURE 24-1. Anterior knee joint.

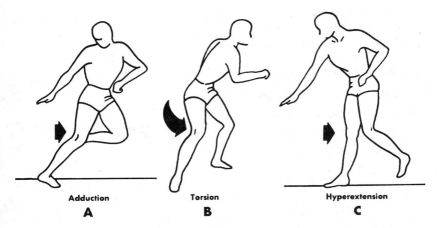

FIGURE 24-2. Mechanisms of knee sprains. **A**, Direct laterial force on knee causes torn medial collateral ligament. **B**, Knee rotation injury may cause lateral, collateral, and medial collateral ligament injury. **C**, Posterior cruciate ligament mechanisms of injury.

■ **COMMON TYPES**
  Medical meniscus injury from rotational trauma
  Collateral ligament injury: medial from valgus stress, lateral from varus stress
  Anterior and posterior cruciate ligament injury from hyperextension trauma
■ **SIGNS AND SYMPTOMS**
  Swelling
  Ecchymosis
  Effusion
  Pain
  Tenderness
■ **THERAPEUTIC INTERVENTIONS**
  Compression bandage
  Elevation
  Cold pack
  No weight bearing
  Orthopedic consult for possible surgical repair

Fingertip Injury
High-pressure paint gun injury

■ **MECHANISM OF INJURY**
  Injection of a stream of paint into fingertip and up into the hand, wrist, and arm. The injury appears only as a small pinhole in the tip of the finger.

■ **THERAPEUTIC INTERVENTIONS**

Keep limb lower than heart level

Check for radial and brachial pulses

Check for neurologic status

Immediate evaluation by a physician for possible surgical intervention

Crush injury of distal phalanx

■ **MECHANISM OF INJURY**

This injury is caused by a crushing force from a heavy object on the distal phalanx.

■ **THERAPEUTIC INTERVENTIONS**

Soft, bulky dressing

Elevation

Nail trephination if a hematoma forms under fingernail (subungual hematoma)

Nail trephination

Equipment

Nail drill, scalpel, or paper clip

Alcohol lamp if paper clip is used

Procedure

1. Prepare the nail with antiseptic solution.
2. Penetrate the nail:
   a. With nail drill
   b. With scalpel, using rotation motion
   c. With paper clip after it is heated red hot
3. Release the pressure caused by the hematoma.
4. Dress with an adhesive bandage.
5. Elevate the fingernail.

Strains

Strains are a weakening or stretching of a muscle at the tendon area.

Mild strain

■ **SIGNS AND SYMPTOMS**

Local pain

Point tenderness

Spasm

■ **THERAPEUTIC INTERVENTIONS**

Compression bandage

Elevation for 12 hours

Cold pack for 12 hours

Weight bearing

Moderate strain

■ **SIGNS AND SYMPTOMS**

Point tenderness

Local pain

Swelling
Discoloration
Inability to use for a short time
■ **THERAPEUTIC INTERVENTIONS**
Compression bandage
Elevation for 24 hours
Cold pack for 24 hours
Analgesia
Light weight bearing

Severe strain

■ **SIGNS AND SYMPTOMS**
Point tenderness
Local pain
Swelling
Discoloration
Snapping noise at time of injury
■ **THERAPEUTIC INTERVENTIONS**
Compression bandage
Elevation for 24 to 48 hours
Cold pack for 48 hours
Analgesia
No weight bearing for 48 hours

Sprains

A mild sprain is a stretching of a ligament that has been forced beyond its normal limit, causing tearing. A moderate sprain is a ligament that has been partially torn. A severe sprain is a ligament that has been completely torn.
  Most common sprains involve ankle, knee, shoulder, and wrist joints.

Mild sprain

■ **SIGNS AND SYMPTOMS**
Slight pain
Slight swelling
■ **THERAPEUTIC INTERVENTIONS**
Compression bandage
Elevation for 12 hours
Cold pack for 24 hours
Light weight bearing

Moderate sprain

■ **SIGNS AND SYMPTOMS**
Pain
Point tenderness
Swelling
Inability to use for a short time

■ **THERAPEUTIC INTERVENTIONS**
Compression bandage/air cast splint
Elevation for 24 to 48 hours
Cold pack for 24 to 48 hours
Crutches
Non–weight bearing gradually progressing to full weight bearing over 5 to 7 days.

Severe sprain (Figure 24-3)

■ **SIGNS AND SYMPTOMS**
Pain
Point tenderness
Swelling
Discoloration

■ **THERAPEUTIC INTERVENTIONS**
Compression bandages, air cast or cast
Elevation for 48 hours (or as long as swelling persists)
Cold pack for 48 hours
Crutches
No weight bearing for as long as moderate pain and swelling persist

Achilles Tendon Rupture

■ **MECHANISM OF INJURY**
This injury usually occurs in stop-and-start sports (such as tennis or racquetball) in which one steps off abruptly on the forefoot with the knee forced into extension.

■ **SIGNS AND SYMPTOMS**
Sharp pain

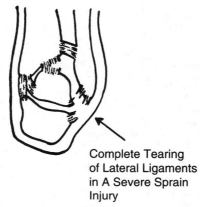

Complete Tearing
of Lateral Ligaments
in A Severe Sprain
Injury

FIGURE 24-3. Ankle sprain, torn ligaments in ankle joint. Posterior view.

Inability to "toe-up" (push off on toes)
Deformity along Achilles (palpable deficit)
Positive Thompson's sign*
■ **THERAPEUTIC INTERVENTIONS**
Compression
Elevation
Cold pack
Crutches
Orthopedic surgery referral

PERIPHERAL NERVE INJURIES

Peripheral nerve injuries (Table 24-1) can be caused by trauma (mechanical, chemical, or thermal), toxins, malignancy, metabolic disorders, or collagen disease. In the emergency situation they are usually associated with lacerations, fractures, dislocations, and penetrating wounds.

Accurate assessment requires an understanding of the distribution of nerves, the origin of motor branches, and the muscles they supply.

Diagnostic tests such as electromyography, nerve conduction tests, and electrical stimulation are of little or no value in the emergency evaluation of peripheral nerve injury.

Repair of peripheral nerves should not be undertaken as an emergency department surgical intervention.

* Positive Thompson's sign: With the leg extended and the foot over the end of a table, squeeze the calf muscle; no heel pull or upward movement will be seen.

TABLE 24-1   Modes for Assessing Common Peripheral Nerve Injuries

NERVE	FREQUENTLY ASSOCIATED INJURIES	ASSESSMENT TECHNIQUE*
Radial	Fracture of humerus, especially middle and distal thirds	Inability to extend thumb in "hitchhiker's sign"
Ulnar	Fracture of medial humeral epicondyle	Loss of pain perception in tip of little finger
Median	Elbow dislocation or wrist or forearm injury	Loss of pain perception in tip of index finger
Peroneal	Tibia or fibula fracture, dislocation of knee	Inability to extend great toe or foot; may also be associated with sciatic nerve injury
Sciatic and tibial	Infrequent with fractures or dislocations	Loss of pain perception in sole of foot

*Test is invalid if extension tendons are severed or if severe muscle damage is present.

FRACTURES

Fractures are divided into two general categories:

Categories

1. Closed (simple)—the skin is not disrupted.
2. Open (compound)—the skin is disrupted by:
   a. A bone puncturing from the inside out
   b. An object puncturing from the outside in, with resultant fracture

Types of Fractures

Transverse

Results from angulation force or direct trauma.

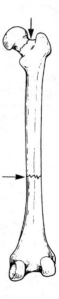

Oblique

Results from twisting force.

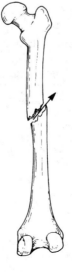

Spiral

Results from twisting force with firmly planted foot.

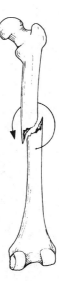

Comminuted

Results from severe direct trauma; has more than two fragments.

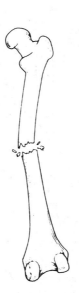

Impacted

Results from severe trauma causing fracture ends to jam together.

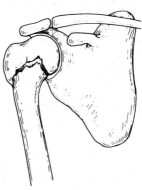

Compressed

Results from severe force to top of head or os calcis or from acceleration/deceleration injury.

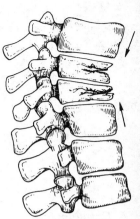

Greenstick

Results from compression force; usually occurs in children under 10 years of age.

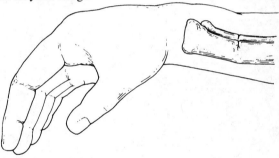

Avulsion

Results from muscle mass contracting forcefully, causing bone fragment to tear off at insertion. Ligament can tear fragment from bone rather than rupturing.

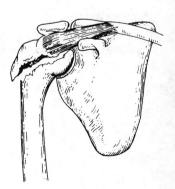

Depression

Results from blunt trauma to a flat bone; usually involves much soft-tissue damage.

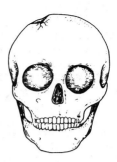

■ **ASSESSMENT**

When treating a patient with a suspected limb fracture, always assess for the "five Ps":

1. Pain and point tenderness
2. Pulse (distal to the fracture site)
3. Pallor
4. Paresthesia (distal to the fracture site)
5. Paralysis (distal to the fracture site)

The following factors should also be included in assessment:

Deformity
Swelling
Crepitus
Discoloration
Open wounds
Other injuries

■ **GENERAL THERAPEUTIC INTERVENTIONS**

Assess the patient as described above.

Determine the mechanism of injury.

Immobilize the limb (above and below the fracture site).

Reassess the neurovascular status.

Apply traction if circulatory compromise is present.

Elevate the injured limb if possible (to decrease swelling and hemorrhage).

Apply a cold pack (to cause vasoconstriction and decrease swelling, spasm, and pain).

■ **COMPLICATIONS OF FRACTURES**

Blood loss causing hypovolemia and shock

Injury to vital organs

Neurologic and/or vascular damage

Infection (in open fractures)

Poor fracture healing may be a result of:

Improper immobilization
Poor reduction
Increased length of immobility
Too much traction
Decreased vascular supply
Decreased neurologic supply
Infection

Fat embolism

Fat embolism may occur 24 to 48 hours after trauma and usually results from a pelvic, tibial, or femoral fracture. Fat embolism may be a life-threatening situation; it has a high mortality.

■ **SIGNS AND SYMPTOMS**
Elevated temperature
Rapid pulse
Decreasing level of consciousness
Ineffective respirations leading to respiratory failure
Restlessness
Cough
Dyspnea
Cyanosis
Pulmonary edema
Petechiae

■ **THERAPEUTIC INTERVENTIONS**
Oxygen at high flow
Supportive therapy
Steroids (in some facilities)
Heparin (in some facilities)

Compartment syndrome

Compartment syndrome is a condition in which circulation to the limb is obstructed. This usually results from pressure within the tissues of the limb and restriction of the expansion of the ''compartment,'' causing tissue hypoxia and eventual necrosis. This is an acute emergency.

Compartment syndrome occurs most commonly when there is massive soft-tissue trauma, when there is a long bone fracture, or in massive burn injuries. Its most frequent location is the anterior compartment and the posterior deep compartment of the lower leg.

■ **SIGNS AND SYMPTOMS**
Pain (especially on dorsiflexion or passive stretch, or after exercise)
Pallor
Pulselessness (or diminished pulse volume)
Paresthesia
Paralysis
Diagnosis is made by compartment pressure monitoring, using a saline-filled manometer. Normal compartment tissue pressure is 12 to 20 cm H_2O.

■ **THERAPEUTIC INTERVENTIONS**
If compartment tissue pressure exceeds diastolic blood pressure, emergency fasciotomy is indicated to decompress compartment pressure.

Specific Fractures

Clavicle Fracture

■ **MECHANISM OF INJURY**
Fall on arm or shoulder
Direct trauma to shoulder laterally

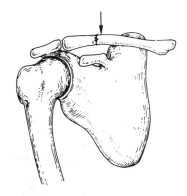

- ■ **SIGNS AND SYMPTOMS**
  Pain in clavicular area
  Point tenderness
  Refusal to raise arm
  Swelling
  Deformity
  Crepitus
- ■ **THERAPEUTIC INTERVENTIONS**
  Assessment of neurovascular status
  Support of arm
  Sling, figure-of-eight bandage or both
  Cold pack
- ■ **COMPLICATIONS**
  Injury to adjacent neuromuscular tissue (rare)
- ■ **SPECIAL NOTES**
  Pad the axillary area well to avoid damage to the brachial plexus and artery.

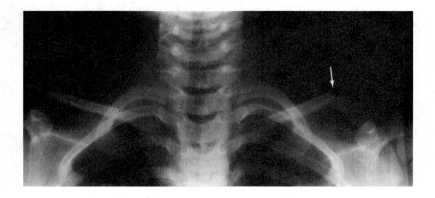

Shoulder fracture (glenoid, humeral head, or humeral neck)

- **MECHANISM OF INJURY**
  Fall on outstretched arm
  Direct trauma to shoulder

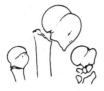

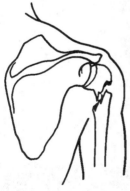

- **SIGNS AND SYMPTOMS**
  Pain in shoulder area
  Point tenderness
  Inability to move arm
  Gross swelling
  Discoloration
- **THERAPEUTIC INTERVENTIONS**
  Assessment of neurovascular status
  Sling and swath
  Cold pack

■ **COMPLICATIONS**

Humeral neck fracture may cause axillary nerve damage.

■ **SPECIAL NOTES**

Shoulder fractures occur in trauma to the shoulder in the elderly because of weaker bone structure; the same mechanisms of injury in a younger person would probably only cause shoulder dislocation.

Scapula fracture

■ **MECHANISM OF INJURY**

Direct trauma

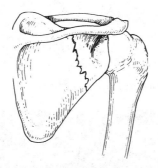

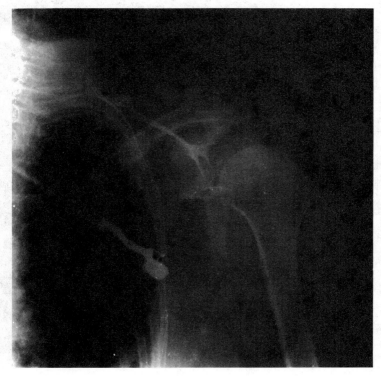

■ **SIGNS AND SYMPTOMS**
  Point tenderness
  Bone displacement
  Pain on shoulder movement
  Swelling
■ **THERAPEUTIC INTERVENTIONS**
  Assessment of neurovascular status
  Sling and swath
  Cold pack
  Axillary care
■ **COMPLICATIONS**
  Underlying injury of ribs and viscera
■ **SPECIAL NOTES**
  Radial nerve damage is demonstrated by decreased sensation in web space and
  inability to extend thumb, fingers, and wrist.

Upper arm (humeral shaft) fracture

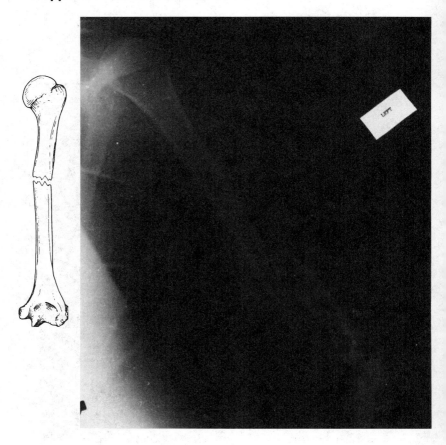

- **MECHANISM OF INJURY**
  Fall on arm and direct trauma
- **SIGNS AND SYMPTOMS**
  Pain
  Point tenderness
  Swelling
  Inability or hesitance to move arm
  Severe deformity or angulation
  Crepitus
- **THERAPEUTIC INTERVENTIONS**
  Assessment of neurovascular status
  Sling and swath
  Traction if there is vascular compromise
  Assessment for other injuries, especially to the chest
  Cold pack
- **COMPLICATIONS**
  Radial nerve damage if fracture occurs in the middle or distal portion of the
     shaft
  Hemorrhage

Elbow fracture

- **MECHANISM OF INJURY**
  Fall on extended arm
  Fall on flexed elbow
- **SIGNS AND SYMPTOMS**
  Pain
  Point tenderness

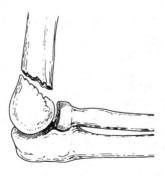

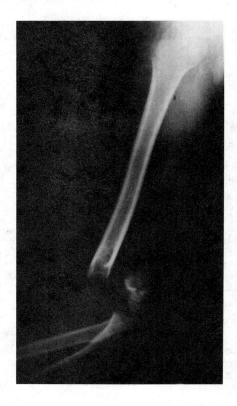

Swelling
Refusal to move elbow
Deformity
Decreased circulation to hand
■ **THERAPEUTIC INTERVENTIONS**
Assessment of neurovascular status
Splinting "as it lies," usually with pillow, blanket, or sling and swath
Cold pack
Flexing of arm to greater degree if there is neurovascular compromise

■ **COMPLICATIONS**
Brachial artery laceration
Median and/or radial nerve damage
Volkmann's contracture*

Forearm (radius or ulna) fracture

■ **MECHANISM OF INJURY**
Fall on extended arm
Direct blow

* In Volkmann's contracture degeneration and contraction of muscles occur as a result of ischemia caused by decreased arterial blood flow.

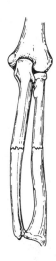

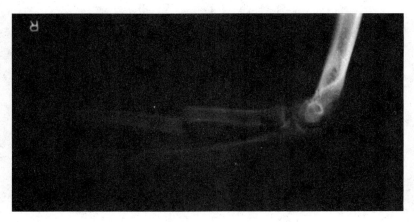

■ **SIGNS AND SYMPTOMS**
  Pain
  Point tenderness
  Swelling
  Deformity or angulation
  Shortening
■ **THERAPEUTIC INTERVENTIONS**
  Assessment of neurovascular status
  Splint
  Sling
  Cold pack
■ **COMPLICATIONS**
  Rare neurovascular compromise
  Volkmann's contracture

Wrist (distal radius, distal ulna, carpal bone) fracture

■ **MECHANISM OF INJURY**
  Fall on extended arm and open hand
■ **SIGNS AND SYMPTOMS**
  Pain
  Swelling
  Deformity
  "Snuff box" tenderness in navicular (scaphoid) fracture
■ **THERAPEUTIC INTERVENTIONS**
  Assessment of neurovascular status
  Splint "as it lies"
  Sling
  Cold pack
  Compression

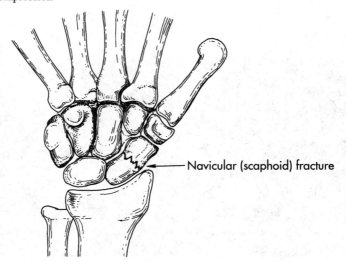

Navicular (scaphoid) fracture

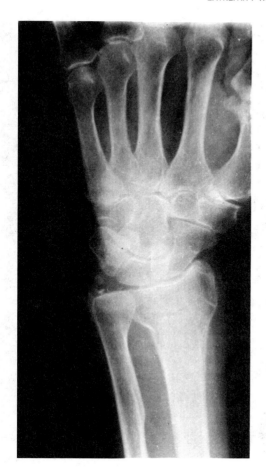

■ **COMPLICATION**
Rare aseptic necrosis

■ **SPECIAL NOTES**
Fracture of the distal radius and ulna is known as a Colles' fracture or silver fork deformity.

Check the mechanism of injury. The patient may have had a fall from a height that originally resulted in a heel (os calcis) fracture, a lumbodorsal compression fracture, and a fall forward into the open hand from the back pain, resulting in a Colles' fracture.

Hand (carpals and metacarpals) fracture or finger fracture (phalanges)

■ **MECHANISM OF INJURY**
Fracture of the fifth metacarpal ("boxer's" fracture)

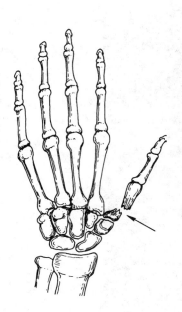

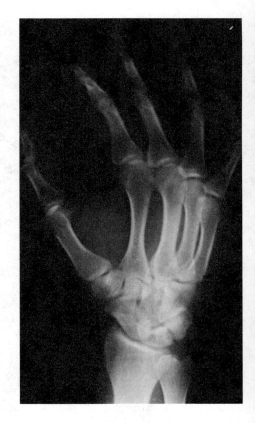

- ■ **SIGNS AND SYMPTOMS**
  Pain
  Severe swelling
  Deformity
  Inability to use hand
  Often open fracture
- ■ **THERAPEUTIC INTERVENTIONS**
  Assessment of neurovascular status
  Control of bleeding
  Dry, bulky dressing on open wounds
  Splint in functional position
  Cold pack
  Pressure

Pelvic fracture

- ■ **MECHANISM OF INJURY**
  Crush injury
  Automobile or motorcycle accident

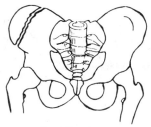

Iliac Wing fx.

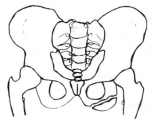

Inferior Pubic Rami fx.

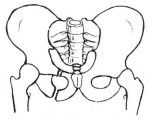

Shear fx. Inferior, Superior
Rami. Sacro Iliac Joint fx.

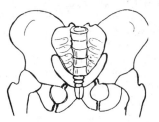

Saddle fx. Billaterial
Inferior Rami fx.

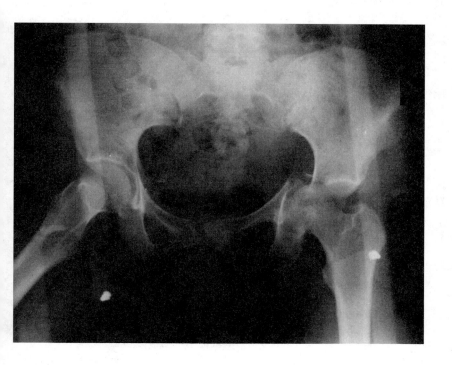

Direct trauma
Fall from height
Sudden contraction of muscle against resistance
■ **SIGNS AND SYMPTOMS**
Tenderness over pubis or when iliac wings are compressed
Paraspinous muscle spasm
Sacroiliac joint tenderness
Paresis or hemiparesis
Pelvic ecchymosis
Hematuria
■ **THERAPEUTIC INTERVENTIONS**
Oxygen/IV fluids
Immobilization of spine and legs (long board)
Flexing knees to decrease pain
Frequent (every 5 minutes) monitoring of vital signs
Check for other fractures and injuries (especially internal)
PASG if indicated
Peritoneal lavage
Type and cross-match
■ **COMPLICATIONS**
Internal bleeding (average blood loss, 2 units)
Bladder trauma
Genital trauma
Lumbosacral trauma
Ruptured internal organs
Shock
Death

Hip fracture

■ **MECHANISM OF INJURY**
In elderly, usually from a fall or minor trauma
In younger people, usually from major trauma
■ **SIGNS AND SYMPTOMS**
Pain in hip or groin area
Severe pain with movement
Inability to bear weight
External rotation of hip and leg
Minimal shortening of limb
If injury is extracapsular and associated with trochanteric fracture:
    Pain in lateral area of hip
    Increased shortening
    Greater external rotation
■ **THERAPEUTIC INTERVENTIONS**
Immobilization
Splint (backboard or one leg to the other)
Check of pulses distal to injury
Frequent (every 5 minutes) monitoring of vital signs

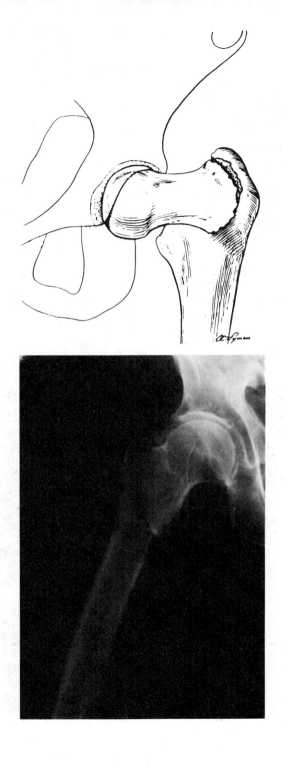

In hospital:
  Early immobilization
  Early surgical intervention
■ **COMPLICATIONS**
  Hypovolemic shock

Femoral fracture

■ **MECHANISM OF INJURY**
  Usually major trauma
■ **SIGNS AND SYMPTOMS**
  Severe pain
  Inability to bear weight on leg
  Swelling
  Deformity

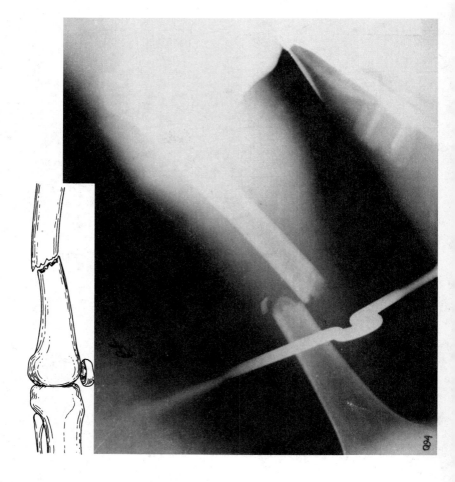

Angulation
Shortening of limb and severe muscle spasm
Crepitus

■ **THERAPEUTIC INTERVENTIONS**
Airway, breathing, and circulation
Traction splint (*do not* use long leg air splint, and *do not* use other leg as splint)
Two large-bore IV lines
Check of distal pulses
Check of distal neurologic status
Check for other injuries
Frequent (every 5 minutes) monitoring of vital signs
Cold pack

■ **COMPLICATIONS**
Hypovolemia (may lose 2 units of blood into thigh)
Severe muscle damage
Knee trauma (overlooked at time of injury)
Shock

Knee fracture (supracondylar fracture of femur, intraarticular fracture of femur or tibia)

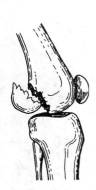

■ **MECHANISM OF INJURY**
Usually automobile, motorcycle, or automobile/pedestrian accident with indirect
    trauma to the knee area
■ **SIGNS AND SYMPTOMS**
Knee pain
Inability to bend or straighten knee
Swelling
Tenderness
■ **THERAPEUTIC INTERVENTIONS**
Long leg splint or one leg splinted to other
Check of distal pulses
Check of distal neurologic status
■ **COMPLICATIONS**
Neurovascular compromise

Patellar fracture

■ **MECHANISM OF INJURY**
Usually direct trauma (fall or impact with dashboard)
Indirect trauma such as a severe muscle pull
■ **SIGNS AND SYMPTOMS**
Pain in knee
Frequently opened fracture
■ **THERAPEUTIC INTERVENTIONS**
Long leg splint
Cover open wound
Cold pack

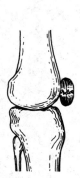

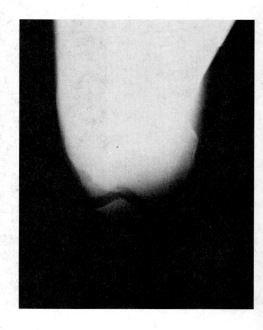

Tibial and/or fibular fracture

- **MECHANISM OF INJURY**
  Direct trauma
  Indirect trauma
  Twisting
- **SIGNS AND SYMPTOMS**
  Pain
  Point tenderness
  Swelling
  Deformity
  Crepitus

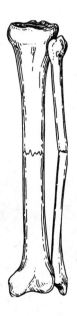

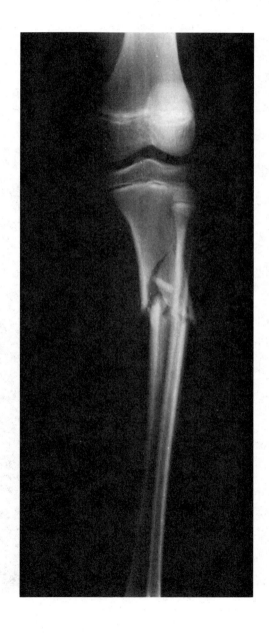

■ **THERAPEUTIC INTERVENTIONS**
Splint as found, if no pulse deficit (long leg splint)
Check of distal pulses; gentle traction only if there is pulse deficit
Sterile dressing over open fracture

■ **COMPLICATIONS**
Soft-tissue damage
Neurovascular compromise

■ **SPECIAL NOTES**
Tibial plateau fractures are usually non-weight-bearing for six months.

Ankle fracture

■ **MECHANISM OF INJURY**
Direct trauma
Indirect trauma
Torsion/inversion/eversion

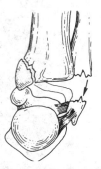

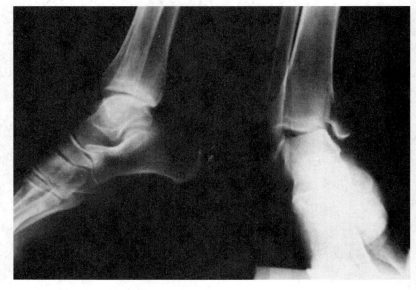

■ **SIGNS AND SYMPTOMS**
Pain
Inability to bear weight
Point tenderness
Swelling
Deformity
■ **THERAPEUTIC INTERVENTIONS**
Splint (soft)
Check of distal pulses; gentle traction if there is pulse deficit
Check of distal neurologic status
Elevation
Cold pack
■ **COMPLICATIONS**
Neurovascular compromise

Foot fracture (metatarsal fracture)

Often associated with ankle injury. *Always* assess foot with ankle.

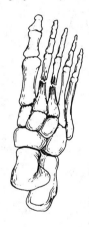

■ **MECHANISM OF INJURY**
Automobile accident
Athletic injury
Crush injury
Direct trauma
■ **SIGNS AND SYMPTOMS**
Pain
Hesitance to bear weight
Point tenderness
Deformity
Swelling
■ **THERAPEUTIC INTERVENTIONS**
Compression dressing
Soft splint

Heel (os calcis) fracture

■ **MECHANISM OF INJURY**
Fall from a height
■ **SIGNS AND SYMPTOMS**
Pain
Swelling
Point tenderness
Dislocation

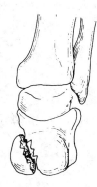

■ **THERAPEUTIC INTERVENTIONS**
Compression dressing
Elevation
Cold pack
■ **COMPLICATIONS**
Often associated with lumbosacral compression fracture

Fracture of toes (phalanges)

■ **MECHANISM OF INJURY**
Kicking hard object
"Stubbing" toe
■ **SIGNS AND SYMPTOMS**
Pain
Swelling
Discoloration
■ **THERAPEUTIC INTERVENTIONS**
Compression dressing
Rigid splint
Elevation
Cold pack

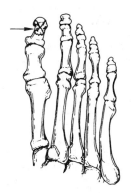

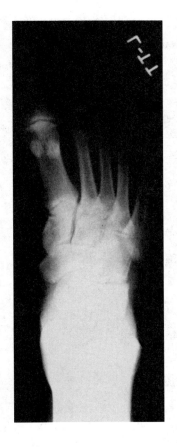
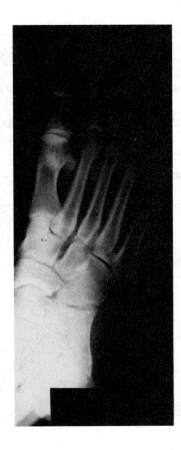

DISLOCATION/SEPARATION

Dislocation occurs when a joint exceeds its range of motion and the joint surfaces are no longer intact. There is usually a large amount of soft-tissue injury in the joint capsule and surrounding ligaments, much swelling, and possible vein, artery, and nerve damage.

■ **SIGNS AND SYMPTOMS**
Severe pain
Deformity at the joint
Inability to move the joint
Swelling
Point tenderness

■ **THERAPEUTIC INTERVENTIONS**
Palpate the joint area carefully.
Splint the joint ''as it lies.''
Do *not* reduce the dislocation in the field.
Early reduction with adequate anesthesia is required in the emergency department.
Check for fractures.
Compare the injured side to the other side.

Specific Dislocations/Separations

Acromioclavicular separation

■ **MECHANISM OF INJURY**
Common athletic injury produced by a fall or a force on point of shoulder.

■ **SIGNS AND SYMPTOMS**
Great pain in joint area
Inability to raise arm or bring arm across chest
Deformity
Point or area tenderness
Swelling
Hematoma

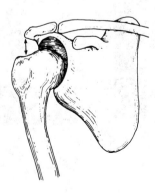

■ **THERAPEUTIC INTERVENTIONS**
   Neurovascular assessment
   Sling and swath
   Cold pack

Shoulder dislocation

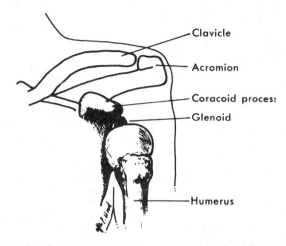

- Clavicle
- Acromion
- Coracoid process
- Glenoid
- Humerus

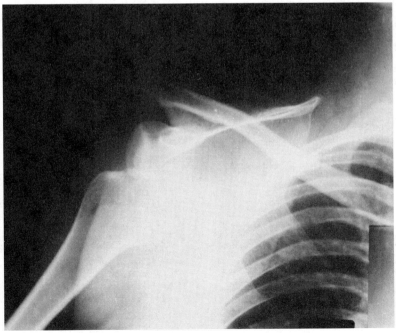

■ **MECHANISM OF INJURY**

Anterior dislocation: usually an athletic injury from a fall on an extended arm that is abducted and externally rotated, resulting in head of humerus locating anterior to shoulder joint. Commonly, this is a recurrent injury.

Posterior dislocation: a rare form of dislocation, usually found in patient with seizure in which extended arm is abducted and internally rotated.

■ **SIGNS AND SYMPTOMS**

Severe pain in shoulder area

Inability to move arm

Deformity (difficult to see in posterior dislocation)

■ **THERAPEUTIC INTERVENTIONS**

Support in position found or position of greatest comfort

Cold pack

Relocation of recurrent dislocation *if* it is easy to do

Check of distal pulses

Check of distal neurovascular status

■ **COMPLICATIONS**

Much soft-tissue damage

Occasional axillary nerve damage

Rare axillary artery damage

Rare brachial plexus damage

Elbow dislocation

■ **MECHANISM OF INJURY**

Fall on an extended arm

Jerking or lifting of a child by a single arm, which causes posterior displacement of the radical head ("nursemaid's elbow")

■ **SIGNS AND SYMPTOMS**

Pain

Swelling

Deformity or lateral displacement

May feel locked

Severe pain produced by movement

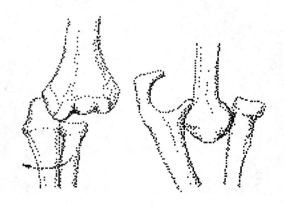

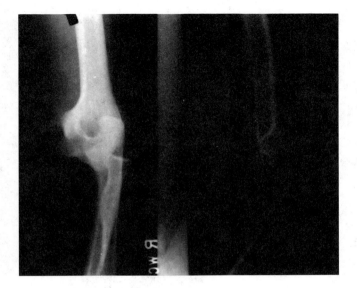

- **THERAPEUTIC INTERVENTIONS**
  Cold pack
  Immobilization
  Check of distal pulses
  Check of distal neurologic status
- **COMPLICATIONS**
  Neurovascular compromise

Wrist dislocation

- **MECHANISM OF INJURY**
  Fall on outreached arm and hand
- **SIGNS AND SYMPTOMS**
  Pain
  Swelling
  Point tenderness
  Deformity
- **THERAPEUTIC INTERVENTIONS**
  Splint
  Sling and swath
  Cold pack
- **COMPLICATIONS**
  Median nerve damage
- **SPECIAL NOTES**
  Median nerve damage is demonstrated by inability to pitch and loss of sensation
  in index and middle fingers.

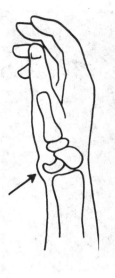
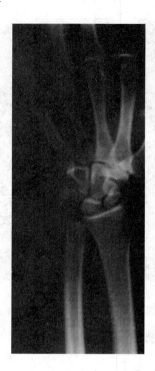

Hand or finger dislocation

- **MECHANISM OF INJURY**
  Fall on outstretched hand or finger
  Direct trauma or ''jamming'' force on fingertip
- **SIGNS AND SYMPTOMS**
  Pain
  Inability to move joint
  Deformity
  Swelling
- **THERAPEUTIC INTERVENTIONS**
  Splint in position of comfort
  Cold pack

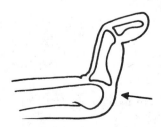

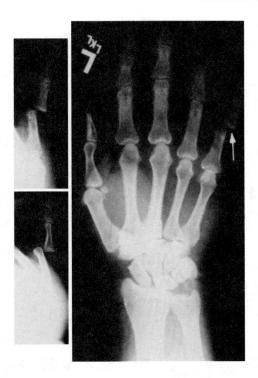

Hip dislocation

- **MECHANISM OF INJURY**
  Usually a major trauma (with extended leg and foot on brake pedal before impact or with knee hitting dashboard)
  Falls
  Crush injuries
- **SIGNS AND SYMPTOMS**
  Pain in hip area
  Pain in knee
  Hip flexed, adducted, and internally rotated (posterior dislocation)
  Hip slightly flexed, abducted, and externally rotated (anterior dislocation)—a rare injury
  Joint feeling locked
  Inability to move leg
- **THERAPEUTIC INTERVENTIONS**
  Splint in position found or in position of comfort.
  Check for distal pulses.
  Check for distal neurologic status.
  Check for other injuries.
  Apply cold pack.

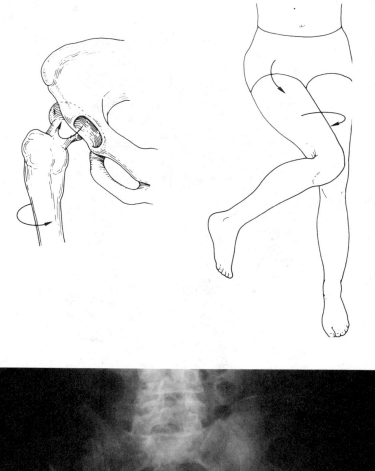

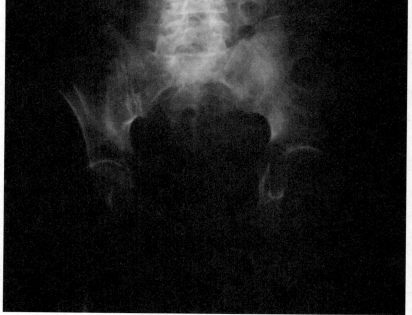

In hospital, relocation within 24 hours or necrosis of femoral head may occur.

■ **COMPLICATIONS**
Sciatic nerve damage
Femoral artery and nerve damage

Knee dislocation

■ **MECHANISM OF INJURY**
Major trauma

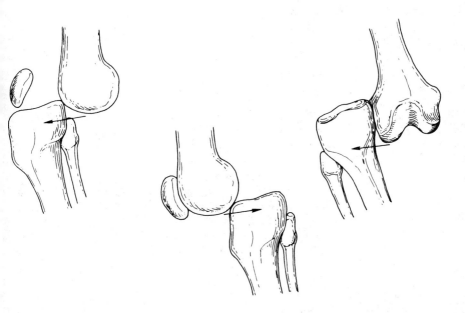

■ **SIGNS AND SYMPTOMS**
Severe pain
Much swelling
Deformity
Inability to move joint

■ **THERAPEUTIC INTERVENTIONS**
Splint in position of comfort.
Check distal pulses.
Check distal neurologic status.
Apply cold pack.
In hospital, early reduction (within 24 hours) to avoid arterial damage.

■ **COMPLICATIONS**
Peroneal nerve damage
Posterior tibial nerve damage
Popliteal artery damage

Patellar dislocation

- **MECHANISM OF INJURY**
  Direct trauma
  Rotation injury on planted foot
- **SIGNS AND SYMPTOMS**
  Pain
  Knee usually in flexed position with inability to function
  Tenderness
  Swelling
- **THERAPEUTIC INTERVENTIONS**
  Splint in position found
  Cold pack

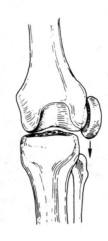

- **COMPLICATIONS**
  Bleeding into knee joint (hemarthrosis)

Ankle dislocation

- **MECHANISM OF INJURY**
  Usually associated with a fracture

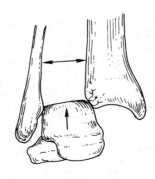

■ **SIGNS AND SYMPTOMS**
Pain
Swelling
Deformity
Inability to move joint
■ **THERAPEUTIC INTERVENTIONS**
Splint in position of comfort
Check of distal pulses
Check of distal neurologic status
Cold pack
■ **COMPLICATIONS**
Neurovascular compromise

Foot dislocation

■ **MECHANISM OF INJURY**
Rare injury
Usually automobile or motorcycle accident
Usually associated with open wound
■ **SIGNS AND SYMPTOMS**
Pain
Tenderness
Swelling
Deformity
Inability to use foot
■ **THERAPEUTIC INTERVENTIONS**
Sterile dressing on open wound
Soft splint
Check of distal pulses
Check of distal neurologic status
Cold pack
■ **COMPLICATIONS**
Neurovascular compromise

PEDIATRIC LIMB TRAUMA

Special attention should be paid to pediatric limb trauma in which fractures occur at the epiphysis, or growth center. A fracture at the epiphysis may cause an early closure of the plate, which results in a shortened extremity as the child grows. If the fracture is only a partial fracture, an angular deformity may result. A child with such a fracture should be followed by an orthopedic surgeon for several months, as it is difficult to predict the outcome at the time of injury.

TRAUMATIC AMPUTATIONS

Traumatic amputations are common to farm workers, factory workers, and motorcyclists; they occur under many different circumstances.

Causes of Traumatic Amputations*

Most amputations are frequently seen with people who work with machines, such as farm workers, industrial workers, and mechanics. However, a substantial number of traumatic amputations are caused by automobile and motorcycle accidents, as well as home accidents caused by lawnmowers or saws. Emergency personnel must take steps to enhance the viability of the severed part so that it can be replanted, if the physician decides on that course of action.

■ **GENERAL THERAPEUTIC INTERVENTIONS**

Ensure airway, breathing, circulation.

Control bleeding.

Support the limb in functional position in partial amputation.

Start two large-bore IV lines, if indicated.

Management of the Severed Part

Intervention in the field

1. Find the severed part (with small digits this is not always easy).
2. Using sterile gloves, debride the part of any gross foreign matter.
3. Wrap the part in a sterile gauze (for digit, ear, etc.), towel, or clean sheet (for larger limbs).
4. Wet the wrapping with sterile normal saline or Ringer's lactate, or rinse part with saline.
5. Place the part in a suitably sized bag or container and seal shut. (Do not immerse part in a solution bath!)
6. Place bag or container inside another container that is filled with ice, if available, or cold water.
7. Transport as soon as the patient's condition is stabilized.
8. A reminder: do not compromise patient care. Life-saving procedures *always* take priority over management of the severed part.

In the emergency department

Assuming the part arrives as outlined above, all that remains to be done is to maintain the temperature of the part at 39° F (4° C). This is easily accomplished by using an ice packing in the outer bag. A hypothermic thermometer will be necessary to monitor the temperature. If the amputated part arrives without prior management, follow the steps previously outlined.

What **not** to do

> *Do not*   place part in tap, distilled, or sterile water
> place in soapy water, formalin, or antiseptic solution
> apply a tourniquet

---

* From Wohlstadter T: Amputations, *JEN* 5(4):36, 1979.

freeze the part

make a judgment as to the viability of the part; this is the physician's decision

immerse part completely in solution bath (this would cause the part to become water-logged)

Survival time

The quality of the preservation of the amputated part will greatly influence its survival time. A well-preserved part without a large amount of muscle tissue (which necroses quickly) can be replanted up to 24 hours after the trauma. However, a nonpreserved part can remain viable for 6 hours at the most.

SPLINTING ORTHOPEDIC INJURIES

Splinting is done to prevent further damage to bone or tissue, prevent damage to nerves, arteries, and veins, and decrease pain. Always splint above and below the injury site.

Splints are divided into four basic types:

Soft splint—soft, not rigid, such as a pillow

Hard splint—firm, rigid surface; such as a board

Air splint—inflatable; provides rigidity without being hard

Traction splint—provides support, decreased angulation, traction

There are many varieties of splint materials and uses, for example:

Thomas, which is used for tibial pin traction

For femoral shaft fractures or fractures of the upper third of the tibia. These should *not* be used on fractures of the hip, lower tibia, fibula, or ankle

Hare

Backboard

Shortboard (or Kendrick extrication device (Figure 24-4)

Longboard

Aluminum long leg

Cardboard

Ladder

Padded board

Air

Vacuum

Improvised

Sling

General Principles of Splint Application

Immobilize the injured part proximal and distal to the injury.

Correct severe angulation only if it is impossible to splint or if vascular compromise is present.

Have a second person place the padding and splint.

Secure the injured part to the splint (do *not* use an elastic bandage).

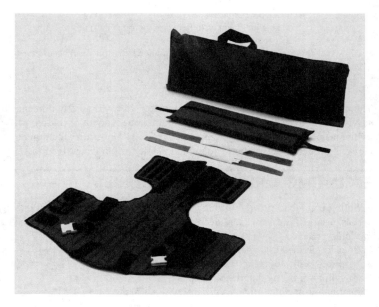

FIGURE 24-4. Kendrick extrication device.

Application of Air Splint (Open on Both Ends*)

Slip the splint over the rescuer's arm backward.
Grasp the distal portion of the injured limb with the arm that has the air splint in place.
Slide the splint onto the injured limb.
Inflate the splint.

PLASTER AND FIBERGLASS CASTS

Refer to a textbook for orthopedic assistants for a complete description of techniques and types of casts.

Application

Ready the plaster or fiberglass impregnated gauze.
Place the stockinette over the casting area and carefully apply cotton roll.
Soak the plaster/fiberglass casting material in warm water.
Apply the cast.
Warn the patient about the "heat" of the casting material.

---

* With a closed-end air splint it is impossible to assess the distal pulses and neurovascular status once the splint is in place.

Allow the cast to dry.

Trim away sharp edges or apply moleskin.

■ **SIGNS AND SYMPTOMS OF PRESSURE SORE**

Elevated temperature

Pain over bony prominences beyond initial few days after injury

Foul odor

Aftercare Instructions for Patients with Casts

Return to the emergency department, the orthopedic clinic, or your private physician in 24 hours for follow-up care.

Keep the cast dry.

Keep the limb elevated above the level of the heart for 24 hours after the injury.

Do not place sharp objects (e.g., coat hangers, knitting needles) down cast.

If skin itches, blow cool air (hairdryer) down cast or scratch other extremity.

If any of the following abnormalities are present, return to the follow-up clinic immediately:

Check the temperature of the digits; it is abnormal if they are very cold or very hot.

Check the color of the digits; it is abnormal if they are blue.

Check if there is feeling in the digits; it is abnormal if there is no feeling.

Wiggle the digits at least once each hour.

If a foreign object is dropped into the cast, call to the follow-up care facility immediately.

Return to the follow-up clinic if cast becomes too tight or if a foul odor is present.

CRUTCH AND CANE FITTING

In fitting crutches, measure with the shoe the patient will be wearing, preferably a low-heeled, tie shoe.

Axillary Crutches (Figure 24-5, A)

Length

Arm piece should be 2 inches from axilla (no weight on axilla)

Tips should be 6 to 8 inches to side and front of foot at 25° angle

Hand piece

Elbow should be at 30° angle of flexion

Loftstrand Crutches (Figure 24-5, B)

Length

Tips should be 6 inches to side and front of foot at 25-degree angle

Hand piece

Elbow should be at 30-degree angle of flexion

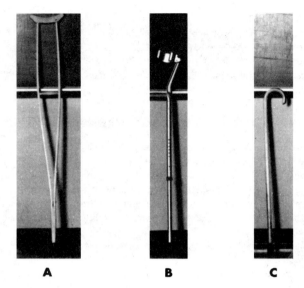

FIGURE 24-5. A, Axillary crutches. The underarm crutch illustrated is not adjustable but is lighter in weight than the adjustable crutch. This type of crutch is available in either wood or metal. **B,** Loftstrand crutch. **C,** Cane with half-circle handle is available in wood or metal.

(From Larson C, Gould M: *Orthopedic nursing,* ed 9. St Louis, 1978, Mosby.)

Cane (Figure 24-5, C)

For assisting balance, offers minimal support; offers assistance in hip injury. Elbow should be at 30-degree angle of flexion with cane next to heel.

GAIT TRAINING

Have the patient stand and balance.

Have the patient hold the crutches 4 inches to the side of the foot and 4 inches in front of the foot.

All weight is carried on the hands by straightening the elbows. Instruct the patient *not* to place any weight on the axillae, even while resting.

In the emergency department, a three-point gait is usually taught, as this type of gait is used when little or no weight bearing is desired.

Be sure to include stair climbing, sitting, and standing instructions (Figure 24-6, *A*).

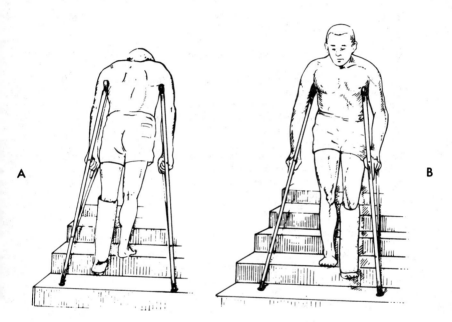

FIGURE 24-6. A, Going upstairs, and **B**, going downstairs, with crutches.
(From Barber J, Stokes L, Billings D: *Adult and child care*, ed 2. St Louis, 1977, Mosby.)

SUGGESTED READINGS

Connolly JF, ed: *DePalma's the management of fractures and dislocations,* ed 3. Philadelphia, 1981, Saunders.

Dobyns JH, Linocheid RL: Athletic injuries of the wrist, *Clin Orthop* 198:141, 1985.

Ferhel RD, Hedley AK, Eckardt JJ: Anterior fracture location of the shoulder: pitfalls in treatment, *J Trauma* 24:363, 1984.

Fisk G: The wrist, *J Bone Joint Surg* 66:396, 1984.

Lombardo JA: Around the elbow, *Emerg Med* 15:14, 1983.

McCarthy JD, Fleishmann J, George WL: Fever, dyspnea, and slurred speech following lower "extremity trauma," *Reviews of Infectious Diseases* 13(1):172, 1991.

Modrall JG, Waver FA, Yellin AE: Vascular considerations in "extremity trauma," *Orthop Clin North Am* 24(3):557, 1993.

Mourad LA: Orthopedic disorders. St Louis, 1991, Mosby.

Newman J: "Nursemaid's elbow" in infants 6 months and under, *J Emerg Med* 2:403, 1984.

O'Brien ET: Acute fractures and dislocations of the wrist, *Orthop Clin North Am* 15:237, 1984.

Parisien JD: Fractures and dislocations of the elbow. In Edlich RF, Spyker DA, eds: *Current emergency therapy '85.* Rockwell, Md, 1985, Aspen.

Patient teaching manual. Springhouse, Pa, 1987, Springhouse.

Schneider FR: *Orthopedics in emergency care.* St Louis, 1984, Mosby.

Simon RR, Koenigsknecht SJ: *Orthopedics in emergency medicine of the extremities.* New York, 1979, Appleton & Lange.

Wadsworth TG, Haddad RJ: Childhood trauma. In Wadsworth TW, ed: *The elbow.* New York, 1982, Churchill Livingstone.

Multiple Trauma

Each year, one out of three Americans sustains a traumatic injury.[1] Trauma is a major cause of disability in the United States and accounts for approximately 140,000 deaths annually.[2] It is the leading cause of death in people under the age of 44,[3] accounts for half the deaths in children under age 4, and 80% of deaths in persons aged 15 to 24 years old.[4] In any emergency department one must be prepared to care for the critically injured trauma patient.

THE ABC⁴ PRIMARY TRAUMA SURVEY

The ABC⁴ Primary Trauma Survey is an organized format for use in the rapid assessment and intervention of the multiply traumatized patient. It provides a systematic approach, whereby a multiply traumatized patient can be initially assessed for life-threatening injuries in approximately 2 minutes. As life-threatening problems are identified, interventions must be initiated.

A = Airway

Assessment of the patient's airway is the first step in the primary trauma survey.

Assessment of the airway should be a "reflex reaction"—it should *always* be done first. The method of airway management should be based on patient findings; treat each patient individually. Airway management includes the following:

Supplemental oxygen

All multiple-trauma patients should receive supplemental oxygen through the appropriate delivery device and at the correct concentration.

Head and neck position

Always assume that the patient has a cervical spine injury until it can be ruled out by a cervical spine x-ray series or other diagnostic tool.

If head and neck position becomes essential in airway management, begin with a modified jaw thrust maneuver, maintaining the cervical spine in a neutral position.

Airway adjuncts

The use of airway adjuncts may become necessary in the management of the patient's airway. Use adjuncts according to their availability, indications, and contraindications.

■ **OROPHARYNGEAL AIRWAY**

Use the oropharyngeal airway only in patients who are unconscious and who do not have a gag reflex.

■ **NASOPHARYNGEAL AIRWAY**

The nasopharyngeal airway may be used on conscious patients who have an intact gag reflex. It is particularly useful in patients with facial trauma, where edema may rapidly ensue and airway obstruction is possible.

■ **ESOPHAGEAL OBTURATOR/ESOPHAGEAL GASTRIC TUBE AIRWAY**

This airway should only be used in patients who are apneic and without a gag reflex. It may be considered when airway management and maintenance are essential and endotracheal intubation cannot be accomplished.

■ **ENDOTRACHEAL TUBE**

Consider placement of an endotracheal tube when total airway management is essential.

In general, orotracheal intubation is recommended in the trauma victim.[5] One must be particularly cautious not to hyperextend the cervical spine in the trauma patient. One method of accomplishing endotracheal intubation without hyperextension of the c-spine is by using a technique known as *tactile* or *digital intubation,* where the epiglottis is palpated with the index and middle fingers of the nondominant hand and the tube is placed with the dominant hand and guided with the fingers of the nondominant hand. This should only be performed on deeply comatose patients.

Nasotracheal intubation may also be considered.

More detail on the use of airway adjuncts can be found in Chapter 4.

■ **CRICOTHYROTOMY**

Cricothyrotomy is a technique that should be used only when airway management by other means cannot be accomplished and the patient has an upper airway obstruction, such as occurs with a fractured larynx.

Two methods used to maintain the airway in this case are:

Needle cricothyrotomy

Surgical incision through the cricoid membrane and tube placement

Suction

Ensure that adequate suction is readily available. As a backup device, a plastic turkey baster is often quite useful for suction when other devices prove to be inadequate.

B = Breathing

The function of ventilation and perfusion is to bring oxygen to the alveoli and to carry carbon dioxide and other waste products from the alveoli. Adequate breathing and ventilation are essential to the trauma victim whose status may be compromised as a result of a ventilation or perfusion defect. Monitor O_2 saturations and blood gases.

Several methods of providing assisted positive pressure ventilation are:

Mouth-to-mask

Using a mask with a non-backflow valve and breathing into the mask rather than directly into the patient's mouth provides a barrier between the rescuer and the victim. This device offers several advantages: It is far more palatable than mouth-to-mouth for most rescuers; it reduces the likelihood of infectious disease transmission; and supplemental oxygen may be added to a port on the mask, increasing the amount of oxygen concentration delivered to the patient.

Bag-valve-mask device

With supplemental oxygen and tubing attached to add a dead space, this device is capable of delivering up to 95% oxygen. The caregiver is also able to sense lung compliance. One of the problems with this device is that it is difficult for one rescuer to achieve an adequate seal.

Demand valve

A demand valve delivers 100% oxygen at 100 L/min. The rescuer must be particularly cautious because there is a possibility of overventilation and development of or further increase of tension pneumothorax. It should not be used on a small child because the flow is too great and may be harmful.

Ventilator

If a ventilator is used, the caregiver should maintain constant observation of the patient and the ventilator. A variety of ventilators can be used on trauma victims, but a volume-cycled ventilator is most commonly used.

C^1 = Circulation

Circulatory status can be assessed by first checking for the presence and quality of a carotid and/or femoral pulse. Peripheral pulses may be absent as a result of direct injury or sympathetic nervous system response as a compensatory mechanism, which causes peripheral vasoconstriction.

Assess the patient's vital signs, including pulse, respirations, blood pressure, temperature, and skin vitals (color, temperature, and moisture) and capillary refill.

Hypovolemic shock

Hypovolemic shock occurs when oxygen and nutrients cannot be transported to the cells and waste products cannot be transported from the cells because blood volume is decreased and adequate pressures cannot be maintained. This results in a reduced amount of available hemoglobin, decreased cardiac output, and low blood pressure.

The average 70 kg (154 lb) person has a blood volume of approximately 5 liters. In a person who was healthy before suffering a traumatic incident and who has normal compensatory mechanisms:

- Mild shock results from a 10% to 20% blood loss (0.5 to 1.0 liters).
- Moderate shock results from a 20% to 40% blood loss (1.0 to 2.0 liters).
- Severe shock results from greater than 40% blood loss (2.0 liters).

■ **SIGNS AND SYMPTOMS**

Restlessness and anxiety
Cool and clammy skin
Tachycardia
Delayed capillary refill
(If greater than 2 seconds, assume shock until proven otherwise.)
Hypotension
Tachypnea
Decreased level of consciousness
Patient complaint of being cold
Patient complaint of being thirsty

■ **COMPENSATORY MECHANISMS**

There are several compensatory mechanisms in shock that will activate an attempt to salvage the brain, heart, and lungs:

Sympathetic nervous system activation. Sympathetic nervous system activation causes the release of epinephrine and norepinephrine, providing alpha and beta stimulation; this causes the heart rate and peripheral resistance to increase. Peripheral vasoconstriction will occur, causing the patient to have cool, clammy skin and cool distal extremities. Because of the peripheral vasoconstriction, the patient, if awake, may complain of being cold.

Renin-angiotensin mechanism activation. When blood flow through the renal arteries decreases, renin angiotensin I and angiotensin II are released. These cause the release of aldosterone, which causes the kidneys to reabsorb sodium and thereby water. As a result of this compensatory mechanism, as well as a decreased renal blood flow, urinary output will decrease.

Antidiuretic hormone release. When hypovolemic shock ensues, antidiuretic hormone (ADH) is released. This causes the kidneys to reabsorb water. This will also be a cause of decreased urinary output.

Intracellular fluid shift. In shock states cell walls become permeable to fluids. Fluids leave the cells and fill the intravascular space. This may also cause the patient, if alert and oriented, to complain of being thirsty, as the cells "dehydrate."

Jugular (neck) veins in shock. If a patient is in shock, assess the jugular veins: Distension may indicate a tourniquet effect on the chest contents, decreasing blood return to the right side of the heart and backflow into the jugular veins. Think about the possibility of a pericardial tamponade or a tension pneumothorax and treat accordingly. Be sure to check neck veins periodically, especially when a cervical collar is in place and the jugular veins are not readily visible.

If neck veins are flat, consider the possibility of hypovolemia and assess further for this condition.

■ **THERAPEUTIC INTERVENTIONS**

100% oxygen. Oxygen may often be required under positive pressure. If positive pressure is used, be attentive to the development of a tension pneumothorax. As soon as possible, obtain arterial blood gases to ensure accurate evaluation of oxygenation status.

Pneumatic anti-shock garment (PASG). The pneumatic antishock garment has fallen out of favor with most providers of trauma care.

IVs

Start two large-bore (14 gauge, if possible) IV lines using a warmed crystalloid solution.

Lines may be started in the antecubital space, jugular veins, or any other large vein site.

Run solutions at a rate that will maintain systolic pressure above 100 mm Hg.

Send a blood specimen for type and cross-match.

Consider using large bore "trauma" tubing or a rapid infusion device.

Control bleeding. Use direct pressure whenever possible. Consider using pressure points and clamping or tourniquets when bleeding is uncontrolled and the situation is life-threatening.

C^2 = Cervical Spine

A cervical spine injury should be considered present in all multiple-trauma patients until it can be proven negative on full cervical spine x-ray series or other diagnostic tools, such as CT. If x-ray is to be used to clear the c-spine, four views are necessary:

Cross-table lateral (must visualize to T-1)

Anterior-posterior

Lateral

Open-mouth odontoid

Flexion/extension views (to check for soft-tissue damage)

Protect the cervical spine by using a stiff cervical collar, rolled blanket, adhesive tape across the eyebrows and onto the backboard, backboard, or other acceptable c-spine protection device. Be sure to protect the thoracic, lumbar, and sacral spine as well by immobilizing from the top of the head to the hips.

C^3 = Chest

There are five types of chest injury that should be ruled out in the primary survey. If they are detected, it is important to initiate *immediate* therapeutic intervention because any of these conditions may be immediately life-threatening. In-depth discussion of each of these conditions can be found in Chapter 22.

Tension pneumothorax

■ **SIGNS AND SYMPTOMS**
Cyanosis
Distended jugular veins
Dyspnea
Deviated trachea (away from the tension)
Cough
Diminished or absent breath sounds
Chest pain
Mediastinal shift (seen on x-ray)
Tachycardia
Decreasing blood pressure

■ **THERAPEUTIC INTERVENTIONS**
Needle thoracostomy or chest tube placement

Flail chest

■ **SIGNS AND SYMPTOMS**
Paradoxical movement of the chest wall
Dyspnea
Cyanosis
Tachycardia

■ **THERAPEUTIC INTERVENTIONS**
Selective endotracheal intubation (if respiratory rate is less than 23, Pao_2 is less than 60 on 50% oxygen, and/or tidal volume is less than 5 ml/kg)
100% oxygen under positive pressure
Careful fluid administration
Analgesia
Consider stabilization of the flail segment

Pericardial tamponade

■ **SIGNS AND SYMPTOMS**
Increased heart rate
Decreased blood pressure ⎤
Muffled heart sounds   ⎬ Beck's Triad
Distended jugular veins ⎦
Dyspnea
Kussmaul's respirations
Paradoxical pulse
Cyanosis (periorbital and peripheral)

■ **THERAPEUTIC INTERVENTIONS**
Oxygen at high-flow rate
High Fowler's position
IV line
Pericardiocentesis or pericardial window

Open chest wound (sucking chest wound)

■ **SIGNS AND SYMPTOMS**
Sucking sound
Dyspnea
Diminished or absent breath sounds
Tachycardia
Hypotension
Signs of tension pneumothorax

■ **THERAPEUTIC INTERVENTIONS**
If the wound is less than two thirds the size of the trachea (the mainstem bronchus), one can safely care for the patient without using an occlusive dressing.
    Cover a larger defect with an occlusive dressing, such as petroleum-impregnated gauze taped on three sides.
    Watch closely for the development of signs and symptoms of tension pneumothorax.
        If signs and symptoms of tension pneumothorax appear, immediately remove occlusive dressing and consider immediate chest tube placement.
    Provide supplemental oxygen.

Massive hemothorax (more than 1500 ml of blood)

■ **SIGNS AND SYMPTOMS**
Same as those for hypovolemic shock (see Chapter 6)

■ **THERAPEUTIC INTERVENTIONS**
Same as those for hypovolemic shock (see Chapter 6)
    Oxygen
    IV lines for fluid and blood replacement
Chest tube(s)
    Large-bore (36 French)
Possible autotransfusion
Possible emergency thoracotomy

C^4 = Consciousness

Assess neurologic status using the Glasgow Coma Scale and DERM mnemonic (see Chapter 9).

Glasgow Coma Scale

BEST MOTOR RESPONSE

Obeys simple commands	6 points
Localizes noxious stimulus	5 points
Flexion withdrawal	4 points
Abnormal flexion	3 points
Abnormal extension	2 points
No motor response	1 point

BEST VERBAL RESPONSE

Oriented	5 points
Confused	4 points
Verbalizes/exclamatory or disorganized	3 points
Moans/groans	2 points
No vocalization	1 point

EYE OPENING

Spontaneously	4 points
To speech	3 points
To noxious stimulus	2 points
No eye opening	1 point

Coma is defined as no response and no eye opening or a score of 7 or less. If the patient is intubated and being ventilated, verbal response should be recorded as a "T" (for tubed). For example, a patient who has flexion withdrawal, is intubated and ventilated, and opens eyes to noxious stimulae would have a GCS of 6T. The Glasgow Coma Scale may not be useful in patients who are severely hypovolemic or intoxicated.

DERM mnemonic

D = Depth of coma

Use stimulus/response. Example: Responds to painful stimulae with flexion withdrawal.

E = Eyes

Check pupillary response.

R = Respiration

Describe rate, rhythm, and depth of respirations

M = Motor/movement

Check extremity movement; if it is present, describe whether it is unilateral or bilateral.

The caregiver may wish to calculate a trauma score for outcome prediction. One that is frequently used is the Champion Trauma Score (CTS).[6] In the Champion Trauma Score the Glasgow Coma Scale and a trauma scoring method are tabulated as follows:

Glasgow coma scale score

Point conversion for use with CTS

14-15	=	5
11-13	=	4
8-10	=	3
5-7	=	2
3-4	=	1

THE SECONDARY SURVEY

Following a primary survey, where life-threatening conditions are identified and treated, a more thorough secondary survey should be performed. Begin by reevaluating the patient's airway and rechecking vital signs. It is also at this point that fractures should be splinted.

Head

Systematically assess and treat the head and neck for lacerations, fractures, and deformities.

Hyperventilate major head trauma patients to lower P_{CO_2} to approximately 28 torr (no less).

Administer mannitol and/or furosemide for major head trauma patients.

Consider computerized axial tomography (CT scan) or skull x-rays.

Suture lacerations.

Check all areas for bruises, discoloration, lacerations, deformities.

Do a rapid systemic evaluation of the following:

Neck

Recheck airway

Check for:

Fractured larynx (anterior neck subcutaneous emphysema)

Wounds/hematomas

Neck vein distension

Pulses

Deformities

Pain

Penetrating objects

Midline trachea

Subcutaneous emphysema

If a c-spine injury is present, administer methylprednisolone (solumedrol in accordance with protocol)

Face

Check for:

Airway problems

Symmetry

Obvious fractures

Dental step-defects or malocclusion

CSF rhinorrhea

Eyes

Check for:

Pupillary response

Trauma

Periorbital ecchymosis

Ears

Check for:

CSF ottorrhea

Ruptured tympanic membrane

Mouth

Check for:

Foreign bodies

Obstruction/lacerations

Chest

Check for wounds/abrasions/deformities/penetrating objects/holes.
Check heart sounds.
Check lung sounds.
Check chest wall symmetry.
Obtain arterial blood gases.
Obtain a 12-lead ECG.
Obtain a chest x-ray, if not already done.

Abdomen

Check for:
Bowel sounds
Rigidity
Pain
Tenderness
Wounds/abrasions/hematomas
Penetrating objects
Eviscerations
Distension

Spine

Check for:
Deformities
Pain on palpation
Abrasions/bruises

Pelvis/Hips

Check for:
Fractures
Deformities
Femoral pulses and distal pulses
Abnormal rotation and/or flexion of legs

Extremities

Check for:
Pulses
Neurologic status distal to injury
Fractures/dislocations/crepitus
Movement
Skin color and temperature
Capillary refill

Perineum

Check for:
Bleeding
Urine extravasation

Buttocks

Check for:
Wounds
Abrasions

General management

Following the completion of systemic assessment:
Cover open wounds.
Repair lacerations.
Administer appropriate IV fluids, blood products, medications.
Ensure that appropriate specimens have been sent to the lab.
Remember tetanus prophylaxis.
Order further appropriate diagnostic tests, such as x-rays, CT scans, peritoneal lavage, pericardiocentesis, serum and urine laboratory tests.
Obtain appropriate consults.
Prepare the patient for possible surgery.
Care for patient and family/significant others' psychological needs.

UNDRESSING THE PATIENT

Undressing the trauma patient is a vitally important step in performing a complete evaluation. Without exposing the patient it is impossible to make a systematic assessment of all of the patient's obvious and occult injuries. While it appears to be a straightforward task, it can be difficult to remove some pieces of clothing, particularly the protective garb that is worn in sports.

Helmets

A variety of helmets are available for those sports that recommend head protection—motorcycle, bicycle, kayak, football, hockey, and auto racing are just a few. The careful removal of this gear is imperative in protection of the potential cervical spine injury.

Procedure

1. Never attempt to remove a helmet alone; airway protection can be achieved with the helmet on, and the potential for complicating an injury with a difficult removal is great.
2. One person should apply inline traction by placing his hands on each side of the helmet with his fingers on the patient's mandible and exerting general pulling; loosen or cut the chin strap to remove.
3. A second person should then receive the weight of the patient's head by placing one hand behind the head, resting on the occiput, and the front hand on the angles of the mandible, thumb on one side, fingers on the other (the second person is now in control of the head and neck).

4. The first person should then remove the helmet by pulling laterally on the sides and sliding it off. NOTE: If the helmet has full face protection, special consideration must be given to the eye covering which must be removed first; if it cannot be removed, tilt the helmet (not the head) back to pass the face protector over the patient's nose.

Boots

Heavy boots create a problem if the patient has sustained an unstable injury to the foot or lower leg. Some simple techniques make the process of removal less painful. REMEMBER: Boots are usually very expensive, and removal without cutting is generally appreciated.

Procedure

1. Inform the patient of each step of the removal process as it is about to occur; employ the patient's cooperation.
2. Place the patient supine; unlace boot and open the boot as freely as possible.
3. Have one person slip both hands on the lateral and medial sides of the patient's lower leg, into the boot; support the ankle and foot as one unit with both hands.
4. Have the second person remove the boot, pulling the toe of the boot in a cephalad direction to gently release the heel (which is being stabilized by the first person).

Rear Entry Ski Boots

To remove rear entry ski boots follow the procedure above, but keep in mind that with the entry in the back the leg must be elevated enough to accommodate the rear flaps opening and the need for pulling before the heel is released is exaggerated.

Neoprene Wet Suit/Stretch One-Piece Ski Racing Suits

Wet suits and one-piece stretch ski racing suits pose a special problem when the patient is a victim of trauma. In most cases the suits can be rolled and pulled off the patient, being turned inside out in the removal (usually requiring more than one undresser). If this is not an option in the emergency setting, they must be cut off. However, consider their great expense and cut along seams if necessary.

Down Clothing

Do not ever cut!
■ **GENERAL GUIDELINES FOR UNDRESSING THE PATIENT**
1. Preserve as much clothing as possible without wasting time.
2. Undress the uninjured extremity first, then the injured limb.
3. Dress in the reverse of #2; injured limb first, uninjured extremity last.

4. Don't forget to look for teeth, contact lenses, and prosthetics.
5. Consider the chain of evidence if foul play was involved with the patient and if the clothes or their contents may be used in court.
6. Remove jewelry and deposit (witnessed) it in a valuables protection envelope in a designated safe, or release it to family. Record this transaction on patient's chart.
7. Consider religious clothing when undressing if situation permits, and consult patient or family about its removal and safekeeping.
8. When clothing must be cut away from patient, try to cut on seams.

TRAUMA FLOW SHEET

It is essential, in trauma, to carefully document all events and findings. Use of a specifically designed flow sheet (Figure 25-1) facilitates this and ensures that important items are not forgotten.

Care of the multiply traumatized patient presents us with an enormous challenge. An organized, systematic, and rehearsed approach will prove most beneficial to the patient.

REFERENCES

1. American College of Surgeons/ Committee on Trauma: *Optimal care of the injured patient.* Chicago, 1993, American College of Surgeons.
2. Department of Health and Human Services: *Healthy people 2000 summary report.* Washington, DC, 1992, U.S. Government Printing Office.
3. U.S. Department of Health and Human Services, Division of Trauma and Transplantation: *Model trauma system care plan.* Washington, DC, 1993, Dept. of Health and Human Services.
4. American College of Surgeons/Committee on Trauma: *Advanced trauma life support manual.* Chicago, 1992, American College of Surgeons.
5. Shea J: Lecture presentation, Emergency Nurses Association Annual Meeting, Orlando, Florida, 1992.
6. Champion HR, Sacco WJ, Carnazzo AJ et al: Trauma score, *Crit Care Med* 9(9): 672, 1981.

SUGGESTED READINGS

Cardona VD et al: Trauma nursing: from resuscitation through rehabilitation, ed 2. Philadelphia, 1993, Saunders.

Emergency Nurses Association: *Trauma nurse care course, student manual.* Chicago, 1994, the Emergency Nurses Association.

Hill DA, Abraham KJ, West PH: Factors affecting outcomes in the resuscitation of severely injured patients. *Australia N Z J Surg* 63(8):404, 1993.

Kidd PS, Neff J: *Trauma nursing: the art and science.* St Louis, 1993, Mosby.

Maloney-Harmon PA: Initial assessment and stabilization of the pediatric trauma patient, *Crit Care Med* 21(supp): S392-1993.

Schmidt J, Moore GP: Management of multiple trauma, *Emerg Med Clin North Am* 11(1): 29051, 1993.

Sheehy SB, Jimmerson CL: *Manual of clinical trauma care: the first hour,* ed 2. St Louis, 1994, Mosby.

EMERGENCY DEPARTMENT TRAUMA CHART

Age:	Sex: ☐M ☐F	DATE:

Approx. Time of Injury:	Other Hospital:

Time of Arrival at DHMC:	MODE: ☐AMB ☐AIR ☐CAR

(Addressograph)

☐ *TRAUMA ALERT*   ☐ *TRAUMA NINE*

MECHANISM _____

FOR MVC:

SAFETY DEVICES:
- ☐ Shoulder Belt ☐ Helmet
- ☐ Lap Belt ☐ Air Bag
- ☐ Lap & Shoulder Belt ☐ Other: _____

- ☐ Driver ☐ Rear Pass Ⓜ
- ☐ FS Passenger ☐ Rear Pass Ⓡ
- ☐ Rear Pass Ⓛ ☐ Pedestrian

E.D. TEAM
Nurse #1 _____
Nurse #2 _____
ED Attending _____
ED Resident _____
Other _____

REVIEW
☐ YES   ☐ NO

SCENE DATA

LOC:	Last vitals	TREATMENTS:
☐ Awake / Alert	BP _____	Airway O2 @ ____ L ☐ PASG
☐ Confused	P _____	☐ OP / NP ☐ C.Collar ☐ IV#1
☐ Responds Pain	R _____	☐ EOA ☐ Backboard ☐ IV#2
☐ No Response	☐ Assisted	☐ ET / NT ☐ Other
☐ > 20 min extrication		☐ Other _____

TRAUMA TEAM	Name	Called	Arrived
Trauma Resident			
Trauma Attending			
Anesthesiologist			
Radiology Tech			
Radiologist			
Social Worker / Chaplain			
Other			
Other			
Other			
Other			
Other			

AIRWAY	TREATMENTS & DIAGNOSTICS	MEDICATIONS
☐ OP / NP	☐ C Collar ☐ Chest Tube	☐ Narcotics
☐ EOA	☐ Backboard ☐ DPL	☐ Paralytics
☐ ET / NT	☐ PASG ☐ CT	☐ Dexamethasone
☐ O2 @ ___ L	☐ IV#1 ☐ XRAYS ☐ C-SPINE	☐ Antibiotics
☐ Assisted	☐ IV#2 ☐ CHEST	☐ Tet Tox
	☐ LABS	☐ Other _____

(PREVIOUS HOSPITAL)

HISTORY

_____
_____
_____
_____
_____

Meds: _____
Allergies: _____ Ht: _____ Wt: _____ Last Tetanus: _____ LMP: _____ Food: _____

Time:	Notes	Time	Notes

RELATIVE NOTIFIED: ☐Yes ☐No	Relationship:	LOCATION:	BELONGINGS GIVEN TO:

DISPOSITION: ☐PACU ☐OR ☐PICU ☐FLOOR	TIME OF DEATH:
☐STEP DOWN_____ ☐ICU ☐MORGUE	ME NOTIFIED: ☐Yes ☐No AUTOPSY: ☐Yes ☐No

TRANSFER TIME:	ORGAN / TISSUE DONATION REQUESTED: ☐Yes ☐No

FIGURE 25-1. Trauma Flow sheet.

Times

O2 Saturation: 75 76 77 78 79 80 81 82 83 84 85 86 87 88 89 90 91 92 93 94 95 96 97 98 99 100

230 220 210 200 190 180 170 160 150 140 130 120 110 100 90 80 70 60 50 40 30 20 10 0

TEMPERATURE
PUPILS R/L
GLASCOW COMA SCALE
Hct / Hgb

● PULSE ○ O2 Sat   **X** RESPIRATIONS   **D** DOPPLER ® BLOOD PRESSURE   ∨ MANUAL BLOOD PRESSURE   ▼ AUTOMATIC BLOOD PRESSURE

GLASGOW COMA SCALE (GCS)

EYE	Spontaneous	4
	To Voice	3
	To Pain	2
	None	1	1 ____
VOICE	Oriented	5
	Confused	4
	Inappropriate Words	3
	Incomprehensible Words	2
	None	1	2 ____
MOTOR	Obeys Commands	6
	Localizes Pain	5
	Withdraws (Pain)	4
	Flexion (Pain)	3
	Extension (Pain)	2
	None	1	3 ____

TOTALS	PTS	GCS TOTAL = 1+2+3 =
13-15	4	GCS T
9-12	3	GCS
6-8	2	GCS
4-5	1	POINTS = A ____
3		

TRAUMA SCORE (TS)

RESP	10 - 29	4
	> 29	3
	6 - 9	2
	1 - 5	1
	NONE	0	B ____
SYS BP	> 90 mm Hg	4
	76 - 89	3
	50 - 75	2
	0 - 49 mm Hg	1
	NO PULSE	0	C ____

ADULTS TS = A + B + C = =

LAB STUDIES

Na | Cl | Gluc.   TIME ___ PT
K | CO2 | Bun/CR   PTT
WBC < Hgb / Hct > Plate.   AMYLASE ___ ETOH

OTHER ____
OTHER ____

BLOOD GASES

TIME	pH	pCO2	pO2	HCO3	FIO2

TIME	E.D. PROCEDURES
	☐ETT ☐NTT SIZE:
	☐ORAL AIRWAY ☐NASAL AIRWAY
	☐CRICOTHYROIDOTOMY
	☐O2 ____ % ☐VENTILATOR
	☐PULSE OXIMETER
	☐CPR
	☐PERICARDIOCENTESIS ☐PERICARDIAL WINDOW
	☐THORACOTOMY
	☐CHEST TUBE R# L#
	☐AUTOTRANSFUSION
	☐MAST TROUSERS TIME INFLATE TIME DEFLATE
	ABD:
	LEGS:
	☐C COLLAR ☐BACKBOARD ☐TIME REMOVED ____
	☐NG
	☐FOLEY
	☐PERITONEAL LAVAGE:
	☐Open Technique
	☐Closed Technique
	☐OTHER ____
	☐GARDNER WELLS TONGS
	☐HARE TRACTION: ☐LLE ☐RLE ☐BOTH

*CRYSTALLOID SOLUTIONS

FLUID TYPE		TOTAL
L.R. 1000ml	1 2 3 4 5 6 7 8	
L.R. BOLUS AMT	1 2 3 4 5 6 7 8	
PRE HOSP. TOTAL:	TOTAL:	

*BLOOD PRODUCTS

TYPE		TOTAL
UNCROSSED PRC	1 2 3 4 5 6 7 8	
CROSSED PRC	1 2 3 4 5 6 7 8	
	1 2 3 4	
PRE HOSP. TOTAL:	TOTAL:	
TOTAL FLUID:		

OUTPUT

TIME			
URINE			
BLOOD			
N.G./O.G.			
CHEST TUBE			
TOTAL OUT:			

LINES

	Gauge	Site
PERIPHERAL IV		
CENTRAL IV		
ARTERIAL LINE		

RADIOLOGY

☐C-SPINE ☐CHEST ☐PELVIS

	TIME LEFT	TIME RETURNED
☐ PLAIN FILMS		

☐HEAD CT
☐ABDOMINAL CT
☐ARTERIOGRAM
☐IVP
☐OTHER

MEDS TIME	MED	DOSE	RT

SIGNATURES

FIGURE 25-1, cont'd.

Burn Trauma

It is estimated that over 60,000 people are hospitalized for burn injuries and 10,000 people die from burn injuries each year. The most common cause of death from burn injuries in the first 48 hours is respiratory problems.

Burns are injuries to the tissues caused by:
- Intense heat or flame (thermal burns)
- Acids or alkalis (chemical burns)
- Electrical current (electrical burns)
- Overexposure to sun or x-rays (radiation burns)
- Friction (friction burns)

The severity of the burn is determined by:
- The amount of body surface area (BSA) involved
- The degree (depth) of the burn (Table 26-1)
- The patient's age
- Previous medical or surgical condition
- Current underlying trauma
- Complications from the original burn injury

CLASSIFICATION OF BURNS

First Degree Burns (Partial Thickness Burn)

Burns through the epithelial layer of skin
Appear as areas of erythema

Second Degree Burns (Partial Thickness Burn)

Burns that include a partial thickness of the dermal layer of the skin
Appear as erythematous areas with blisters

Third Degree Burns (Full Thickness Burn)

Full thickness burns of the dermal layer of the skin

TABLE 26-1 Classification of Burn Injury

DEPTH OF BURN	SENSITIVITY	APPEARANCE	HEALING TIME AND RESULTS	TREATMENT
Partial thickness				
First degree				
Epidermal	Hyperalgesia	Erythema	3-5 days; no scarring	Moisturizers
Superficial dermal	Hyperalgesia to pink	Blisters, red, moist	6-10 days; minimal slurring	Topical antibacterial agents or biologic dressings required
Second degree				
Moderate dermal	Normal algesia	Blisters, pink, moist	10-18 days; some scarring	Topical anitbacterial agents or biologic dressings required
Deep thermal	Hypoalgesia or anal-gesia	Blisters, opaque, with less mois-ture	>21 days; maximal scarring if not excised and grafted	Topical anitbacterial agents and early excision and grafting
Full thickness				
Third degree				
Loss of all dermal elements with extension into fat, muscle, and bone	Analgesia	White, opaque, brown, or black, occasionally deep red; very dry, leathery; may or may not have blisters or thrombosed veins	Never heals if area is larger than 3 cm². The longer the wound is open, the more hypertrophic the scar	Topical antibacterial agents and early excision and grafting

(From Sheehy SA, Marvin JA, Jimmerson CL: *Manual of clinical trauma care: the first hour*, St. Louis, 1989, Mosby.)

Appear white and leathery and may or may not blister
Thrombosed vessels can sometimes be visualized beneath these burns
Some burns extend to muscle and bone
May have a charred appearance

Rule of 9s

Burns are categorized as major, moderate, or minor. The extent of burns may be assessed using the Rule of 9s (Figure 26-1) and/or the Lund and Browder Chart (Figure 26-2).

Major burns

A second degree burn over more than 25% of BSA *or*
A third degree burn over more than 10% of BSA in an adult

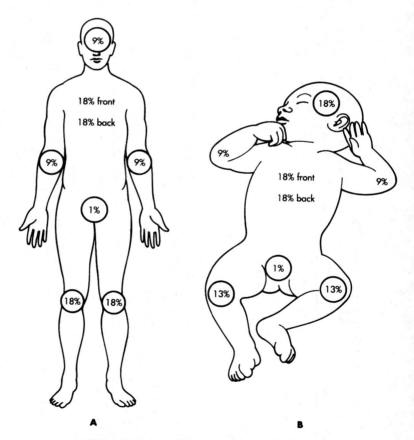

FIGURE 26-1. Rule of Nines. **A**, Adult. **B**, Children.

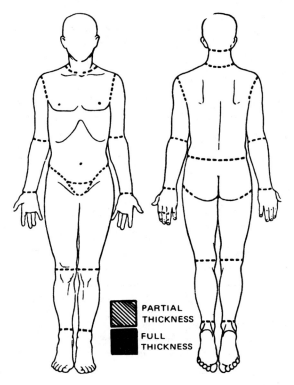

PARTIAL THICKNESS

FULL THICKNESS

Percent Surface Area Burned

AREA	1 YEAR	1-4 YEARS	5-9 YEARS	10-14 YEARS	Y 15 YEARS	ADULT	2"	3"
Head	19	17	13	11	9	7		
Neck	2	2	2	2	2	2		
Ant. Trunk	13	13	13	13	13	13		
Post Trunk	13	13	13	13	13	13		
R. Buttock	2½	2½	2½	2½	2½	2½		
L. Buttock	2½	2½	2½	2½	2½	2½		
Genitalia	1	1	1	1	1	1		
R. U. Arm	4	4	4	4	4	4		
L. U. Arm	4	4	4	4	4	4		
R. L. Arm	3	3	3	3	3	3		
L. L. Arm	3	3	3	3	3	3		
R. Hand	2½	2½	2½	2½	2½	2½		
L. Hand	2½	2½	2½	2½	2½	2½		
R. Thigh	5½	6½	8	8½	9	9½		
L. Thigh	5½	6½	8	8½	9	9½		
R. Leg	5	5	5½	6	6½	7		
L. Leg	5	5	5½	6	6½	7		
R. Foot	3½	3½	3½	3½	3½	3½		
L. Foot	3½	3½	3½	3½	3½	3½		
TOTAL								

FIGURE 26-2. Lund and Browder formula.
(From Artz CP, Moncrief JA: *The treatment of burns*, ed 2. Philadelphia, 1969, Saunders.)

A second degree burn over more than 20% of BSA in a child
Any third degree burn in a child
Burns involving the hands, face, eyes, ears, feet, or perineum
All inhalation burns
All electrical burns
Any deep, circumferential burn
Burns with associated major trauma
Burns in any poor-risk patient (age >55 years old, underlying medical problems, e.g., diabetes, heart diseases, renal failure)

Moderate burns

A second degree burn over 15% to 25% of BSA in an adult
A second degree burn over 10% to 20% of BSA in a child

Minor burns

A second degree burn over less than 15% of BSA *or*
A third degree burn over less than 2% of BSA in an adult
A second degree burn over less than 10% of BSA *or*
A third degree burn over less than 2% of BSA in a child
Hospital admission is recommended for patients with:
  Second or third degree burns over greater than 10% of BSA
  Burns of hands, feet, and perineum
  Circumferential burns
  Electrical or chemical burns
  Burns associated with multiple or significant trauma
  Burns associated with suspected child abuse

BURN CARE

Burn care should be initiated by the first person to arrive at the scene of the incident.

Care of Minor to Moderate Burns

Remove smoldering material.
Remove restrictive clothing and jewelry.
Initiate cooling efforts (saline soaked dressings).
Assess extent of burn.
Shave hair surrounding wound, but do not shave eyebrows.
Debride devitalized tissue.
Leave blisters intact.
Cover wound with antimicrobial agent and bulky dressing.
Check for tetanus prophylaxis.
Consider antibiotics.
Provide aftercare instructions.
  Keep dressing clean and dry.

Elevate burned extremity for 24 to 48 hours.
Give prescriptions or instructions for analgesia.
Provide follow-up care; check wound in 2 days.

Care of Moderate to Major Burns

Prehospital

Rescuer should protect self against flames, noxious gases, smoke, explosions, falling debris, etc.
Flush chemicals from the surface or remove victim from electrical source.
ABCs (especially in those with facial and neck burns).
Check for signs of smoke inhalation (flames in a closed space, carbonaceous sputum, facial and neck burns, hoarse voice, coughing).
Check for other injuries (especially victims involved in explosions, motor vehicle accidents, or jumping from a burning building).
Remove smoldering clothing (if nonadherent to skin).
Control bleeding.
Remove restrictive clothing and jewelry.
Make brief neurologic exam (include level of consciousness, pupils, motor and sensory function).
Splint fractures.
Initiate an intravenous line of Ringer's lactate (if the burn is less than 30% of body surface area, run at a rate of 3 to 4 ml/lb/hr; if burn is greater than 30% body surface area, run at rate of 6 to 8 ml/lb/hr). Later, use Baxter's formula.
Control pain (if burn is not associated with trauma, administer morphine sulfate or meperidine hydrochloride intravenously).
Estimate extent of burn.
Cover burned area with clean, dry, sterile (if possible) sheet. Do not wrap large burns in saline-soaked dressings because cool dressings will reduce body temperature.
Check vital signs (do not avoid taking blood pressure because the limb is burned).
Administer humidified oxygen at 100% concentration.
Pay strict attention to airway and suctioning.

In the emergency department

Continue fluid resuscitation.
Repeat vital signs every 15 minutes.
Obtain arterial blood gases.
Endotracheal intubation if P_{O_2} is less than 50 mm Hg.
Consider analgesia.
Use nasogastric tube to decompress stomach; avoid possible aspiration of gastric contents.
Have the patient assume a comfortable position.
Obtain chest x-ray film.
Start additional IV lines.

Insert Foley catheter; send urine to lab to check for myoglobulinuria and/or
hemoglobinuria.

Initiate hourly urine measurements.

Start arterial line if blood pressure is difficult to obtain.

Lab: Complete blood count, prothrombin time, electrolytes, calcium, magnesium, blood urea nitrogen, creatinine, glucose, bilirubin, phosphorus, alkaline
phosphatase, total protein, carboxyhemoglobin, and toxicology screen, if
indicated

Get type and cross-match if indicated.

Monitor cardiac rhythm.

Take 12-lead ECG.

Weigh.

Consider burn unit admission or referral to burn center.

Airway Management

Inhalation injuries occur frequently with burn injuries. They may occur in three
phases. Most inhalation injuries are a combination of these types:

Carbon monoxide toxicity

Upper airway obstruction

Injury of lower airway and lung parenchyma by chemicals

Because of the potential for obstructive edema, establish a patent airway.

It may be necessary to initiate a nasopharyngeal or endotracheal tube.

If there is airway obstruction, it may be necessary to perform emergency cricothyrotomy.

Sometimes pulmonary damage is not evident in the early prehospital and emergency department phases. Always anticipate pulmonary complications and have
equipment readily available so that intervention can take place readily and rapidly.

When a patient gives a history of exposure to smoke or other toxic products
of combustion, assume and anticipate pulmonary complications and pulmonary
damage until it is proven otherwise.

■ **SIGNS AND SYMPTOMS OF SMOKE INHALATION**

Soot in the nostrils

Singed nasal or facial hair

Carbonaceous sputum

Hoarse voice

Drooling

Stridor

Cough

Burns around mouth

■ **THERAPEUTIC INTERVENTION**

Oxygen at high flow by mask or nasopharyngeal or endotracheal tube

Obtain a carboxyhemoglobin level; this may help to predict pulmonary complications and allow for preventive therapeutic interventions early in the course of
treatment.

Pain Management

Remember *not* to cool the entire burn area all at once if extensive surface area is burned; doing so may cause severe hypothermia.

If an analgesic is given, administer it through the IV route to ensure uniform, timely distribution throughout the body. The most common analgesic agent administered is morphine sulfate, given in 2 to 4 mg increments slowly and titrated to achieve the desired analgesic effect. Pay close attention to respiratory status, morphine sulfate may cause respiratory depression.

An alternative to morphine sulfate administration is nitrous oxide gas, which the patient can self-administer.

IV Fluid Replacement

Problems with fluid and electrolyte balances are directly proportional to the extent of the burn injury.

Place a Foley catheter and carefully measure hourly urine output.

Calculate fluid replacement in accordance with the extent of the burn, using one of the major burn formulas as a guideline.

The Baxter (Parkland) formula

First 24 hours—give Ringer's lactate 4ml/kg of body weight multiplied by the percentage of burned BSA:

Give half the calculated amount in the first 8 hours.

Give the remaining half over the next 16 hours.

Second 24 hours—give D_5W to maintain serum sodium at less than 140 mEq/L.

Give potassium supplement to maintain normal serum potassium level.

Give plasma or plasma substitute to maintain adequate circulating volume.

The modified Brooke formula

First 24 hours—give 2 ml/kg of body weight multiplied by the percentage of burned BSA.

Give half of the calculated amount in the first 8 hours.

Give the other half over the next 16 hours.

Second 24 hours—D_5 and NS or NS to maintain adequate urine output.

Give colloids—0.3 ml/kg of body weight multiplied by the percentage of burned BSA.

Blood and blood products are not given in the initial phases of the burn injury unless the patient is hypovolemic from associated trauma.

Fluid amounts may be adjusted in accordance with pulse, blood pressure, urine output, urine glucose, level of consciousness, and the presence of nausea and vomiting or a paralytic ileus.

Standard fluid guidelines are not used when an electrical injury has occurred. Ringer's lactate should be administered at a rate of 1 to 2 L/hr until the patient demonstrates that he or she is being adequately resuscitated. This is evidenced by a urine output two to three times normal (so that myoglobin can be excreted rapidly).

Escharotomy

Escharotomy is performed if circumferential burns are constricting the chest wall, causing respiratory compromise or constriction of arteries and venous structures of the extremities and impairing circulation. The most common sites for escharotomies are:

Fingers   Chest
Hands   Legs
Arms   Toes

These may be performed in the early phases of emergency department care if there is a threat to life or limb from the impairment. Escharotomy is done by simply cutting through all the layers of the skin with a sterile scalpel and blade, allowing for separation of the tissue and for circulation to be reestablished. Incisions are made in the areas shown in Figure 26-3.

Special Management of Specific Burns

Chemical Burns

All chemical burns should be flushed with copious amounts of water or normal saline solution immediately after exposure. All clothing and jewelry should be removed. Powdered chemicals should be brushed from the skin before irrigation. Consult a Poison Control Center should you encounter any unusual or unfamiliar chemical. Neutralizing agents are contraindicated since the chemical reaction may produce more heat. Resultant burns should be treated as thermal burns.

If there are chemical burns of the eye, irrigate the eyes with copious amounts of normal saline solution or water for at least 20 to 30 minutes. Immediately after irrigation, but before fluorescein staining and slit-lamp examination, obtain results of visual acuity examination. Chemical burns of the eyes usually require ophthalmologic consultation.

Electrical burns

Sometimes an electrical burn may appear very minor because of the lack of ability to visualize the damage. Entrance and exit sites may be small, but destruction of underlying tissue may be extensive. This destruction is caused by the intense heat that results from the passage of electrical current through the tissues. The direction and the extent of electrical burns may not be evident for 7 to 10 days.

A common complication of an electrical burn injury is ventricular fibrillation caused by the passage of electrical current through the myocardium. If ventricular fibrillation occurs, initiate cardiopulmonary resuscitation immediately and accomplish defibrillation as soon as possible. In this instance prolonged resuscitation efforts are often successful.

Other important considerations in management of electrical burn victims include:

Avoid direct contact with the victim.

Remove the victim (carefully) from the source of the current.

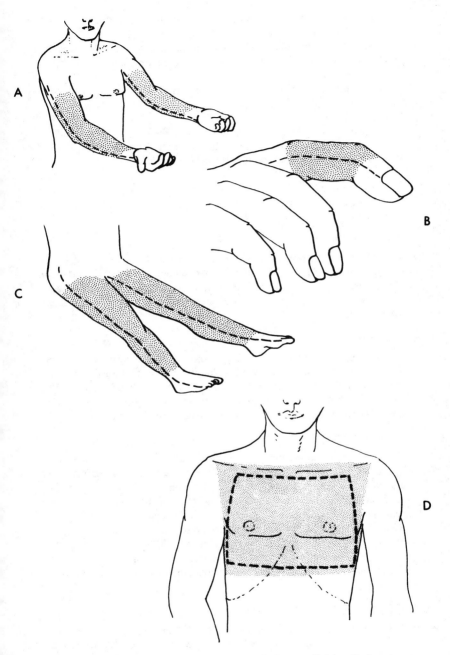

FIGURE 26-3. Proper sites for escharotomy. **A**, Arms. **B**, Fingers. **C**, Legs. **D**, Anterior thorax.

Use a nonconductive object to remove the source of the electrical current *or*
Turn off the electrical current.
Initiate ABCs immediately if patient has no pulse and is not breathing.
Check for concurrent trauma and apply appropriate life-saving therapeutic
    intervention.
Notify the receiving hospital as soon as possible, as they may have to make
    arrangements for:
    A burn-unit bed *or:*
    Transfer of a patient to a burn center once the patient is stabilized
    An ECG is indicated if the current appears to have passed through the chest.
Hospital admission is essential for electrical burn victims who have demon-
strated:
    Major burn injury
    Loss of consciousness
    Cardiac dysrhythmias

Radiation burns

Radiation burns are usually caused by overexposure to the sun. Sunburn cases
are typically first degree and sometimes second degree burns. The most com-
forting measure for this patient is the application of cool, moist compresses. If
fever and chills are present, administer antipyretic agents such as aspirin or
acetaminophen.

Tar burns

Tar burns usually result from roofing tar or asphalt and usually involve the face,
head, neck, hands, and arms. Cooling should be initiated immediately. No
attempts should be made to peel off the tar. Instead, it should be softened and
loosened with mineral oil, vaseline, or a solvent made especially for this purpose. The resultant burns should be treated as thermal burns.

Friction burns

Friction burns are also known as "brush burns," "floor burns," and "road
burns." This type of burn is caused by heat produced by friction. Friction burns
are frequently seen in athletes who fall on gymnasium floors, tennis courts, or
artificial-surface football fields or running tracks, and in motorcycle riders not
wearing protective clothing who are involved in accidents.
Remove foreign bodies or debris (cinders, dirt particles, etc.). This often
    requires administration of a topical local anesthetic or nitrous oxide gas.
Scrub the wound with a surgical soap solution and a soft brush.
Ensure that all particles are removed to avoid permanent scarring known as tat-
    tooing.

SUGGESTED READINGS

Froman P: Wound care—burns. In Hamilton G, ed: *Presenting signs and symptoms in the
    emergency department: evaluation and treatment.* Baltimore, 1993. Williams and Wil-
    kins.

Kravitz M: Thermal injuries. In Cardona V, Hurn P, Mason P et al, eds: *Trauma nursing from resuscitation through rehabilitation.* Philadelphia, 1988, Saunders.

Marvin JA: Burns. In Sheehy SA, Marvin JA: *Manual of clinical trauma care: the first hour,* ed 2. St Louis, 1993, Mosby.

Marvin J: Burns and thermal injuries. In Sheehy S, ed: *Emergency nursing: principles and practice.* St Louis, 1992, Mosby.

Meyer A, Salber P: Burns and smoke inhalation. In Saunders C, Ho M, eds: *Current emergency diagnosis and treatment,* ed 4. E. Norwalk, Conn, 1992, Appleton and Lange.

PART FOUR

FOUR

Special Populations

Sexual Assault

Anyone of either sex can be sexually assaulted at any age. Sexual assault is one of the four most violent and frequent crimes occurring in the United States each year, and women and girls are most often the victims. During the assault victims often fear for their lives and thus may submit to the demands of the assailant. After the assault, victims often have a feeling of disbelief, followed by a period of shock. Victims may also have feelings of guilt or self-blame, fear, extreme vulnerability, helplessness, personal violation, shame, and embarrassment. Emergency departments should develop a specific protocol for the treatment of—and collection of evidence from—the sexual assault victim. The primary focus is:

1. To minimize the physical and psychological trauma to the victim.
2. To maximize the probability of collecting and preserving the physical evidence for potential use in the legal system.

It is not the responsibility of the emergency department staff to decide whether a patient has been sexually assaulted: their responsibility is to ensure the physical well-being of the victim, collect evidence, and provide emotional support and follow-up.

As with any other violent crime, in many states hospital staff are required to report sexual assault to the police. The victim is *not* required to give information or evidence to the police.

TRIAGE

When a victim of sexual assault arrives at the emergency department, place the victim in an area away from the noisy routines of the department. Emergency department registration of the victim should take place in a private environment as well. A general consent for medical treatment should be signed at this time.

Every attempt should be made not to leave the victim alone. The importance of having a support person available cannot be overemphasized. Well-trained support personnel from the area rape crisis center can provide the intervention necessary during the patient's evaluation and treatment in the emergency department. They can assist emergency department personnel in explaining procedures, and can provide counseling for the victim, family members, and significant others. The advocate can also provide information regarding referrals and the availability of any compensatory programs in the area. The advocate on call should be called to the emergency department and introduced to the victim. At all times the victim must be given the choice whether or not to speak to the advocate. A list of rape crisis centers should be readily available in the emergency department.

If possible, for continuity the person taking the initial history should be the one to remain with the victim throughout the stay in the emergency department.

Do not have the victim undress until evidence collection is in progress.

Never discourage a sexual assault victim from seeking evaluation, as evidence can be obtained for days after the assault has taken place.

Do not prohibit the victim from voiding, but carefully obtain a specimen for pregnancy test, UA, and possibly to check for sperm. A midstream specimen is NOT obtained, as this could wash away evidence.

NURSING ASSESSMENT

Assess the general physical appearance of the patient. Serious trauma should *always* be treated before evidence collection. Minor injuries can wait until after evidence collection.

Assess general emotional state.

Obtain a complete set of vital signs. Consider last tetanus immunization if appropriate.

SEXUAL ASSAULT EVIDENCE COLLECTION

The collection of forensic evidence may be completed by a certified nurse examiner, physician, nurse practitioner, or police examiner in accordance with department policy. Written informed consent for examination and collection of evidence should be obtained as well as permission to release the information to the appropriate law enforcement agencies.

Kits made specifically for sexual assault evidence collection are available and should be utilized in evidence collection.

All supplies should be gathered and available in the room *prior* to the start of evidence collection to avoid interruption of the procedure and maintain the chain of evidence.

Prior to Vaginal Exam
History

Obtain history of assault (pertinent details, i.e., oral, rectal, anal, vaginal penetration. Penetration with fingers, penis, foreign object, oral contact by assailant, by victim, ejaculation [if victim knows]).

Date and time of assault
Physical surroundings
Weapon(s) or restraint(s) used

Did victim douche, defecate, brush teeth, bathe, vomit, change clothes, urinate, eat, or drink prior to exam?

Was the victim using contraception?

Did the assailant use contraception or lubricant?

Obtain significant past medical history.

Age at menarche

Gyn infections

Gravity/parity

Presently pregnant

Most recent coitus within the last 5 days (were contraceptives used?)

Current mode of contraception prior to assault

Present illness

Present medications

Drug allergies?

Explain all procedures of evidence collection to the victim.

All evidence should be placed in paper, not plastic, containers, as plastic promotes mildew and destruction of evidence.

After each step, the evidence is sealed in an envelope and labeled with the victim's name, site of collection, date and time of collection, and name of the collector.

Clothing collection

Place a large sheet on the floor, then the paper sheet provided in the kit. Have the victim step onto the center of the sheet and carefully undress, one item at a time. DO NOT SHAKE CLOTHES, AS VALUABLE MICROSCOPIC EVIDENCE COULD BE LOST. Collect each piece and place it in a separate paper bag. Give the victim a gown, fold the paper and the sheet in such a manner as to preserve the evidence, and place both in a paper bag. Staple all bags shut and label as above.

Foreign material collection

Collect any foreign material such as leaves, dirt, fiber, hair, etc., and place in center of a piece of paper and fold paper to preserve the evidence. Debris such as dried semen, blood, or saliva from a bite mark should be collected by lightly moistening cotton swabs with distilled water and thoroughly swabbing the area. Allow swabs to air dry and return them to the original paper sleeve. Write description on the paper sleeve, e.g., ''suspected semen from left anterior thigh.'' Place the swabs in an envelope, seal it, and label as above. The entire body should be inspected at this time for less conspicuous injuries such as bruises, abrasions, or lacerations.

Some states also obtain scrapings from underneath the nails. This is analyzed for blood and tissue. Use a wood stick, place it in an envelope, seal and label as above.

Oral specimen collection

Obtain oral swabs and smear. Using two swabs, swab the buccal area and gum line. Using both swabs, prepare one smear. Allow both smear and swab to dry. Place them in an envelope, seal and document as above.

Hair specimen collection

To obtain hair shed by the assailant or crime scene debris, use a paper towel and comb. Place paper towel under head, and comb hair so that any loose hair or debris will fall onto the towel. Fold towel and comb to preserve evidence, place them in envelope, seal and document as above. Some states require that at least 15 head hairs be pulled from all areas of the head. The root structure is used in the forensic lab for analysis and identification of loose hairs.

Obtain pubic hair shed by the assailant in the assault. Use a paper towel placed under victim's buttocks, and with gloved hand comb or brush any loose hairs or debris from the pubic area. Fold towel carefully to preserve any evidence, place it in an envelope, and seal and document as above. If you used a comb, include the comb in the envelope. Some states require the collection of 15 to 25 pubic hairs plucked by the root from all areas of the pubis.

Saliva specimen collection

Obtain "known saliva sample." Using filter paper, have victim either drop a sample of saliva (from the mouth only), or fold the filter paper in half and have victim place folded edge in the mouth and saturate it this way. NOTE: The victim should not have anything to eat or drink for 30 minutes prior to obtaining the sample. Allow disk to air dry, return to envelope, seal and document as above.

Blood specimen collection

Obtain blood for typing, DNA testing, and VDRL or any other testing necessary for medical clearance at this time. Place the blood tubes required by the state in the envelope, seal and document as above.

Vaginal/Rectal Examination

Vaginal specimen collection

Obtain vaginal swabs and smear. Using both swabs together, swab the vaginal vault, then prepare the smear using both swabs. Allow both specimens to air dry, place them in the envelope, seal and document as above. This is also the time to obtain gonorrhea and/or chlamydia cultures to send to the hospital lab.

Penile specimen collection

To obtain a penile collection, slightly moisten two cotton swabs with distilled water, thoroughly swab the external surface of the penile shaft and glans. Prepare smear as above, air dry, place in an envelope, and seal and document as above.

Rectal specimen collection

Obtain rectal swab and smear. Using both swabs together, gently swab the rectal canal. Prepare smear as above, air dry, and place in an envelope. Document as above.

Documentation and Follow-up

Document findings on the exam on anatomic drawings; if photographs are indicated, they should be included in the evidence kit.

An information sheet should be given to the victim at the end of the examination. This should include all information regarding treatment that was done and follow-up plans. For example, additional tests such as blood for syphilis, or gyn smears for gonorrhea or chlamydia. Pregnancy test—to determine preexisting pregnancy only! Was any antibiotic treatment given to the victim? Name of medication and what dosage. If antibiotic treatment was not given, what was the reason. If pregnancy prophylaxis was given, a whole list of expected reactions and a medication schedule should be given to the victim. For information on AIDS counseling and confidential testing centers, the best source is the AIDS hotline (1-800-752-2437).

If at all possible, an appointment should be made with a gyn physician or nurse practitioner in 3 to 6 weeks for follow-up of test results or reculture if necessary. The victim should acknowledge receipt or refusal of this information by signing the bottom of the form.

SECURING THE EVIDENCE

All medical and forensic specimens collected should be kept separate. When all evidence has been collected, forensic specimens should be placed back in the kit. The kit should then be sealed and labeled appropriately. The complete kit and clothing should be kept together and stored in a safe place. Victims should not be allowed to handle evidence once it has been collected. Only a law enforcement official or authorized agent should transfer physical evidence from the hospital to the crime lab.

If the victim does not agree to release the evidence to law enforcement, emergency department personnel should not react negatively to this decision. They should inform the victim that the release of the evidence is not a commitment to prosecute. If permission is not gained, the kit and clothing should be kept in a secure refrigerated area for a period of time. The evidence will not spoil if kept refrigerated for up to 2 weeks. Inform the victim of the length of time the evidence will be kept prior to destruction, thereby providing the victim with an opportunity to reconsider.

NOTES OF INTEREST

Wet or damp clothes should be air dried before packing.

All swabs for evidence collection should be air dried.

If the victim is not wearing the clothing worn at the time of the assault, collect only those items in direct contact with the genital area. Inform the police so that clothing actually worn during the assault can be collected. DO NOT CUT THROUGH ANY EXISTING HOLES, RIPS, OR STAINS.

If bite marks are found, the local authorities can bring in a forensic odontologist to make bite mark impressions.

When obtaining swab specimens from the oropharanyx and rectum, appropriate cultures for gonorrhea and chlamydia can be obtained.

Smears should NOT be chemically fixed or stained.

For treatment of sexually transmitted disease, see Chapter 16.

For emergency department nurses the process of evidence collection can be time-consuming, frustrating, and stressful. Successful prosecution of sexual offenders requires accurate collection and documentation of evidence. It is not always necessary for the attending nurse or doctor to be present during court proceedings. If testimony is required, accurate and thorough documentation will help staff members to recall the events. Care must be taken to assure that no subjective opinions or conclusions are drawn as to whether or not a crime has occurred. Terms such as ''rape'' or ''sexual assault'' in medical documentation indicate a conclusion has been reached and may prejudice legal proceedings.

Evidentiary collection is only one part in the total care of the patient. Total patient care involves evaluation for and treatment of injuries, STDs, risk of pregnancy, and crisis intervention concurrently.

SUGGESTED READINGS

Ledray L: The sexual assault examination: overview and lessons learned in one program, *JEN* 18(3):223, 1992.

Ledray L: The sexual assault nurse clinician: a fifteen-year experience in Minneapolis, *JEN* 18(3):217, 1992.

Lipscomb G et al: Male victims of sexual assault, *JAMA* 267(22):3064, 1992.

Osborn M, Bryan S: Evidentiary examination in sexual assault, *JEN* 15(3):284, 1989.

Satin A et al: Sexual assault in pregnancy, *Obstetr Gynecol* 77(5):710, 1991.

Sexual assault aftercare instructions, *JEN* 18(2):152, 1992.

The State of New Hampshire office of the Attorney General: *Sexual assault: A hospital/community protocol for forensic and medical examination.*

Domestic Violence

Domestic violence has only recently (within the last 10 to 15 years) been treated with the seriousness that it deserves. The AMA declared that domestic violence against women is a true epidemic. Domestic violence is rampant. Healthcare workers have to be retrained to believe domestic violence with a fist is as important as violence with a gun.

Domestic violence generally (in ≥ 90% of the cases) involves women being abused by their male partners. However, violence against men by their female partners, violence against one partner in a gay or lesbian relationship, and violence against the elderly can also occur.

The abuse in domestic violence can be physical, sexual, and/or psychological. Generally psychological abuse accompanies all forms. The victims are made to feel responsible, alone, lonely, and without a means of help. Abuse can include controlling behaviors, which leaves the victim without money, food, clothing, and family at the whim of the abuser.

It is important to understand that domestic violence can occur in all socioeconomic groups. Typically those who abuse are often well educated, and may have experienced some form of abuse in their childhood. "Three to four thousand women in the United States are battered to death by their partners each year; three to four million are beaten. Battering is the single greatest cause of injury to women in the United States, more than mugging, car crashes and rapes combined!"[1]

INDICATIONS OF DOMESTIC VIOLENCE

1. The patient admits to past or present physical or emotional abuse as a victim or *witness.*
2. The patient denies physical abuse, but presents with unexplained bruises, whiplash injuries consistent with shaking, areas or erythema consistent with slap injuries, grab marks on arms or neck, lacerations, burns, scars, fractures or multiple injuries in various stages of healing, fractured mandible, or perforated tympanic membranes.
3. Common sites of injury in battering are areas hidden by clothing or hair

(i.e., face, head, chest, breasts, abdomen, and genitals). Accidental injuries usually involve the extremities, whereas domestic violence often involves both truncal and extremity injuries.

4. Extent or type of injury is inconsistent with the explanation offered by the patient.
5. The woman is pregnant. Violence often begins with the first pregnancy and with injuries to the breasts or abdomen.
6. The patient presents evidence of sexual assault or forced sexual actions by her partner.
7. The partner (or suspected abuser) accompanies the patient, insists on staying close to the patient, and may try to answer all questions directed to her.
8. The patient indicates fear of returning home and concern for the safety of children.
9. Substantial delay exists between the time of injury and presentation for treatment. The patient may have been prevented from seeking medical attention earlier or may have had to wait for the batterer to leave.
10. The patient describes the alleged "accident" in a hesitant, embarrassed, or evasive manner, or avoids eye contact.
11. The patient has "psychosomatic" complaints such as panic attacks, anxiety, choking sensation, or depression.
12. Complaints of chronic pain (back or pelvic pain) with no substantiating physical evidence often signify fear of impending or actual physical abuse.
13. Psychiatric, alcohol, or drug abuse history in the patient or partner; e.g., eating disorder, self-mutilation.
14. History of suicide attempts or suicidal ideation. Battering accounts for one in every four suicide attempts by all women and half of all suicide attempts by black women.
15. Review of medical records reveals repeated use of emergency department or other medical and/or social services. Medical history reveals many "accidents" or remarks by nurse or physician indicating that previous injuries were of suspicious origin.

NEED TO EDUCATE; ESTABLISH PROTOCOL

According to the latest information, conservative estimates show that *at least* 20% of the women who present to the emergency room are victims of domestic violence. Those same estimates show that ≤5% of those women are identified accurately as being victims of domestic violence.

The victims may present to the emergency department with a variety of complaints. Physical injuries are most easily related to domestic violence, but less obvious are the complaints of headaches, abdominal pain or cramps, fatigue, etc. (signs of stress). The economic impact from visits ultimately caused by domestic violence is significant.

The need to establish protocols to identify, treat, support, and follow victims of domestic violence is critical (to begin to deal with the medical conditions that victims of domestic violence experience). For only then, when we begin to identify, can we begin to help.

Conservative estimates generated by the National Crime Survey project that the annual medical cost incurred because of family violence totals $44 million each year. Indirect costs include the productivity lost from 175,000 days missed from paid work. Morbidity due to family violence causes 21,000 hospitalizations, 99,800 days of hospitalization, 28,700 emergency department visits, and 39,900 visits to a physician each year.[2]

ASSESSMENT

It is imperative to provide a quiet, safe, private environment to assess the victim. It is advisable to interview and assess the patient without the significant other present. Have the patient undress completely so that any hidden injuries will be exposed. Assess mental and emotional status also (including substance abuse, suicidal ideations, or homicidal ideations).

It is important to understand the psychological effect of being battered. The victim usually is made to feel ignorant and worthless by the abuser. She may have been repeatedly told that no one cares or wants to hear, and that if she reveals the abuse, more violence will follow. Therefore, it can be extremely difficult for victims to take that first step. Breaking through that barrier of silence and denial begins the process of effective healing (physically and psychologically).

Take a careful medical/physical history.

Ask nonthreatening questions:

1. You seem frightened of your partner. Has he ever hurt you?
2. Sometimes patients tell me they have been hurt by someone close to them. Could this be happening to you?
3. Does your partner consistently control your actions or put you down?
4. Your partner seems very concerned and anxious. Was he responsible for your injuries?
5. I noticed you have a number of bruises. Could you tell me how they happened? Did someone hit you?[3]

The acronym SAFE will help recall questions to ask in a nonjudgmental way. Here are some examples of questions:

Stress/Safety: What stress do you experience in your relationships? Do you feel safe in your relationship/marriage? Should I be concerned for your safety?

Afraid/Abused: Are there situations in your relationships where you have felt afraid? Has your partner ever threatened or abused you or your children? Have you been physically hurt or threatened by your partner? People in relationships/marriages often fight. What happens when you and your partner disagree?

Friends/Family: Are your friends aware that you have been hurt? Do your parents or siblings know about the abuse? Do you think you could tell them and do you think they would be able to give you support? (Assess the degree of social isolation.)

Emergency Plan: Do you have a safe place to go and the resources you (and your children) need in an emergency? If you are in danger now, would you like help in locating a shelter? Would you like to talk with a social worker/counselor/me to develop an emergency plan?[4]

It is *very* important to assess the patient's safety to help reduce the danger she might face after discharge. Let the patient know that domestic violence is against the law and that she can choose to make a police report. She can also get a temporary restraining order.

Questions to ask:

1. Where is the abuser now?
2. Does he know that you are here?
3. Has the abuser ever used or threatened to use weapons?
4. Are weapons available to the abuser?
5. Has the abuser been drinking or taking drugs?
6. Has the abuse been increasing in severity and/or frequency?
7. Do you have children?
8. Are they safe now?
9. Are they being abused? (Refer to your child abuse protocol.)
10. Does the abuser verbally threaten you?
11. Has the abuser threatened your friends or relatives?
12. Has the abuser threatened to commit suicide if you leave?

Explain to the patient the physical and emotional sequelae of chronic battering.

Stress the importance of follow-up for medical, legal, and social support.

Emphasize to the patient that she *can* break the cycle of violence.[5]

ADVOCACY/SUPPORT SERVICES

The role of the advocate is an important one. Advocates receive special training and are usually volunteers. Their role is to be available to help and support the patient when needed, from the initial visit in the emergency department through the critical days or months ahead.

The advocate's role is to offer the victim opportunities to explore the various options available (e.g., crisis intervention, safe home network, and legal advocacy). Advocates make no judgments and work with the victim in *support* of choices she makes, regardless of whether the advocate agrees with the choice. There are many times when the victim/patient actually returns home to an unsafe and potentially violent environment. Victims are frequently not prepared to separate from violent partners for a variety of complex, psychosocial reasons (i.e., low self-esteem, guilt, fear, loneliness, lack of support systems, lack of money, etc.). It is the role of the advocate to provide *unconditional* support so that the victim can feel that she is no longer alone.

When someone presents to the emergency department as a victim of domestic violence, local women's advocacy/support services should be notified to initiate contact and support while the patient is in the emergency department. Know your area's hotline numbers for abused women/children. Often social services will be contacted to assist the patient through the various programs/options available to her.

KNOW YOUR LEGAL OBLIGATIONS

It is important to know the law in the state in which you live regarding the reporting of domestic violence injuries:

1. Do you report life-threatening injuries (i.e., gunshot wounds, strangulation, etc.)?
2. Do you report if the patient has been drinking or has a history of alcohol or drug abuse?

Many times domestic violence includes sexual assault and a history of alcohol or drug abuse. Often the victim's own sexual history could possibly be used against her. Know the laws of reporting!

CHARTING

I. Accurate and concise documentation is essential for future medical and legal assessments. Clearly document:
  A. 1. Time, date, place, and witnesses to assault/"accident"
     2. Name, badge number, and telephone number of law enforcement officer accompanying the patient
     3. Assessment of the patient's safety
  B. Avoid long descriptions and quotes that deviate from the medical problem (e.g., "He was angry at me because I let the kids go to the movies."). This type of information is inadmissible in court and could be counterproductive if inconsistent with court testimony.
  C. If the patient states abuse as the cause of injury, prepare patient's explanation by writing: "Patient states . . ." This protects the patient and yourself since you cannot be held liable for recording a patient's statement or the medical facts of your expert medical opinion. For example you would record, "Patient states she was hit in the face by her mate's fist, punched in the stomach two times and hit with a screwdriver he grabbed off the table."
II. Avoid subjective data that might be used against the patient (e.g., "It was my fault he hit me because I didn't have the kids in bed on time.").
III. If patient denies being assaulted, write, "The patient's explanation of injuries is inconsistent with physical finding" or "injuries are suggestive of battering."
IV. Record size, pattern, estimated age, description, and location of all injuries.
  A. Use body injury map to locate injuries.
  B. Be specific, e.g., "multiple contusions and lacerations" will not convey a clear picture to a judge or jury, but "contusions and lacerations of the throat" will back up allegations of attempted strangling. Record nonbodily evidence of abuse, such as torn clothing and jewelry (Domestic Violence protocol, Dartmouth-Hitchcock Memorial Hospital).

REFERENCES

1. *National women's health report,* 13(4), Fall 1991.
2. Randall T: Medical News and Perspectives, Domestic violence intervention calls for more than treating injuries, *JAMA* 939, 1990.
3. Dartmouth-Hitchcock Domestic Violence Protocol, May, 1993.
4. Ashur ML: *Asking about domestic violence SAFE* questions, *JAMA* 269(18):2367, 1993 (letter).
5. Campbell JC, Sheridan DJ: Emergency Nursing Interventions with battered women *Clinical Articles* 15(1):12, 1989.

Obstetric and Gynecologic Emergencies

Patients with obstetric and gynecologic emergencies are frequent visitors to the emergency department, particularly because of the increasing difficulty of finding OB/GYN physicians who are accepting new patients. There are many varieties of OB/GYN emergencies; some of the more common ones are referenced in this chapter. For additional information, the reader is referred to one of the many OB/GYN reference texts listed at the end of this chapter.

CHILDBIRTH

Although usually one of the most natural occurrences on earth, the imminent birth of a baby can frighten the best of us. The most important thing to remember is to keep calm and organized.

■ **DEFINITIONS**

labor The process by which the fetus, placenta, and membranes are expelled from the uterus. This usually occurs 40 weeks after conception.

gravida The number of pregnancies, including the present.

para The number of pregnancies that have gone to at least 20 weeks of gestation, regardless of whether the infant was dead or alive at birth.

primigravida Pregnant for the first time.

nullipara Woman who has not carried a pregnancy to viability.

primipara Woman who has carried one pregnancy to viability.

multipara Woman who has carried more than one pregnancy to viability.

■ **EXAMPLES**

Gravida 3, Para 1 Woman in her third pregnancy; she has delivered one viable child.

Gravida 4, Para 0   Woman in her fourth pregnancy; she has carried none of them to viability.

Gravida 2, Para 2   Woman in her second pregnancy; she has delivered two viable children (twins).

COMPLICATIONS OF PREGNANCY

Bleeding in Pregnancy

Placenta Previa

Placenta previa accounts for 85% of cases of hemorrhage in the last trimester of pregnancy. This occurs when part or all of the placenta covers the cervical os.

■ **SIGNS AND SYMPTOMS**

Sudden *painless* bleeding (usually after 7 months of gestation)
Bright red blood from the vagina
Shock (decreased blood pressure and elevated pulse)

■ **THERAPEUTIC INTERVENTIONS**

Place the patient in shock position.
Begin IV therapy with Ringer's lactate.
If bleeding is heavy, transport for cesarean section.
Do not perform vaginal examination when vaginal bleeding is present prior to an ultrasound to determine placental placement.

Abruptio Placentae

Abruptio placentae is one of the major causes of bleeding in the last trimester of pregnancy. It is caused by separation of the placenta from the uterine wall prior to the actual birth process. This usually occurs after 20 weeks of gestation.

■ **SIGNS AND SYMPTOMS**

Uterine pain or tenderness
Bleeding may be frank, bright red vaginal bleeding or it may be concealed, with no bleeding apparent
Sudden colicky pain
Decreased blood pressure
Increased pulse
Diaphoresis
Cold, clammy skin
Uterine rigidity
If a large area of the placenta is separated, fetal heart tones may not be present

■ **THERAPEUTIC INTERVENTIONS**

Administer oxygen at 8 L/min by nasal cannula.
Begin IV therapy with Ringer's lactate.
Mark the level of the uterus on the abdomen.
Transport the patient rapidly for obstetrical care.
Do not perform vaginal examination without knowing the location of the placenta.

Pregnancy-Induced Hypertension (PIH)

Preeclampsia

One form of PIH is preeclampsia. Preeclampsia is a hypertensive, multisystem disorder associated with hypertension, proteinuria, edema, CNS irritability, and at times coagulation or liver function abnormalities.

■ **SIGNS AND SYMPTOMS**

Elevated blood pressure (systolic pressure of 140 to 200 mm Hg, diastolic greater than 90 mm Hg)

Albuminuria (2+ dipstick on catheter specimen or clean catch)

Oliguria

Edema of face, hands, sacrum

Increased weight gain

Visual changes

Facial puffiness

Headaches

Nausea

Epigastric or URQ pain

Increased DTRs with clonus

■ **THERAPEUTIC INTERVENTIONS**

Give supportive care.

Schedule obstetric consultation immediately.

Initiate magnesium sulfate therapy as ordered.

Transfer for obstetrical care.

Eclampsia

Eclampsia represents the convulsive phase of preeclampsia. Approximately 5% of preeclamptic patients will become eclamptic. There is significant maternal and fetal mortality associated with eclampsia.

■ **SIGNS AND SYMPTOMS**

Seizures

Symptomatology of preeclampsia

Elevated blood pressure (systolic pressure of 140 to 200 mm Hg, diastolic greater than 90 mm Hg)

Albuminuria (2+ dipstick on catheter specimen or clean catch)

Oliguria

Edema of face, hands, sacrum

Increased weight gain

Vision changes

Facial puffiness

Headaches

Nausea

Epigastric or URQ pain

Increased DTRs with clonus

Decreased fetal heart tones particularly during seizure and postictal for as long as 15 to 20 minutes

■ **THERAPEUTIC INTERVENTIONS**
For seizure condition
Maintain the airway.
Give oxygen at 8 L/min by nasal cannula.
Give magnesium sulfate (2 to 5 g) by *slow* IV push.
Provide supportive care.
Assess for pulmonary edema.

Gestational Trophoblastic Disease

Gestational trophoblastic disease includes hydatidiform mole and gestational trophoblastic tumors.

■ **SIGNS AND SYMPTOMS**
Bright red or brownish bleeding/spotting
Enlarged uterus
Very high HCG levels
Often absence of FHT at 12 weeks or greater
"Snowstorm" pattern with ultrasound
Signs of preeclampsia at an early gestational age

■ **THERAPEUTIC INTERVENTIONS**
Monitor vital signs carefully if bleeding is heavy.
Prepare for D & C/uterine evacuation if bleeding is heavy.
Monitor pulmonary status carefully if D&C is performed.
Observe for signs and symptoms of preeclampsia.

Ectopic Pregnancy

An ectopic pregnancy follows implantation of a fertilized egg outside the endometrial cavity, usually in the fallopian tube. Of all ectopic pregnancies, 98% are tubal, with cervical, abdominal, and ovarian implantations accounting for the remaining 2%. As the fetus grows, the fallopian tube will tear and eventually rupture.

■ **SIGNS AND SYMPTOMS**
Abnormal uterine bleeding
Severe sudden onset of unilateral pelvic pain
Abdominal tenderness and guarding
Positive pregnancy test
Suspected pregnancy (full breasts, late period, etc.)
Missed menstrual period or "late" for period
Syncope
Woman feels that she would feel better if she could have a bowel movement
Adnexal mass
Shoulder pain
If ruptured
Decreasing blood pressure
Elevated pulse

Decreasing level of consciousness
Cold, clammy skin
Delayed capillary refill

■ **DIAGNOSIS**
HCG levels
Hematocrit and hemoglobin
Pregnancy test
Ultrasound
Culdocentesis

■ **THERAPEUTIC INTERVENTIONS**
Administer oxygen at 8 L/min by nasal cannula.
Initiate IV therapy with Ringer's lactate.
Administer antibiotics.
Consider applying the PASG if indicated and in accordance with local protocol.
Prepare the patient for surgery.
Give $Rh_o(D)$ immune globulin (RhoGAM) if indicated.

Ruptured Ovarian Cyst

Ovarian cysts may be asymptomatic until hemorrhage, rupture, or torsion occur. A ruptured ovarian cyst may be confused with an ectopic pregnancy because signs and symptoms are quite similar.

■ **SIGNS AND SYMPTOMS**
Lower abdominal pain—sudden, sharp, unilateral
Nausea and vomiting
Peritoneal irritation
Irregular menstrual cycle
Adnexal mass
Low-grade temperature
Hemoperitoneum

■ **THERAPEUTIC INTERVENTIONS**
Administer oxygen at 8 L/min by nasal cannula.
Initiate IV therapy with Ringer's lactate.
Place the patient in shock position.
Consider applying the PASG if indicated and in accordance with local protocol.
Give antibiotics.
Surgery is required for removal of the cyst.

STAGES OF LABOR

Stage 1—Dilatation Stage
From the onset of regular uterine contractions to complete cervical dilation.
Average time: 12.5 hours in a primipara; 7 hours in a multipara.
Stage 2—Expulsion Stage
From the time of complete dilation until the baby is delivered. Average time:
80 minutes in a primipara; 30 minutes in a multipara.

Stage 3—Placental Stage
> From the time immediately following delivery of the baby until the expulsion of the placenta. Average time: 5 to 15 minutes.

EMERGENCY DELIVERY

■ **SIGNS AND SYMPTOMS OF IMPENDING DELIVERY**
If the following signs and symptoms are present, prepare for immediate delivery. When assisting with a delivery, attempt to maintain sterile technique if possible. If delivery is imminent, do not delay to maintain sterility at the risk of endangering both the mother and the infant.
> Heavy, bloody show
> Frequent contractions
> Desire to ''bear down'' by the mother
> Mother stating that she is going to defecate or that the ''baby is coming''
> Bulging membranes from the vulva
> Crowning of the fetal head (Figure 29-1, *A, B*)
> Fetal bradycardia

■ **EQUIPMENT**
Basin or plastic bag
Scissors or scalpel (sterile) to cut cord
2 cord clamps or 2 Kelly clamps
1 bulb syringe
Sterile gloves
Heated Isolette (if possible) or warm blankets
Identification bands for mother and infant

■ **PROCEDURE**
1. Be calm.
2. Prepare the mother by placing her in a prone position with her knees bent or in a side lying position (Figure 29-2). Delivery of the anterior shoulder is often easier if mom is side lying. This implies someone supporting her upper leg.
3. Take vital signs (including fetal heart tones) if time permits.

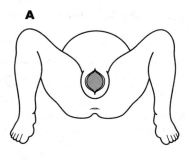 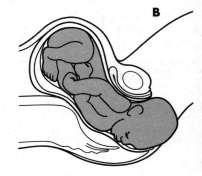

FIGURE 29-1. Childbirth sequence. **A,** Crowning. **B,** Cross-section view of crowning.

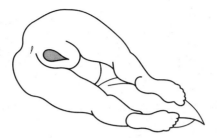

FIGURE 29-2. Side lying position.

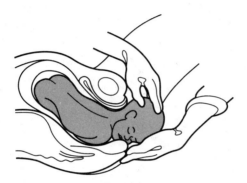

FIGURE 29-3. Perineal support.

4. Offer much verbal support; explain what is going on.
5. Put on sterile gloves.
6. Place a fluid-absorbent pad under mother.
7. Have the mother pant with each contraction or push gently.
8. Place gentle pressure on the fetal head when it crowns to avoid rapid expulsion of the fetus. Support the perineum with a towel (Figure 28-3).
9. Support the head with both hands, but allow it to rotate naturally (Figure 29-4, Figure 29-5, *A* and *B*).
10. Check for the cord around the infant's neck.
    If it is there, attempt to slip it over the infant's head.
    If it is too tight, immediately clamp the cord in two places and cut the cord between the clamps.
11. Suction the infant. Suction mouth first in order to clear the oropharynx. Suction nose second. Suctioning the nose often stimulates the baby to gasp—you want the mouth cleared when this happens. (Remember that newborns are obligate nose breathers.)
12. Deliver the shoulders by guiding the head downward to deliver the anterior shoulder and then upward to deliver the posterior shoulder.

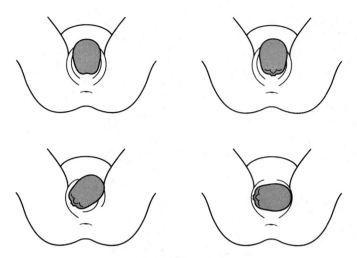

FIGURE 29-4. Birth and rotation.

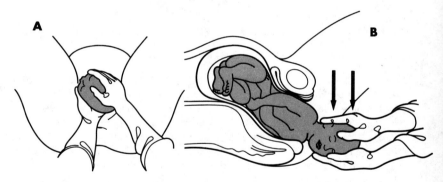

FIGURE 29-5. **A**, Delivery of head. **B**, Cross-section view of delivery of head.

13. The remaining parts of the infant may deliver quickly. You may need to apply gentle traction (Figure 29-6, *A*).
14. Note the time of birth.
15. If the membranes are still intact, quickly snip them at the nape of the neck and peel them away from the face.
16. Hold the infant along the length of your arm with the head dependent and suction the mouth and nose once again or place the infant on the surface of the bed (Figure 29-6, *B*).
17. Clamp the cord and cut between the clamps using sterile scissors.
18. Dry the baby immediately and thoroughly. Assess for evidence of respiratory effort as you are drying the baby.

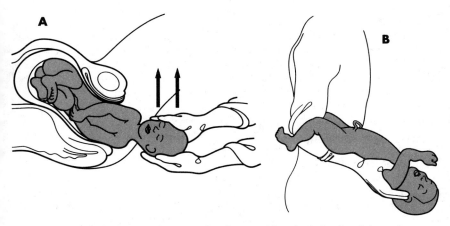

FIGURE 29-6. **A**, Delivery of the rest of body. **B**, Holding the baby, head dependent.

TABLE 29-1   Apgar Score Chart

	0	1	2
Heart rate	0	Less than 100	More than 100
Muscle tone	Limp	Some flexion	Well flexed
Reflexes (catheter in nose)	No response	Grimace	Cough or sneeze
Color	Blue, pale	Pink body, blue extremities	Pink

19. The infant should make a first effort to breathe by crying spontaneously. If spontaneous breathing still does not occur, initiate positive pressure ventilation.

    Check heart rate after 30 minutes of positive pressure ventilation. If heart rate is below 80, initiate chest compressions and neonatal CPR.

20. Determine an Apgar score at 1 minute and again at 5 minutes (Table 29-1).

21. Keep the infant warm by wrapping it in a blanket and/or placing it in a heated Isolette. If an Isolette is not available, have the mother hold the infant, using skin-to-skin contact.

Delivery of the Placenta

■ **SIGNS AND SYMPTOMS OF IMPENDING DELIVERY OF THE PLACENTA**

The umbilical cord advances 2 to 3 inches farther out of the vagina.

The fundus rises upward in the abdomen.

The uterus becomes firm and globular.

A large gush of blood comes from the vagina.

■ **PROCEDURE**
1. Instruct the mother to "bear down."
2. Apply *gentle* traction on the cord; do *not* pull on the cord.
3. Massage the fundus immediately after delivery of the placenta.
4. Once the placenta is delivered, inspect it for missing sections.
5. Save the placenta in a basin or plastic bag and send it with the mother to the obstetrical unit.

Care of the Mother

Wipe the perineal area gently with a clean dry towel.
Place a sanitary napkin or towel in the perineal area.
Massage the fundus while applying suprapubic pressure.
Initiate IV therapy (usually Ringer's lactate or Ringer's lactate with 5% dextrose) at approximately 150 ml/hr (faster if bleeding is excessive).
Administer oxytocic agents in accordance with the facility policy or in accordance with physician's orders (usually pitocin).
Keep the mother warm.
Observe closely; monitor the vital signs frequently (every 15 minutes) until they are stable.
Put an infant identification band on the mother's wrist.

Care of the Infant

Keep the infant warm.
Maintain the infant's airway by placing the infant on its side.
Apply erythromycin or silver nitrate eye prophylaxis (in accordance with facility policy).
Administer phytonadione (Aquamephyton) for hypoprothrombinemia prophylaxis (in accordance with facility policy).
Observe the cord for bleeding.
Put an identification band on both the wrist and ankle.
Observe closely and monitor vital signs.

NORMAL NEWBORN VITAL SIGN RANGE		
Pulse: 100-160	Respirations: 40-60	Temperature: >36.5° C

COMPLICATIONS OF DELIVERY

Nonreassuring Fetal Heart Rate

■ **SIGNS AND SYMPTOMS**
Meconium stained amniotic fluid. (Fluid will be green or dark yellow. It can also be very thick.)

■ **THERAPEUTIC INTERVENTIONS**

Apply oxygen.

Attempt to have mother blow with contractions as if she were "blowing out a candle."

Prepare equipment to intubate the baby at birth. (A size 3.0 or 3.5 tube is needed.) If possible, have a pediatrician present.

When equipment is available, encourage mother to push with contractions if she feels pressure or the urge to push.

Suction the baby's mouth and nose thoroughly after delivery of the head and before delivery of the body.

If intubation is possible, visualize the vocal cords immediately after birth. If meconium is visible below the cords, insert an ET tube and apply suction as the ET tube is removed. This requires the use of a meconium aspirator.

Repeat this procedure before encouraging the baby to breathe (hopefully no longer than 20 to 30 seconds).

■ **SIGNS AND SYMPTOMS**

Decreased fetal heart tones (less than 100 beats per minute)

■ **THERAPEUTIC INTERVENTIONS**

Encourage mother to push if she feels the urge to push.

Administer oxygen at 8 L/min via nasal cannula or mask.

Place the mother in a side lying position.

Check for prolapsed cord.

Initiate IV therapy with Ringer's lactate.

Follow steps for normal vaginal delivery or rapid transport for cesarean section.

Be prepared to administer neonatal resuscitation.

Breech Position of Fetus

In 3% of all births the fetus presents in the breech position, with either the buttocks first or a foot first (known as a footling breech). These positions are dangerous for the fetus because of the increased likelihood of a prolapsed cord and of a difficult delivery. Delivery of the fetus in these states is best accomplished by cesarean section. If delivery is progressing, apply the following therapeutic interventions:

Support the legs and buttocks of the baby.

When the mother has a contraction, pull gently on the baby. Placing a towel around the baby helps to grasp the infant..

Insert your finger into the vagina—deliver one shoulder, then the other (Figure 29-7, *A* and *B*).

DO NOT PULL ON THE BABY. This may cause the cervix to clamp tighter around the baby's head. Work with the mother's contractions.

Deliver the head by supporting the baby's chest with your arms and hands.

Place your finger into the vagina and find the baby's mouth.

As mother pushes with contractions, reach into baby's mouth, grasp the chin and apply gentle upward pressure to head and shoulders (Figure 29-8).

It may be necessary to apply suprapubic pressure as well.

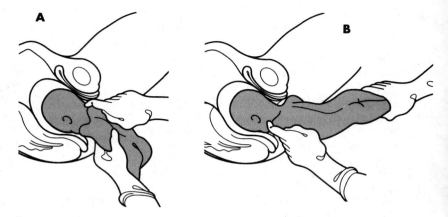

FIGURE 29-7. **A**, Extraction of anterior arm. **B**, Extraction of posterior arm. Breech-shoulder delivery.

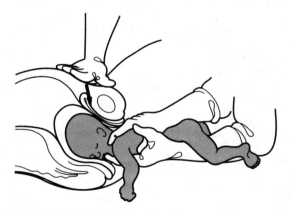

FIGURE 29-8. Delivery of arms and shoulders. Breech-head delivery.

Prolapsed Cord

A prolapsed cord is a state in which the cord precedes the infant. This is an absolute emergency (Figure 29-9, *A* to *C*).

■ **SIGNS AND SYMPTOMS**

Visible cord protruding from vagina

Fetal heart rate less than 100

■ **THERAPEUTIC INTERVENTIONS**

Elevate the mother's hips or place in knee-chest position.

Administer oxygen at 8 L/min by nasal cannula.

Keep the mother warm.

Place a gloved hand into the vaginal canal and elevate the fetus's head to

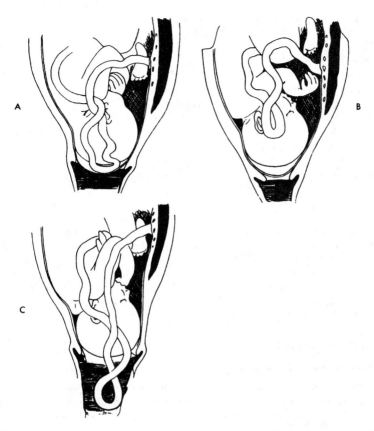

FIGURE 29-9. A, Cord prolapsed at the inlet. **B,** Cord prolapsed into the vagina. **C,** Cord prolapsed through the introitus.

(From Dickason E: *Maternal-infant nursing care*, ed 2. St Louis, 1994, Mosby-Year Book.)

relieve pressure on the cord; once this has been accomplished, leave your hand in place.

Leave the cord as it is; do not attempt to place it back in the vagina.

Feel the cord for pulsations.

Notify the appropriate personnel and transport the patient so that an immediate cesarean section can be performed. If transport time is prolonged, keep cord moist with saline-moistened towels.

Postpartum Hemorrhage

Normal bleeding after delivery is 300 to 500 ml. More than this amount is excessive. Hemorrhage is considered to be 750 ml or more.

■ **SIGNS AND SYMPTOMS**

Steady flow of bright red blood

Decreasing blood pressure
Increasing pulse
Pale, clammy skin
Nausea
Signs of hypovolemia
■ **THERAPEUTIC INTERVENTIONS**
Give oxygen at 8 L/min by nasal cannula.
Place the mother in Trendelenburg's position.
Begin IV therapy with Ringer's lactate with oxytocin (Pitocin, Syntocinon).
Apply manual pressure to tears.
Massage the uterus while applying suprapubic pressure.
If hypovolemic shock occurs, consider application of the PASG.

ABORTION

The term *abortion* is applied to a pregnancy that fails to survive to 20 weeks, with the products of conception weighing less than 500 grams. The frequency of abortion is 10% to 15% of known pregnancies. The major complications of abortion are hemorrhage and infection. Pregnancy loss in the first trimester is largely due to developmental defects of the embryo. Later loss is more frequently associated with infections or endocrine or anatomic abnormalities within the maternal reproductive organs.

Types of Abortions
Threatened abortion

A threatened abortion is said to occur in cases where early symptoms of abortion, such as episodic, painless uterine bleeding and mild cramping are present. The cervical os is closed, the uterus is enlarged and soft, and the pregnancy test is positive.
■ **THERAPEUTIC INTERVENTIONS**
Bed rest

Inevitable abortion

Bleeding becomes moderate, cramping becomes moderate, and the cervical os is open. Loss of the pregnancy cannot be prevented or stopped.
■ **THERAPEUTIC INTERVENTIONS**
Bed rest
Analgesics/narcotics
Patient may have D & C at provider's and patient's discretion
RhoGAM if indicated

Incomplete abortion

In an incomplete abortion, bleeding is heavy, cramping is severe, and the cervical os is open. The uterus is enlarged and the pregnancy test is positive. Some tissue has been passed, but some products of conception have been retained.

■ **THERAPEUTIC INTERVENTIONS**
Oxygen at 8 L/min by nasal cannula
IV therapy with Ringer's lactate
Oxytocic agents
Surgery for curretage
RhoGAM if indicated

Complete abortion

In complete abortion there is a small amount of bleeding, cramping is mild, all tissue has been passed, and the cervical os is closed.

■ **THERAPEUTIC INTERVENTIONS**
Observation

Missed abortion

A loss of pregnancy in which the products of conception remain in the uterus for an extended period after the fetus has died. In addition, the characteristic symptoms of bleeding and cramping are absent.

■ **THERAPEUTIC INTERVENTIONS**
Some providers may send the patient home for expectant management
Possible dilation and curettage

Septic abortion

Infection after abortion occurs occasionally in patients who had a complete abortion without dilation and curettage. More frequently it occurs in patients with delayed treatment of incomplete abortion or as a result of an earlier elective termination of pregnancy. The organisms most frequently responsible are alpha- and beta-hemolytic strep, gram-negative aerobes such as *E. coli,* and occasionally *Clostridium welchii,* all of which are often the normal flora of the vagina.

Particular concern must be directed toward *Clostridium,* an anaerobic organism capable of producing gas gangrene, tissue necrosis, and tissue sloughing in the uterus. Prompt treatment is essential and if improvement does not occur after dilation and curettage, hysterectomy is indicated.

■ **SIGNS AND SYMPTOMS**
Foul discharge
Constant pain
Temperature elevation
Chills
Uterine tenderness

■ **THERAPEUTIC INTERVENTIONS**
To avoid significant morbidity and mortality the treatment of septic abortion
    must be immediate and aggressive antibiotics appropriate to infecting agent
Oxytocin infusion
Dilation and curettage
Observe for signs of endotoxic shock: hypotension, renal failure, and tachy-
    cardia

Postabortion Considerations

The patient should be given the following information after abortion.

Vaginal bleeding may last 1 to 2 weeks. The bleeding should get progressively lighter until it subsides.

Slight cramping is normal for several days.

No douching, tampons, and intercourse for at least 2 weeks or until her follow-up visit.

Rest for 2 to 3 days.

Take temperature morning and evening for 5 days.

Contact provider for:

Temperature above 100° F

Excessive bleeding

Severe cramps

Chills

Severe nausea and vomiting

If the patient receives a dilation and curettage with anesthesia, give appropriate information regarding effects of medication.

Many women and men find the loss of their child, even very early in pregnancy, devastating. Comfort as appropriate, reassure that feelings of grief and loss are to be expected. Refer for appropriate counseling as needed. The obstetrical/maternity unit may have a list of resources to help the woman or couple with their grief—such as Compassionate Friends, SHARE.

VAGINAL BLEEDING

Abnormal uterine bleeding is one of the most common gynecologic complaints. Causes of uterine bleeding are many and varied. Particular concern for the welfare of the fetus exists if the patient is pregnant.

To assist in establishing a firm diagnosis, it is important to obtain a good history from the patient. Important questions to answer are:

Are the vital signs stable? Is the hematocrit stable? If not:

Initiate IV therapy with Ringer's lactate.

Have the PASG standing by.

Is the patient pregnant? Do a 2 minute and 2 hour pregnancy test.

If the patient is pregnant, is she aborting?

Do *not* do a vaginal examination if the patient is more than 20 weeks gestation.

Before doing a vaginal exam on a pregnant patient who is bleeding, it is important to rule out placenta previa by ultrasound.

If the patient is not pregnant or is under 20 weeks, a vaginal exam should be performed.

Is the cervical os open or closed? If it is closed, abortion may be threatening. Patients may experience bleeding caused by trauma, cervical or vaginal lesions, or cervical or vaginal polyps. Treatments center around the immediate concern for the patient's well-being with a recommendation for follow-up gynecologic consultation.

Dysfunctional Uterine Bleeding (DUB)

The most common cause of DUB is a disturbance in the cyclic pattern of the endometrium. This can be caused by a variety of abnormalities in the patient's hormonal patterns.

■ **THERAPEUTIC INTERVENTIONS**

Treatment for immediate concerns related to bleeding

IV therapy/volume support

Long-term therapy: either progestin alone, oral high-dose estrogen–progestin birth control pills, or estrogen alone

Recommendation for follow-up gynecologic consultation

GYNECOLOGIC INFECTIONS

Pelvic Inflammatory Disease (PID)

The term *pelvic inflammatory disease* is a commonly used term that implies infection in the pelvis: the uterus, fallopian tubes, ovaries, pelvic peritoneum, or some combination of these sites. The term can obscure diagnosis and treatment. Three clinically identifiable subgroups of PID are: (1) endometritis-salpingitis, (2) pelvic peritonitis, and (3) tuboovarian abscess.

Pelvic inflammatory disease occurs as a result of upward migration of bacteria. The bacteria most often isolated are *gonorrhea, streptococci, E. Coli, Proteus, Klebsiella-enterobacter, Clostridia,* and *chlamydia.* There are several predisposing factors. Among these are an IUD, trauma, multiple intercourse partners, or history of recent abortion. PID may be the cause of chronic abdominal pain, ectopic pregnancy, or infertility. The presenting symptoms and treatment options are outlined in Table 29-2.

Toxic Shock Syndrome

Toxic shock syndrome is characterized by the abrupt onset of pyrexia, myalgias, and a diffuse rash with edema, and blanching erythema. Less frequent symptoms are vomiting, diarrhea, and hypotension. The etiologic bacteria is usually *Staphylococcus aureus,* which can be isolated from local sites of skin disruption.

Menstrual toxic shock syndrome is most often associated with use of tampons and the contraceptive sponge. However, it has also been associated with tubal ligation, hysterectomy, and carbon dioxide laser vaporization of genital condyloma.

■ **THERAPEUTIC INTERVENTIONS**

Supportive therapy for septic shock

Blood pressure support

Respiratory support

Eliminate source of toxin

Penicillin

Corticosteroids

Contact isolation

TABLE 29-2   Diagnosis and Management of Symptomatic Pelvic Inflammatory Disease

HISTORY AND PELVIC EXAMINATION	LABORATORY TESTS	TREATMENT
Pain and tenderness	Gram stain and culture genital tract Complete blood count Possible culdocentesis or laparoscopy	Oral antibiotics Pain medication
Pain, tenderness, and fever <102.5° F	As above	As above; may need hospitalization and intravenous antibiotics
Pain, tenderness, and fever >102.5° F or nausea and vomiting	As above plus blood culture	Hospitalization and intravenous antibiotics
All the above plus pelvic mass	As above plus culdocentesis if cul-de-sac is bulging	Surgery if mass does not resolve on antibiotics
Septic shock in addition to any of the above	As above plus central venous pressure monitor	As above plus steroids and cardiovascular medications

(From: Kase N, Weingold A, Gershenson O: *Principles and practice of clinical gynecology.* New York, 1990, Churchill Livingstone, p. 588.)

Infections of External Genitalia

Recognition and diagnosis of external genitalia infections are made through visual observation. Some of the more common ones are:

INFECTION	THERAPEUTIC INTERVENTIONS
Scabies	Kwell lotion or shampoo
Vulvar abscess	Incision and drainage Antibiotics Sitz baths
Simple cyst	Sitz baths
Bartholin's cyst (infected)	Antibiotics Sitz baths Later, incision and drainage Urination via Foley catheter Check for gonorrhea
Condyloma (genital warts)	Local application of podophyllin Trichloracetic acid Large lesions surgically removed or treated with laser
Herpes	Acyclovir Analgesics

Vaginal Infection

If the ecology of the vagina is disturbed, vaginal infection may occur. Vaginal infection is not usually an emergency situation but is a frequently seen com-

TABLE 29-3 Gynecologic Emergencies
Differential diagnosis of common vaginal infections

ORGANISM	OCCURRENCE	COLOR	ODOR	CONSISTENCY	OTHER	LAB TEST(S)	THERAPEUTIC INTERVENTION
Hemophilus vaginalis	31% of all vaginal infections	Whitish-gray	Foul	Watery		Wet mount culture and Gram's stain to exclude other organisms	Sultrin, 1 applicatorful 2 times a day for 4 to 6 days .
Bacterial (nonspecific) vaginitis	27% of all vaginal infections	Yellow	Foul	Water/creamy	May be caused by retained foreign body	Wet mount culture and Gram's stain to exclude other organisms	Antibiotics (type-specific); remove foreign body
Candida albicans	26% of all vaginal infections	White	Odorless	Cheesey; heavy flow	Causes monilial vaginitis	Pseudohyphae from KOH wet mount	Nystatin (Mycostatin) vaginal tablets 1 to 2 times daily for 7 to 14 days or clotrimazole (Gyne-Lotrimin) vaginal tablets once a day for 7 days
Trichomonas vaginalis	16% of all vaginal infections	Yellowish-gray	Fishy	Creamy; bubbly	Frequently, erythema around cervical os	Wet mount shows motile protozoa	Metronidazole (Flagyl) 250 mg po 3 times daily for 7 days. Male partner must also be treated with same drug and dosage. If woman's pregnant, substitute Tricofuron

From Budassi SA: JEN 6(3):35, 1980.
Other causes of vaginal discharge include: (1) cancer of cervix or uterus, (2) IUD, (3) pelvic inflammatory disease, (4) rectal or bladder fistula, and (5) senile vaginitis.

plaint in the emergency department because it is an annoyance to the patient. The four most common types of vaginal infections are described in Table 29-3.

ABDOMINAL/PELVIC PAIN

Endometriosis

The condition in which endometrial tissue cells are found growing outside the uterus is known as endometriosis. This tissue reacts to hormonal changes just as normal endometrial tissue does. As menstruation occurs, endometrial tissue sloughs; this may be the cause of the chief complaint of pelvic pain.

■ **SIGNS AND SYMPTOMS**
Depends on the extent of the disease
Dysmenorrhea
Episodic pelvic pain
Dysuria/hematuria
Dyspareunia
Infertility

■ **DIAGNOSIS**
Clinical visualization by laparoscopy
Biopsy

■ **THERAPEUTIC INTERVENTIONS**
Hormone (exogenous)
Danazol (Danocrine)
Oral contraceptive agents
Consider surgery

SEXUAL ASSAULT

Sexual assault is covered in detail in Chapter 27.

CONTRACEPTIVE EMERGENCIES

Occasionally a patient with a contraceptive emergency will present to the emergency department. Table 29-4 lists some of the more common contraceptive emergencies.

Due to increasingly difficult access to care for some women, the emergency department serves as the only option for health care. When emergencies arise around pregnancy, it is a stressful and frightening time for families. Your capable skills and caring approach make a tremendous impact and difference to the family.

SUGGESTED READINGS

Avant RF: Spontaneous abortion and ectopic pregnancy, *Primary Care* 10:161, 1983.
Benrubi G, Harwood-Nuss D: *Obstetrical emergencies.* New York, 1990, Churchill Livingstone.
Bobak I, Jensen M: *Maternity and gynecologic care: the nurse and the family.* St Louis, 1993, Mosby.

TABLE 29-4   Contraceptive Emergencies

TYPE	PROBLEM	THERAPEUTIC INTERVENTION
Diaphragm	Unable to remove	Remove with ring forceps
IUD	Unable to remove	Remove with ring forceps
	Lost string	X-ray or ultrasound to determine position; may be removed with IUD hook
	Partial expulsion	Remove; consider alternate form of contraception
	Migration to abdominal cavity	X-ray or ultrasound to determine position; may require exploratory laparotomy
Oral contraceptives	Thrombophlebitis	Bed rest; local heat; anticoagulation
	Pulmonary embolus	ABCs; oxygen, IV, analgesia, bronchodilators, heparin, reassurance
	Cerebrovascular accident	ABCs; oxygen IV

Blackburn S, Loper D: *Maternal, fetal, and neonatal physiology: a clinical perspective.* Philadelphia, 1992, Saunders.

Comeau J et al: Early placenta previa and delivery outcome, *Obstet Gynecol* 61:577, 1983.

Danforth DN: *Obstetrics and gynecology,* ed 4. Philadelphia, 1982, Harper & Row.

Droegemueller W, Bressler R: Clinical management of IUD complications, *Drug Therapy,* 1982.

Holman JF, Tyrey EL, Hammon CB: A contemporary approach to suspected ectopic pregnancy with use of quantitative and qualitative assage for the B-subunit of HCG and Sonography, *Am J Gynecol Obstet* 150:151, 1984.

Kase N, Weingold A, Gershenson D: *Principles and practice of clinical gynecology.* New York, 1990, Churchill Livingstone.

Ledger WJ: The management of pelvic inflammatory disease, *Hosp Phys* 10:45, 1982.

Oxorn H, Foote W: *Human labor and birth.* New York, 1988, Appleton-Century-Crofts.

Pritchard JA et al: *Williams obstetrics,* ed 17. New York, 1985, Appleton-Century-Crofts.

Quan M, Johnson R, Rodney WM: The diagnosis of acute pelvic pain, *West J Med* 139: 110, 1983.

Quan M, Rodney WM, Johnson RA: Pelvic inflammatory disease, *J Fam Prac* 16:131, 1983.

Schacter J: Sexually transmitted chlamydia trachomatis infection: management of the most common venereal disease, *Postgrad Med* 72:60, 1982.

Sound Reiner SJ: Lower abdominal pain. In Cohen AW, ed: *Emergencies in obstetrics and gynecology.* New York, 1981, Churchill Livingstone.

Weckstein LN et al: Current perspective on ectopic pregnancy, *Obstet Gynecol Surv* 40: 259, 1985.

Wilson JR, Carington ER, Ledger WJ: *Obstetrics and gynecology,* ed 7. St Louis, 1983, Mosby.

Wingate MB: Geriatric gynecology, *Primary Care* 9:53, 1982.

CHAPTER 30

Pediatric Medical Emergencies

This chapter presents a broad overview of pediatric problems commonly seen in the emergency department. Because there is not enough space to detail every possible emergency condition, the reader is referred to the list of suggested readings at the end of the chapter.

GENERAL APPROACH TO THE PEDIATRIC PATIENT

Most health care personnel are not used to working with large numbers of sick children on a daily basis. As a result, it is normal to feel a bit anxious when a pediatric patient arrives in the emergency department, especially a very sick child. It is important to remain calm and to have self-confidence. There are a few basic rules to follow when dealing with a sick child:

- Be gentle but firm.
- Use common sense.
- Speak directly to the child.
- Be honest with the child; if something is going to hurt, say that it is going to hurt.
- Tell the child what is about to be done.
- Tell the child what is being done while it is being done.
- Remember that parents may be very anxious, too:

   Allow the parents to be with the child whenever possible.

   If for some reason the parents cannot be with the child, be sure that someone is available to stay with them or at least to keep them informed periodically about the child's condition.

   Some procedures are more easily accomplished if the parent holds the child (e.g., examinations of a child's ear).

   Between examinations, allow the child to sit in the parent's lap if possible.

See Table 30-1 for a description of theories of child development and emergency department interventions according to age.

PEDIATRIC TRIAGE

Pediatric triage begins with the visual assessment: "Does the child look sick?" The level of activity, skin color, and breathing pattern are the key signs to consider in the initial visual assessment. Is the child extremely pale, ashen, or mottled? Is the child markedly tachypneic with grunted or shallow respirations? Visual triage must be more than a simple peek through the blankets.

Triage Criteria

I. Primary Survey
  A. Airway
    1. Patency
  B. Breathing
    1. Rate—tachypnea/slow respirations
    2. Quality
    3. Breath sounds—wheezing, stridor
    4. Mechanics—retractions, grunting
  C. Circulation
    1. Skin color: mottled, ashen pallor, cyanotic, dusky, flushed
    2. Capillary refill time—delayed >2 seconds
    3. Skin temperature
    4. CNS perfusion—response to parents, response to threatening stimuli (nurse), response to pain
II. Vital Signs (Table 30-2)—note any deviation from normal
  A. Age of child
  B. Temperature—any temperature associated with abnormalities of activity, respiration pattern, or dermal warning signs
    1. Fever, greater than 105° F
    2. Hypothermia
      a. Less than 96° F (infant)
      b. Less than 95° F (toddler, child)
  C. Heart rate
    a. Greater than 200 beats/minute (infant)
    b. Greater than 180 beats/minute (toddler)
    c. Greater than 160 beats/minute (child)
    d. Profound bradycardia in any age group
    (Note that sinus arrhythmia is normal in most pediatric patients.)
  D. Respiratory rate
    a. Greater than 60 breaths/minute (infants)
    b. Greater than 40 breaths/minute (toddlers)
    c. Greater than 30 breaths/minute (child)
  E. Blood pressure—any BP associated with poor capillary refill
    1. Systolic

TABLE 30-1   Theories of Child Development and Suggested Interventions

	BIRTH-18 MO	19 MO-2 YR	3 YR-5 YR	6 YR-11 YR	12 YR-18 YR
Theories of child development					
Erikson	Trust vs mistrust	Autonomy vs shame and doubt	Initiative vs guilt	Industry vs inferiority	Identity vs role confusion
Freud	Oral-sensory	Anal	Phallic	Latency	Genital
Piaget	Sensorimotor egocentrism	Preoperational, beginnings of perceptual constancy	Preoperational, prelogical reasoning	Concrete operations	Formal operations
Task mastery	Differentiate self and nonself	Toilet training	Use of language	Logic	Abstract thinking
Pain perception	Physical but possibly not cognitive pain perceived, in younger patients	Primarily egocentric: "Here and now" May see pain as punishment	Pain as punishment Overextension of causality Fear and fantasy	Beginning of understanding of true causality Fear of destruction and death	Concept of emotional and physical pain Understanding of root causes of pain

Suggested interventions				
1. Involve caretaker in care of child.	1. Prepare caretaker for procedures.	1. Explain procedure *immediately before* performing it.	1. Explain procedure beforehand.	1. Give *full* explanations.
2. Keep child warm.	2. Tell caretaker that he or she may assist in normal care.	2. Allow child to see and touch samples of equipment.	2. Enlist cooperation.	2. Encourage child's participation.
3. Keep room quiet.	3. Give child a familiar toy or blanket as a transitional object.	3. Be honest: "This will sting."	3. Ask about simple preferences.	3. Allow time for questions.
4. Provide comfort measures (e.g., pacifier).	4. Use child's name.	4. Use simple distractions and talk to child.	4. Give alternatives (e.g., child may yell but not move).	4. Provide *privacy.* Child may want to exclude parents.
5. Keep child on caretaker's lap during physical examination.	5. Restrain child as little as possible.	5. Allow child to see under bandages.	5. Identify sensations and personnel.	5. Avoid teasing and embarrassing child.
6. Return child to caretaker as soon as possible after procedures; allow caretaker to comfort child.	6. Avoid covering child's face.	6. Use praise, adhesive bandages, and small rewards.	6. Use distraction and counting games.	6. Allow as much control as possible.
	7. Describe sensations and talk with child during the procedures.		7. Include child in discharge instructions.	7. Provide discharge instructions to patient.
	8. Praise, smile, and have a cheerful attitude.		8. Use rewards, stickers, badges, and praise.	8. Reassure child that his or her behavior was appropriate.

From Barkin R: *Pediatric emergency medicine.* St Louis, 1992, Mosby.

TABLE 30-2 Average Vital Signs and Weight by Age

AGE	HEART RATE AVERAGE (beats/min)	HEART RATE RANGE	SYSTOLIC BLOOD PRESSURE AVERAGE (mm Hg)	SYSTOLIC BLOOD PRESSURE RANGE	RESPIRATORY RATE (breaths/min)	WEIGHT (kg)
Preterm	140	120-180	50	40-60	55-65	2
Term newborn	140	90-170	72	52-92	40-60	3
1 mon	135	110-180	82	60-104	30-50	4
6 mon	135	110-180	94	65-125	25-35	7
1 yr	120	80-160	94	70-118	20-30	10
2 yrs	110	80-130	95	73-117	20-30	12
4 yrs	105	80-120	91	65-117	20-30	16
6 yrs	100	75-115	96	76-116	18-24	20
8 yrs	90	70-110	99	79-119	18-22	25
10 yrs	90	70-110	102	82-122	16-20	30
12 yrs	85	60-110	106	84-128	16-20	40
14 yrs	80	60-105	110	84-136	16-20	50

From Barkin R: *Pediatric emergency medicine*. St Louis, 1992, Mosby.

    a. Less than 50 systolic (infants)
    b. Less than 60 systolic (toddlers)
    c. Less than 70 systolic (child)
F. Weight, less than third to fifth percentile for age

MEDICATION ADMINISTRATION

Pediatric dosages of medications are given in accordance with the child's weight (refer to Table 30-2). Total pediatric dosage should never exceed adult dosage. It is important to be able to estimate a child's weight quickly and accurately.

INTRAVENOUS THERAPY IN PEDIATRICS

The most difficult aspects of starting an IV on an infant or child are finding a vein, controlling the patient during puncture, and anchoring the needle to prevent infiltration and mechanical irritation to the vessel. The most significant aspect of the procedure is supporting the patient and the parents emotionally and performing so efficiently that little pain results. The most underrated aspect of this procedure is the fear and discomfort the clinician experiences when establishing an IV on a tiny child, particularly when the clinician has not used the skill frequently enough to be precise and efficient.

Young children tend to have deep veins well covered with subcutaneous tissue, and in the presence of volume depletion may not evidence peripheral veins even with a tourniquet applied. If the volume is severely depleted and the child is thus compromised, do not attempt peripheral extremity lines. Such cases are emergencies of the highest magnitude; to avoid a time delay, intraosseus access, central lines, or a cutdown by an experienced clinician would be best.

In cases where time is not of the essence, scalp veins or veins on the dorsum of the hand or foot may be used to place a 22-gauge or larger over-the-needle catheter.

Sites to Avoid

Antecubital fossa (clinical lab technicians will need access to these areas)
Veins over joints
Veins that might need to be used for cutdown (femoral, saphenous)
Bruised, fractured, or burned areas

Criteria for Selection of Large Veins

Large quantities of fluid must be administered
Blood products must be administered
Solution is hypertonic

Equipment Needed for Peripheral Vein IV

22-gauge or larger over-the-needle catheter (with syringe attached)

Alcohol or iodinated solution (CAUTION: may obscure vein in poor light)

IV extension tubing attached to a 100 ml volume control chamber, connected to an IV solution and properly flushed, attached to infusion pump

Armboard

Tourniquet

Silk tape, cut in strips

Technique for Inserting Over-the-Needle Catheter into Peripheral Vein (Figure 30-1)

Explain the procedure to the child and parents.

Select a vein and restrain all extremities before beginning. You will probably need assistance, especially with an infant or toddler. If time permits, apply a warm compress over selected insertion site to promote vasodilation.

Make the puncture with the bevel away from the vein and the point toward the vein; the indirect method is preferred (entering from the side and at a slight angle to the vein) when using an over-the-needle catheter to avoid flattening the vein or piercing the posterior wall.

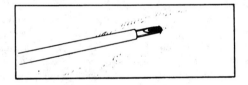

FIGURE 30-1. To insert an over-the-needle catheter the needle should be properly aligned with the bevel up.

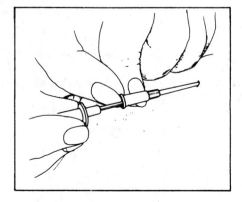

Withdraw the needle before advancing the catheter.

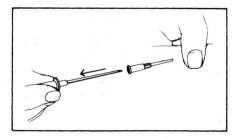

Remove the needle before attaching an infusion set.

Once the skin and vein are entered, realign the needle and advance slightly. Blood will generally appear in the flashback chamber. If a small syringe is attached before puncture, slight negative pressure can be applied to the plunger to elicit a flashback of blood.

On flashback of blood, stop advancing the needle. Stabilize with one hand while the thumb and forefinger of the other hand disengage the catheter from the needle and advance it into the vein as far as possible.

Release the tourniquet, remove the needle, and begin the flow of IV fluid.

Apply adhesive bandage over insertion site, apply tape in chevron pattern over catheter. Place three rows of tape over site, add tension loop of tubing. Wrap rolled gauze dressing over IV site for added protection.

INTEROSSEOUS INFUSION

See Chapter 5.

AIRWAY

Hypoxia is not an uncommon finding in children. Children have higher metabolic rates than adults. Oxygen consumption is 50% greater in a child than in an adult. With each degree of temperature increase there is an associated oxygen consumption increase of 7%. Pay close attention to this and to the patency of the child's airway.

The most common cause of respiratory distress in children is airway obstruction. The four main areas of airway obstruction are the basopharynx, the oropharynx, the larynx and upper trachea, and the lower airway. If the child is in respiratory distress but is moving some air, try to identify the cause of the obstruction. Perform a rapid assessment for:

Level of consciousness	Skin vital signs (color, temperature, moistness)
Signs of hypoxia	Use of accessory muscles of respiration
Breath odor	Tidal volume
Lung sounds	Vital signs (be sure to include temperature)
Midline trachea	Dehydration
Distended neck veins	

Nasopharynx Obstruction

Nasopharynx obstruction may occur as a result of foreign bodies, edematous adenoids, edema from trauma, or carcinomas.

■ **SIGNS AND SYMPTOMS**

Mouth breathing (remember that very small infants are obligate nose breathers; a nasal obstruction in an infant may be life-threatening)

Cyanosis

■ **THERAPEUTIC INTERVENTIONS**

Turn the child on his or her side.

Insert an oropharyngeal airway.

Administer oxygen.

Oropharynx Obstruction

Obstruction of the oropharynx may be caused by facial trauma with swelling of the tongue or by foreign body aspiration.

■ **SIGNS AND SYMPTOMS**

Noisy breathing (gargling or snoring sounds) or absence of breath sounds

Neck extended ''like a turtle''

Insistence on sitting up

Cyanosis

Difficulty speaking

Difficulty swallowing

■ **THERAPEUTIC INTERVENTIONS**

Insert an oropharyngeal or nasopharyngeal airway if epiglottitis has been ruled out.

Administer oxygen therapy.

If the patient is moving air, do not attempt to remove the foreign body and do not change the patient's position.

If there is no air movement, hold the infant prone with head lower than the trunk, administer five back blows, followed by up to five downward chest thrusts (Figure 30-2).

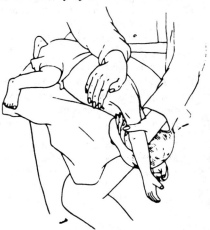

FIGURE 30-2. Child is placed in head-down position while up to 5 firm back blows are applied.

Once again, attempt to ventilate the infant.

If the child is unable to cough or breathe effectively, a series of up to five subdiaphragmatic abdominal thrusts is recommended.

LARYNX OBSTRUCTION

Epiglottitis

Epiglottitis is a life-threatening bacterial infection of the epiglottis and the surrounding structures. The diagnosis is made by ''thinking of it''—the child ''looks sick.''

■ **SIGNS AND SYMPTOMS**

Massive swelling of epiglottis (usually from a bacterial infection)

Commonly seen in 2- to 5-year-old children, but may be seen even in adults

Elevated temperature (above 103.1° F [39.5° C])

Abrupt onset

Anxious appearance

Tachycardia

Sore throat

Respiratory difficulty

Muffled voice

Refusal to change to other than a sitting position (Never place a child on his or her back.*)

Neck extended (like a turtle)

Profuse salivation

Dysphagia

No cough

Hypoventilation

History of infection, ingestion of a hot beverage, or steam inhalation

■ **THERAPEUTIC INTERVENTIONS**

Do not attempt to look into the child's mouth; doing so may cause respiratory arrest.*

Give oxygen therapy as tolerated (this usually requires intubation).

Make ENT/anesthesia evaluation—most safely done in operating room with intubation/tracheostomy equipment available.

Consider an emergency needle cricothyrotomy.

Administer steroids.

Croup

Croup is a viral infection of the trachea and larynx—it may extend to the bronchi—that causes edema and inflammation of the lining of the trachea and larynx.

■ **SIGNS AND SYMPTOMS**

Child usually 3 months to 3 years of age

History of increasing nocturnal distress for several days resulting from an upper respiratory infection

*Inserting a tongue blade into the mouth or having the child lie down may induce respiratory arrest.

Usually active, appears well
Low-grade fever
Loud "barking" cough
Hoarse voice
Inspiratory stridor
Sternal retraction
Tachypnea
Tachycardia
■ **THERAPEUTIC INTERVENTIONS**
Administer humidified oxygen.
Administer humidified cool air.

Laryngospasm

Laryngospasm is not common, but when it occurs, it can be life-threatening. It is difficult to distinguish from a foreign body airway obstruction. It may be caused by anaphylaxis.

■ **SIGNS AND SYMPTOMS**

Vomiting	Bronchospasm
Urticaria	Hypotension
Periorbital edema	Absence of breath sounds

■ **THERAPEUTIC INTERVENTIONS**
Ensure airway management, consider intubation.
Administer oxygen therapy.
Perform emergency needle cricothyrotomy if the airway cannot be opened.
Administer epinephrine if caused by anaphylaxis.
Administer antihistamines if indicated.
Administer bronchodilators if indicated.
Administer steroids if indicated.

Lower Airway Obstruction

Asthma

Asthma is a recurrent reactive airway disease associated with reversible airway obstruction caused by bronchospasm mucus gland hypertrophy and mucus plugging.

■ **SIGNS AND SYMPTOMS**
Expiratory wheezes (sometimes inspiratory also)
Possibly no expiratory sounds if there is no air movement
Coughs
Retractions
Prolonged expiration
Tachycardia
Dyspnea
■ **THERAPEUTIC INTERVENTIONS**
Administer oxygen as tolerated to maintain transcutaneous oxygen saturation above 95%.

Administer beta-2 specific nebulized bronchodilator.
Administer antibiotics if needed.
Administer corticosteroids for moderate to severe episodes.
Consider epinephrine.

Status asthmaticus

Status asthmaticus is asthma that fails to respond to conventional therapy. It
will lead to respiratory failure if therapeutic intervention is not applied.

■ **THERAPEUTIC INTERVENTIONS**

Administer beta-2 specific nebulized bronchodilator every 20 minutes until reso-
lution of bronchospasm.
Administer humidified oxygen therapy according to arterial blood gas values/
transcutaneous oxygen saturation.
Establish an IV line—consider hydration to maintain adequate volume status.
Administer corticosteroids.
Consider IV aminophylline for patients who do not respond to inhaled beta ago-
nists.
Treat fluid and electrolyte imbalances according to laboratory values.
Be prepared to handle respiratory arrest.

Bronchiolitis

Bronchiolitis is a viral infection of the lower respiratory tract that occurs in children less than 2 years old, most often in children under 1 year. It is most often
caused by respiratory syncytial virus.

■ **SIGNS AND SYMPTOMS**

History of mild upper respiratory infection
Respiratory difficulty
Wheezing, dyspnea
Intercostal retractions
Frequent coughing
Prolonged expiratory phase

■ **THERAPEUTIC INTERVENTIONS**

Monitor transcutaneous oxygen saturation.
Administer beta-2 specific nebulized bronchodilator.
Humidified oxygen
Corticosteroids
Respiratory isolation of patient with RSV
Put on another line, hydrate as necessary, avoid overhydration.

Pneumonia

Pneumonia is an inflammation of the lung parenchyma caused by a variety of
infectious agents, including viruses and bacteria.

Viral

Most commonly respiratory syncytial and parainfluenza viruses.

- **SIGNS AND SYMPTOMS**
  Gradual onset over a few days, preceded by upper respiratory infection
  Cough
  Low-grade fever
  Rales
  Tachypnea
  Wheezing
  Apnea episode in infant
- **THERAPEUTIC INTERVENTIONS**
  Hydration as necessary
  Antipyresis
  Oxygen as needed
  Nasal aspiration for RSV titer

Bacterial

- **SIGNS AND SYMPTOMS**
  More abrupt onset
  Fever
  Tachypnea, tachycardia
  Grunting respirations
  Decreased breath sounds
  Meningismus with upper lobe pneumonia
- **THERAPEUTIC INTERVENTIONS**
  Same as with viral
  Antimicrobial therapy

FEVERS

An elevated temperature is probably the single most common cause for which a parent brings a child to the emergency department. Fevers have various causes, most commonly infection, but also can be due to poisonings, dehydration, and collagen–vascular diseases.

- **SIGNS AND SYMPTOMS**

Rapid pulse	Flushed skin
Tachypnea	Agitation
Diaphoresis	

- **THERAPEUTIC INTERVENTIONS**
  Give forced fluids (clear liquids).
  Dress the child in lightweight clothing.
  Give antipyretic medication: acetaminophen (Tylenol), 15 mg/kg initially. Do not use aspirin in a child under 12 years of age.
  Give tepid bath or shower.
  Treat the cause of the fever.
  Fever without a known cause in the infant under 3 months of age should receive fever work-up, including lumbar puncture, blood cultures, and urine culture.

SEIZURES

The most common etiology of seizures in children is fever. Febrile seizures usually occur between the ages of 3 months and 5 years. They occur in association with a febrile illness, most often of viral etiology. Two thirds of children who have had seizures will not have another. Frequent causes of seizures are central nervous system infections, poisoning, epilepsy, and head injury.

Refer to Chapter 9, Neurologic Emergencies, for further information on seizure disorders.

POISONING

Pediatric poisoning can be difficult to diagnose in the field and the emergency department. It is important, on the telephone as well as in person, to obtain a good history from the child's parents, relatives, friends, or neighbors.

What drug or product did the child take?

How much did the child take?

When did the child take it?

Is the child having any symptoms at present?

Is the child having difficulty breathing?

What medication does the child take routinely?

Has the child ever done this before?

Request that the product or product container, even if empty, be brought to the emergency department.

Calls concerning poisoning should be referred to the nearest poison control area for management. Pediatric signs and symptoms and therapeutic interventions for poisoning are similar to those in adults. Please refer to Chapter 13, Toxicological Emergencies, for this information.

Poisoning Statistics

According to the annual report of the American Association of Poison Control Centers, children younger than 3 years of age were involved in 44% of the cases; and 59% occurred in children less than 6 years.[1] A male predominance is found among poison exposure victims younger than 13 years, but the gender distribution is reversed in teenagers. Children younger than 6 years of age comprised only 4.1% of the fatalities. Children younger than 6 years are more likely to ingest nontoxic substances or minute amounts of toxic substances. The majority of preschoolers' ingestions are done because they are curious; adolescents' ingestions are most often suicidal gestures.

"Red Flag" Drugs and Products

The following drugs and products can cause serious toxicity in children (often with a very small dose or amount).

Clonidine—signs and symptoms occur within 30 minutes. Decreased blood pressure, decreased respirations (apnea), bradycardia, and coma.

Clozapine (Clozari)—one half tablet has caused respiratory arrest in a child.

Cyclic antidepressants.

Lomotil (Diphenoxylate)—requires 24 hour hospitalization in children.

Isoniazid causes seizures—causes pyridoxine deficiency. Pyridoxine (Vitamin B_6) is antidotal.

Chloroquine (antimalarial drug) has a quinidine-like effect on the heart and vasodilatory properties.

Super nail glue removers—contain a product converted to cyanide.

Oil of wintergreen—contains methyl salisalate 98% 1 ml—1365 mg of salycylate.

Propoxyphene (Darvon) causes CNS and cardiovascular decrease, coma, and seizure. Sudden respiratory arrest within 15 to 30 minutes.

Nicotine causes sudden onset seizures in 15 to 90 minutes.

Camphor-containing products cause sudden onset seizures within 5 minutes.

Organophosphate pesticides cause CNS decrease, dyspnea, and coma.

Calcium channel blockers—children with one tablet of the sustained-release variety have developed bradycardia and hypotension 16 to 24 hours after ingestion. Admit.

Chloral hydrate—deep coma occurs rapidly.

Highest frequency of substances ingested by children.

1. Over-the-counter drugs
2. Prescription drugs
3. Cleaners
4. Cosmetics
5. Plants

Button Battery Ingestion

There are several hundred button battery ingestions by children in the United States every year. X-ray localization should be done in all button battery ingestions, regardless of whether the child is symptomatic or not. If the battery is retained in the esophagus, removal is indicated to prevent esophageal burns and more serious sequelae, such as death. If the battery is not in the esophagus and child has no peritoneal signs, discharge to home. Parents are instructed to search stool to recover battery and to contact Poison Control Center for further information.

Iron Ingestion

Iron ingestion is the primary cause of pediatric poisoning deaths. It is rapidly absorbed in the small intestine. Excess iron is directly caustic to the gastrointestinal mucosa, causing hemorrhage with resulting hypovolemia and shock.[2]

Aftercare Instructions for Parents (Table 30-3)

Discuss:
   Follow-up care
   Prevention
See Table 30-3 for key prevention concepts compiled by the New Hampshire Poison Information Center.

TABLE 30-3 Key Prevention Concepts Compiled by the New Hampshire Poison Information Center

POISON PROOF YOUR HOME	MEDICINE SAFETY	PESTICIDE SAFETY	PROTECT YOUR CHILD
Throw away antidote charts. Most charts are outdated. Call the Poison Center for information instead.	Do not take medicines in front of children. They tend to mimic adults.	Read and follow label directions before using a pesticide.	Put products away immediately after they are used.
Ammonia—mix with water only.	Do not refer to medicine as candy.	Remove food and dishes before treating a kitchen area. Wait for shelves to dry before replacing items.	Do not leave a child and poison alone "for a second." A considerable number of poisonings occur while a parent is on the telephone.
Perfumes, colognes, and after-shaves—store them as you would medicine.	Do not give medicine in the dark or without reading the label.	Keep children and pets away from sprayed area for 24–48 hours.	If you have young children, crawl on your hands and knees to see if there are any hazards. This puts you at their eye level and you may spot a possible hazard. Brightly colored containers and objects, especially red, attract a child's attention.
Insecticides, weedkillers, gasoline, and turpentine—lock up in a cabinet.	Lock medicines in a cabinet.	Avoid breathing the fumes.	
Ashtrays—empty and keep cigarettes and butts out of the reach of children.	Clean out medicine cabinet twice a year. Flush old or outdated medicine down the toilet.	Ventilate the inside of the house well before re-entering.	Destroy berries and mushrooms from any areas on your property that are accessible to children.
Medications and vitamins—keep safety caps securely on and out of the reach of children.		Wear washable clothing that covers your arms, legs, and feet. (Suede, leather, boots and jewelry cannot be decontaminated.)	
Know the names of your plants both indoors and outdoors.		Never spray outdoors on a windy day.	
		Avoid breaks, spills, and splashes from container.	
		Store pesticides in their original container in a locked cabinet.	
		When finished, take a thorough shower, washing hair and skin twice with soap. Wash contaminated clothing separately.	
		Mixing or diluting should be done outside in a well-ventilated area.	
		Lock up poisons in a specific cupboard or in a tackle box!	

THE UNCONSCIOUS CHILD

Evaluation of the unconscious child must be rapid, systematic, and thorough. Ensure ABCs.

Monitor transcutaneous oxygen saturation by pulse oximetry; administer oxygen as necessary; consider intubation.

Make neurologic assessment, including Pediatric Glascow Coma Scale (Table 30-4).

Obtain history from family.

Initiate IV, nasogastric tube, Foley catheter.

Laboratory evaluation: CBC, lytes, BUN, CR. Consider when indicated LFTs, ammonia and toxicology screen, ABG, ETOH level, lumbar puncture, CT scan of head.

TABLE 30-4   Pediatric Glasgow Coma Score (PGCS)

GLASGOW COMA SCORE (GCS)	PEDIATRIC MODIFICATION	
Eye opening	**Eye opening**	
≥1 year	*0-1 year*	
4 Spontaneously	Spontaneously	
3 To verbal command	To shout	
2 To pain	To pain	
1 No response	No response	
Best motor response	**Best motor response**	
≥1 year	*0-1 year*	
6 Obeys command		
5 Localizes pain	Localizes pain	
4 Flexion withdrawal	Flexion withdrawal	
3 Flexion abnormal (decorticate)	Flexion abnormal (decorticate)	
2 Extension (decerebrate)	Extension (decerebrate)	
1 No response	No response	
Best verbal response	**Best verbal response**	
>5 years	*2-5 years*	*0-2 years*
5 Oriented and converses	Appropriate words and phrases	Cries appropriately, smiles, coos
4 Disoriented and converses	Inappropriate words	Cries
3 Inappropriate words	Cries/screams	Inappropriate crying/screaming
2 Incomprehensible sounds	Grunts	Grunts
1 No response	No response	No response

A score is given in each category. The individual scores are then added (range 3-15). A score <8 indicates severe neurologic injury.
From Barkin R: *Pediatric emergency medicine.* St. Louis, 1992, Mosby.

Causes of Unconsciousness in a Child

Central nervous system

Trauma
Infection
Seizures

Cardiovascular

Congestive failure
Congenital heart disease
Infection

Respiratory

Acute respiratory failure/obstruction/hypoxia
Trauma
Allergy
Infection

Shock

Septic
Hypovolemic
Neurogenic
Cardiogenic
Anaphylactic

Gastrointestinal

Vomiting and diarrhea
Dehydration

Metabolic

Ketoacidosis
Hypoglycemia
Toxic ingestions
Reye's syndrome

Endocrine

Addisonian crisis

MENINGITIS

Meningitis is an inflammation of the meninges of viral or bacterial etiology. The most common bacterial organisms are *H. influenzae, S. pneumoniae,* and *N. meningitidis.* The clinical presentation of meningitis varies with the age of the child and the severity of the illness.

■ **SIGNS AND SYMPTOMS**

Neonate

Irritability
Lethargy

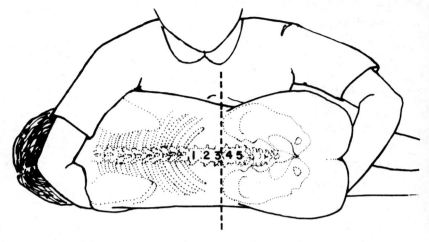

FIGURE 30-3. Position for pediatric lumbar puncture.
(From Barkin R: Pediatric emergency medicine. St Louis, 1992, Mosby.)

Bulging anterior fontanelle
Poor feeding
Seizures
Infants
Fever
Vomiting
Seizures
Nucchal rigidity
Lethargy
Children
Fever
Vomiting
Nucchal rigidity
Headache
Altered mental status
■ **THERAPEUTIC INTERVENTIONS**
Ensure ABCs.
Lumbar puncture—see Figure 30-3 for positioning child LP.
Administer antimicrobial therapy as indicated promptly.

MENINGOCOCCEMIA

Meningococcemia is caused by *Neiseria meningitidis* and death can result within hours.
■ **SIGNS AND SYMPTOMS (rapid onset)**
Fever
Chills
Rash—maculopapular, petechial, or purpuric

Possible headache
Hypotension
Disseminated intravascular coagulation
■ **THERAPEUTIC INTERVENTIONS**
Immediate treatment
LP, septic work-up, CBC, electrolytes, glucose, ESR
Urinalysis, DIC screen
IV access
Prompt initiation of appropriate antibiotic therapy

GASTROINTESTINAL COMPLAINTS

Vomiting

Antiemetics have no place in the management of vomiting in the pediatric patient. Vomiting can have many causes, most often self-limiting viral gastroenteritis. Intractible vomiting may be a sign of:
Increased intracranial pressure
Reye's syndrome
Gastrointestinal reflux
Viral gastroenteritis
Bowel obstruction

Diarrhea

Diarrhea is usually self-limited and due to viral gasteroenteritis. In most cases diarrhea can be controlled with dietary change, such as eliminating milk temporarily and having the child eat the BRAT diet (bananas, rice, applesauce, toast, and clear liquids).

If serious episodes of diarrhea occur, they may be accompanied by voluminous stools, bloody diarrhea, and/or concomitant vomiting.

Dehydration

Vomiting and diarrhea are the most common causes of dehydration in a child.

Approximately 60% of a child's body weight and 78% of a newborn's weight is fluid, 25% of which is extracellular and thus unstable. This fact, coupled with the child's high metabolic rate (with a high fluid turnover) and kidneys that are inefficient (producing a large amount of dilute urine), predispose the child to dangerous dehydration when large amounts of fluid are lost rapidly through fever, vomiting, or diarrhea.

See Table 30-5 for estimation of dehydration.
■ **SIGNS AND SYMPTOMS**
Dry mucus membranes
Decreased urination
Weight loss
Depressed anterior fontanelle

TABLE 30-5   Estimation of Dehydration

CLINICAL MANIFESTATIONS	DEGREE OF DEFICIT			
	5%	10%	15%	20%
Heart rate	Normal range	Compensatory tachycardia	Noncompensatory tachycardia	Morbid tachycardia Bradycardia
Blood pressure	Normal range	Normal range	Low normal	↓ Blood pressure
Quality of pulses	Normal	2+ peripheral 3+ central	1+ peripheral 2+ central	0 peripheral 1+ central
Capillary refill	2-3 sec.	>3 sec.	>4 sec.	>5 sec.
Urinary output	<2 ml/kg/h	<1 ml/kg/h	<0.5 ml/kg/h	None
Level of consciousness	Irritable	Irritable/lethargic	Obtunded	Obtunded/coma
Color/temperature	Pink/warm	Pale/cool	Cyanotic/cold	Ashen/cold
Mucous membranes	Moist	Dry	Dry	Parched
Fontanel	Flat	Slightly depressed	Sunken	Sunken
Weight	↓ 5%	↓ 10%	↓ 15%	↓ 20%

From Jackson DB, Saunders R: *Child health nursing.* Philadelphia, 1992, Lippincott.

Reduced skin turgor
Listlessness
Sunken eyeballs
Orthostatic hypotension
■ **THERAPEUTIC INTERVENTIONS**
Obtain electrolytes, BUN, urine specific gravity. Give initial bolus of 20 ml/kg
RL or NS over 20 minutes. If no improvement, repeat 20 mg/kg bolus or RL or
NS, then hydrate according to weight and percentage of dehydration.

ABDOMINAL PAIN

A definite cause for abdominal pain in the ambulatory pediatric patient is not
always found. The most common cause of abdominal pain in children is viral
gastroenteritis. Constipation is a frequent cause. Other causes of pediatric
abdominal pain include pneumonia, lead intoxication, diabetic ketoacidosis, poisoning, and foreign body ingestion. Children should be evaluated appropriately
to rule out the more serious causes of abdominal pain. Abdominal surgical
emergencies will be discussed in the next chapter. Common tests to evaluate
abdominal pain are complete blood count and urinalysis.

VARICELLA (CHICKENPOX)

Varicella is caused by the same organism that causes herpes zoster. There is a
14- to 21-day incubation period. Varicella is contagious from 1 day before the
appearance of the rash until all lesions begin to crust, approximately 5 days.
Children with varicella appear mildly sick. The level of illness seems to parallel
the amount of rash involved. The rash, which consists of macules, papules, and
vesicles, occurs primarily on the trunk and extremities, although it is not
uncommon to find some amount of rash on the face. Children with varicella
usually develop a rash as the first sign of the disease. Occasionally they will
have a slight fever for 1 or 2 days before the rash appears. If a child is immuno-
suppressed, danger of severe illness is great. Hospital admission is required.

Therapeutic intervention includes administration of antipyretics, antihistamines, and lots of oral fluids as well as other supportive therapy. Avoid aspirin.
Oatmeal baths may help relieve itching. The caregiver should be sure that the
child's fingernails are short to avoid bacterial infection when the child scratches
the lesions.

SUDDEN INFANT DEATH SYNDROME

Sudden infant death syndrome (SIDS), or crib death, is the sudden, unexpected
death of an apparently healthy baby for which no adequate cause of death can
be found on autopsy. It usually occurs in infants between the ages of 1 month
and 1 year, with peak incidence being at 2 to 4 months. There are several theories as to why SIDS occurs. The most prominent, though unproved, of these are
that SIDS is caused by:
Disorder (apnea) of sleep

Nasal congestion (infants are obligate nose breathers)

Laryngeal spasms

On postmortem examinations of SIDS victims, some of the more common findings are:

Frothy sputum in the mouth and nose

Emesis

Small height and weight for age

Empty bladder and rectum

Intrathoracic petechiae

Pulmonary congestion

Dilated right heart

■ **THERAPEUTIC INTERVENTIONS**

Usually nothing can be done to save the infant despite rigorous resuscitation efforts. Most therapeutic intervention will be directed toward the grieving parents. The most common reaction by parents of a child who dies of SIDS is complete devastation. There are many guilty feelings and much self-blame or blame of one parent by the other parent, especially if one parent is away at the time of the infant's death. The incidence of divorce is very high among parents with infants who have died from SIDS.

It is important, after some preparatory counseling, to state that the baby is dead and has died from SIDS. Let the parents know that SIDS is a common cause of death in infancy and that there was nothing they could have done to prevent it. It is important to let them know that it is *not* a hereditary disease.

Arrange for an autopsy and inform the parents that they will be notified of the cause of death within 48 hours. Once the parents receive notification of the official cause of death, schedule another counseling session with them. If this is beyond the capabilities of your staff, refer the family to the National Foundation for Sudden Infant Death Syndrome, 8240 Professional Place, Landover, MD 20785. The number of a local SIDS parent group can be obtained from the national group or local phone directory.

REFERENCES

1. Litovitz TL: 1992 Annual report of the American Association of Poison Control Centers National Data Collection System, *Am J Emerg Med* 9:497, 1993.
2. Barkin R et al: *Pediatric emergency medicine.* St Louis, 1992, Mosby.

SUGGESTED READINGS

Barkin R et al: *Pediatric emergency medicine.* St Louis, 1992, Mosby.

Fuhrmann B, Zimmerman J: *Pediatric critical care.* St Louis, 1992, Mosby.

Gugguan Greene M: *The Harriet Lane handbook,* ed 12. St Louis, 1991, Mosby.

Grossman M, Dieckmann R: *Pediatric emergency medicine.* Philadelphia, 1991, Lippincott.

Haddad L, Winchester JF: *Clinical management of poisoning and drug overdose,* ed 2. Philadelphia, 1990, Saunders.

Hall CG, McBride JT: Respiratory syncytial virus, *N Engl J Med* 325:1, 1991.

Hazinski M: *Nursing care of the critically ill child,* ed 2. St Louis, 1992, Mosby.

Jackson D, Saunders R: *Child health nursing.* Philadelphia, 1993, Lippincott.

Korin G: Medications which can kill a toddler with one tablet or teaspoonful, *J Toxicol* 31(3):407, 1993.

Litovitz TL et al: 1992 Annual Report of the American Association of Poison Control Centers National Data Collection System, *Am J Emerg Med* 494:9, 1993.

Pellock J, Myer E: *Neurologic emergencies in infancy and childhood,* ed 2. Boston, 1993, Butterworth-Heinemann.

Sheehy S: *Emergency nursing principles and practice,* ed 2. St Louis, 1992, Mosby.

Skoner DP, Fisher TJ et al: Pediatric predictive index for hospitalization with acute asthma, *Am J Emerg Med* 16:25, 1987.

Pediatric Trauma and Surgical Emergencies

PEDIATRIC TRAUMA

Over 50% of all pediatric deaths result from trauma. The number one cause of traumatic injury is motor vehicles, followed by burns and falls. Although the basic principles of trauma management are the same in an infant or child as in an adult, there are a few issues specific to the infant and child with which one should be familiar. The child is most often a victim of blunt trauma, whereas penetrating trauma is most often the primary cause of adult trauma. The injured child should be cared for in an emergency department prepared for the unique needs of the child, with pediatric-specific equipment and supplies. See Pediatric-specific Equipment, Table 31-1.

Primary Survey

The initial assessment is divided into four steps: airway, breathing, circulation, and disability. It is used to identify and treat life-threatening injuries.

Airway/with cervical spine immobilization

Children have smaller airways than adults. The child's relatively large tongue, and the obstruction of infant's nares, who are nasal breathing, can be causes of airway compromise.

■ **ASSESSMENT**
Patency of airway
Oral foreign bodies
Alignment of cervical spine

■ **THERAPEUTIC INTERVENTIONS**
C-spine immobilization is imperative for all children who have sustained trauma.

TABLE 31-1 Pediatric-specific Equipment

	AIRWAY MANAGEMENT	VASCULAR ACCESS	MISCELLANEOUS
Premature to 6 mo			
	ET tubes	Overneedle type catheters	Feeding tubes
	2.5	24 gauge	5 French
	3.0	22 gauge	8 French
	3.5	Scalp veins	Blood pressure cuff
	Stylettes	25 gauge	Neonate
	6 French	23 gauge	Chest tubes
	Laryngoscope blades	Cook single-lumen catheter set	10 French
	0 straight	3 French	12 French
	1 straight	Pediatric side-arm set	16 French
	Tracheostomy tubes	5.5 French	
	00	Umbilical catheters	
	1	5 French	
	Nasopharyngeal airways	3.5 French	
	12 French	Umbilical tape	
	14 French		
	De Lee suction trap		
	Bulb syringe		
	Neonatal self-inflating bag		
	Premie and newborn masks		
	Oropharyngeal airways		
	1		
	2		
	Suction catheters		
	5/6		
	8		
6 Mo to 2 yrs			
	ET tubes	Overneedle type catheters	Foley catheter
	3.5	24 gauge	8 French
	4.0	22 gauge	Feeding tubes
	4.5	Scalp veins	8 French
	5.0	25 gauge	Nasogastric tubes
	Stylette	23 gauge	8 French
	6 French	21 gauge	10 French
	Suction catheters		
	8 French		
	10 French		
	Pediatric bag		
	Infant mask		
	Nasopharyngeal airways		
	14 French		

Continued.

Additional pediatric surgical instrumentation may be required.
From Barkin R: *Pediatric emergency mnedicine.* St Louis, 1992, Mosby.

TABLE 31-1 Pediatric-specific Equipment—cont'd.

	AIRWAY MANAGEMENT	VASCULAR ACCESS	MISCELLANEOUS
	Tracheostomy tubes	Single-lumen catheter set	Blood pressure cuffs
	1	3 French	Infant
	Laryngoscope blades	Side-arm set	Child
	1 straight	5.5 French	Chest tubes
	1.5 straight	Double-lumen catheter set	16 French
		5 French	20 French
			24 French
3 to 6 yrs			
	ET tubes	Overneedle type catheters	Foley catheters
	5.0	23 gauge	10 French
	5.5	20 gauge	12 French
	6.0	Scalp veins	NG tubes
	Stylettes	25 gauge	10 French
	6 French	23 gauge	12 French
	14 French	21 gauge	Blood pressure cuff
	Laryngoscope blades	Single-lumen catheter set	Child
	1.5 straight	4 French	Chest tubes
	2 straight	Side-arm sheaths	20 French
	2 curved	5.5 French	24 French
	Tracheostomy tube	7.5 French	28 French
	2	Triple- or double-lumen catheter set	
		7.0 French	
	Suction catheter		
	14 French		
	Pediatric nonrebreather mask		
	Pediatric bag		
	Nasopharyngeal airways		
	16 French		
	18 French		
	22 French		
	Oropharyngeal airways		
	3		
	4		
	Oropharyngeal airways		
	Infant 1		
	Child 2		
	16 French		
	18 French		

7 to 10 yrs

ET tubes	Suction catheter	Overneedle type catheters	Foley catheter
6.0	14 French	20 gauge	12 French
6.5	Adult nonrebreather mask	18 gauge	NG tubes
7.0 (Cuffed/noncuffed)	Small adult mask	Scalp veins	16 French
Stylette	Adult bag	25 gauge	18 French
14 French	Nasopharyngeal airways	23 gauge	Chest tubes
Laryngoscope blades	24 French	20 gauge	28 French
2 straight	26 French	Single-lumen catheter sets	32 French
2 curved	28 French	3 French	36 French
3 straight	Oropharyngeal airways	5 French	
3 curved	4	Side-arm sheaths	
Tracheostomy tube	5	7.5 French	
3		Triple- or double-lumen catheter set	
		7.0 French	

Additional pediatric surgical instrumentation may be required.

From Barkin R: *Pediatric emergency medicine*. St Louis, 1992, Mosby.

■ **AIRWAY MANAGEMENT**

The airway should be cleared of any obstructing matter, such as blood and emesis. A jaw thrust should be used to open the airway. An oral airway is used in the unconscious child. In the conscious child a nasal airway is utilized. The oral airway should not be rotated into position, since this can cause trauma to teeth and soft-tissue structures in the oral pharynx. The oral airway should be inserted visually; pull the tongue forward and insert gently over the tongue. When oxygenation, ventilation, and airway control are inadequate, intubation is required. An uncuffed endotracheal tube is used for the child under 8 years of age to decrease vocal cord trauma, subglottic edema, and ulceration. The narrowest portion of the airway of a child under 8 years of age is at the cricoid cartilage below the vocal cords. The vocal cords are the narrowest portion of the older child's airway.

Breathing

The pediatric patient is further compromised by a high metabolic rate (oxygen consumption is 6 to 8 ml/kg/min in a child compared to 3 to 4 ml/kg/min in an adult)[1] When breathing becomes inadequate, hypoxemia occurs more rapidly.

■ **ASSESSMENT**

Observe respiratory rate, depth, and quality.
Observe for any abnormal breathing pattern—grunting, retractions.
Auscultate breath sounds.
Observe position of trachea.
Check integrity of chest wall.

■ **THERAPEUTIC INTERVENTIONS**

Administer O_2 by non-breather mask at 100% initially. If breathing is compromised, assist ventilations with bag-valve-mask or positive pressure ventilation.

Circulation

The child's circulating blood volume is 80 mg/kg. The child has a smaller absolute circulating blood volume and cardiac output than the adult.[2] Consequently, significant reductions in the child's circulating blood volume can compromise systemic perfusion.[2] Hypotension is a late-occurring sign, usually after a circulating blood volume loss of 20%.

■ **ASSESSMENT**

Capillary refill
Areas of external hemorrhage
Pulse-quality, effectiveness
Skin color and temperature

■ **THERAPEUTIC INTERVENTIONS**

If pulseless, initiate CPR, pediatric advanced life support.
If cardiovascular function present, but ineffective:

1. Initiate vascular access with two large-bore IVs; give 20 ml/kg bolus of warmed RL or NS; repeat if necessary. If no response, repeat 20 mg/kg bolus. Administer type specific or O-negative packed cells 10 ml/kg if shock persists. Exploratory laparotomy to identify the bleeding site if more than 50% of the child's blood volume must be replaced.[3] The use of

PASG (pneumatic antishock garment) is controversial as an adjunct to fluid therapy in the child. It can be a consideration for use in a pelvic fracture if there is ongoing hemorrhage.

2. Apply direct pressure to areas of external hemorrhaging.

Disability—neurologic evaluation

The child's large head size in relation to body size, accompanied by weak neck muscles, make the pediatric patient more susceptible to head injury. Head injury is the leading cause of death due to trauma in children.

■ **ASSESSMENT**

Pupillary size and response

Level of consciousness

Neurologic responsiveness—Glasgow Coma Scale or AVPU scale

    A—alert and oriented

    V—responsive to verbal stimuli

    P—responsive to painful stimuli

    U—unresponsive

■ **THERAPEUTIC INTERVENTIONS**

Consider pharmacologic intervention to improve mental status in selected cases, such as Narcan or $D_{25}W$.

Secondary Survey

Upon completion of primary survey and resuscitation, the secondary survey is started.

■ **ASSESSMENT AND THERAPEUTIC INTERVENTIONS**

Any remaining clothing is removed so that a complete assessment can be obtained.

The pediatric patient should be covered in warm blankets, in a warm room, and given warm IV fluids. "Children have large surface area/volume ratios, so they lose more heat to the environment through evaporation, conduction and convection than adults."[4]

Trauma labs are sent.

X-rays are done.

Obtain complete vital signs (temperature, pulse, respirations, blood pressure).

Obtain history of injury, past medical history including allergies, present medications, and immunization status.

Obtain a detailed head-to-toe assessment, anteriorly and posteriorly.

Administer additional interventions as needed: chest tube placement, wound care, splint fractures, etc.

COMMON TRAUMA LAB TESTS IN CHILDREN

CBC + differential	Prothrombin time
Serum electrolytes	Partial thromboplastin time
BUN	Glucose
Type and cross-match	Arterial blood gases
Amylase	

(Should be able to run all the specimens listed above with 10 to 20 ml of blood.)

STANDARD TRAUMA X-RAYS

Cervical spine
Chest
Pelvis
CT scan as indicated

PEDIATRIC SURGICAL EMERGENCIES

Appendicitis

Appendicitis is common in adolescents and young adults. It is the most common cause of abdominal surgery in children. It is often difficult to diagnose in the early stages of inflammation in infants and toddlers. The incidence of rupture in children under 6 years of age exceeds 50%, possibly due to the thickness of the appendiceal wall in these younger patients.[5]

■ **SIGNS AND SYMPTOMS**
Starts as periumbilical pain, then localizes in right lower quadrant—McBurney's point
Anorexia—if not present, appendicitis unlikely
Vomiting
Decrease in activity level
Guarding of right lower quadrant
Pain with movement
Mild temperature elevation
With rupture—high fever, rigid abdomen, tachycardia, dehydration

■ **THERAPEUTIC INTERVENTIONS**
Maintenance of NPO
Hydration
Abdominal x-ray film
CBC
Urinalysis to rule out other causes
Abdominal ultrasound if difficulty obtaining diagnosis
Antibiotic therapy
Early operative intervention

Intussusception

Intussusception is the telescoping of one segment of bowel into another. It most commonly occurs between the ages of 3 to 12 months with a male predominance. The usual location is the ileocecal valve.

■ **SIGNS AND SYMPTOMS**
May have had respiratory infection or viral gastroenteritis
Episodic abdominal pain, comfortable between episodes

Vomiting occurs in 50% of cases, after onset of pain

Passage of "currant jelly" stool with bloody mucus in ⅓ of children with intussusception

Early exam may be normal except colic

Later in course: fever, tachycardia, dehydration, lethargy

■ **THERAPEUTIC INTERVENTIONS**

Maintenance of NPO

CBC, BUN, electrolytes

IV hydration

Abdominal x-ray film

Barium enema for attempted reduction for hemodynamically stable child

Operative intervention if barium enema reduction failed, or unstable child

Incarcerated Inguinal Hernia

An inguinal hernia become incarcerated when viscera becomes entrapped in the hernial pouch. It occurs most often in infants under 1 year of age. With prolonged incarceration, there is increased edema and pressure, causing strangulation.

■ **SIGNS AND SYMPTOMS**

Cramping abdominal pain

Irritability

Vomiting

Firm to fluctuant mass in groin

Edema, erythema over mass with strangulated hernia

■ **THERAPEUTIC INTERVENTIONS**

Reduction in emergency department if not strangulated

If strangulated, operative intervention

Malrotation with Midgut Volvulus

Malrotation is a congenital anomaly in which abnormal rotation and attachment of bowel to the mesentery occurs. The midgut, which consists of the duodenum, small intestine, and ascending to midtransverse colon, then becomes vulnerable to twisting (volvulus) and infarction.

■ **SIGNS AND SYMPTOMS**

Bilious vomiting

Abdominal pain, distension

Bloody stools

Hematemesis

Later—shock, sepsis

■ **THERAPEUTIC INTERVENTIONS**

Stable—hydration, upper GI series, then operative intervention

Unstable—antibiotic therapy, emergency operative intervention

Testicular Torsion

Testicular torsion is the twisting of the spermatic cord causing venous obstruction, swelling, arterial ischemia, and testicular infarction. It often occurs in patients with a congenital abnormality of the spermatic cord, most often a bell clapper deformity. The adolescent age group is most commonly affected.

■ **SIGNS AND SYMPTOMS**
Usually acute onset of pain
Swelling, tenderness, erythema of scrotum
Enlarged testes
Possible association with nausea, vomiting
No urinary symptoms
"Blue dot" sign

■ **THERAPEUTIC INTERVENTIONS**
Doppler ultrasound if diagnosis uncertain
Timely surgical correction to prevent testicular infarction

AIRWAY AND GASTROINTESTINAL TRACT FOREIGN BODIES REQUIRING SURGICAL INTERVENTION

Ingestion and aspiration of foreign bodies occurs most frequently among infants, toddlers, and preschool children. Symptoms vary; the child can be asymptomatic or have acute airway compromise.

Airway Foreign Bodies

■ **SIGNS AND SYMPTOMS**
Witnessed episode of choking
Dyspnea
Cough
Decreased breath sounds
Stridor
Wheezing
Cyanosis

■ **THERAPEUTIC INTERVENTIONS**
Ensure ABCs.
Obtain chest x-ray film.
Consider lateral decubitus view by fluoroscopy.
Depending on location of foreign body, removal by laryngoscopy or bronchoscopy.

Esophageal Foreign Bodies (Figure 31-1)

■ **SIGNS AND SYMPTOMS**
Can be asymptomatic
Drooling

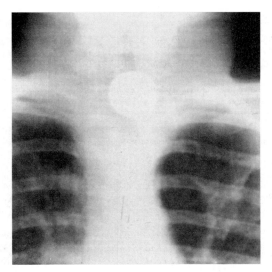

FIGURE 31-1. Coin in esophagus appears round. If lodged in trachea, it would look like a slit.
(From Silverman F, Kuhn J: *Coffey's pediatric x-ray diagnosis: an integrated imaging approach*, vol 1, ed 9. St Louis, 1993, Mosby.)

Inability to swallow food
Vomiting
Pain in neck or throat
■ **THERAPEUTIC INTERVENTIONS**
Ensure ABCs.
Check lateral soft tissue of neck and obtain chest x-ray film.
All esophageal foreign bodies must be removed, usually by esophagoscopy.
If recent ingestion, some esophageal foreign bodies can be removed under fluoroscopy.

Gastrointestinal Foreign Bodies

■ **SIGNS AND SYMPTOMS**
History of ingestion
Usually asymptomatic
Exam usually benign
Rare perforation
■ **THERAPEUTIC INTERVENTIONS**
Chest x-ray film
Most often conservative treatment
If ingested object is very large or has sharp edges, child will require hospitalization.
Operative intervention is required when there is significant bleeding, peritoneal signs are present, and there is failure to progress through GI tract.

REFERENCES

1. Chameides L: *Textbook of pediatric advanced life support.* Dallas, 1988, American Heart Association.
2. Hazinski MF: *Nursing care of the critically ill child,* ed 2. St Louis, 1992, Mosby. p 833.
3. Eichelberger M: *Pediatric trauma prevention, acute care, rehabilitation.* St Louis, 1993, Mosby.
4. Hazinski MF: *Nursing care of the critically ill child,* ed 2. St Louis, 1992, Mosby, 1992. p 835.
5. Ashcraft K, Holder T: *Pediatric surgery,* ed 2. Philadelphia, 1993, Saunders, p 472.

SUGGESTED READINGS

Ashcroft K, Holden T: *Pediatric surgery,* ed 2. Philadelphia, 1993, Saunders.

Barkin R et al: *Pediatric emergency medicine.* St Louis, 1992, Mosby.

Eichelberger M: *Pediatric trauma prevention, acute care, rehabilitation.* St Louis, 1993, Mosby.

Fuhrman B, Zimmerman J: *Pediatric critical care.* St Louis, 1992, Mosby.

Gugguan Greene M: *The Harriet Lane handbook,* ed 12. St Louis, 1991, Mosby.

Grossman M, Dieckmann R: *Pediatric emergency medicine.* Philadelphia, 1991, Lippincott.

Hazinski M: *Nursing care of critically ill child,* ed 2. St Louis, 1992, Mosby.

Jackson D, Saunders R: *Child health nursing.* Philadelphia, 1993, Lippincott.

Kaufmann CR, Rivera FP: Pediatric trauma: need for surgical management, *J Trauma* 29(8): 1120, 1989.

Stringel G: Appendicitis in children: a systematic approach for a low incidence of complications, *Am J Surg* 154:625, 1987.

Silverman F, Kuhn J: *Caffey's pediatric x-ray diagnosis: an integrated imaging approach.* St Louis, 1993, Mosby.

Child Maltreatment

Child maltreatment was not recognized as a common cause of trauma in children for many years. It is now estimated that there are 652,000 cases of child maltreatment in the United States each year.[1] Of the *known* cases 49% are reported by hospitals (personnel in emergency departments and pediatric units) and physicians, 23% by police, 12% by schoolteachers, nurses, and guidance counselors, and 16% by others (neighbors, friends, and even parents themselves).[2]

Child maltreatment/abuse is any harm that occurs to a child as a result of physical and/or emotional abuse. It can take many forms. Many children are the victims of more than one type of abuse.

TYPES OF ABUSE

Physical Neglect

Failure to provide basic needs, such as food, shelter, clothing, schooling, and medical care

Emotional Neglect/Abuse

Failure to provide a secure, loving, trusting, nurturing environment[3]
Actions or words by another that cause damage to a child's psychological well-being

Physical Abuse

Non-accidental trauma inflicted on a child

Sexual Abuse

Molestation of a child by an older child, an adolescent, or an adult, which can include violent acts and "nontouching" acts such as pornographic photography.

DUTY TO REPORT

The duty to report actual or suspected child maltreatment exists in all 50 states. It must be reported to the local police or social service agency. Anyone who reports child maltreatment is immune from prosecution, provided that the report is made in good faith. Remember: The reporter does not have to prove child maltreatment to report it. If there is a suspicion, it should be reported.

FACTORS THAT MAY CONTRIBUTE TO CHILD MALTREATMENT

Sociologic Situations

Unemployment
Inadequate housing
Profound poverty[4]
Low self-esteem

Parental/Significant Other Stressors

Single-parenting
Young mother[5]
Illness (especially chronic illness)
Many small children
Premature child
Child with feeding difficulty
Hyperactive child
Psychiatrically ill parent[6]
Child with developmental disability
Child with physical disability
Addicted child (mother abused drugs during the prenatal period)

Situational Responses

Substance abuse of parent or significant other of parent
Parent/significant other competing with child for attention
Lack of impulse control

Parental Expectations

Many abusers were themselves abused
Belief that corporal punishment is an acceptable form of punishment
Inability to provide nurturing love

SIGNS AND SYMPTOMS OF CHILD MALTREATMENT

Neglect

- Appearance of not being cared for
  - Dirty
  - Malnourished
  - Poor dentition
  - Inappropriate dress for weather conditions
  - Failure-to-thrive
  - Severe cradle cap
  - Severe diaper rash
  - Bald patches on scalp
  - Psychological dwarfism
- Lack of parental concern
- Attention-seeking behavior
- Passive/aggressive behavior

Physical Injury

Pay attention to

- Confusing/conflicting stories
- Unexplained injury
- Evasive answers to questions
- Nonbelievable history
- History that does not fit the growth and development level of the child
- Frequent or repeated injuries
- Frequent emergency department visits for nonspecific problems
- Little concern for the child
- No volunteering of information regarding the injury
- Anger toward the child for being injured
- Use of many different emergency departments (to prevent discovery)
- The child thinks that punishment is deserved
- The child is very afraid of adults
- The child's self-esteem is very low
- The child is very manipulative
- The child has a blank stare
- The child seeks and accepts affection from anyone and everyone

Look for

- **BRUISING** abrasions/ecchymosis/lacerations (old and new), hand prints, marks that take on the shape of the object, such as an extension cord, a rope, or a belt buckle
- **BITE MARKS** (human bite marks)
- **FRACTURES**
  - Especially in children less than 3 years old

- When the story is inconsistent with the type of fracture
- Fractures in various stages of healing

■ **HEAD INJURIES**
- Unexplained unconsciousness
- Unexplained cardiopulmonary arrest
- Subgaleal hematoma
- Traumatic alopecia
- Hair growing in various lengths in different spots
- Subdural hematoma
  - If a subdural is found, it must be assumed to be caused by child maltreatment until proven otherwise
  - If a subdural is found in an infant, it was most likely caused by severe shaking
- Displaced nasal cartilage
- Bleeding from nasal septum
- Fractured mandible

■ **MOUTH**
- Lacerated frenulum of upper lip
- Loosened or missing teeth not age appropriate
- Burns of lips or tongue

■ **EYE**
- Hyphema
- Periorbital ecchymosis (''black eye'')
- Retinal hemorrhage
- Detached retina

■ **EARS**
- Ruptured tympanic membrane

■ **PETECHIAE**
- Choking may cause petechiae to form on the face and head
- May be caused by twisting the skin

■ **TRUNCAL INJURIES**
- Bruising
- Burns
- Lacerations

■ **GENITALIA AND PERINEAL INJURIES**

■ **LIMB INJURIES**
- Fractures
- Dislocations

■ **BURNS**
- Unusual burn patterns
  - Cigarette burns
  - Submersion burns
  - Scald burns
  - Iron burns

■ **POISONING**
- The story does not fit the findings
- The child has ingested alcohol or illegal drugs

■ **MUNCHAUSEN'S-BY-PROXY**
  • The history and symptoms have been fabricated to gain medical attention

Emotional Abuse

By the parents

  • Verbal abuse
  • Verbal threats
  • Constant criticism
  • Expectations that are outrageous
  • Use of a child to play husband against wife and vice versa
  • Behavior that is in excess
  • No affection shown toward the child

The child may demonstrate

  • Withdrawal
  • Eating disorders
  • Head banging
  • Rocking
  • Learning disorders
  • Enuresis
  • Suicidal behavior

Sexual Abuse

There are between 50,000 and 100,000 children who are sexually abused each year in the United States.[7,8]

These are some of the signs in a child who has been sexually abused:
  • Social withdrawal
  • Bladder/bowel problems
  • Complaints of pain in the rectal or perineal area
  • Bruised or swollen genitalia
  • Rectal bleeding
  • Bruised or lacerated penis or scrotum
  • Sleep disorders
  • Blood or stains on underwear
  • Frequent urinary tract infections
  • Encopresis/enuresis
  • Complaint of frequent stomach aches
  • Bites/petechiae on nipples, genitalia, or thighs
  • Sexual knowledge beyond what is appropriate for age

In older children:
  • Change in eating habits
  • Change in school behavior
  • Delinquency
  • Runaway problem
  • Childhood pregnancy

THE INTERVIEW

The initial interview in the emergency department will most likely set the tone for the entire evaluation process. The primary goal of therapeutic intervention is to care for the immediate medical needs of the child, to prevent further harm to the child, and to assist the child and the family to deal with this crisis.

The parent(s) and child should be interviewed separately. This will allow for the parents to become emotional without worrying about what their child will think while this is going on. Methods to interview a child will vary, depending upon the child's growth and development age. It is always best to have one single interviewer talk to a child. One should attempt to make the child feel comfortable.

- Ask open ended questions, at first.
- Avoid questions that deal directly with the assault, at first.
- If the situation is one of possible sexual assault, ask questions that are specific about the sexual act
  - Ask if oral, anal, vaginal, or other sex has occurred.
  - Be sure to use language that the child can understand.
  - It may prove to be very useful to have an anatomically correct doll in the exam room so that the child can point to specific areas.
- If the child does not speak with you, see if role reversal will help. Ask the child to pretend that he or she is the nurse and you are the child.
- Ask how many times this has happened before.
- Ask when this happened this time.
- Ask if this has happened to his or her brothers or sisters or any other children.
- Ask if the child knows the person who did it and who that person is.
- If the child is female and has started menstruating, determine if there is a possibility of pregnancy.

THE EXAMINATION

Undress the child completely, providing for the child's modesty needs. Always take the time to explain what you are about to do. Perform:

- A primary and secondary survey
- A skeletal survey
- A hematological survey
- A visual acuity examination
- An eye examination
- A neurological examination
- A chest examination
- An abdominal examination (including a rectal examination)
- An assessment of growth and development level
- Check for other physical injuries.

If there is a suspicion of sexual assault, also check for:

- Injuries to the oral area
- Vaginal tears, bleeding, discharge

- A torn hymen
- Rectal tears
- Relaxed rectal muscles
- Send lab specimens for
    - Cultures:
  - Throat
  - Vagina
  - Rectum
  - Urethra
    - Smears:
  - Motile sperm
  - Old sperm
    - Serum syphilis screen
    - Forensic use
  - Imprint of teeth marks
  - Sample of wet or dried secretions

Be sure to carefully document all findings and to preserve evidence so that the chain of custody of the evidence is not broken. Be sure to record facts only—no speculation! Include quotes from the child and describe behaviors of the child. Document any strange reactions of the child. Use body maps to locate and document injuries or findings. Describe any diagnostic tests that were done and any treatments that were given.

If photographs are taken, they must be labeled with the date and time they were taken, the child's name and medical record number, and the name of the person taking the photograph.

Following the examination, ask the child if he or she has any questions. Keep the parents informed of the physical findings. Make sure to emphasize that follow-up appointments are very important to keep.

THE REPORT TO AUTHORITIES

The report will depend upon your institution's policies and procedures. In general, the following should be reported:

- The child's name (and possible other names used)
- The child's address and phone number
- The child's birth date
- Where the assault occurred
- The reason for your suspicion
- The cause of the injury
- The extent of the injury
- The circumstances surrounding the injury
- The name of the child's mother and father
- The name of the suspect
- The suspect's address and phone number
- Your name, work address, and work phone number
- A description of the child
- The location of the child

Be sure to document to whom this information was reported and the date and time it was reported.

OTHER CONDITIONS THAT MIMIC CHILD MALTREATMENT

There are several other conditions that may mimic child maltreatment. Among these are:

- Sudden infant death syndrome
- Failure to thrive
- Several coagulation disorders
- Petechiae of unknown etiology
- Mongolian spots
- Ethnic practices that produce physical marks
  - Cupping and moxibustion (Chinese)
  - Coin rubbing (Vietnamese)
  - Scarring (East African)

PREVENTION OF CHILD MALTREATMENT

The key to a reduction in child maltreatment is prevention. Prevention can be accomplished by intensive education. Children must know that it is not OK to hurt anyone. Teenagers must know this also. And, most important, parents and other adults must understand that it is not OK to hurt a child. Families who are at high risk must receive education to learn how to cope with stress, to understand normal growth and development patterns, to know where to find help and support. Schoolteachers and guidance counselors should receive special education to identify families and children at risk and to identify a child who has been maltreated. An objective of the *Healthy People 2000* project is to reduce the incidence of child maltreatment to less than 25.2 per 1000 children.[9]

Hospital personnel, and emergency care personnel in particular, must be familiar with identification of the maltreated child and must be encouraged to report all suspected cases for the welfare of the child.

REFERENCES

1. U.S. Department of Health and Human Services 2000: *Summary Report.* Washington, DC, 1992, U.S. Government Printing Office.
2. Ards S, Harkell A: Reporting of child maltreatment: a secondary analysis of the National Incidence Surveys, *Child Abuse and Neglect* 17(3):337, 1993.
3. Garbino J: Psychological child maltreatment: a developmental view, *Primary Care: Clinics in Office Practice* 20(2):307, 1993.
4. U.S. Department of Health and Human Services: National Center on Child Abuse and Neglect. *National Study of the Incidence and Severity of Child Abuse and Neglect: Executive Summary.* Washington, DC, 1982, U.S. Government Printing Office.
5. Stier DM, Leventhal JM, Berg AT et al: Are children born to young mothers at increased risk of maltreatment? *Pediatrics* 91(3):642, 1993.

6. Helfer RE, Kempe CH: *Child abuse and neglect.* Cambridge, Mass, 1970, Harper and Row.

7. DeFrancis V: *Protecting the child victim of sexual crimes.* Denver, 1969, American Humane Society.

8. U.S. Department of Health and Human Services: National Center on Child Abuse and Neglect. Denver, 1984, American Humane Society.

9. U.S. Department of Health and Human Services 2000: *Summary Report.* Washington, DC, 1992, U.S. Government Printing Office.

SUGGESTED READINGS

American Association of Pediatrics: Guidelines for the evaluation of sexually abused children, *American Association of Pediatrics News,* Nov. 1990.

Ayoub CC, Willett JB, Robinson DS: Families at risk of child maltreatment: entry-level characteristics and growth in family functioning during treatment, *Child Abuse and Neglect.* 16(4):495, 1992.

Garbino J, Kostelney K: Child maltreatment as a community problem, *Child Abuse and Neglect* 16(4):455, 1992.

Johnson M: Child abuse and neglect. In Sheehy SB: *Emergency nursing,* ed 3. St Louis, 1992, Mosby.

Kelley SJ: Child abuse and neglect. In Kelley SJ: *Pediatric emergencies.* Norwalk, Conn, 1988, Appleton & Lange.

Kelley SJ: Interviewing the sexually abused child. *JEN* 11:5, 234, 1985.

Kelley SJ: The use of art therapy with sexually abused children, *J Psychosocial Nurs* 22: 12, 1984.

Kelley SJ: Critical communications for the sexually abused child, *Pediatr Nurs* 11:421, 1985.

Kelley SJ: Child maltreatment, stressful life events, and behavior problems in school aged children in residential treatment, *J Child and Adolescent psychiatr mental health nursing* 5(2):5, 1992.

Miller EL: Interviewing the sexually abused child, *Maternal-Child Nursing* 10:103, 1985.

33

CHAPTER

Psychiatric Emergencies

The goal of emergency care of the mentally incapacitated patient is to describe that patient in accordance with perceived or real behavior and to intervene in terms of short-term management or referral. Determine whether the problem is organic in nature or is a functional impairment.

GENERAL MANAGEMENT TECHNIQUES

Identify the nature and severity of the patient's presenting problem. Often one must rely on the patient's family or friends for this information. There are certain key questions that should be answered:

Is the patient a danger to himself, herself, or others?

What were the events that led up to this condition?

Was there some thing or event that triggered it?

Why is this person coming for help *now*?

Who brought the patient in?

What does the patient expect from this visit?

In the interview of the patient:

Appear calm and collected.

Set firm limits.

Do not allow the patient to ramble.

Be sure that help is nearby should the patient become physically dangerous; do not allow the patient to come between you and the door.

Try to decrease the patient's anxiety.

Accept the patient's behavior as fact; do not agree or disagree with the patient.

Be clear in your explanations to the patient.

Be honest with the patient about your therapeutic plan.

MENTAL STATUS EXAMINATION

Patients who come to the emergency department with a chief complaint that may represent a psychiatric problem should have a mental status examination that should include the following parameters:

General

Level of consciousness
Motor behavior
Age
Sex
Marital status
Relationship to others
Orientation to time, place, person, reason for being there

Mood

What is the predominant emotion the patient is displaying?

Affect

Does the patient have a flat, normal, or increased affect?

Associations

Does the patient have normal progression of ideas? Are ideas and thoughts
loose or illogical?

Intellect

Is the patient slow? Normal? Bright?

Memory

Is the patient's memory poor? Good?

Thought processes

Are thought processes normal? Is the patient having hallucinations or delusions?
Is the patient confused?

Content of thoughts

Does the patient have phobias? Is the patient constantly repetitious? Is the
patient obsessive? Compulsive? Suicidal? Preoccupied?

Abstract thinking

Can the patient interpret proverbs correctly?

Insight and judgment

Can the patient answer questions of judgment normally?

STRESS

Stress is a state that is intensified when there is a change or threat with which
the individual must cope. Stress as a motivating force can help both the patient
and the health care provider. Unchanneled stress can be inhibiting and
debilitating.
 Stress is:
 Essential for life and growth

Always present to some degree, since every individual is continually adapting to internal and external environmental changes

A response to living

Subject to individual response and stimulus specificity

Displayed as specific signs and symptoms

Measurable qualitatively and quantitatively

Growth-promoting or growth-impeding

Considered psychological when it focuses on the meaning of a stimulus and its anticipated capacity to produce harm

Considered physiological when it focuses on the harm or disturbance to tissue structure or function that has *already* occurred

A stressor is a factor or agent that is perceived as a threat to existence or lifestyle and thereby causes an increase in the stress state. Assumptions regarding stressors include that they are:

A source of motivation for change

Categorized by origin: social, psychological, or physical

Uniquely perceived by each individual

The product, and not the cause, of perception

A condition that imposes a demand on the individual for adjustment

Some generalized sources of stressors can be identified:

Sense of helplessness

Sense of hopelessness

Diminished ability to meet expectations of self or others

Diminished ability to function

Sense of isolation or alienation

Threat to identity through altered body image (real or imagined)

Loss of control (real or imagined)

Pain (emotional or physical)

Change in status (real or imagined)

Loss of someone or something important (a person, pet, home, job, or health)

Factors that influence stress response include:

Cognitive activity	Genetic influences
Personality traits	Past coping patterns
Past experiences	Situational factors
Cultural learning	Environmental factors
Present level of energy	Biological variables

Classes of response to stressors include:

Affective

Motor-behavioral

Alteration of cognitive functioning

Physiological changes

All responses to stressors (mental, emotional, cognitive, and somatic) consume energy. There is no correlation between the intensity of the stressor and the coping behavior used by an individual.

Assessment of Stress Level

Assessment of an individual's stress state is made by observation, interaction data, and clinical data. People respond to stress in a holistic manner, but the central nervous system and endocrine system create the most specific physiologic indices. Baseline information about blood pressure, pulse rate, and respiratory rate provide parameters for assessment of stress level, but an ongoing comparison of these parameters is needed, since none of them shows an absolute increase or decrease during periods of increased stress.

Observational and interaction data

■ **IDENTIFICATION OF STRESSOR**
Origin
Number
Duration
■ **ASSESSMENT OF PATIENT**
Degree of perceived threat
Past experience with comparable stressor
Physical and psychological energy reserve
Resources, capabilities, and potential
Personality variables
Levels of anxiety
Appearance and physical history
■ **EVALUATION OF ENVIRONMENT**
Situational constraints
Cultural restraints
Social controls
Support system available

ANXIETY

Anxiety is a diffuse response that alerts an individual to an impending threat, real or imagined. Fear is a natural psychological and physiological response to an actual threat. Fear is object-focused, but anxiety is ''faceless fear''—no identifiable object can be isolated.

The cause of anxiety is any perceived threat to the security of an individual. The origin may be the result of:
• Biological factors:
　Alteration in homeostasis
　Lack of food, water, shelter, clothing
　Fear of illness, injury, surgery, old age, pain
• Psychological factors:
　Decreased self-esteem
　Death or loss of a loved one or thing
　Pain
　Real or imagined rejection or abandonment
• Sociological factors:

Inability to meet expectations of role, status, values
Inability to maintain sense of belonging

■ **THERAPEUTIC INTERVENTIONS**

The goal is to promote an environment in which the patient can achieve an adequate degree of self-control.

To decrease the patient's feelings of anxiety:
Provide general support.
Have the patient talk.
Keep calm and appear calm.
Direct the patient toward reality.
Assist the patient in setting priorities.
Help the patient identify the source of anxiety.
Let the patient have some control of the situation.
Use consultations and referrals when necessary.

Levels of Anxiety

Mild

Mild anxiety is usually a productive state; use this situation as an information-sharing relationship.

Moderate

Moderate anxiety may be productive, but expends more energy than is necessary; use this as a directive-supportive relationship.

Serious

Serious anxiety is usually nonproductive and even counterproductive; the caregiver must take control of the situation. Give direct commands in short, simple sentences, and focus on intellectual functioning.

Severe

Severe anxiety is crippling to witness and experience, and rapidly becomes contagious. Isolate the individual from others (use physical restraints if needed). Do not leave the patient alone. Be supportive but firm.

Terror

Terror is "do-or-die" situation; assume total responsibility for the patient. Take over total care.

Psychiatric and Psychological Emergencies

The health team's most important function is to establish the feeling that capable assistance to establish self-control is available. Some individuals lack self-control and are out of contact with reality. The primary concern of the emergency physician is not to specify an etiology or give a label to the presenting syndrome, but to facilitate an evaluation of the degree of dysfunction and amount of contact with reality so that immediate treatment is made or referral to another resource for more extensive treatment is accomplished.

Management Strategies to Use with the Angry/Belligerent Patient*

1. Why do people get angry?
   A. *The helpless child*: Under stress (such as pain or illness), many people feel as helpless a child. They then become angry with "parental" figures (e.g., physicians and nurses), who they see as not taking care of them.
      Strategy: Decrease the stress by telling the patient that you are interested in taking care of him or her.
   B. *The temper tantrum*: Many persons have learned that anger will get them what they want. For example, a child throws a temper tantrum to get ice cream, and his mother gives it to him just to stop the screaming. The child learns he will get his ice cream if he yells loud enough. (You can see how this might apply to the patient who demands pain medication.)
      Strategy: Point out to the patient that his anger will not get him what he wants, but will in fact make it more difficult for those trying to help him.
   C. *Scapegoating*: Sometimes when you are feeling angry with one person, you end up taking it out on another. Patients do the same thing.
      Strategy: If the patient's anger seems out of proportion to the situation, you might ask who he is really angry at.
   D. *Inadvertent provocative behavior*: Sometimes without realizing it, you may be talking in such a way as to provoke someone's anger toward you (especially with nonverbal gestures, facial expressions, or tone of voice).
      Strategy: Be aware of both verbal and nonverbal communications.
2. Additional tools.
   A. *Bullfight technique*: Agree with the reality aspects of the patient's anger. ("Yes, you really have a point there, you have been waiting for the doctor for a long time.")
   B. *Engage the patient as an ally in his own treatment.* ("Given the realistic limitations we are under, how do you think we can best help your situation?") Ask the patient for suggestions.
   C. *Show your jugular.* ("I'm just as upset by this impersonal emergency room as you are.")
   D. Make yourself a person, not an impersonal target. ("It really upsets me when you get angry like this, and makes it harder for me to help you.")
   E. *Suggestion box technique*: ("Could you write down your complaints?")
   F. *Set firm limits and expectations of behavior.* Point out clearly the consequences to the patient of not keeping within those limits. ("You know, if you keep acting like this, we will have to call the security guards.")
   G. *Time-out*: Give the person a private place to get angry and hostile and tell him to come back when he has cooled off.

*Courtesy Dr. Regina Pally, Los Angeles.

GENERAL APPROACH TO THE MENTALLY DISTURBED PATIENT

Remember that illness has three components:
- Physical
- Psychological

• Sociological

In dealing with the patient with mental illness:

Establish good rapport.

Establish eye contact.

Appear relaxed.

Let the patient know he or she is really cared about as a patient.

Listen well, but establish parameters to questions; do not project thoughts.

Establish a chief complaint.

What is the patient asking for?

Why is the patient asking for it at this time?

What precipitated this visit?

What usually precipitates it?

What has helped in the past?

Use questions carefully and intentionally.

Observe and record critically.

Speak so the patient can understand.

Recognize regression—regression causes increased suggestibility; be careful about what is said and do not allow lengthy regressions.

Be honest.

Expect proper behavior.

Anticipate the emotional component.

Explain each thing that is done for the patient.

Take the patient seriously.

Do not cut corners; be thorough.

Validate behaviors.

Do not be afraid to ask for help.

Do not be afraid to admit to not knowing something.

Include the family whenever possible.

NONPSYCHOTIC SITUATIONS

Acute Anxiety Attack

An acute anxiety attack typically lasts from a few minutes to several hours. The individual does not have loss of contact with reality, but judgment and insight are impaired. The major management focus is on preventive aspects through teaching self-management.

■ **SIGNS AND SYMPTOMS**

Hyperactivity

Dry mouth

Fidgety movement of hands

Precordial discomfort (sense of pressure in chest)

Choking sensation

Dysphagia or inability to swallow

Feelings of "impending danger"

Literal attempts to escape

Hyperventilation: breathlessness, paresthesias, and acute restlessness

Sweaty palms
Tachycardia
Tremors
Profuse sweating
Urinary frequency

■ **THERAPEUTIC INTERVENTIONS**

Rule out hyperventilation syndrome.

After a thorough physical examination with attention to the cardiopulmonary system, if no physical cause is found, emphasize to the patient the importance of seeking mental health treatment on a nonemergency basis to work on the underlying cause of anxiety.

Avoid false or excessive reassurance; give supportive, reassuring attention during the attack.

Acute Brain Syndrome

An acute brain syndrome is caused by intoxication with or withdrawal from alcohol or other drugs, metabolic toxins, or direct trauma to the brain, which produces changes in the cerebral chemistry or tissues.

■ **SIGNS AND SYMPTOMS**

Clouded sensorium, ranging from confusion to disorientation
Memory deficit
Loss of judgment
Ataxia
Inability to attend to the environment
Slurred speech
Visual or auditory hallucinations
Deviant vital signs

■ **THERAPEUTIC INTERVENTIONS**

Observe the patient carefully.
Monitor and record vital signs frequently.

Acute Delirium

■ **CAUSES**

Biochemical disturbances, for example, electrolyte imbalance, hypoglycemia, uremia, porphyria, or hepatitis
Metastatic neoplasm
Systemic infection
Cerebral hypoxia
Drug withdrawal
Heavy metal toxicity

■ **SIGNS AND SYMPTOMS**

Delusions
Illusions
Disorientation
Frightening dreams

Outbursts of rage
Difficulty in retention and recall
Hyperventilation
Tachycardia
Tremors
Restlessness

■ **THERAPEUTIC INTERVENTIONS**

Identify and remove any toxic substance.
Orient the patient to reality by making simple repetitive statements.
Simplify the environment.
Maintain normal lighting (keep lights on at night).
Have a responsible person stay with the patient.
Avoid physical restraints, which only increase confusion, disorientation, and
    general agitation.

Acute Grief

Acute grief is caused by loss of a significant object or person within a recent
time.

■ **SIGNS AND SYMPTOMS**

Dazed, confused state
Emotional lability with overt tears or moaning
Diminished and slowed speech
Inability to concentrate
Narrowed intellectual functioning
Thought content focused on "lost object"
Feelings of helplessness
Vital signs within normal limits
Anorexia or change in appetite
Weight change

■ **THERAPEUTIC INTERVENTIONS**

Accept the individual's behavior and provide supportive dialogue.
Encourage expression of feelings, especially sadness and loss.
Provide privacy in a room with normal lighting, but decreased environmental
    stimuli.
Teach the importance of proper nutrition and fluid intake, even if the desire to
    eat is diminished.
Encourage the individual to seek out a close friend or family member or
    bereavement group to discuss feelings of grief.

Depression

Depression is generally perceived by health professionals as anger turned
inward. It is considered dysfunctional after an actual loss if it extends beyond a
4 to 6 week period or renders the individual incapable of normal coping behavior. Feelings of sadness accompanied by feelings of guilt without reason may be
present.

■ **SIGNS AND SYMPTOMS**

Feelings of worthlessness, loneliness, helplessness, and sadness

Need for self-punishment and self-blame

Lack of impulse control

Diminished interest

Physical fatigue, especially in the morning

Psychomotor retardation or agitation

History of sleep disturbance

Indecisiveness

Auditory hallucinations

Weight change, loss of appetite, and easy fatigability

Reduced facial animation

Abnormal electrolyte values (sodium and potassium)

Possible diuretic, antidepressant drug, and minor tranquilizer side effects

Wringing of hands

Suicidal ideation

Decreased libido

Constipation

Pacing

■ **THERAPEUTIC INTERVENTIONS**

Do not isolate the patient.

Avoid excessive environmental stimuli or forced decision-making.

Provide safety and psychological security.

Reality test while encouraging the expression of feelings, especially underlying anger.

Help the patient express grief at loss of a loved one; point out that this is normal.

Explore sources of emotional support.

Prescribe antidepressant medications.

Involve family members and social network for continued support.

Assess the risk of suicide.

Suicide

There are over 30,000 successful suicides a year, or 80 each day. In addition to successful suicides, there are over half a million unsuccessful attempts each year—1,300 each day, or 1 each minute.

Assessing Suicide Potential

SEX   Males are more serious suicide risks than females.

Females attempt suicide three times more often than males.

Males are three times more successful at suicide than females.

There are 6 suicides per 100,000 females.

There are 18 suicides per 100,000 males.

Females tend to use drugs.

Males tend to use firearms.

AGE	Suicide potential increases with age.
	Younger people try more often.
	Older people are more often successful on the first attempt.
RACE/ETHNIC GROUPS/ MINORITIES	Suicide rate in the United States is higher in foreign-born people.
	There is a high rate of suicide among homosexuals.
	Moslems have the lowest suicide rate of any religious group, followed by Catholics, Jews, and Protestants.
MARITAL STATUS	Married people have the lowest rate.
	Risk is high in the widowed or divorced group.
	Singles commit twice as many suicides as married people.
FAMILY HISTORY	If family history of suicide attempts is high, there is increased risk of suicide.
	Risk is high if there have been previous attempts (40% to 80% of people who are successful at suicide have made previous attempts).
SEASONAL	More suicides occur in spring and fall.
	More suicides occur on Wednesdays and Saturdays; fewest on Sundays.
OTHER	Substance abuse (alcohol, drugs) greatly increases risk.
	Risk is more serious if the plan is well thought out or the patient has a weapon.
	Do not be afraid to ask if the patient is planning suicide.
	Mental illness increases the risk.
	Debilitating physical illness increases the risk.
	History of serious emotional loss increases the risk (at the time of the loss or on anniversary of the loss).

■ **SIGNS AND SYMPTOMS**

Feelings of worthlessness, hopelessness, helplessness, confusion
Restlessness
Agitation
Irritability
GI complaints
Insomnia
Fatigue
Indifference
Decreased physical activity
Actual suicide attempt that was unsuccessful

Approach to the Suicidal Patient

The approach to the suicidal patient has as its goal establishing a psychologically and physically protective environment. It is also important to establish an empathetic rapport.

■ **PROBLEM SOLVING**

Suicidal thoughts are attempts by the patient to solve problems. Try to find out what the patient thinks the problem is. This must be done after intervention for the crisis, such as care for the patient after overdose or wrist slashing. Common areas for problems include:

Love life	Interpersonal problems
Job situation	Illness (mental and physical)
Work problems	Alcohol abuse
Financial problems	Drug abuse
Family problems	

■ **EVALUATE WITH THE PATIENT**
Look for alternatives for the patient.
If the patient is unsure of possible alternatives or has no alternatives, hospitalization is mandatory.
If there are alternatives, be specific about them.
Try to involve the family or friends whenever possible in the decision-making and/or planning.
When in doubt, obtain a psychiatric consultation.
If this is not available, admit the patient to the hospital for observation.
The patient may require sedation.

POSTTRAUMATIC STRESS DISORDER

Posttraumatic stress disorder is a reaction to a witnessed or experienced catastrophic event, such as war, rape, injury, etc. These individuals usually demonstrate emotional, physical, behavioral, and psychological impairment.

■ **SIGNS AND SYMPTOMS**
Guilt/blame/self-punishment
Experiencing flashbacks of the event
Dissociation
Depersonalization
Psychogenic amnesia
Psychogenic fugue
Difficulty in concentrating and problem solving
Emotional lability
Sleep disturbances
Sexual dysfunction
Suicide ideations
Substance abuse
Impaired relationships: relating to mistrust, betrayal, or rejection

■ **THERAPEUTIC INTERVENTIONS**
Remain calm and relaxed.
Develop and utilize a support system.
Identify traumatic event.
Prescribe antidepressant medications.
Prescribe antianxiety medications.
Assess the risk of suicide.

Assess the potential for violence.

Consider consultations and referrals.

HOMICIDAL AND ASSAULTIVE BEHAVIOR

Homicidal and assaultive behavior is experienced in acute intoxication, paranoia, or mania, or is seen in sociopathic individuals. Extreme caution should be used to protect oneself and others in the environment.

■ **THERAPEUTIC INTERVENTIONS**

Approach the individual with an obvious show of force (group of people).

Confiscate all real or potentially harmful objects.

Physically restrain and establish psychological and physical controls on behalf of the individual.

Establish one person as a liaison who assumes a calm, authoritative, and unhurried manner.

Speak in simple, direct sentences.

Separate the individual from the family and/or the intended victim; if the victim is not present, emergency personnel are responsible for making sure that the person is warned of the patient's ideations.

Observe for suicidal as well as homicidal attempts, since suicide may follow homicidal attempts because of generally impaired judgment.

HOMOSEXUAL PANIC

Homosexual panic is a behavior seen in those who have a reaction to latent homosexuality (usually males). The individual has misperceived a recent male- or female-centered association that may have provided visual stimulation of homoerotic fantasies.

■ **SIGNS AND SYMPTOMS**

Obsessive thinking focused on sexual activity

Inability to isolate fact from fantasy

■ **THERAPEUTIC INTERVENTIONS**

Provide an opportunity for the patient to express his or her fears in a nonjudgmental environment.

Avoid physical contact.

Avoid physical techniques such as injections of medicine and rectal examinations.

Offer referral for follow-up counseling.

ORGANIC BRAIN SYNDROME

Organic brain syndrome is diffuse disruption and impairment of the functioning capacity of brain tissue from a variety of causes, e.g., Alzheimer's disease, brain tumor, etc.

■ **SIGNS AND SYMPTOMS**

Decreased orientation

Decreased memory

Decreased judgment
Decreased ability to calculate and figure
Shallow affect

Acute organic brain syndrome is usually rapid in onset, temporary in nature, and very reversible.

Chronic organic brain syndrome is very slow in progression and is usually non-reversible. Signs and symptoms of chronic brain syndrome include:
   Dementia
   Delirium
   Stupor, coma, or death
Whenever a caregiver comes into contact with a patient who has organic brain syndrome, he or she should ask about the possibility of a medication-induced syndrome (many medications may cause this).

ACUTE PSYCHOTIC REACTIONS

A psychosis is the deterioration of a person's thought process, affective response, and ability to be in touch with reality, to communicate, and to relate with others. Deterioration continues to the point at which the patient cannot deal with the processes of daily living and loses contact with reality. Do not agree with reality distortion, but avoid arguing in your approach to guiding the individual in reality testing. This patient should be treated in a quiet, sparsely decorated room. If the patient is extremely violent or has the potential to become so, restraints or a locked room may be considered. Undress the patient and place him or her in a hospital gown (remove clothing or other objects that may conceal weapons).

Schizophrenic Reactions

■ **SIGNS AND SYMPTOMS**
   Delusions
   Auditory hallucinations
   Difficulty with associations
   Disordered thought with clear sensorium
   Combative or assaultive behavior
   Withdrawn or catatonic behavior
   Bizarre gesturing
■ **THERAPEUTIC INTERVENTIONS**
   Establish a history of previous hospitalization and/or use of major tranquilizers
      that the patient voluntarily stopped or was requested to stop taking.
   Use simple, concrete expressions and brief sentences.
   Avoid figures of speech that are subject to misinterpretation.
   Use an authoritative manner to help assure the patient of your ability to control
      yourself and the environment.
   Listen as the patient talks of delusions to gain clues about any thinking disorder.

If the patient is paranoid, avoid closed doors or blocked doorways; allow the patient to feel "uncornered."

If phenothiazines are given, observe for postural hypotension and pseudoparkinsonism side effects.

Consider hospital admission.

Paranoia

Paranoia is a syndrome within the schizophrenic classification. A paranoid person demonstrates a loss of reality contact through a delusional system, generally of persecution or excessive religious statements. The paranoid patient can be dangerous because of feelings that either specific people or unnamed forces are "out to get me."

■ **SIGNS AND SYMPTOMS**

Delusions of a projective nature

Feelings of uniqueness going toward grandiosity

Auditory hallucinations

Difficulty with association

Illogical thought process

Obsessive thinking

Combative or assaultive behavior

Restlessness

Agitation

■ **THERAPEUTIC INTERVENTIONS**

Avoid psychological and physical threats or challenges while providing limits and reality testing.

Use simple, concrete expressions.

Remain calm and authoritative.

Move slowly and quietly to avoid appearing intrusive.

Sit or stand on the same level with the patient to avoid a "power" position.

Allow the patient to be close to the slightly ajar door.

Allow the patient to verbalize distorted or illogical thinking.

If the patient threatens violence or aggression against a particular person or group, notify them.

Avoid trying to convince the patient that the delusions are erroneous and avoid adding validity to any false belief.

Hypomania/Manic Psychosis

Hypomania or manic psychosis patients usually have recurrent episodes of either mood elevation or depression. Serum lithium level should be measured immediately in those patients who have been on lithium therapy.

■ **SIGNS AND SYMPTOMS**

Elation or increased mental excitement that is unstable

Irritability, sometimes irrational anger

Pressured speech (delivered rapidly through tight lips)

Increased motor activity (talks easily and endlessly)

Demanding or euphoric manner
Grandiose ideas
Loud voices
Sexual acting out or content focused on sex
Loud-colored clothing, bright-colored makeup (overdone)

■ **THERAPEUTIC INTERVENTIONS**
Assume an authoritative, nonthreatening manner.
Guard the patient, caregivers, and environment against physical harm.
Decrease environmental stimulation.
Provide an unencumbered, safe, and private room to allow pacing or ritualistic
    motor activity.
Do *not* encourage the patient to talk; ask succinct questions.
Respond in an unhurried, simple speech pattern.
Avoid mechanical restraints if possible.

DRUG-RELATED PSYCHIATRIC EMERGENCIES

The function of emergency personnel in an acute drug-induced crisis is one of
clinical intervention, critical observation, and supportive therapeutic communication.

■ **SIGNS AND SYMPTOMS**
Respiratory depression
Increased temperature, pulse, and respirations, and decreased BP
Increased or decreased pupil size
Decreased muscle tone
Tremors
Gastrointestinal symptoms
Decreased level of consciousness
Distortion of mood/thought patterns
Track marks

■ **QUESTIONS TO ASK**
What type of drug was taken?
How much?
What has happened since the drug was taken?
What other drugs have been used (drug history)?
At what time was the last dose of the drug taken?
At what time did the patient start abusing the drug?
How was the drug taken (orally, subcutaneously, by injection, by inhalation)?
Where was the drug obtained?
Was alcohol consumed?

Categories of Drugs

Belladonna alkaloids

Over-the-counter hypnotic drugs such as Nytol and Sominex contain scopol-
amine. Taken in large amounts, they produce an atropine-like psychosis. Phenothiazines, tricyclic antidepressants, and antihistamines are potent anticholinergic

drugs. Some plants also contain belladonna alkaloids. The classic description of belladonna effects is "blind as a bat, dry as a bone, red as a beet, and mad as a hatter."

■ **SIGNS AND SYMPTOMS**
Delirium
Mental confusion
Intense thirst and dry mouth
Dysphagia
Restlessness
Talkativeness
Thought blockade
Dilated pupils
Inability to visually accommodate
Flushed, hot, and dry skin
Rapid and weak pulse
Hoarse, raspy voice
Urinary retention or slow, painful urinary stream

■ **THERAPEUTIC INTERVENTIONS**
Give frequent sips of water.
Use a saline flush to moisten the eyes.
Insert urinary bladder catheter if needed.
Provide a calm environment in subdued lighting.
Serve as a calm, nonjudgmental listener, but *do not* encourage talking.

Opiates and related compounds

Included in the opiate group are heroin, morphine, hydromorphone (Dilaudid), pentazocine (Talwin), methadone (Dolophine), and propoxyphene (Darvon). The list is in order of intensity of euphoria and diminished sensorium.

■ **SIGNS AND SYMPTOMS**
State of sluggishness
State of euphoria
Somnolence
Track marks (popliteal fossa, ankles, forearm veins, sublingual)
Constricted pupils
Decreased blood pressure
Decreased heart rate
Decreased body temperature

■ **THERAPEUTIC INTERVENTIONS**
ABCs
Dextrose 50%
Naloxone 0.8 mg IV or IM
Observe for withdrawal syndrome: coryza, yawning, lacrimation, increased pulse and respiratory rate, perspiration, and tremors (these start 6 to 12 hours after the last dose).
Observe in addition for insomnia, severe abdominal cramps, vomiting and diarrhea, tachycardia, and hypertension (these start 12 to 48 hours after the last dose).

Observe for respiratory depression and impending heroin pulmonary edema if that drug is suspected.

If naloxone (Narcan) has been given, be alert for agitation and aggressive behavior as the patient withdraws from the opiate.

Hallucinogens

Hallucinogens are psychedelic drugs such as LSD and DMT (acid), peyote, mescaline, STP, psilocybin, and phencyclidine (PCP, angel dust). Individuals on a ''bad trip'' are especially sensitive to the environment and are suspicious of people. Subjective symptoms wax and wane.

■ **SIGNS AND SYMPTOMS**

Grossly impaired judgment
Intense visual or auditory hallucinations
Unusual changes in self-perception
Rapid mood swings
Flight of ideas
Lack of coordination
Loss of control that comes in waves
Panic state
Increased blood pressure and pulse rate
Pupil dilation
Chills and shivering
Increased muscle tension
Tremors
Nausea (especially with mescaline)
Convulsions

■ **THERAPEUTIC INTERVENTIONS**

1. Provide a constant vigil by a supportive person (a trusted, responsible friend or one particular staff person).
   a. Give simple, repetitive statements.
   b. *Do not* challenge the patient's values, beliefs, life-style, or distorted thinking.
2. Use ''talk down'' techniques. (*Do not* use ''talk down'' with PCP.)
   a. Establish verbal contact to allay fears.
   b. Encourage the patient to talk.
   c. Encourage expressions of perceptions and feelings.
3. Reality test on a continuous basis.
   a. Focus on physical characteristics of the room.
   b. Repeatedly identify person(s) in the room.
   c. Have the patient focus on inanimate, stationary objects in the room as a center of orientation.
   d. Encourage the patient to keep his or her eyes open.
4. Provide a protective, quiet, and nonthreatening room.
   a. Normal lighting.
   b. Decreased visual and auditory stimuli.
5. Guard yourself against spontaneous aggressive behavior.
6. Be alert for suicidal behavior.

Phencyclidine (angel dust)

It is classified as an analgesic and a hallucinogenic agent. It can be taken by inhalation, ingestion, or intravenously.

■ **SIGNS AND SYMPTOMS**

Severe anxiety, agitation, drowsiness, or coma
Psychosis (acute onset)
Constricted pupils
Increased then decreased respirations, followed by respiratory arrest
Elevated then decreased blood pressure
Vertical nystagmus
Ataxia
Euphoria
Increased then decreased deep tendon reflexes
Nausea and vomiting
Clonus
Increased then decreased urinary output
Tremors followed by seizures
Amnesia
Opisthotonos
Distorted images and thought processes
Depersonalization
Hallucinations
Dysrhythmias

■ **THERAPEUTIC INTERVENTIONS**

Reduce external stimuli (quiet, dim room).
Decrease the number of people present.
Use restraints and total observation.
Do not attempt to talk the patient down.
Give haloperidol (Haldol) IV (but remember that haloperidol has a shorter half-life than PCP) *or* Diazepam (Valium).
Consider hospital admission.

Central nervous system stimulants

All psychostimulants produce excitation of the central nervous system. Tolerance develops rapidly and is sometimes accompanied by psychological dependence. A physical withdrawal syndrome is unlikely, but a real let-down feeling accompanies discontinuation of the drug.

Amphetamines

■ **SIGNS AND SYMPTOMS**

Increased rate of speech
Extraordinary hyperactivity
Rapid flight of ideas
Mood swings
Irritability and hostility
Aggressiveness
Unexplained fear and jitteriness

Talkativeness
Hallucinations (auditory or visual)
Clear sensorium and memory
Delusions of persecution
Increased blood pressure, pulse rate, and temperature
Dilated pupils
Insomnia
Twitching muscles
Nausea or vomiting
Severe abdominal pain
Grand mal seizures

Cocaine or crack

■ **SIGNS AND SYMPTOMS**
Euphoria and feeling of mental agility
Formication (sense of insects crawling under skin)
Loose association
Paranoid delusions
Perforated nasal septum
Elevated body temperature
Dilated pupils
Skin pallor

■ **THERAPEUTIC INTERVENTIONS**
Place the patient in a quiet, secure, large room.
Reduce environmental stimuli.
Allow the patient to move about.
Observe vital signs, especially temperature.
Allow the patient to "talk down."
Be alert to violent or aggressive tendencies and protect caregivers and the environment.
Be aware of repetitive compulsive behavior.
A period of "crash" is followed by marked depression, which can lead to suicidal behavior; therefore, use precautions to prevent suicide.

Central nervous system depressants

Depressants are most dangerous in terms of acute overdose and withdrawal morbidity. Withdrawal represents a medical emergency of the first order. Tolerance develops rapidly; the shorter the half-life, the more physiologically addicting the drug. Alcohol and barbiturate intoxication are similar in signs and symptoms.

Acute alcohol intoxication

■ **SIGNS AND SYMPTOMS**
Slowed thinking
Impaired memory and judgment
Labile emotions
Uninhibited behavior

Inattention and distractibility
Euphoria or depression
Slurred speech
Agitation or extreme compliance
Unsteady gait
Smell of alcohol on the breath
Nausea and vomiting
Tremors
Flushed or pale face
Systolic hypertension
Tachycardia
Muscle weakness

■ **THERAPEUTIC INTERVENTIONS**

Observe the patient carefully.
Monitor vital signs, especially blood pressure and heart rate.
Place patient in a quiet, protected area.
Guard against aspiration and physical injury.
Speak in a calm, authoritative manner.
If a sedative or barbiturate drug is given, be alert to respiratory depression.
If a major tranquilizer is given, be alert to hypotension.
Obtain an ingestion history, including alcohol, in combination with other drugs.
  See Chapter 12 for measurement of alcohol withdrawal symptoms, as the
    patient who stops drinking may precipitate a withdrawal crisis in increas-
    ingly serious stages.
  See Chapter 12 for medical management.

Barbiturates

The main danger of overdose is stupor and cardiorespiratory collapse. Because
of their ability to depress CNS functioning, there is an extremely high incidence
of barbiturate use for intended or gestured suicide.

■ **SIGNS AND SYMPTOMS**

Muscular incoordination	Postural hypotension
Slurred speech	Hypothermia
Paranoid ideation	Depressed respiration
Restlessness	Nausea
Clouded sensorium progressing to coma	Convulsions
Wide-based ataxic gait	Tremors
Irritability	Hyperreflexia
Dilated pupils	Muscular weakness

■ **THERAPEUTIC INTERVENTIONS**

Management generally includes withdrawal of the abused drug under inpatient
    conditions for close monitoring of misuse of drugs.
Provide a quiet, secure room.
Carefully observe and record signs and symptoms.
Be especially alert for convulsions, which can progress to status epilepticus, and
    respiratory distress.

Avoid physical restraints.

A withdrawal syndrome appears within 10 to 15 hours: apprehension, muscle weakness, hypotension, seizures, and psychosis may occur.

Bromides

Bromides are more likely to produce chronic poisoning than an acute overdose.

■ **SIGNS AND SYMPTOMS**

Gradual increase in drowsiness without release by sleep

Depression

Confusion

Hallucinations (visual)

Delusions of paranoid nature

Hypomanic state

Acneform skin eruptions (especially on the face and around the hair roots)

Serum drug level above 75 mg/100 ml

Heavily fixed tongue

Foul breath

■ **THERAPEUTIC INTERVENTIONS**

Provide a quiet, secure room.

Ascertain the source of bromide intake; many patients are unaware of the poison-like effect of over-the-counter sleep agents.

Reality test regarding delusions and hallucinations.

Marijuana

The most common complication of marijuana is that the user experiences an anxiety attack.

■ **SIGNS AND SYMPTOMS**

Elevated blood pressure	Apprehension
Tachycardia	Restlessness
Tachypnea	Feeling of doom

■ **THERAPEUTIC INTERVENTIONS**

Psychological support

Reassurance

Diazepam by mouth if the reaction is severe

Phenothiazine dystonic reactions

Phenothiazine dystonic reactions may be caused by prochlorperazine (Compazine), trifluoperazine (Stelazine), chlorpromazine (Thorazine), fluphenazine (Prolixin), and haloperidol (Haldol), all of which are phenothiazines. Signs and symptoms of phenothiazine dystonic reactions are often mistaken for hypocalcemia, seizure disorders, and tetany. Be sure to ask about a medication history when a patient comes to the emergency department with these signs and symptoms.

■ **SIGNS AND SYMPTOMS**

Signs and symptoms usually appear 4 to 5 days after ingestion.

Oculogyric crisis	Facial grimaces
Protruding tongue	Opisthotonos
Torticollis	Tortipelvic crisis

■ **THERAPEUTIC INTERVENTIONS**

Diphenhydramine (Benadryl) IV or

Benztropine (Cogentin) or

Trihexyphenidyl (Artane)

Adverse central nervous system reactions to antipsychotic drugs

Sometimes the drug of choice in treating a psychiatric condition produces more stress than relief for the patient. One such instance is the severe extrapyramidal side effects of some major tranquilizers. These reactions are more likely to occur during the *initial* phase of psychotropic drug therapy. The appearance of undesirable side effects can be anxiety-provoking for the patient and the family. The potential hazard and the sudden onset of the symptoms can cause the patient to refuse to take any type of prescribed medicine that could be effective in decreasing psychotic symptoms. Emergency personnel can do much to help the individual realize that use of antipsychotic drugs requires patience in obtaining a satisfactory therapeutic response.

Medical management to counteract adverse reactions is quickly achieved in most instances by anticholinergic drugs such as diphenhydramine (Benadryl) or antiparkinsonian drugs such as benztropine mesylate (Cogentin) or trihexyphenidyl (Artane).

Parkinsonism usually develops within 20 days of the initial drug therapy. Symptoms include muscular rigidity, resting tremors, a masklike face, and drooling. Dystonia usually develops within 1 hour to 5 days.

■ **THERAPEUTIC INTERVENTIONS**

Educate the patient to the fact that untoward symptoms will disappear rapidly with proper medication, usually go away even if untreated, and usually are completely reversible.

Provide a quiet, darkened room for the patient to lie down until the antagonist drug takes effect.

Have a nonthreatening person stay with the patient until the undesirable symptoms have subsided (generally within 1 hour after administration of an antagonist drug IM).

Disposition of the patient

The major question that arises with the therapeutic intervention of the psychiatric patient is whether he or she should be hospitalized. One important factor is the presence or absence of a solid support system in terms of family or friends and their willingness to observe or supervise the patient.

When to hospitalize the patient involuntarily:

If the patient is a physical threat to himself or herself (suicidal)

If the patient is a physical threat to others (homicidal)

(Involuntary hold criteria differ in each state, but most states have included these two criteria)

If the patient is addicted to alcohol or drugs

The hold is usually placed by a psychiatrist or psychiatric consultant. These holds are usually for a limited time (72 hours in most states).

SUMMARY

By definition, a psychiatric emergency occurs when a person's adaptive capacity is ineffective in coping with life's stressors. Psychiatric emergencies require careful listening and a great deal of common sense. It is not easy to remain calm, appear authoritative, and thereby be therapeutic when the entire situation is anxiety-provoking. Self-sufficiency and self-control should be the goal of any intervention. The most powerful strategy in helping the individual establish a sense of self-control (power) is to show an attitude of decisive action (authority) and compassion (care).

In psychiatric emergencies the signs and symptoms of the health problem are sometimes so obvious in the individual's bizarre behavior or thinking that it is often easier to evaluate what is wrong than to assess what is right. The strengths to build on are as important as isolating the impairments causing the dysfunction. A complete evaluation includes the patient's healthy as well as the unhealthy parts. The treatment process is based on the individual's strengths that have been identified and validated through the assessment process. Emergency personnel need to develop an understanding of people and their coping behaviors. This basic knowledge of human behavior synthesized with medical and surgical knowledge should provide the needed tools of sensitivity and knowledge to meet the patient's immediate needs.

SUGGESTED READINGS

Haber J, McMahon AL, Price-Hoskins P, Sideleau BF: *Comprehensive psychiatric nursing*, ed 4, St Louis, 1992, Mosby.

Keltner NL, Schwecke LH, Bostrom CE: *Psychiatric nursing: a psychotherapeutic management approach.* St Louis, 1991, Mosby.

Pasquali EH, Arnold HM, DeBario N: *Mental health nursing: a holistic approach*, ed 3. St Louis, 1989, Mosby.

Puskar KR, Obus NL: Management of the psychiatric emergency, *Nurse Practitioner* 14: 7, 1989.

Sheehy SB: *Emergency nursing principles and practice,* ed 3. St Louis, 1992, Mosby.

Special Considerations for the Geriatric Patient

Elderly persons (over age 65) represent a growing population in the United States today. Currently they comprise 11% of the population, and that number is expected to reach 20% by the year 2020.[1] This is of significance to emergency nursing as perhaps one out of every four patients seen could be aged 65 or over. Caring for these patients requires not only knowledge surrounding the ABCs of emergency care, but an understanding of the normal physiological changes associated with aging. For the purpose of this text, geriatric or elderly will be defined as those patients over the age of 65.

A thorough history and physical assessment are important. Special attention should be given to the patients' past medical and surgical history, preexisting conditions, and medications they are currently taking. A family member or spouse may be needed to assist in obtaining a history if the patient is not an accurate or reliable witness, and all medical records should be obtained if available. The hallmark of aging is the loss of reserve capacity. There is an overall decrease in the ability to compensate for stress and a slower return to normal function, or homeostasis, after an untoward event.[2] Table 34-1 reflects the physiological changes associated with aging. These changes will directly affect the patient's ability to recover and recuperate from untoward events. They are essential to providing quality of care and must be incorporated into the nursing process. This will ensure the best outcomes for the geriatric emergency department patient.

PHYSIOLOGICAL CHANGES ASSOCIATED WITH AGING

PHYSICAL ASSESSMENT

A head-to-toe assessment needs to be accomplished on any emergency patient, but it is of particular importance to the elderly patient. Observation, auscultation, and palpation are sometimes the only ways an abnormality can be determined.

TABLE 34-1   Structural and Functional Changes as a Result of Aging

BODY SYSTEM	ALTERATION
Tissues	Decreased number of active cells
	Reduced tissue elasticity
Cardiovascular	Decreased distensibility of blood vessels
	Increased systolic blood pressure
	Increased systemic resistance
	Decreased cardiac output
	Slow response to stress
Pulmonary	Decreased strength of respiratory muscles
	Limited chest expansion
	Decreased number of functioning alveoli
	Decreased elastic recoil, small airway collapse
	Decreased resting oxygen tension
	Diminished protective mechanisms
Neurological	Decreased number of functional neurons
	Decrease in nerve conduction velocity
	Short-term memory loss
	Reduced cerebral blood flow
	Decreased visual acuity and speed of dark adaptation
	Decreased pupillary response and accommodation
	Increased auditory tone threshold
	Diminished sensation and touch acuity
Gastrointestinal/genitourinary	Decreased peristalsis
	Diminished acid secretion and thickened mucosa
	Decreased total nephron count
	Decreased glomerular filtration rate
	Diminished concentrating ability
Musculoskeletal/integumentary	Narrowing of intervertebral disks
	Bone loss, increased risk for fracture
	Increased wear on joints
	Decreased number of muscle cells
	Loss of muscle strength
	Loss of skin thickness

From Andrews JF: Trauma in the elderly, *Forum Medicum, Postgraduate Studies in Trauma Nursing,* 1990.

General Observations/Pertinent Questions

The nurse should observe for and discuss the following when performing the assessment:

Speech or hearing impairments

Mood disturbance or difficulty with thought processes

Differences between patient's chief complaint and that of the family

Living arrangements, activities of daily living, socioeconomic circumstances and the physical layout of the home, i.e., if stairs are present, etc.

Thorough review of all of the patient's medications. Look for possible adverse reactions, drug interactions, and toxic or subtherapeutic levels. Many elderly patients are on numerous medications and this "polypharmacy" may be the cause of their present problem. Proper medication dosing, interactions, and scheduling should be discussed with the patient, or if appropriate a visiting nurse association referral made to set up such a schedule.

Dietary history—what the patient eats, how often, who shops, if there are difficulties associated with shopping, and smell or taste impairments, any problems with chewing, swallowing, and presence or absence of dentures and how well they fit.

Urinary incontinence

Depression or anxiety. Poor appetite, change in sleep patterns and constipation are common in the elderly, but may also be symptoms of depression. Ask about suicidal thoughts and crying spells. Ask about over-the-counter medications and alcohol intake. Alcohol and over-the-counter medications can interact together and/or with prescribed medications to cause psychological and physiological problems.

Sexual problems or difficulties. Elderly men may have a problem with impotence or unreliable erections and women may have vaginal dryness. Remind them that it is not abnormal to still have sexual feelings.

A thorough physical exam should be performed with the patient unrobed and in a hospital gown.[3]

Head

Observation
Palpation for pain, bleeding, or fractures
Elicit history of a fall, recent or weeks ago
Elicit history of neurological changes, changes in mental status, or history of loss of consciousness
Subdural hematomas are more frequent in the elderly as a result of anatomic changes associated with aging and may be acute or chronic.
Prepare patient for CT and/or operating room.

Chest

Observation for equal, bilateral expansion, and observable abnormalities
Auscultation for bilateral breath sounds and presence or absence of adventitious breath sounds
Palpation for pain, fractures, crepitus
Monitor O_2 sat (low 90s may be their normal)
Monitor ability to handle and clear secretions
Check for gag reflex and coughing ability
Hypoventilation may be the patient's normal

Observe for use of accessory muscles
Observe for nasal flaring
ABGs and oxygen saturation levels may be indicated
If ETT placement is warranted monitor for the development of pneumonia.

Abdomen

Observe for surgical scars, distended abdomen.
Auscultate for bowel sounds
Elicit bowel elimination pattern; slowed peristalsis associated with aging tends
   to predispose these patients to constipation.
Prepare for KUB—flat and upright.
Elicit urination pattern; men are predisposed to urinary dribbling and women to
   stress incontinence. Note amount, color, specific gravity, and any odor of
   urine.
Obtain urinalysis/urine culture.
Check skin around perineum for evidence of excoriation and breakdown.
■ NURSING INTERVENTIONS
Keep clean and dry.
Offer bedpan or walk to bathroom frequently.

Extremities

Observe for deformities, bruising, normal and abnormal coloring.
Look for shortening of leg and external rotation of the foot when a fall has
   occurred or hip fracture is suspected.
Palpate pulses.
Assess range of motion.
Monitor vital signs frequently as fractures cause bleeding in the bones, which
   can cause shock in the elderly.
Assess for fractures with no history of trauma—suspect elder abuse.

Skin

Observe for turgor, intact skin, skin tears, bruising—old and new, burns—old
   and new, rashes, areas of breakdown, temperature, and color.
■ NURSING INTERVENTIONS
Inquire about bruises, skin tears, and burns.
Give diphtheria/tetanus inoculation if needed.
Dress tears using paper tape and nonstick dressings.
Gently clean areas of breakdown and apply protective ointment.
Take temperature. Less body fat and muscle mass makes the elderly more prone
   to hypothermia. Warm IV fluids, apply warmed blankets, pad bony promi-
   nences.
Inquire as to who cares for the patient if bruising and tears are not caused by
   falls or bumps. Suspect elder abuse. Use nonjudgmental approach and con-
   tact social services if suspicion is high.

GERIATRIC EMERGENCIES

Falls

Falls are the leading cause of death in elderly trauma victims, and more than half of all deaths as a result of falls involve persons aged 75 or older. Predisposing factors include: poor vision and hearing, gait disturbances, diminished muscle strength, osteoporotic bones, and associated frailty. Medical conditions contributing to falls include cardiac arrhythmias, dizziness, seizure disorder, and arthritis. Environmental factors such as loose carpets, awkward stairways, poor lighting, and unfamiliar surroundings can contribute to seemingly minor falls.[3] These falls contribute to fractures, head injuries, and internal injuries such as splenic rupture, and are compromising to both the previously healthy and not so healthy patient.

■ **PREVENTION OF FALLS** (please refer to the following box):
1. Removal or securing of loose carpeting
2. Improved lighting
3. Handrails and siderails where needed
4. Moving furniture with sharp edges or padding the sharp edges
5. Shoes that are "sensible" with flat heels
6. Assistance in the home if possible
7. Knowledge of 9-1-1 access

Injury Prevention Activities for the Elderly

Remove or tack down all scatter rugs.
Check all staircases for stability, and install handrails whenever possible.
Apply nonslip strips on stairways.
Carpet areas that are prone to spills or slipperiness.
Reduce clutter and open clear pathways through all rooms.
Pad wooden or metal edges on furniture.
Install bright lights in hallways and entrances.
Place nonslip mats in bathtub and shower.
Install grab bars near all bathrooms.
Install smoke detectors and check them at regular intervals.
Investigate assistive cooking devices, such as burner shields, long-handled utensils, and protective hand gear.
Do not wear loose-fitting garments while cooking.
Use rear stove burners rather than front ones, and avoid storing goods you may need over the stove.
Check central furnace and space heaters frequently to ensure proper functioning.
Reduce thermostatic setting on water heater, and clearly label all hot water faucets.
Review directions for operating major appliances annually.

From Andrews JF: Trauma in the elderly, *Forum Medicum, Postgraduate Studies in Trauma Nursing*, 1990.

Burns

Diminished neurological sensation, impaired vision and hearing, and psychomotor delay may leave the elderly unable to avoid the hazards of heat and flames. The elderly are four times more likely to experience scalding or contact burns.[3]

Treatment can be found and is the same as treatment discussed in Chapter 26, however careful consideration must be made for the elderly burn victim as physiological changes do compromise their healing and recovery.

■ **PREVENTION**

1. Short sleeved, non-nylon shirts and pajamas
2. Discourage smoking, especially while resting
3. Smoke detectors and fire extinguishers easily accessible with ease of operation
4. Assistance with cooking, as needed; extra care when cooking with gas
5. Discourage use of hot water bottles and heating pads, or have patient monitor temperature with a thermometer or set at the low setting
6. Knowledge of 9-1-1 access

Motor Vehicle Crash

Visual and hearing disturbances, decreased reaction time, and increased traffic all play a part in motor vehicle events involving the elderly. One third of all pedestrian fatalities occur in persons aged 65 and over.[4]

Trauma management essentially remains the same for these patients as trauma management for younger patients. Structural and functional changes associated with aging will have an impact on care and patient recovery, however. See Chapter 25 for treatment.

■ **PREVENTION**

1. Minimal night driving if patient has "night blindness"
2. Encourage seat belt use
3. Have patient drive only in familiar areas, avoiding highly congested areas or areas under construction
4. If they or others are concerned with their driving abilities encourage contacting state licensing agencies to inquire about "Over 75 Refresher Courses."

Elder Abuse

Awareness and understanding of elder abuse is becoming more apparent. Although assessment of elder abuse is often difficult and time consuming, its role cannot be stressed enough. Emergency nurses can play a large part in this role. They are usually the first persons the elderly patient encounters in the emergency department setting. Knowledge of a sympathetic, nonjudgmental approach often will elicit information from the patient.

■ **CLUES**

Unexplained fractures or bruising, burns, or internal injuries can be the presenting problems.

Unexplained delays in seeking treatment and differing accounts of what happened, by the patient and family members can be reason to suspect elder abuse, as are unusual injury locations and unusual patient-family interactions.

The patient may be hesitant to speak about abuse as he or she relies on that family member for care and shelter. Frustration, economic difficulties, lifestyle changes, and inability to care for the elderly patient are some reasons that elder abuse exists.

If suspected, the social services division of the hospital needs to be notified to offer information and follow-up or referral.

Elder Abandonment—"Granny Dumping"

This is an alarming and growing phenomenon in emergency departments. We are now experiencing a rapidly growing elderly population that requires various amounts of care and attention.[5]

Family members are usually the caregivers and may find it frustrating and difficult to fulfill the role of caring for a chronically ill or disabled family member. They turn to the emergency department for help when they become overwhelmed. The emergency department is the place for this abandonment because it is open 24 hours a day, 7 days a week. They come to the emergency department for support, compassion, and for a break from their caregiving role.

With the advent of DRGs, hospitals are less likely to admit patients for "social disposition," yet with abandonment they may have little other choice. Social services must then intervene to discuss other options for the caregiving families, or to provide services to give them a respite from care, and possibly placement of these patients.

As improvements are made in health care and preventive services, people are now living longer and more active lives. People over the age of 65 are more mobile and productive, thus putting them at higher risk for experiencing health care emergencies.

As emergency care providers, we need to have the knowledge, skills, and understanding necessary to provide quality emergency nursing care to this growing population.

REFERENCES

1. U.S. Bureau of the Census: Projections of the population of the United States by age, sex and race 1983 to 2080, *Current Population Reports* Series P-25, No 952. Washington, DC, Government Printing Office, 1984, pp 1-23.
2. Andrews J: Trauma in the elderly, *Postgraduate Studies in Trauma Nursing*, 1990.
3. Schroeder SA, Krupp MA, Tierney LM et al: *Current Medical Diagnosis and Treatment*, 22, 1991.
4. Rossman I: Mortality and morbidity overview. In Rossman I: *Clinical geriatrics*, ed 3, vol 1. Philadelphia, 1986, Lippincott.
5. Meredith M: Elderly abandonment, *Top Emerg Med*, 3:65, 1992.

SUGGESTED READINGS

Bloom J, Ansell P, Bloom M: Detecting elder abuse: a guide for physicians, *Geriatrics* 44(6):40, 1989.

Goldstein S, Reichel W: Physiological and biological aspects of aging. In *Clinical Aspects of Aging*. Baltimore, 1983, Williams and Wilkins.

Petro J, Belger D, Salzberg A et al: Burn accidents and the elderly, *Geriatrics* 44(3):26, 1989.

Rossman I: The anatomy of aging, *Clinical Geriatrics*, 1986.

CHAPTER 35

Organ and
Tissue Donation

Each year thousands of life-saving and life-enhancing organ and tissue transplants are performed. These patients receive gifts of life, sight, mobility, and independence. Yet each year one third to one half of all patients waiting for a vital organ transplant die before an organ becomes available. Many attempts have been made to ease the profound shortage of donor organs and tissues.

In 1968 the passage of the Uniform Anatomical Gift Act (UAGA) allowed persons to indicate their intent to donate after death by signing an organ donor card. If there was no indication of prior intent, the UAGA permitted the legal next of kin to give consent after death. The Omnibus Budget Reconciliation Act of 1986 (OBRA) required that hospitals write policies and protocols to assure that families were given information regarding their right to donate and that potential donors would be identified and referred to a local Organ Procurement Organization (OPO).

Regardless of efforts being made to increase the supply of organs and tissues available for transplant, it is important to reflect on the needs of a grieving family. Many families find comfort in making a donation and feel strongly about their right to make that choice for their loved one.

ROLE OF THE EMERGENCY DEPARTMENT NURSE

Become familiar with donation criteria and the hospital's policy on determination of brain death.

Contact the local Organ Procurement Organization to determine medical suitability whenever a death is imminent.

Discuss the possibility of donation with the primary physician.

Look for an organ donor card among patient's belongings.

Obtain permission for donation from medical examiner or coroner.

Offer family the option of donation in conjunction with Organ Procurement Organization.

Assist with donor management.

Provide bereavement support to family members.

TISSUE DONATION (CARDIORESPIRATORY DEATH)

Almost anyone who dies can be a tissue donor. Eye, heart for valve, and skin recovery can be performed in the morgue. Bone and saphenous vein recovery must be done in an operating room. Donor criteria vary. Avoid ruling someone out prior to making a referral.

General Tissue Donor Criteria

Eyes	Age 0-72 (>72yo tissue may be recovered for research)
Heart for valves	Age 0-55
Bone	Age 17-70
Skin	Age 17-70
Saphenous vein	Age 17-55 (males only)

Minimum Exclusion Criteria

Unresolved septicemia

Metastatic cancer (not a rule out for eye donation)

Injectable drug abuse

HIV positive or history of high-risk group for HIV (per U.S. Public Health Service guidelines)

Management

If the patient is to be an eye donor, follow this procedure prior to sending the body to the morgue:

Elevate the head of the bed.

Tape the eyelids shut with paper tape.

Apply ice packs to the eyelids.

Other tissue donations do not require specific management by nursing staff.

ORGAN DONATION (BRAIN DEATH)

A potential organ donor is a previously healthy individual who has suffered "irreversible cessation of all brain functions, including the brain stem."[1] Brain death criteria are determined by state legislation based on standard medical practice.

General Organ Donor Criteria

Age: newborn to 80 years

Brain death (see brain death criteria below)

Intact cardiorespiratory system

Apneic, on ventilator (see apnea test below)

Avoid ruling out a potential donor prior to discussing the case with the donation coordinator who is on call at the local Organ Procurement Organization. Donor criteria may vary and change frequently based on current medical practice and the day-to-day needs of critically ill patients on the waiting list.

The following are general criteria. Each hospital has its own policy and procedure based on state law and accepted medical practice.

Brain death criteria[1]

Known cause of condition

Diagnosis made in absence of hypothermia (temperature $<32.2°$ C) and central nervous system depressants

Cerebral unresponsiveness

Areflexic, except for simple spinal cord reflexes

Pupillary, extraocular, gag, and cough reflexes are absent

No spontaneous respiration

Condition irreversible (duration of observation depends on clinical judgment)

Flat EEG (if performed)

Absence of blood flow by cerebral radionuclide scan or arteriogram (if performed)

Apnea test[1]

- Preoxygenate.
- Disconnect ventilator, give O_2 at 8 to 12 L/min by tracheal cannula.
- Observe for spontaneous respirations.
- After 10 minutes, draw ABG.
- Reconnect the ventilator.
- The patient is apneic if the P_{CO_2} >60 mm Hg and there is no respiratory movement.
- If hypotension and/or dysrhythmias develop, immediately reconnect the ventilator. Consider other confirmatory tests.

Minimum Exclusion Criteria

Metastatic cancer

HIV positive or AIDS

Management*

In the majority of cases organ donor evaluation and management will be carried out in an intensive care unit due to the amount of time that it takes to complete the process. However, there will be those instances when the donation process

*Courtesy of Katie Dunn, RN, BS, CPTC, Donation Coordinator, New England Organ Bank.

will be initiated in the emergency department setting. Your local Organ Procurement Organization is your primary and most valuable resource at this time.

In general the initial evaluation of a potential organ donor includes the following data:

- Age and past medical history
- Assessment of family dynamics
- Accurate bedscale weight
- Blood type
- CBC with differential, full chemistry profile including liver function tests
- ABGs on current ventilator settings
- Frequent monitoring of vital signs including urine output
- Monitoring for evidence of septicemia

While individual organ systems are being evaluated, the donor's care must be carefully managed to optimize organ perfusion and to minimize the development of infection. Thus sterile technique, when applicable, should be maintained.

The "Rule of 100's" can be used as a guideline for management:

- Maintain a systolic blood pressure of 100.
- Maintain an arterial Po_2 of 100 on the minimal Fio_2
- Maintain an hourly urine output of 100 cc.

With the loss of cerebral function comes the potential for complications. Some of the most common complications seen in the brain dead individual include:

Neurogenic diabetes insipidus

- Due to pituitary dysfunction and loss of endogenous ADH
- Diagnosed by hypernatremia, hypokalemia, urine outputs of greater than
- 500 cc per hour, hyperosmolar serum, hypo-osmolar urine
- Treatment includes the use of low-dose vasopressin infusion or DDAVP

Neurogenic pulmonary edema

- Frequently seen in donors with a traumatic cause of death
- Mechanism of injury not well understood
- Diagnosed by CXR and deteriorating ABGs
- Treatment includes use of PEEP, of colloids vs. crystalloids, and lasix

Neurogenic shock

- Due to loss of vasomotor tone and dehydrational therapy
- Treatment includes volume restoration and use of vasoconstrictors. Dopamine usually the drug of choice for hypotension. Other drug therapies may include: dobutamine, neosynephrine, and epinephrine.

Neurogenic hypothermia

- Due to loss of hypothalamic temperature control
- May lead to EKG changes, cardiac dysrhythmias
- Proactive treatment the best choice: use of warming blankets, lights, blood and fluid warmers

BODY DONATION

Most people who desire body donation have made prior arrangements with a medical school.

Call the local Organ Procurement Organization for instructions.

HOW TO REFER A POTENTIAL DONOR

Call the Organ Procurement Organization (OPO) assigned to your area to refer a potential donor or to ask questions regarding medical suitability. A donation coordinator will assist you with the evaluation of a potential donor and, if requested, will provide on-site services that may include obtaining consent, donor management, and organ and tissue recovery. "It is important to note that, before a declaration of death, the Organ Procurement Organization coordinator will provide advice consistent with the medical and nursing goals (i.e., survival of the patient.)."[2]

If you do not know the name or telephone number of the local Organ Procurement Organization, call the United Network for Organ Sharing (UNOS) at 1-800-292-9537. There are 11 designated regions in the United States and within those regions there are one or more Organ Procurement Organizations providing service (Figure 35-1).

Call the Organ Procurement Organization every time a death occurs to assure that all families are given the option of choosing donation.

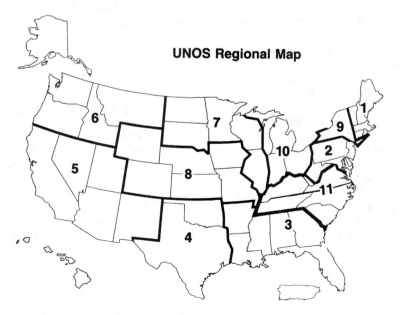

FIGURE 35-1. UNOS regional map.

When you call the Organ Procurement Organization be prepared to give the following information:
- Patient's name, age, sex, race, and medical record number
- Diagnosis and hospital course
- Status of brain death determination
- Whether or not the family has been approached about donation and their response

The importance of an early referral cannot be overemphasized. Placing the call when death is imminent allows you to give the family the most accurate information about the donation possibilities, decreases the time required to complete the process, and therefore increases the likelihood of a successful outcome.

Some hospitals have in-house coordinators or donor nurses whose responsibility it is to act as liaison with the local Organ Procurement Organization and to facilitate one or more stages of the donation process. Find out what your hospital's policy and protocol are on organ and tissue donation. (Refer to the box below.)

DHMC Protocol

Dartmouth-Hitchcock Medical Center Organ and Tissue Donor Program

Protocol for initiating organ & tissue donation

The purpose of this protocol is to assure that all patients and their families are made aware of their option to either donate or decline to donate organs or tissues for transplantation, education or research and to demonstrate our compliance with New Hampshire law and JCAHO regulations.

If a patient has a severe illness/injury that will likely progress to death, a member of the health care team will page the organ donor nurse on call—beeper –9653—to determine the patient's medical suitability for donation should death occur.

A. Tissue donation (cardiorespiratory death: not on ventilatory support)

1. The organ donor nurse will return the call and determine whether or not the patient is medically suitable to donate eyes, heart valves or bone. The organ donor nurse will obtain permission from the medical examiner when appropriate.
2. After consultation with a physician on the patient's primary service, a member of the health care team offers the family of a potential donor the opportunity to choose donation.
3. The family is supported, whether or not they choose donation.
4. The family wishes are documented in the medical record.
5. Informed consent by the legal next-of-kin may be obtained by the nurse, physician, social worker or clergy member if the patient will donate eyes. The organ donor nurse will obtain consent for donation of heart for valves or bone.* There is a consent form in each death packet.

---

*Permission for organ or tissue donation must be obtained from the first available next of kin in the following order: spouse; adult son or daughter; either parent; adult brother or sister; other next of kin; legal guardian; person authorized to dispose of the body.
From Dartmouth-Hitchcock Medical Center, Lebanon, N.H., 1993.

Continued.

DHMC Protocol—cont'd

6. The organ donor nurse will arrange all tissue recoveries and follow-up with the patient's family.
7. If eyes are to be donated:
a. Elevate the head of the bed
b. Tape eye lids shut with paper tape
c. Apply light ice packs to each eye
Before the body is transferred to the morgue.
B. Organ donation (brain death: on ventilator)
1. The organ donor nurse will review the medical record for specific exclusion criteria. (No laboratory tests or procedures are used to determine medical suitability, at this time, without the express permission of the family and the patient's primary physician.)
2. After consultation with a physician on the patient's primary service (not CCS), the organ donor nurse will be available for a family discussion regarding donation, when appropriate. Prior to this discussion, the organ donor nurse will consult the medical examiner to obtain permission for donation.
3. Once brain death has been pronounced, if the family desires donation, informed consent will be obtained by the organ donor nurse.
4. The donor will then be transferred to the Donor Service and the attending physician will be the transplant surgeon on call.
5. The donation process will be coordinated by the organ donor nurse in collaboration with New England Organ Bank and the transplant surgeon.

MEDICAL EXAMINER CASES

In certain cases you must ask the medical examiner or coroner to release the body for donation. It is wise to obtain this permission prior to speaking to the patient's family, as the medical examiner may restrict the donation or may refuse to allow any organs or tissues to be recovered.

A medical examiner's or coroner's case may include:
• Homicide or suspicion of homicide
• Suicide or suspicion of suicide
• Death by accident, trauma, or poisoning

CONSENT

"A thorough evaluation of donor potential before discussion with the family can prevent the situation in which a family readily embraces the opportunity to donate only to be informed later that this option does not exist for them."[2]

By Whom

Any health care professional who is caring for the patient, who has a positive attitude about donation, and who is familiar with the process. This may be the Organ Procurement Organization's donation coordinator or the donor hospital's physician, nurse, pastoral caregiver, or social worker.

Those family members authorized to give consent, and the order in which they have this authority, is specified in each state's Uniform Anatomical Gift Act. The Health Care Proxy's ability to direct care on the patient's behalf ends at the death of the patient. He or she therefore may not consent to donation unless authorized to do so under the UAGA.

How

Give the family time to acknowledge the loss of the loved one.
Provide a private space for grieving and discussion.
Assess the family's understanding of what the physician has told them.
Identify the patient's legal next-of-kin and key support persons.
Assess the family's understanding of brain death.
Explain brain death in terms they can understand.
Ask the family to reflect on what their loved one would have wanted.
Provide facts about donation essential to helping them make their decision.
Give them as much time as possible to discuss it among themselves.
Allow time to say good-bye to their loved one.
Provide support whether or not they choose to donate.
Document your discussion with the family in the patient's medical record.

Facts

The patient will be tested for HIV and other transmissible diseases.
There is no cost to the donor family.
The family should contact the donor hospital or Organ Procurement Organization if there is a question about billing.
All major religions support organ and tissue donation.
The Organ Procurement Organization will provide general follow-up information about the recipients.
There is no disfigurement as a result of a donation.
The quality of medical care will not be compromised if donation is considered.

BEREAVEMENT SUPPORT

Some Organ Procurement Organizations provide bereavement support services. Contact your hospital's Social Service Department to inquire about what services are available locally.

WHY SHOULD WE OFFER FAMILIES THE DONATION OPTION

Many health care professionals worry that offering the option of donation to a grieving family causes them to suffer more than they already have. However, most families take comfort in making this gift and they have the right to make that decision. *If we do not ask, we have made that decision for them.*

The best reason for offering families the donation option is expressed eloquently by Maggie Cooligan, a critical care nurse and donor mother: "It is true that in the sudden or traumatic death of our loved one, we are experiencing one of the most difficult types of loss. You observe us in a state of shock, a state of anger and/or guilt, and a state of denial. You do not want to increase the hurt. You do not want to expose your own feelings of mortality. You do not want to ask. However, your request presents us with hope when we have lost all hope. You present us with an option when we have no other options. We have already experienced the pain of death. What more can you say to hurt me when you have already said, 'your child has died.' Potential donor families have a right to be offered the option to donate. We have a right to alleviate some of the pain we will experience in grieving. We have the right to make some sense out of a usually senseless death. We have the right to be part of allowing another person to live."[3]

REFERENCES

1. Report of the medical consultants on the diagnosis of brain death to the President's Commission for the Study of Ethical Problems in Medicine and Biomedical and Behavioral Research: guidelines for the determination of death, *JAMA* 246:2184, 1981.
2. Willis R, Skelley L: Serving the needs of donor families: the role of the critical care nurse, *Crit Care Nurs Clin North Am* 4(1):63, 1992.
3. Cooligan M: Katie's legacy, *Am J Nurs* 87:483, 1987.

SUGGESTED READINGS

Cate FH:. Health care decision-making and organ and tissue donation, *J Transplant Coordination* 2:84, 1992.

McNally-Pederson ME: Tissue and organ donation. In Sheehy SB, ed: *Emergency nursing principles and practice.* St Louis, 1992, Mosby.

Norton DJ, Nathan HM, Hamilton BT et al: Current practices of determining brain death in potential organ donors, *Transplant Proc* 22:308, 1990.

Peele A: The nurse's role in promoting the right of donor families, *Nurs Clin North Am* 24:939, 1989.

Index